KU-242-511

BIOMECHANICS and ESTHETIC STRATEGIES in
Clinical Orthodontics

WOLLO MAN

ORDINARY

DAW 251606
L97

BIOMECHANICS and ESTHETIC STRATEGIES in *Clinical Orthodontics*

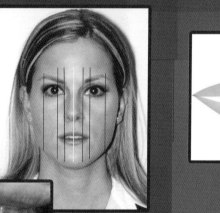

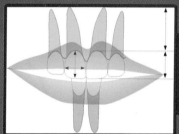

Ravindra Nanda, BDS, MDS, PhD
UConn Orthodontic Alumni Endowed Chair
Professor and Head
School of Dental Medicine
University of Connecticut
Health Center
Farmington, Connecticut

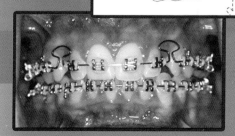

ELSEVIER
SAUNDERS

ELSEVIER
SAUNDERS

11830 Westline Industrial Drive
St. Louis, Missouri 63146

BIOMECHANICS AND ESTHETIC STRATEGIES IN CLINICAL ORTHODONTICS
Copyright © 2005, Elsevier Inc.

All rights reserved. No part of this publication may be reproduced or transmitted in any form or by any means, electronic or mechanical, including photocopying, recording, or any information storage and retrieval system, without permission in writing from the publisher.

Permissions may be sought directly from Elsevier's Health Sciences Rights Department in Philadelphia, PA, USA: phone: (+1) 215 238 7869, fax: (+1) 215 238 2239, e-mail: healthpermissions@elsevier.com. You may also complete your request on-line via the Elsevier homepage (http://www.elsevier.com), by selecting 'Customer Support' and then 'Obtaining Permissions'.

NOTICE

Clinical orthodontics is an ever-changing field. Standard safety precautions must be followed, but as new research and clinical experience broaden our knowledge, changes in treatment and drug therapy may become necessary or appropriate. Readers are advised to check the most current product information provided by the manufacturer of each drug to be administered to verify the recommended dose, the method and duration of administration, and contraindications. It is the responsibility of the licensed prescriber, relying on experience and knowledge of the patient, to determine dosages and the best treatment for each individual patient. Neither the publisher nor the author assumes any liability for any injury and/or damage to persons or property arising from this publication.

International Standard Book Number 0-7216-0196-0

Executive Editor: Penny Rudolph
Senior Developmental Editor: Jaime Pendill
Publishing Services Manager: Karen Edwards
Senior Designer: Kathi Gosche

BARTS & THE LONDON QMSMD	
CLAS	WU440 NAN
CIRC	ORDINARY
SU.	DAW E97 25/5/06
READ	
OLD ED	

Printed in China

Last digit is the print number: 9 8 7 6 5 4 3 2 1

In memory of Dr Surender Kumar Nanda

A wonderful husband, father, brother, educator, philosopher, mentor, and friend,
Whose life was dedicated to the advancement of practice and science of orthodontics.
He continually sought truth in what is good and helping others reach their full potential.
Our profession will forever be grateful for his contributions.

CONTRIBUTORS

Frank H. Chang, DDS
Department of Orthodontics
School of Dentistry
National Taiwan University
Taipei, Taiwan

Jenny Z. Chang, DDS
Department of Orthodontics
School of Dentistry
National Taiwan University
Taipei, Taiwan

R. Scott Conley, DMD
Assistant Professor
Division of Orthodontics
Vanderbilt University Medical Center
Nashville, Tennessee

Tarisai C. Dandajena, DDS, MS
PhD Fellow
Department of Cell Biology
Research Fellow
Department of Orthodontics
College of Medicine and College of Dentistry
University of Oklahoma Health Sciences Center
Oklahoma City, Oklahoma

Nejat Erverdi, DDS, PhD
Professor and Chairman
Department of Orthodontics
Marmara University
Istanbul, Turkey

John C. Huang, DMD, DMedSc
Assistant Professor
Director of Curriculum
Division of Orthodontics
School of Dentistry
University of California at San Francisco
San Francisco, California

Sunil Kapila, DDS, MS, PhD
Professor and Chair
Department of Orthodontics and Pediatric Dentistry
School of Dentistry
University of Michigan
Ann Arbor, Michigan

Robert G. Keim, DDS, EdD
Associate Dean, Advanced Studies
University of Southern California
School of Dentistry
Editor, Journal of Clinical Orthodontics
Associate Professor
University of Southern California
Rossier School of Education
Los Angeles, California

Ahmet Keles, DDS, DMSc
Associate Research Investigator
The Forsyth Institute
Boston, Massachusetts

Gregory J. King, DMD, DMSc
Professor and Chairman
Department of Orthodontics
School of Dentistry
University of Washington
Seattle, Washington

Vincent G. Kokich, DDS, MSD
Professor
Department of Orthodontics
School of Dentistry
University of Washington
Seattle, Washington

Vincent O. Kokich, DMD, MSD
Affiliate Assistant Professor
Department of Orthodontics
School of Dentistry
University of Washington
Seattle, Washington

Andrew Kuhlberg, DMD, MDS
Assistant Professor
Department of Orthodontics
School of Dental Medicine
University of Connecticut Health Center
Farmington, Connecticut

Harry L. Legan, DDS
Professor and Director
Division of Orthodontics
Vanderbilt University Medical Center
Nashville, Tennessee

Ram S. Nanda, DDS, MS, PhD
Professor and Endowed Chair
Department of Orthodontics
College of Dentistry
University of Oklahoma Health Sciences Center
Oklahoma City, Oklahoma

Ravindra Nanda, BDS, MDS, PhD
UConn Orthodontic Alumni Endowed
Chair
Professor and Head
School of Dental Medicine
University of Connecticut Health Center
Farmington, Connecticut

Jill Bennett Nevin
Doctoral Candidate
Annenberg School for Communication
University of Southern California
Los Angeles, California

Junji Sugawara, DDS, PhD
Associate Professor
Department of Orthodontics and Dentofacial Orthopedics
Tohoku University
Sendai, Japan

Flavio Andres Uribe, DDS, MDS
Assistant Professor
Department of Orthodontics
School of Dental Medicine
University of Connecticut Health Center
Farmington, Connecticut

Bjørn U. Zachrisson, DDS, MSD, PhD
Professor
Department of Orthodontics
University of Oslo
Oslo, Norway

PREFACE

Within the past two decades, interest in esthetics from orthodontists, medical professionals, and the general population has increased dramatically and continues to rise. While esthetics can be very subjective and variable between different ethnicities, specific characteristics of attractive people can be defined. These characteristics should be considered during diagnosis, treatment planning, and design of mechanics to correct dentofacial malocclusions.

For the first time, an orthodontic textbook combines two very important aspects of orthodontic treatment: esthetics and biomechanics. Biomechanics is the most important aspect of the design of an orthodontic appliance, and this book highlights how the esthetic objectives of orthodontic treatment can be successfully achieved with biomechanically based orthodontic appliances. This book describes the design of simple appliances which can be easily incorporated in any prevailing orthodontic technique and philosophy.

This book complements our book, "Biomechanics in Clinical Orthodontics", published in 1996. It expands on and updates two chapters from this book, and adds 16 new chapters. It draws on the expertise of authors who are considered leaders in their field. The topics range from diagnosis and treatment planning to biomechanic principles and finishing of various malocclusions.

Drs Huang, King, and Kapila discuss the state of the art in biologic mechanisms of tooth movement. Dr Keim discusses the social psychology of facial esthetics, an important subject that has probably never been this comprehensively discussed before in the orthodontic literature. Dr Zachrisson succinctly describes how a carefully designed treatment can enhance esthetic results. Drs Ram Nanda and Dandajena give a critical report on various

Class II treatment methodologies. This book devotes three chapters to the subject of Class III malocclusion by Drs Sugawara and Chang. The contemporary subject of skeletal implants and absolute anchorage is covered in two chapters by Drs Erverdi, Keles, and Sugawara. Drs Legan and Conley address biomechanical considerations in surgical orthodontics. Drs Kokich and Kokich Jr discuss the important role of periodontics and restorative dentistry in the esthetic outcome of orthodontic cases. My colleagues, Drs Kuhlberg and Uribe, have made excellent contributions in coauthoring seven chapters with me.

This book takes a sequential approach to diagnosis and treatment planning with emphasis on esthetic objectives, combined with occlusion as well as functional esthetics. It gives numerous case reports using hundreds of color illustrations of varying malocclusions and appliances. Furthermore, this book encompasses the expertise of some of the most eminent clinicians and scientists in the field of contemporary orthodontics. The esthetic parameters and biomechanically designed appliances presented here can be applied to achieve predictable results.

Orthodontic residents, faculty, and private practitioners alike will find useful information on the most important aspects in orthodontics. After 3 years of continuous work, I am very delighted and proud to present you with this textbook. I am very grateful to all the contributors and hope that the orthodontic community enjoys reading this textbook as much as we have enjoyed writing it.

Ravindra Nanda
December 2004
Farmington, CT

ACKNOWLEDGMENTS

First of all, I want to thank my fellow contributors for taking time out of their busy schedules to write some of the best reading in orthodontics. Their expertise is highly appreciated.

My heartfelt thanks to my colleague, Dr Flavio Uribe, for helping me throughout the process in developing this book. Working closely with him ensures me that our profession has excellent young talent who will provide a bright future for all those in our field. Dr Andy Kuhlberg did a superb job in contributing to three chapters. His skillful computer artwork appears in more than 10 chapters.

My special thanks to Dr Erin Kazmierski-Furno, my chief resident, who never said no to any request. She spent innumerable hours scanning hundreds of photographs and helping me compile illustrations for this book.

My personal thanks to Perry Haque, Lindsay Brehm, and Paul Blanchette for their help at various levels during the last few years.

I also want to express my gratitude to more than 125 alumni for their unselfish support. I want to take this opportunity to acknowledge and thank them for their financial support in establishing the UConn Orthodontic Alumni/ Ravi Nanda chair in Orthodontics. It is quite an honor and no teacher can ask for more.

I also want to recognize Penny Rudolph, Executive Editor at Elsevier, who felt it was worthwhile to have a follow-up book to *Biomechanics in Clinical Orthodontics*. Also, my sincere thanks to Jaime Pendill, Senior Developmental Editor at Elsevier, for constantly pushing me and my co-authors to finish this project on time.

Lastly, special thanks to my wife, Catherine, for supporting me at every stage to complete this project.

Ravindra Nanda

CONTENTS

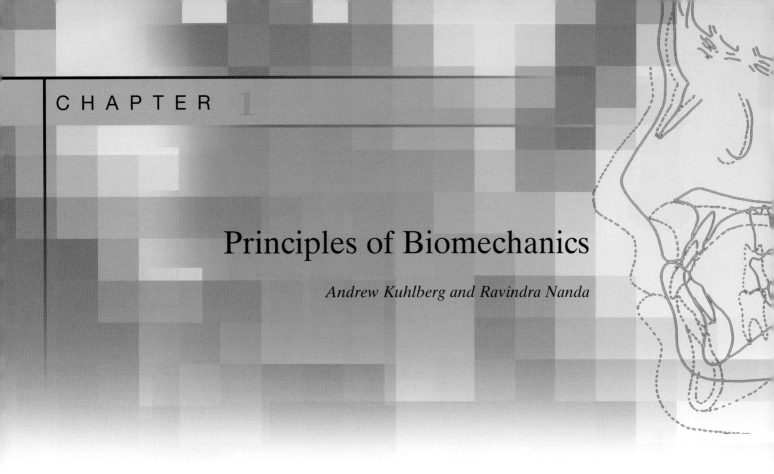

CHAPTER 1

Principles of Biomechanics

Andrew Kuhlberg and Ravindra Nanda

Orthodontic tooth movement results from the application of forces to teeth. The orthodontic appliances that are selected, inserted, and activated by the clinician produce these forces. The teeth and their associated support structures respond to these forces with a complex biologic reaction that ultimately results in the teeth moving through their supporting bone. The cells of the periodontium, which respond to the applied forces, are insensitive to the bracket design, wire shape, or alloy of the orthodontic appliances—their activity is based solely on the stresses and strains occurring in their environment. To achieve a precise biologic response, precise stimuli, mechanical or otherwise, have to be applied. The complexity and variability associated with biologic systems encourages clinical precision in the application of any stimulus. Reducing the unknown factors related to the delivery of treatment can reduce the variability in treatment response. Knowledge of the mechanical principles governing forces is necessary for the control of orthodontic treatment.

The basis of orthodontic treatment lies in the clinical application of biomechanic concepts. Mechanics is the discipline that describes the effect of forces on bodies; biomechanics refers to the science of mechanics in relation to biologic systems. Orthodontic treatment applies forces to teeth; the forces are generated by a variety of orthodontic appliances. An analogy is the use of pharmaceutical agents in medicine. Medications are used to achieve a specific biologic response aimed at resolving or relieving a patient's problems or symptoms. Judicious prescription of medication

requires an understanding of the mechanisms of action of the therapeutic agents in order to obtain the desired clinical results. Orthodontists depend on a similar application of mechanical force systems for treatment success.

The duration of orthodontic treatment still approaches 2 years; arguably because of the time it takes to correct the unintended side effects (undesirable tooth movements) that occur during treatment. Inefficient care may arise as much from technical imprecision as from factors such as poor patient compliance. If biomechanic principles are applied to mechanotherapy, not only may treatment time be reduced, but more individualized treatment plans could be developed to achieve more predictable results. The proper application of biomechanic principles increases treatment efficiency through improved planning and delivery of care.

Mechanical Concepts in Orthodontics

An understanding of several fundamental mechanical concepts is necessary in order to understand the clinical relevance of biomechanics to orthodontics.

The first concept is *center of resistance*. All objects have a center of mass. This is the point through which an applied force must pass for a free object to move linearly without any rotation, i.e., the center of mass is an object's "balance point." Figure 1-1A depicts the center of mass of a generic free body. A tooth within a periodontal support system is

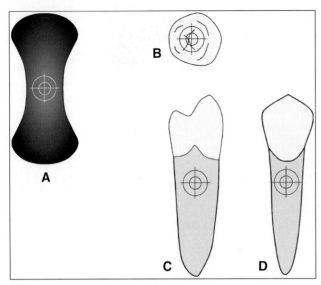

Fig. 1-1 Center of resistance. **A** Center of mass of a free body. **B** Frontal, **C** occlusal, and **D** mesial views of the center of resistance of a single tooth.

not a free body because it is restrained by the periodontium. The center of resistance is analogous to the center of mass for restrained bodies and is the equivalent "balance point" for restrained bodies. Figure 1-1B-D shows the approximate location of the center of resistance for a single tooth. Note that the center of resistance can be described in each plane of space. Single teeth, units of teeth, complete dental arches, and the jaws themselves each have center(s) of resistance. Figure 1-2 shows the approximate center(s) of resistance for a two-tooth segment and for a maxilla.

The center of resistance of a tooth is dependent on the root length and morphology, the number of roots, and the level of alveolar bone support (Fig. 1-3). The exact location of the center of resistance for a tooth is not easily identified; however, analytic studies have determined that the center of resistance for single-rooted teeth with normal alveolar bone levels is about one-fourth to one-third the distance from the cementoenamel junction (CEJ) to the root apex.[1–6] The center of resistance of facial bones (i.e. the maxilla), entire teeth arches, or segments of teeth may also be estimated.[7] Experimental and analytic studies report the center

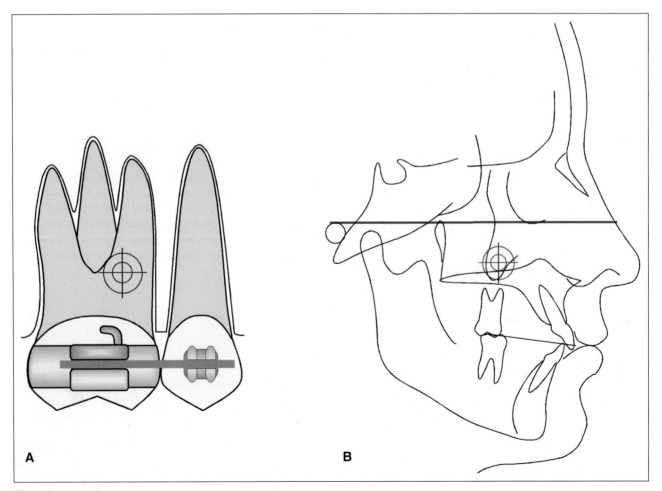

Fig. 1-2 Center of resistance for **A** a two-tooth segment and **B** a maxilla.

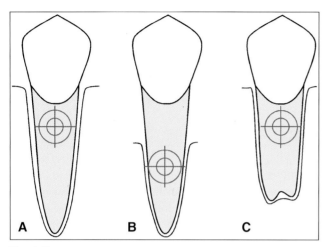

Fig. 1-3 Location of the center of resistance depends on the alveolar bone height and root length. **A** Location of the center of resistance with alveolar bone loss and **B** with a shortened root.

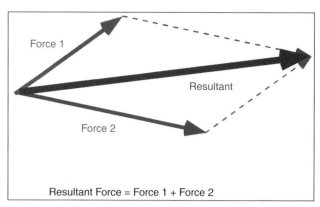

Resultant Force = Force 1 + Force 2

Fig. 1-5 Vector addition. The sum of two or more vectors is the resultant. It is found by connecting the vectors "head-to-tail" while maintaining the length and direction of the line of action.

of resistance for a maxilla to be slightly inferior to the orbitale for the maxilla, and distal to the lateral incisor roots for intrusive movements of maxillary anterior teeth.[5,6]

Although its precise location is typically unknown, it is important to have a conceptual awareness of the center of resistance of a tooth (or teeth) when selecting and activating an orthodontic appliance. The relationship of the force system acting on the tooth to the center of resistance determines the type of tooth movement expressed. This relationship is discussed in more detail later in the chapter.

It is the application of a *force* that results in orthodontic tooth movement. Forces are the actions applied to bodies. A force is equal to mass multiplied by acceleration ($F = ma$). Its units are Newtons or gram × (millimeters/second).[8] Grams are often substituted for Newtons in clinical orthodontics because the contribution of acceleration (m/s^2) to the magnitude of the force is clinically irrelevant. A force is a vector and is defined by the characteristics of vectors.[9] Vector quantities are characterized by having both magnitude and direction (Fig. 1-4). The magnitude of the vector represents its size. Direction is described by the vector's line of action, sense, and point of origin (or point of application). Orthodontic forces are produced in a variety of ways—the deflection of wires, activation of springs, and elastics are common methods.

Multiple vectors can be combined through vector addition (Fig. 1-5). Since vectors have both magnitude and direction, simple addition of vector quantities arithmetically is impossible. The sum of two or more vectors is termed the *resultant*. Vectors may be added by placing the origin of one vector at the head of another, while maintaining the vectors' lines of action (in both length and direction). The resultant vector is found by connecting the origin of the first vector to the head of the final vector. Quantitative determination of resultants requires trigonometric calculations.

Vectors can also be resolved into components. Decomposition of a force into components along the *x, y,* and *z* axes can aid in vector addition (Fig. 1-6). Clinically the determination of the horizontal, vertical, and transverse components of a force improves the understanding of the direction of tooth movement. Again trigonometry must be applied to calculate the values of the vector components.

Orthodontic forces are most commonly applied at the crown of a tooth. Therefore the application of the force is generally not through the center of resistance of the tooth.

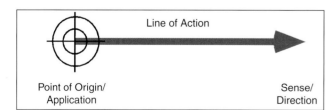

Fig. 1-4 Force vectors are characterized by magnitude, line of action, point of origin, and sense.

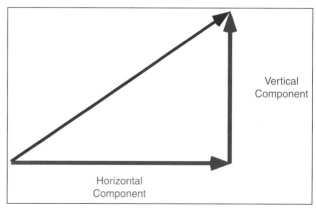

Fig. 1-6 Vector components. A vector can be analyzed by its components along reference axes.

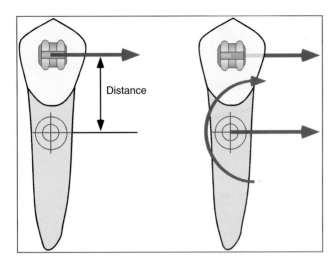

Fig. 1-7 Moment of a force. A force that does not pass through the center of resistance produces a rotational movement as well as linear movement.

Forces not acting through the center of resistance do not solely produce linear motion. The *moment of the force* results in some rotational movement also. The moment of the force is the tendency for a force to produce rotation. It is determined by multiplying the magnitude of the force by the perpendicular distance of the line of action to the center of resistance (Fig. 1-7). Its direction is found by following the line of action around the center of resistance toward the point of origin (Fig. 1-7). The units of measurement of moments are in gram-millimeters (Newton-millimeters). The importance of the moment of a force is often not recognized in clinical orthodontics, but awareness of it is needed to develop effective and efficient appliance designs.[9]

Two variables determine the magnitude of the moment of a force—the magnitude of the force and the distance (Fig. 1-8). Either can be effectively manipulated by the clinician to achieve the desired force systems.

Another method of achieving rotational movements is through the *moment of a couple* (Fig. 1-9). A couple is two parallel forces of equal magnitude acting in opposite directions and separated by a distance (i.e. different lines of action). The magnitude of a couple is calculated by multiplying the magnitude of force(s) by the distance between them; the units are also in gram-millimeters. The direction of the rotation is determined by following the direction of either force around the center of resistance to the origin of the opposite force. Couples result in pure rotational movement about the center of resistance *regardless of where the couple is applied on the object* (Fig. 1-10). Couples are often referred to as the applied moment in orthodontics. Torque is a common synonym for moment (both moments of forces and of couples). Torque is erroneously described in terms of degrees by many orthodontists. The degrees of wire bending or the

angulation of bracket slot design are methods to produce moments, i.e., they describe the shape of the wire or bracket. The appropriate unit for the applied torque is gram-millimeters (force × distance). It is the description of the moments that more accurately describes the rotational components of a force system and appliance design.[9]

Equivalent Force Systems

The application of forces or couples (moments, torque) usually occurs at the bracket. Wires, elastics, and springs are attached to the tooth at the bracket. A useful method for predicting the type of tooth movement that will occur with appliance activation is to determine the *equivalent force system* at the tooth's center of resistance. Equivalency is a concept that describes or defines an alternative but equal combination of forces and moments to the applied force and moments at their point of application, usually the bracket itself. This analysis finds the force system at the center of resistance that is equivalent to the applied force system. The force system at the center of resistance accurately reflects the type of movement. A pure force at the center of resistance results in linear movement (no rotation), while a pure couple results in rotation.[7]

Determining the equivalent force system at the center of resistance is a simple procedure (Fig. 1-11). First the force vectors are replaced at the center of resistance. The linear quality of the force vector is independent of its location on the body; the vector is simply placed at the center of resistance, maintaining its magnitude and direction. The moment of the force is also determined (as described above); since the force at the bracket also generates a moment of a force, this moment is equal to the magnitude of the force multiplied by the distance of the point of application to the center of resistance. The magnitude and direction of a couple are independent of their location. Couples are also known as free vectors, their effect on the object is the same regardless of their location, and they always produce rotation about the object's center of resistance. Therefore both the moment of force and the applied moment can be placed at the center of resistance. Finally the moment of the force and the applied moment are added to determine the net moment. The resulting force system describes the expected tooth movement. By determining the equivalent force systems, it becomes apparent that achieving desired and predictable tooth movements requires an awareness of both applied forces and moments.

Types of Tooth Movement

Tooth movement can be described in many ways; however the essentially infinite variety of movements can be categorized into four basic types: tipping, translation, root movement, and rotation. Each type of movement is the result of a different applied moment and force (in terms

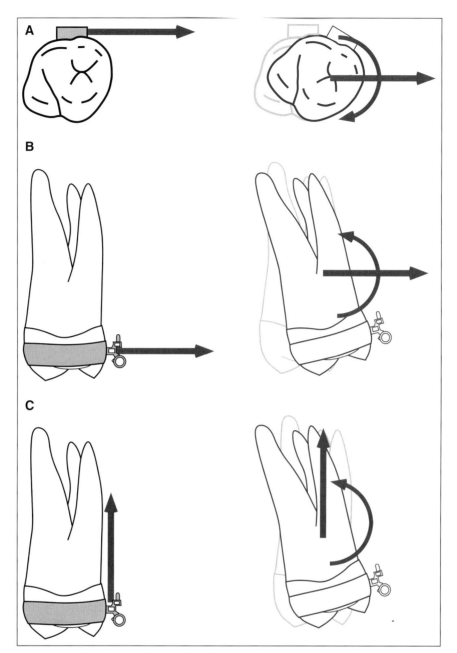

Fig. 1-8 Clinical examples of moments of a force. **A** Mesial force at the molar bracket creates a moment tending to rotate the tooth "mesial-in." **B** Expansion force on a molar creates a moment tipping the crown buccally. **C** Intrusive force at the molar bracket creates a moment tipping the crown buccally. (Reproduced with permission from Nanda R. Biomechanics in clinical orthodontics. Philadelphia: WB Saunders, 1996.)

of magnitude, direction, or point of application). The relationship between the applied force system and the type of movement can be described by the *moment/force ratio*. The moment/force ratio of the applied force and moment determines the type of movement or the center of rotation.[2,3,9–12] The movement that occurs is dependent on the moment/force ratio and the quality of the periodontal support: shorter roots or reduced alveolar bone height alter the type of movement that occurs based on the moment/force ratio.

Tipping

Tipping is tooth movement with greater movement of the crown of the tooth than of the root. The center of rotation of the motion is apical to the center of resistance. Tipping can be further classified on the basis of the location of the center of rotation into uncontrolled and controlled tipping. Uncontrolled tipping includes tipping with a center of rotation between the center of resistance and the apex. Controlled tipping is tipping with the center of rotation at the root apex.

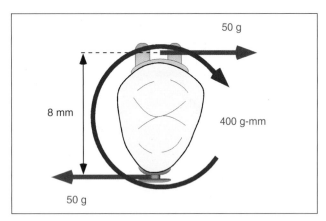

Fig. 1-9 Moment of a couple. A couple produces pure rotation about the center of resistance.

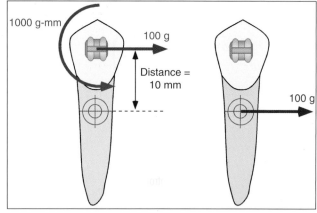

Fig. 1-11 Equivalent force system at a tooth's center of resistance. **A** Force system applied at the bracket. **B** Force system at the center of resistance. The force system at the center of resistance describes the expected tooth movement.

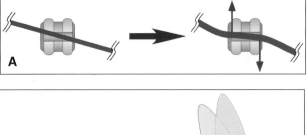

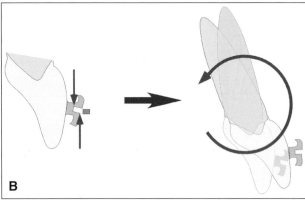

Fig. 1-10 Clinical examples of couples. **A** Engaging a wire in an angulated bracket. **B** Engaging a rectangular (edgewise) wire in a bracket slot.

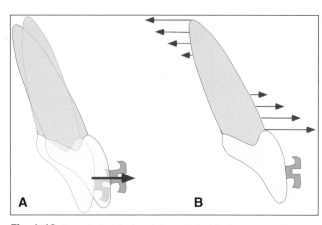

Fig. 1-12 Uncontrolled tipping. **A** Uncontrolled tipping produced by a single force (no applied moment). **B** Stress pattern in the periodontal ligament. Notice the root apex moves in the opposite direction from the movement of the crown.

Uncontrolled Tipping

A single, horizontal, lingually-directed force at the level of a bracket will cause movement of the root apex and crown in opposite directions. This is the simplest type of tooth movement to produce (the tooth's crown simply needs to be pushed or pulled), but it is often undesirable. It is frequently termed uncontrolled tipping (Fig. 1-12A). Figure 1-12B shows a typical stress pattern generated by uncontrolled tipping. The stresses are nonuniform, and maximum stresses are created at the root apex and crown. The moment/force ratio for this type of tooth movement is 0:1 to approximately 5:1.[1,9] (Note: moment/force ratios are for average root lengths and 100% alveolar bone height.)

In certain circumstances uncontrolled tipping can be useful, such as with Class II, Division 2 and Class III malocclusion patients where the excessively upright incisors often need to be flared.

Controlled Tipping

Controlled tipping is a very desirable type of tooth movement. It is achieved by the application of a force to move the crown, as done in uncontrolled tipping, *and* application of a moment to "control" or maintain the position of the root apex. Figure 1-13A shows tipping movement with the center of rotation of the tooth at the root apex. A moment/force ratio of 7:1 is generally necessary for controlled tipping.

Figure 1-13B shows the pattern of stresses produced in the periodontal ligament for this type of tooth movement. The stress at the root apex is minimal, which helps to maintain the integrity of the apex, and the concentration

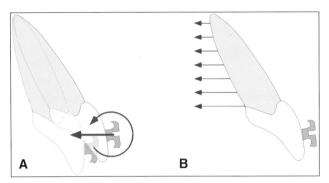

Fig. 1-13 Controlled tipping. **A** Controlled tipping with the center of rotation at the root apex. **B** Stress pattern in the periodontal ligament with controlled tipping. The stresses are greatest at the cervical margin.

of stresses at the cervical area allows timely tooth movement.[1,9] In patients with protrusive maxillary incisors, the root apex is often in a good position and does not need to be moved. The only major movement is of the crown.

Translation

Translatory tooth movement is also known as "bodily movement." Translation of a tooth takes place when the root apex and crown move the same distance and in the same horizontal direction. The center of rotation is infinitely far away.

Figure 1-14A shows parallel movement or translation of an incisor. A horizontal force applied at the center of resistance of a tooth will result in this movement. However the point of force application at the bracket is away from the center of resistance. As with controlled tipping, bodily movement requires the simultaneous application of a force and a couple at the bracket. Compared to controlled tipping, the magnitude of the applied couple must increase in order to maintain the tooth's axial inclination. A moment/force ratio of 10:1 typically produces translation. Figure 1-14B

shows that this type of tooth movement produces uniform stresses in the periodontium.[1,9]

Root Movement

Changing a tooth's axial inclination by moving the root apex while holding the crown stationary is termed root movement (Fig. 1-15A). The center of rotation of the tooth is at the incisal edge or bracket. Root movement requires further increasing the magnitude of the applied couple. Moment/force ratios of 12:1 or greater result in root movement.[9] Figure 1-15B shows the stress distribution in the periodontium with this type of tooth movement. Stress levels in the apex area require significant bone resorption in this area for tooth movement to take place. This concentration of stresses may produce undermining resorption, which causes a significant slow down in the rate of movement. This slower pace of root movement can be used advantageously to augment anchorage.

Root movement in orthodontic treatment is frequently described as "torque." Torque is the application of forces that tend to cause rotation. Placing twists in a rectangular wire, or the angle of the bracket slot with the long axis of the tooth and the occlusal plane, is often called torque. It is usually quantified by measuring the angle of the degree of twist placed in the wire. Angular measurements are poor descriptors of the mechanical characteristics of the spring design or the stresses influencing tooth movement. The torque magnitude is dependent on the slot size, wire dimension, amount of play between the two, as well as the actual tooth position. For example stating that a 0.018" × 0.025" wire has 17° of torque for four maxillary incisors gives no indication of the magnitude of the moment or the measurable stress placed on the teeth.

Rotation

Pure rotation of a tooth requires a couple. Since no net force acts at the center of resistance, only rotation occurs. Clinically this movement is most commonly needed

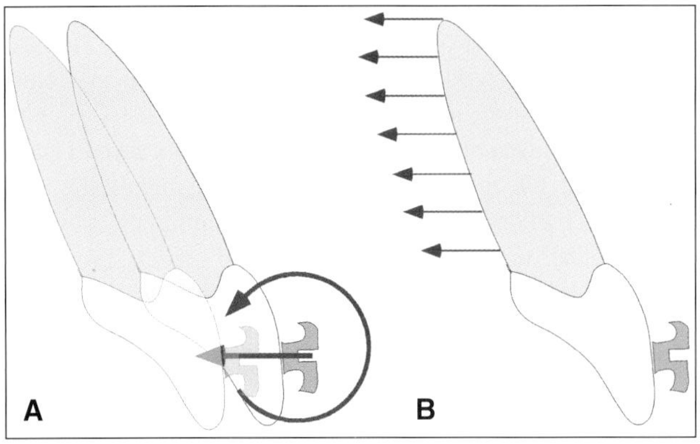

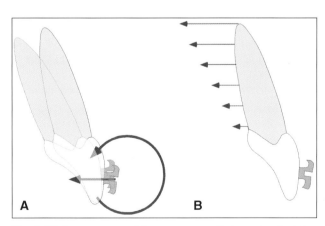

Fig. 1-14 Translation. **A** Translational or bodily tooth movement. **B** Stress pattern in the periodontal ligament with translation. Uniform stresses occur throughout the periodontal ligament.

Fig. 1-15 Root movement. **A** Root movement with the center of rotation at the incisal edge. **B** Stress pattern in the periodontal ligament with root movement. The stresses are greatest at the apex.

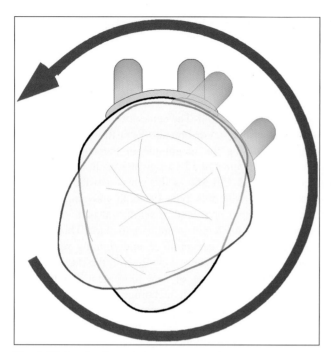

Fig. 1-16 Rotation. Pure rotation occurs around a tooth's center of resistance.

for movement as viewed from the occlusal perspective (Fig. 1-16).

Static Equilibrium

Statics is a field of mechanics that examines forces acting on bodies at rest. Static equilibrium is a valuable application of Newton's laws of motion to the analysis of the force system delivered by an orthodontic appliance.[9,13,14] Newton's laws underlie some of the fundamental concepts of mechanics. The three laws are:

1. *Law of inertia.* Every body continues in its state of rest or uniform motion in a straight line unless it is compelled to change by the forces impressed on it.
2. *Law of acceleration.* The change in motion is proportional to the impressed motive force and is made in the direction of the straight line in which the force is impressed.
3. *Law of action and reaction.* To every action there is always an opposing and equal reaction.

To understand the application of these laws to orthodontics, consider what is happening when a wire is inserted into poorly aligned brackets. The wire must be deflected or activated in order for it to be tied into the brackets. Once the wire is inserted, both the first and third laws of motion are apparent. First the wire and the teeth are both at rest; the wire is not moving, and neither are the teeth (although the periodontal structures feel a stress that will elicit the biologic reactions necessary for tooth movement). Thus the law of inertia is demonstrated. Similarly the third

law, the law of action and reaction, is demonstrated. The deflected wire is applying a force to the teeth, and the teeth are applying an equal and opposite force on the wire. With the "active" (on the teeth) and "reactive" (on the wire) forces being equal and opposite, no net force is acting and the resting state is maintained.

A more important application of the law of action and reaction is through the concept of static equilibrium. Static equilibrium implies that, at any point within a body, the sum of the forces and moments acting on a body is zero; i.e. if no net forces or moments are acting on the body, the body remains at rest (static). The "body" may be defined as the wire or spring and all the teeth to which the wire or spring is attached. Statics is a field of mechanics that considers the effects of sets of forces acting on bodies at rest.

Applying the fundamentals of static equilibrium to the analysis of the force system produced by orthodontic appliances aids in predicting tooth response to tooth movement. The analysis of equilibrium can be stated in equation form:

- Horizontal forces = 0
- Vertical forces = 0
- Transverse forces = 0

and

- Moments (horizontal axis) = 0
- Moments (vertical axis) = 0
- Moments (transverse axis) = 0

This formulation is most easily demonstrated in a cantilever-type orthodontic appliance.[8,15–17] Figure 1-17A depicts the buccal view of an intrusion arch inserted into the molar tube, but not tied to the incisors; Figure 1-17B depicts the appliance tied to the incisors. The wire is inserted into the auxiliary tube of the molar and tied to an anterior segment (overlaid) such that it is not inserted into the incisor bracket slot.

As stated above the sum of the forces must equal zero. Therefore the vertical intrusive forces acting on the incisors must be opposed by vertical extrusive forces acting on the molar. For the vertical forces, the state of equilibrium is readily seen. The vertical forces also establish a couple (they are equal and opposite, non-colinear forces). Figure 1-18 shows the force system. The vertical forces could be considered to be an *interbracket couple*, as each force is acting on a single bracket. The moment of this couple must be opposed by another moment equal in magnitude and acting in the opposite direction. This moment must be acting at the molar. It is an *intrabracket couple*, produced by the forces applied by the wire inside the bracket or tube. This moment's direction compels the molar to tip the crown distally. The magnitude of the moment is equal to the distance between the points of application of the paired vertical forces.

Figure 1-19 shows another clinical situation that allows further examination of the equilibrium state of an appliance. Two incisors are tipped toward one another;

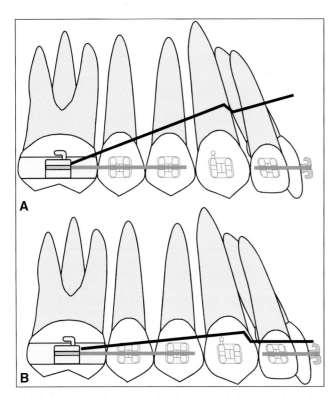

Fig. 1-17 Schematic diagram of an intrusion arch. **A** Passive form: the intrusion arch inserted in the molar tube but not engaging the incisor(s). **B** Intrusion arch activated by tying it to the anterior segment.

the incisors, equal and opposite moments are needed. The brackets are "figure of eight" tied to hold the interbracket distance, and a straight wire is inserted. The resulting force system is shown in Figure 1-19B. The figure of eight tie produces a small horizontal force on each incisor. These forces act in opposite directions (pulling each crown toward the other) and in the same line of action; thus the rules of equilibrium are satisfied. The wire produces moments acting on each tooth. In this example the moments are equal in magnitude and opposite in direction (the moments acting on both teeth tend to move the roots mesially).

The simple examples above demonstrate how to determine an appliance's equilibrium state. The application of unequal moments results in more complex force systems, as may occur with bracket malalignment (in any plane), the placement of eccentric "V"-bends[18–20] or gable bends, or the use of auxiliary space closure springs. Whenever the applied moments are unequal in magnitude, "additional" forces must be present to oppose moment difference. In many cases these "additional" forces are vertical in direction (extrusive/intrusive). The vertical forces could result in extrusive tooth movements (deepening of the overbite or eruption of posterior teeth and an increase in the lower facial height/vertical dimension) or a change in the occlusal plane. Determination of the complete force system in equilibrium aids in the recognition of these side effects.

Being aware of the force system produced by an orthodontic appliance in equilibrium aids in the prediction of the response to treatment. The desired, beneficial movements of the teeth can be foreseen along with potential negative side effects. Prior knowledge of any mechanical side effects makes compensation possible before these effects occur. These side effects cannot be eliminated! They should be dealt with through alternative designs or additional appliances (i.e. use of headgear) in order to negate or minimize side effects.

the crowns contact near the incisal edge, but the axial inclination of the incisors is poor, with excessive root divergence. This situation may arise with initial closure of a midline diastema. For the purpose of demonstration assume that the incisors are tipped equally mesially and that the brackets are accurately positioned. To upright

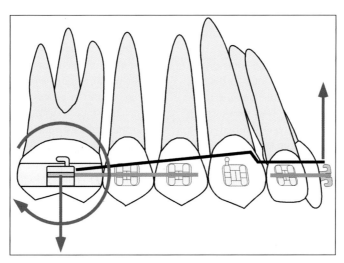

Fig. 1-18 Force system from an intrusion arch in equilibrium. The vertical forces (blue) are "balanced" by the tipback moment (red) acting on the molar.

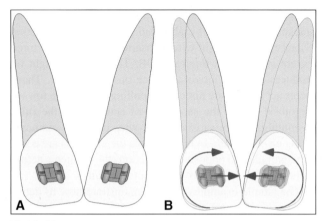

Fig. 1-19 Diastema closure by mesial tipping of the incisors. **A** Crowns contact but there is excessive divergence of the roots. **B** Force system for uprighting the incisors; the forces and moments are equivalent in magnitude, opposite in direction.

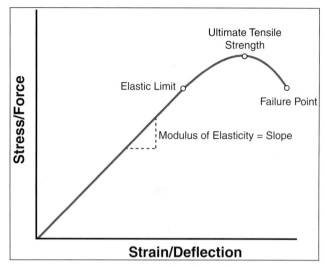

Fig. 1-20 Stress–strain curve for an orthodontic wire. See text for further description of the material characteristics demonstrated.

Material Considerations

Orthodontic Wires and Springs

Archwires, springs, and elastics are the primary means of generating forces for orthodontic treatment. Wires and springs are fabricated from a myriad of alloys.[21] Stainless steel, long the standard material, has been joined by nickel–titanium alloys,[22] titanium–molybdenum alloys,[23] and a variety of other alloys. Understanding the basic material characteristics is essential in selecting wires for use in treatment.[24] The bottom line is that wires act as springs in clinical orthodontics.

The mechanical characteristics of a material are determined by several factors. Intrinsic properties are inherent qualities of the wire. These properties are determined by the material composition at a molecular or crystalline level. Variation of intrinsic properties alters the nature of the alloy itself. Extrinsic properties are macroscopic features of the material, such as wire diameter or length. These features can be determined by the clinician.

The fundamental characteristics describing a material's properties are depicted by a stress–strain or load–deflection curve (Fig. 1-20). A few key features of this curve express the clinical characteristics of a wire. The stress–strain diagram relates the load or force (stress) exerted on a material to the distortion (strain) of that material. Two areas of the curve can be described: the elastic region and the plastic region. The elastic region is the linear portion of the curve. Deformation of the material in this region is temporary—i.e. the material will return to its original shape with removal of the stress (load). Distortion of the material beyond the elastic range results in permanent deformation of the material—i.e. the material changes shape. Orthodontic wires and springs are generally used in the elastic region for tooth movement.

The *modulus of elasticity* is the slope of the elastic region of the stress–strain curve. It represents the stiffness or flexibility of a wire. Stress–strain is an intrinsic property of the alloy, i.e., the modulus of elasticity is an inherent quality of the alloy. The clinical analog to the modulus is the load–deflection rate of a wire. The load–deflection rate depends on both the intrinsic and extrinsic properties of the wire (diameter, length, loading condition, etc).

A flexible wire would demonstrate a flatter curve (low modulus) in the elastic range, whereas a stiff wire would have a steep curve (high modulus). The lower the modulus, the less the force per unit deflection, and the more flexible the wire. Conversely stiffer wires demonstrate a higher modulus with a greater force per unit deflection.

The *elastic limit*, also called the proportional limit or yield strength, is the point at which any greater force will produce permanent deformation in a wire. Technically it is a difficult point to measure precisely. For practical purposes the yield strength is identified as the point where 0.1% of deformation is measured. Beyond the elastic limit is the plastic range. Distortion or deflection of a wire beyond the elastic limit is necessary to place a bend in a wire.

The amount of deflection in a wire up to the elastic limit represents a wire's *elastic range*. This characteristic is clinically useful because it determines the allowable amount of activation of a wire or spring. Wires with greater elastic ranges can be activated further than wires with smaller ranges.

The *ultimate tensile strength* of the wire is the peak of the curve (in the plastic range). It is the maximum stress of force a material can withstand. Deflection beyond the ultimate tensile strength shows a weakening of the material. If a wire is deflected far enough, the failure point is reached and the wire breaks. The extent to which the material will return to its original shape after the removal of the load is the material's spring back (unless the failure point is reached).

Each of the above characteristics of the stress–strain curve is determined by the intrinsic properties of the material. The clinically important load–deflection curve for an individual wire is determined by both the intrinsic and extrinsic conditions. Wire diameter, length, and loading condition all affect the load–deflection characteristics of a wire. For tooth movement the elastic characteristics of a wire are most relevant. Generally decreasing the wire diameter results in reduced load–deflection rates. Increasing the span of the wire also tends to decrease the load–deflection rate. Increasing the length of the wire by increasing the inter-bracket distance is a common method of increasing the range of activation, as well as decreasing the load–deflection rate. Lower load–deflection rates are typically associated with greater force constancy over the activation range.

Orthodontic Brackets

In fixed appliance therapy, brackets and tubes are the primary means of engaging the active forces with the teeth. The majority of bracket designs can trace their ancestry to the original edgewise appliance developed by Edward H Angle in the early 1900s. An especially notable advance in the basic edgewise bracket occurred with Andrew's intro-duction of the "straight wire appliance." Since then many others have offered refinements to the straight wire con-cepts, resulting in an enormous number of variations on the theme; these designs are broadly described as preadjusted appliances.

Fundamentally, the orthodontic bracket acts as a handle, i.e., it is the mechanism through which the clinician attaches wires, springs, elastics, or other devices that exert forces on the teeth. The edgewise-style brackets utilize a rectangular wire slot that allows the application of a combination of multiple, simultaneous forces (i.e. couples), giving the orthodontist a high degree of three-dimensional clinical control.

The bracket slot in the original, standard edgewise bracket lay roughly perpendicular to the facial/labial surface of the tooth. In addition the depth of these brackets was constant, regardless of the tooth to which it was attached. Three-dimensional control of tooth movement was achieved by precise wire bending. Buccal–lingual inclination required twist-type bends in the rectangular wire to generate the torque needed for this movement.

Preadjusted appliances differ from the standard edgewise brackets primarily by incorporating design features aimed at reducing or eliminating the need for wire bending. The specific angulations of the slots to the occlusal plane are described by the appliance's prescription. The "straight wire appliance," pioneered by Andrews, emphasizes bracket design and placement over wire bending. An independent but key development in orthodontic technology that enhanced the use of preadjusted brackets was the use of

alternative wire alloys. Rather than progressing through a sequence of wire sizes, "variable modulus orthodontics" allows the use of large dimension wires that better capitalize on the bracket prescription by advancing through materials of increasing elastic modulus. In other words the wire's material properties, instead of its dimension, become the driving feature in its selection. A focus on wire alloy and bracket design shifts much of the technical element of treatment away from historically traditional "wire bending" toward material science, and appliance (bracket prescription) selection and placement.

An orderly sequence of treatment stages (i.e. first-, second-, and third-order movements) aids treatment efficiency. A typical approach addresses the malocclusion with a primary emphasis toward one plane at a time. First rotations of teeth relative to the occlusal view (first order) are corrected. The key feature of the bracket in this dimension is its mesiodistal width. Engaging a flexible wire into the bracket facilitates rotational control. Second occlusogingival leveling and mesiodistal root parallelism are achieved (second order). The bracket width, its position on the tooth, the vertical dimension of the bracket slot, and increasing wire stiffness contribute to achieving these corrections. Finally rectangular wires are used to express the buccal–lingual couples (torque) aimed at aligning the roots in their proper third-order inclinations. While not necessarily sufficient for optimal results, careful attention to the bracket positions on each tooth, and progressing through a selection of wires of different sizes, dimensions (round versus rectangular), and/or alloys, often enhances treatment effectiveness. Failure to attend to the details of bracket placement may even result in detrimental movements due to bracket position errors.

An important consideration in bracket prescription selection is the "snugness" of fit of rectangular wires in the slots. Smaller dimension square or rectangular wires are less efficient in exerting torque on the bracket than wires of greater dimension. Bracket designs with lower "torque" values require larger archwires in order to produce the tooth inclination for which the bracket was intended. In a further progression of these concepts, attention is increasing toward the selection of bracket prescriptions on the basis of individual patient needs and computer-aided design and machining (CAD/CAM) in appliance manufacturing.

A comparison of the springiness or stiffness of wires based on diameter reveals the effect of wire size on the relative force values the wires express on the teeth (Fig. 1-21). For the purposes of comparison, 0.014" and 0.016" diameter wires are used as baseline standards (the springiness of each is weighted at 1.00). The springiness of a wire varies with the fourth power of the change in diameter ($[d/2d]^4$). For instance the stiffness and therefore the applied force levels increase 71% when moving from a 0.014" wire to a 0.016" wire, while moving from a 0.016" wire to a 0.020" wire represents a 144% increase in stiffness.

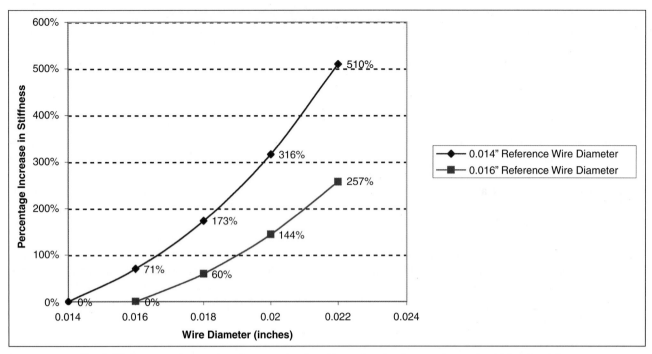

Fig. 1-21 Percentage increase in stiffness as a function of increasing wire diameter. See text for detailed description.

It is readily apparent that selecting larger or smaller wires has a significant effect on the relative stiffness or springiness of a wire. An important consideration is the magnitude of force of the wire used for comparison. For example if the force from a 0.014" wire is 50 g, a 71% increase only increases the force to 85 g (assuming equivalent deflections). However increasing the wire diameter to 0.018" brings the force levels to 137 g. The magnitude of force and the desired increase in force should be considered when increasing wire dimension.

Nature of Tooth Movement Along an Orthodontic Wire

The role of the orthodontic wire in treatment is to act as a spring and/or a guide. The force required to deflect the wire into the bracket slot provides the activation energy that will produce the tooth movement. In the elastic range, the strain within the wire is the reciprocal of the strain on the periodontal tooth support. A wide range of factors interact and influence the clinical response.

Imagine an archwire in the slot of a bracketed tooth. Using a stretched coil-spring or elastic, a force is applied at the level of the bracket, parallel to the wire. This force will pull the tooth, causing it to tip, as described above. As it tips, the bracket will contact the wire. The bracket will be exerting forces on the wire, and the wire will be exerting equal and opposite forces on the bracket. Because the tooth is restrained by the periodontal support structures,

no further movement will occur (until the biologic reactions remodel the bone). The moment of the applied force is the product of the force magnitude multiplied by its distance to the center of resistance of the tooth. At the bracket, this moment will be "twisting" the wire. The bracket's twist on the wire will continue until the bending moment of the wire equals the moment of the applied force. The bending moment of the wire is determined by the properties of the wire (e.g. wire size, alloy, interbracket distance). If the wire is of very low stiffness, it will deflect considerably before this equilibrium is reached. For a very stiff wire, little or no deflection will occur. From this point the bracket will slide along the wire.

Sliding mechanics can become rather complicated. Frictional forces resist the sliding movement. The force of friction equals the product of the normal force (the force pushing the two surfaces together) and the coefficient of friction. The coefficient of friction varies depending on the materials/surfaces in contact and the presence of lubrication, and is different in static (nonmoving) and kinetic (moving) situations. The magnitude of the force of friction is independent of the surface area in contact. The frictional forces retard or reduce the applied force, decreasing the effective force acting to produce motion. As long as wires are used as rails for sliding the teeth into position, friction cannot be eliminated. Reducing either the normal forces or the coefficient of friction will decrease the frictional force.

The analysis of the clinical situation in orthodontics is thus quite complex. However several useful clinical concepts can be derived. For effective sliding, stiffer wires will prevent more tipping than more flexible wires (assuming equal surface characteristics). When attempting to slide along very flexible wires, very light retraction-type forces must be used to maintain axial inclination control. For similar conditions a wider bracket will exert lower normal forces compared to a narrow bracket; therefore the frictional forces will be lower with wider brackets.

Finally the effect of the mobility of the tooth and the degree of play between the wire and its attachment must be considered. Friction acts as long as the surfaces are in contact. Play between the wire and the bracket sides, ligation techniques, and the inherent mobility of the tooth within the periodontal ligament all contribute to altering the wire–bracket interface and therefore lead to frequent changes in the loading condition. Chewing and biting produce a form of vibration or jiggling of the teeth, potentially breaking or disrupting the instantaneous contact of the wire and bracket. Whenever this occurs, the effect of friction is lost, and the tooth is free to move consistent with the forces acting upon it (including the orthodontic forces and the constraints of the periodontal support).

Considerations in Appliance Design

Ideal orthodontic care achieves specific, individualized, predetermined treatment objectives. The three major components of treatment are: (1) diagnosis—identifying a patient's specific problems that need treatment; (2) treatment planning—establishing treatment goals that identify precise objectives for treatment outcome; and (3) delivering treatment—the course of action (treatment) selected that addresses the patient's problems and is directed toward meeting the individualized goals. These components imply that different patients require different treatments, i.e., one appliance design (bracket prescription, archwire sequence, etc.) will not solve all patients' problems. Applying the concepts of biomechanics to the selection and design of orthodontic appliances improves the precision of treatment.[13] No bracket design or prescription can automatically deliver individualized treatment objectives. Only the orthodontist can control the specific characteristics of the force system used in treatment.

Specific Considerations

Force magnitude is the "lightness" or "heaviness" of the force. Ideal treatment requires forces to be within an appropriate range to elicit an efficient biologic response without detrimental side effects. Frequently the term "optimal force" is used. An optimal force is the lightest force that will move a tooth to a desired position in the shortest possible time and with no iatrogenic effects. Unfortunately an accurate measure of the optimal force eludes deter-

mination.[25] Force magnitudes as small as 2 g have been shown to produce tooth movement,[26] whereas forces from headgear and orthopedic appliances often exceed 500 g.

Force constancy is the consistency of the applied force over the range of activation of the appliance. For tooth movements over large distances, continuity of the force levels throughout is often desired. Force constancy can be obtained by reducing the load–deflection rate in one or more of the following ways: (1) reducing the cross-section of a wire; (2) increasing the interbracket distance; (3) incorporating loops in the wire; and (4) using memory alloys.

Reducing the Wire Cross-Section

This method is commonly used. The advantage of using small-diameter wires is that flexibility eases ligation into the brackets, especially in the early stages of the treatment of malaligned teeth. However the smaller the cross-section of the wire, the less the control expressed on a tooth in three planes of space.

A large cross-section wire provides better bracket engagement and control in tooth positioning, but at the same time the load–deflection rate and magnitude of force generated may be too high. Larger cross-sections and rectangular (edgewise) wires permit greater expression of the three-dimensional control designed into modern brackets. But as stiffness increases, the range of activation decreases as the load–deflection rate increases. This provides excellent control in the final stages of treatment when small, detailed tooth movements are necessary. Large-dimension wires can also be used to anchor units in the early stages of treatment.

Increasing the Interbracket Distance

A large interattachment distance reduces the load–deflection rate and helps deliver constant force magnitude, providing better directional control of the tooth movement. The wire length results in greater wire flexibility. Many bracket and auxiliary spring designs integrate increased interbracket distances to achieve improved force constancy. A practical application of the principle of large interbracket distance is to bypass the teeth or tooth in need of major movement using a simple spring or a cantilever from an auxiliary tube on the first molar.

Incorporating Loops in the Wire

Prior to the introduction of memory alloys, one of the most common methods to reduce the load–deflection rate was to incorporate loops into the appliance system. Most of the loops used in orthodontics are simple loops, which only increase the amount of wire material, thereby reducing the load–deflection rate. However for a biomechanically sound appliance system, it is important to understand the loop design to effectively reduce the load–deflection rate and wire deformation. With a carefully designed loop shape and by placing more wire in the area of loop deformation, the loop efficiency can be increased.

Memory Alloys

One of the most significant advances in the practice of clinical orthodontics over the past 15 years has been the introduction of memory alloys, such as nickel–titanium, to effectively reduce the load–deflection rate.[22] Now large-dimension memory alloy wires can be used much earlier in treatment for better tooth motion control. The nickel–titanium wire has a significantly lower modulus of elasticity than stainless steel wires. A reduction in the modulus of elasticity translates into an almost 1:1 reduction in the load–deflection of the archwire.

The magnitude of the moment and its constancy should also be considered. Control of both force and moment magnitudes establishes the moment/force ratio. As discussed above, the moment/force ratio determines the type of tooth movement. A pure force applied at the tooth crown or bracket produces an "uncontrolled" tipping, resulting in the crown and apex moving in opposite directions. The application of a pure moment (couple) rotates a tooth about its center of resistance. A combined moment and force must be simultaneously applied to achieve other types of tooth movement. In many clinical situations, the moment is produced by the wire–bracket combination, whereas the force is obtained from elastics or springs.[27]

The *point of force application* is a very important, yet often overlooked, fundamental consideration in appliance design. The point of force delivery and the direction of force relative to the center of resistance of the tooth have a significant effect on the type of tooth movement. Forces acting at a distance from the center of resistance generate moments of the force, potentially producing unwanted tooth movements.

Several simple examples illustrate the concept. Figures 1-22A-D show four different inclinations of the central incisors: ideal inclination; upright; significantly flared; and lingually inclined, respectively. In all four examples the same vertical intrusive force is applied to the incisors. Figures 1-22A-C show that the farther the line of force is labial to the center of resistance, the larger the moment which would move the root lingually and the crown labially. Thus in this example, although the force direction and amount are similar, the type of tooth response would be quite different.

Conversely Figure 1-22D shows that a vertical intrusive force applied to a severely lingually tipped incisor would have the opposite moment as compared to the moments shown in Figures 1-22A-C. The force direction would further lingually tip the incisor instead of improving it since the line of force is lingual to the center of resistance of the incisors.

An example of an appliance using these principles in its design is the intrusion arch. An intrusion arch is an auxiliary appliance for incisor intrusion and/or molar tipback. The intrusion arch is ligated to an anterior segment. It exerts a vertical force through a "point attachment" to the anterior teeth. The large interbracket distance increases the range of activation, thereby reducing the force magnitude while increasing the force constancy. The point of force application can be varied depending on the axial inclination of the incisors. The simple, two-tooth design allows measurement of the force magnitude. The tipback moment acting on the molars equals the force multiplied by the interbracket distance. This basic appliance is typical of all cantilever-type designs. Figure 1-23 shows a cantilever design for extrusion of an impacted maxillary canine.

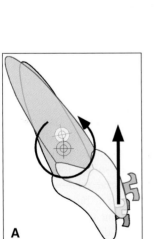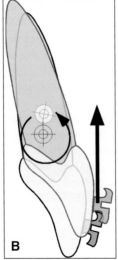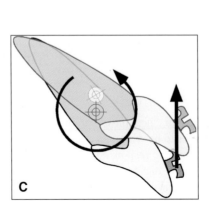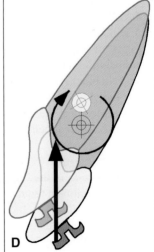

Fig. 1-22 Effect of axial inclination and location of the point of force application on tooth movement. An intrusive force on an incisor with **A** normal axial inclination, **B** upright incisor, **C** flared incisor, and **D** lingually inclined incisor.

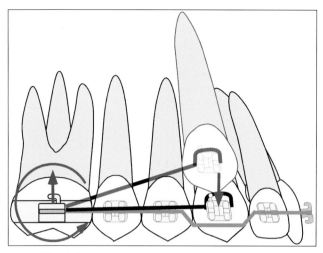

Fig. 1-23 Cantilever force for the extrusion of a canine.

Biomechanic considerations are also useful in the comparison of cervical versus occipital (high-pull) headgear. The line of action of the force produced by a cervical headgear lies inferior to the center of resistance of the molar and/or maxilla. Thus a moment of the force is

produced, tending to tip the crowns distally. Furthermore the force vector can be decomposed into horizontal and vertical components. The vertical component is extrusive (inferiorly directed) and the horizontal force is distal (posteriorly directed).

This is similar to the force of an occipital headgear. The line of action passes through the estimated center of resistance. Therefore no moment of the force is produced. The vertical and horizontal components of the force are distal (posteriorly directed) and intrusive (superiorly directed).

Although both appliances are headgears, their biomechanic characteristics are quite different. Depending on the particular requirements of a patient's treatment, either of these appliance designs can be selected.

Summary

Biomechanic principles explain the mechanism(s) of action of orthodontic appliances. They are of fundamental importance to understanding orthodontic treatment. Cognitive application of biomechanic concepts in the delivery of orthodontic care can be beneficial in achieving efficient and effective treatment.

REFERENCES

1. Andersen K, Mortensen HT, Pedersen E, Melsen B. Determination of stress levels and profiles in the periodontal ligament by means of an improved three-dimension finite element model for various types of orthodontic and natural force systems. J Biomed Eng 1991;13:293–303.
2. Tanne K, Koenig HA, Burstone CJ. Moment to force ratios and the center of rotation. Am J Orthod Dentofacial Orthop 1988;94:426–431.
3. Tanne K, Nagataki T, Inoue Y, Sakuda M, Burstone CJ. Patterns of initial tooth displacements associated with various root lengths and alveolar bone heights. Am J Orthod Dentofacial Orthop 1991;100:66–71.
4. Tanne K, Sakuda M, Burstone CJ. Three-dimensional finite element analysis for stress in the periodontal tissue by orthodontic forces. Am J Orthod Dentofacial Orthop 1987;92:499–505.
5. Vanden Bulcke MM, Burstone CJ, Sachdeva RC, Dermaut LR. Location of centers of resistance for anterior teeth during retraction using the laser reflection technique. Am J Orthod Dentofacial Orthop 1987;91:375–384.
6. Vanden Bulcke MM, Dermaut LR, Sachdeva RC, Burstone CJ. The center of resistance of anterior teeth during intrusion using the laser reflection technique and holographic interferometry. Am J Orthod Dentofacial Orthop 1986;90:211–220.
7. Nanda R, Goldin B. Biomechanic approaches to the study of alterations of facial morphology. Am J Orthod 1980;78:213–226.
8. Andersen K, Pedersen E, Melsen B. Material parameters and stress profiles within the periodontal ligament. Am J Orthod Dentofacial Orthop 1991;99:427–440.
9. Smith RJ, Burstone CJ. Mechanics of tooth movement. Am J Orthod 1984;85:294–307.
10. Burstone CJ, Pryputniewicz RJ. Holographic determination of centers of rotation produced by orthodontic forces. Am J Orthod 1980;77:396–409.
11. Christiansen RL, Burstone CJ. Centers of rotation within the periodontal space. Am J Orthod 1969;55:353–369.
12. Kusy RP, Tulloch JFC. Analysis of moment/force ratio in the mechanics of tooth movement. Am J Orthod Dentofacial Orthop 1986;90:127–131.
13. Burstone CJ. The mechanics of the segmented arch techniques. Angle Orthod 1966;36:99–120.
14. Demange C. Equilibrium situations in bend force systems. Am J Orthod Dentofacial Orthop 1990;98:333–339.
15. Burstone CJ. Deep overbite correction by intrusion. Am J Orthod 1977;72:1–22.
16. Nanda R. The differential diagnosis and treatment of excessive overbite. In: Nanda R, ed. Symposium on orthodontics. Dental Clinics of North America. Philadelphia: WB Saunders, 1981:69–84.
17. Shroff B, Lindauer SJ, Burstone CJ, Leiss JB. Segmented approach to simultaneous intrusion and space closure: Biomechanics of the three-piece intrusion arch. Am J Orthod Dentofacial Orthop 1995;107:136–143.
18. Burstone CJ, Koenig HA. Creative wire bending—the force system from step and V bends. Am J Orthod Dentofacial Orthop 1988;93:59–67.
19. Burstone CJ, Koenig HA. Force systems from the ideal arch. Am J Orthod 1974;65:270–289.
20. Koenig HA, Vanderby R, Solonche DJ, Burstone CJ. Force systems from orthodontic appliances: An analytical and experimental comparison. J Biomech Eng 1980;102:294–300.

21. Burstone CJ. Variable-modulus orthodontics. Am J Orthod 1981;80:1–16.
22. Burstone CJ, Qin B, Morton JY. Chinese NiTi wire—a new orthodontic alloy. Am J Orthod 1985;87:445–452.
23. Burstone CJ, Goldberg AJ. Beta titanium: A new orthodontic alloy. Am J Orthod 1980;77:121–132.
24. Kapila S, Sachdeva R. Mechanical properties and clinical applications of orthodontic wires. Am J Orthod Dentofacial Orthop 1989;96:100–109.

25. Quinn RS, Yoshikawa DK. A reassessment of force magnitude in orthodontics. Am J Orthod 1985;88:252–260.
26. Weinstein S. Minimal forces in tooth movement. Am J Orthod 1967;53:881–903.
27. Issacson RJ, Lindauer SJ, Rubenstein LK. Moments with edgewise appliance: Incisor torque control. Am J Orthod Dentofacial Orthop 1993;103:428–438.

SUGGESTED READING

Burstone CJ. The segmented approach to space closure. Am J Orthod 1982;82:361–378.

Dermaut LR, Vanden Bulcke MM. Evaluation of intrusive mechanics of the type "segmented arch" on macerated human skull using the laser reflection technique and holographic interferometry. Am J Orthod 1986;89:251–263.

Faulkner MG, Fuchhuber P, Haberstock D, Mioduchowski A. A parametric study of the force/moment systems produced by T-loop retraction springs. J Biomech 1989;22:637–647.

Jacobson A. A key to the understanding of extraoral forces. Am J Orthod 1979;75:361–386.

Kloehn SJ. Guiding alveolar growth and eruption of teeth to reduce treatment time and produce a more balanced denture and face. Angle Orthod 1947;17:10–33.

Melsen B, Fotis V, Burstone CJ. Vertical force considerations in differential space closure. J Clin Orthod 1990;24:678–683.

Melsen B. Adult orthodontics: Factors differentiating the selection of biomechanics in growing and adult individuals. Int J Adult Orthod Orthognath Surg 1988;3:167–177.

Nanda R. Biomechanic and clinical considerations of a modified protraction headgear. Am J Orthod 1980;78:125–139.

Nagerl H, Burstone CJ, Becker B, Kubein-Messenburg D. Centers of rotation with transverse forces: An experimental study. Am J Orthod Dentofacial Orthop 1991;99:337–345.

Nikolai RJ. On optimum orthodontic force theory as applied to canine retraction. Am J Orthod 1975;68:290–302.

Pedersen E, Andersen K, Melsen B. Tooth displacement analyzed on human autopsy material by means of a strain gauge technique. Eur J Orthod 1991;13:65–74.

Pryputniewicz RJ, Burstone CJ. The effect of time and force magnitude on orthodontic tooth movement. J Dent Res 1979;58:1754–1764.

Roberts WW, Chacker FM, Burstone A. Segmental approach to mandibular molar uprighting. Am J Orthod 1982;81:177–184.

Romeo DA, Burstone CJ. Tip-back mechanics. Am J Orthod 1977;72:414–421.

Ronay F, Kleinert W, Melsen B, Burstone CJ. Force system developed by V bends in an elastic orthodontic wire. Am J Orthod Dentofacial Orthop 1989;96:295–301. [Published erratum: Am J Orthod Dentofacial Orthop 1990;98:19A.]

Wood MG. The mechanics of lower incisor intrusion: Experiments in nongrowing baboons. Am J Orthod Dentofacial Orthop 1988;93:186–195.

Yoshikawa DK. Biomechanic principles of tooth movement. In: Nanda R, ed. Symposium on orthodontics. Dental Clinics of North America. Philadephia: WB Saunders, 1981:19–26.

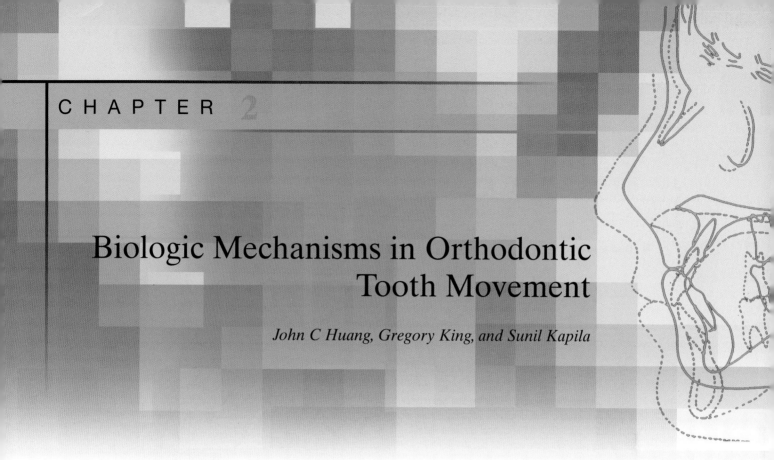

CHAPTER 2

Biologic Mechanisms in Orthodontic Tooth Movement

John C Huang, Gregory King, and Sunil Kapila

The goal of this chapter is to examine the relationships between orthodontic biomechanics and the underlying biologic processes. The topics discussed include the factors affecting the rate of tooth movement, anchorage considerations, causes of relapse, and root resorption. All the relevant biologic principles underlying orthodontic tooth movement can be characterized as tissue remodeling. The process of orthodontic tooth movement is a resultant dynamic change in the shapes and composition of the investing bone and soft tissues. The dental and peridental tissues (dentin, cementum, periodontal ligament [PDL], and alveolar bone) all have active reparative mechanisms and will adapt under the normal forces of orthodontic appliances. At the most basic level extrinsic forces set up localized areas of "pressure" and "tension" in the tissues adjacent to teeth and the subsequent responses satisfy the principles of Wolff's law of bone remodeling.[1] When orthodontists use fixed appliances to apply forces on teeth, predictable tooth movement is anticipated. This is accompanied by transiently increased tooth mobility and, occasionally, radiographic evidence of mild root resorption. Experienced clinicians also expect a certain amount of relapse to occur following orthodontic treatment. Other types of natural tooth migration commonly encountered are eruption of primary and succedaneous teeth, as well as mesial or distal drifting of teeth. These physiologic processes are not necessarily stimulated by biomechanic signals. In rare instances teeth fail to erupt or move in response to forces (i.e. ankylosis). Each of these common clinical findings can be explained with a better understanding of the underlying biologic principles that determine tooth movement.

Tooth Movement

Clinical Responses

Kinetics of Orthodontic Tooth Movement

From a clinical perspective orthodontic tooth movement has three distinct phases: (1) displacement phase; (2) delay phase; and (3) acceleration and linear phase (Fig. 2-1).

Displacement phase. The initial reaction of a tooth following force application is almost instantaneous (within a fraction of a second) and reflects the immediate movement of the tooth within the viscoelastic PDL cradle. These movements are generally predictable by biophysical principles and typically do not involve extensive amounts of tissue remodeling or deformation of the investing alveolar bone.[2] The fluid compartments within the PDL play an important role in the transmission and damping of forces acting on teeth.[3] The magnitude of the displacement response is also dependent on root length and alveolar bone height, which are factors that determine the location of a tooth's center of resistance and center of rotation (see Ch. 1).[4,5] For example loss of alveolar bone results in a more apically positioned center of resistance, which affects the nature of both the initial displacement and net tooth movement (Fig. 2-2). Age is another factor affecting displacement. Young's modulus of the PDL has been shown to be greater in adults than in adolescents, and this

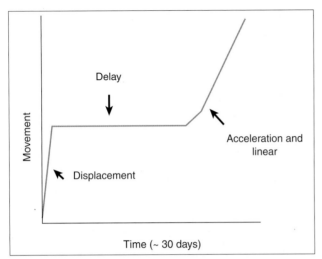

Fig. 2-1 Phases of orthodontic tooth movement. The classic curve has three phases: an initial displacement that reflects the viscoelastic properties of the tooth supporting structures; a delay or lag period characterized by no movement; and a postlag phase with linear tooth movement. Minimal tooth movement occurs during the first two phases, and most of the tooth movement occurs during the acceleration and linear phase when alveolar bone remodeling occurs. The time line is approximate with considerable individual variation due to mechanical and biologic differences.

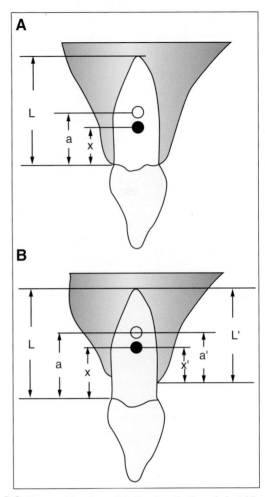

Fig. 2-2 Degree of freedom within the viscoelastic periodontal ligament apparatus (displacement) is affected by root lengths and alveolar bone heights. **A** Varying root length (L) will cause shifts in the positions of the distance of the center of rotation (CRo) to the cervix (a) and the distance of the center of resistance (CRe) to the cervix (x). **B** Shows how alveolar bone height changes can affect CRo and CRe. (L = average root length; a = distance of the CRo to the cervix; x = distance of the CRe to the cervix; L' = varying alveolar bone heights; a' = distance of the CRo to the alveolar crest; and x' = distance of the CRe to the alveolar crest.) Ultimately the patterns of tooth displacement will be determined by the change in the position of CRe produced by changes in alveolar bone height or root length. (Modified with permission from Tanne K, Nagataki T, Inoue Y, Sakuda M, Burstone CJ. Patterns of initial tooth displacements associated with various root lengths and alveolar bone heights. Am J Orthod Dentofacial Orthop 1991;100:66–71.)

difference in biomechanic properties correlates to an equivalent or somewhat increased stress level in the PDL in adults. It is suggested that this might reduce the biologic response of the PDL and thus delay tooth movement in adults.[6] The displacement capacity of a tooth can change even within the same individual; the elasticity of the PDL and alveolar bone has the potential to be substantially reduced at the end of tooth movement.[7]

Delay phase. The second phase of the orthodontic tooth movement cycle is characterized by the absence of clinical movement and is generally referred to as the delay or latency phase. During this period there is no tooth movement but extensive remodeling occurs in all tooth-investing tissues. The absolute amount of force applied is not as relevant as the relative force applied per unit area. Depending on the localized compression of the PDL, there can be either (1) a partial occlusion of the blood vessels in the area; or (2) an absolute occlusion of blood vessels when high excessive forces have been applied. In cases of partial blockage, the blood vessels delivering nutrients to the area have the capacity to adapt to the new environment and can undergo angiogenesis to bypass occluded areas. However complete occlusion of vascular flow leads to temporary necrosis of the immediate area and follows a completely different pathway of tooth movement, which is slower to be initiated, starting after approximately 1–2 weeks. In either situation structural and biochemical changes initiate a cascade of cellular mechanisms required for bone remodeling.

Aging has been shown to substantially affect the proliferative activity of the PDL cells and subsequent tooth movement, particularly during the delay phase.[8] However some studies on molar movement in animal models have shown faster initial tooth movement in young subjects than in adults. Yet, once tooth movement had reached the linear phase, the rate of tooth movement became equal in both groups. This indicates that the clinically observed increase in orthodontic treatment time for adults can be primarily attributed to the delay phase prior to the onset of tooth movement, but the rate of migration is equally efficient once tooth movement has started.[9]

Acceleration and linear phase. The third phase of the cycle is characterized by rapid tooth displacement. Tooth movement is initiated in deference to the adaptation of the supporting PDL and alveolar bone changes. Studies on the bone-resorptive osteoclast response following orthodontic appliance activation indicate that when appliance reactivation occurs during the appearance of reactivation osteoclasts, a second cohort of osteoclasts can be recruited immediately. This causes immediate, significant tooth movement with no greater risk of root resorption.[10] The force magnitude directly affects the rate of tooth movement. High forces in excess of 100 g used in conventional orthodontic therapy to retract canine teeth have been shown to produce a lag phase of up to 21 days before tooth movement. Lower forces can induce tooth translation without a lag phase at rates that are still clinically significant.[11] The difference in rates of tooth movements can be explained by the different biologic responses (frontal resorption versus undermining resorption) discussed later in the chapter. Equally as important as magnitude, however, is the timing of the force application. The force regimen has more influence on the rate of orthodontic tooth movement than the force magnitude.[12] Light continuous forces are much more conducive to orthodontic tooth movement because the cell biology system remains in a constantly responsive state. Conversely the application of intermittent forces creates a fluctuating environment of cellular activity/quiescence (Fig. 2-3A). Additionally it is recognized that very low forces produce lower rates of tooth movement then higher forces (Fig. 2-3B) up to a specific optimal threshold. Exceeding this optimal force does not result in substantially greater rates of tooth movement. This threshold may differ between individuals as demonstrated in experiments on beagle dogs where it was noted that 25 cN of force caused greater tooth movement then 10 cN of force in one animal, but not in another (Fig. 2-3B and C).

Ankylosis

In rare cases a tooth may not move at all, regardless of the amount of external force applied on it. A likely cause of this is a phenomenon known as "ankylosis" where the PDL fibers are conspicuously absent and therefore cannot serve as an intermediary between the root structure and the alveolar bone. The contact point is a direct fusion of the cementum layer to the cortical bone of the tooth socket. Apart from idiopathic ankylosis, the primary cause of ankylosis is extrinsic localized trauma.[13] In cases of severe dental trauma, such as avulsion or intrusion, there is injury to the periodontal membrane resulting in a direct fusion of the alveolar bone with the tooth. Consequences of this condition include progressive resorption of the root with replacement by bone (replacement resorption) and arrested growth of the alveolar process in growing patients. Individuals with congenitally missing succedaneous permanent teeth characteristically exhibit infraocclusion and over-retention of ankylosed deciduous teeth.[14] Partial ankylosis can also occur when only limited areas of the teeth are fused to the bone. If these localized regions of bone–tooth attachment can be overcome with sufficient force application, the remainder of the tooth that does have PDL support can

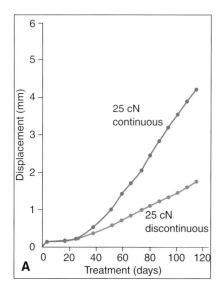
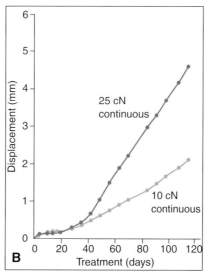
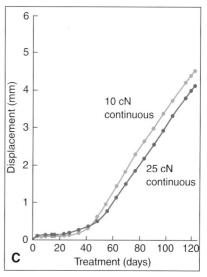

Fig. 2-3 Time displacement curve for premolar tooth movement in a beagle dog experimental model demonstrating that light continuous forces of 25 cN are more effective in tooth movement than discontinuous forces (**A**), and continuous forces of 25 cN produce greater movement than 10 cN in one animal (**B**), while in another animal the two forces produce equal amounts of tooth movement (**C**), demonstrating individual variation and a plateau effect in the latter animal. (Reproduced with permission from van Leeuwen EJ, Maltha JC, Kuijpers-Jagtman AM. Tooth movement with light continuous and discontinuous forces in beagle dogs. Eur J Oral Sci 1999;197:468–474).

proceed towards a normal pattern of tissue remodeling and tooth movement.

Principles of Anchorage in Orthodontics

The biomechanics of orthodontics are not always designed for the purpose of moving teeth. For certain cases the intent of the clinician may be to hold the position of certain teeth in the arch, or to use groups of teeth comprising an "anchor unit" to serve as a foundation for pushing or pulling other teeth. Several types of anchorage are used in orthodontics: (1) extraoral anchorage appliances (e.g. headgear) where external skeletal structures are used; (2) intraoral implants and miniscrews that are osseointegrated within the bone and therefore are extremely stable; and (3) dental anchorage, which is essentially the preparation and consolidation of teeth into units for use in pushing or pulling the rest of the dentition.

Dental anchorage is a term applied to the intentional minimization of migration of specific teeth through the supporting alveolar bone structure. The following section elaborates on dental anchorage since it is based on the premise of biologic adaptation to orthodontic forces. Dental anchorage can be increased either by increasing the number of teeth consolidated into the anchor unit or by intentionally angulating specific teeth to better resist movement or both. In general, teeth with greater root surface area will tend to move less when used to move teeth with less root surface area. This occurs because the ability to resist movement is directly related to the periodontal fibers and bone surface area engaged in withstanding tooth movement. When forces are light and distributed over large surface areas, the compression on underlying periodontal structures leads to a partial vascular occlusion of the system and a transient ischemia. Although limited, there is still oxygenation to the area, enabling the microsystem to adapt and recruit new blood vessels for initiation of frontal resorption to occur. Movement of teeth with frontal resorption occurs within 3–4 days. However when hyalinization of bone occurs in areas of periodontal compression during force application, there is a significant retardation of tooth movement while undermining resorption occurs. In this case the resistance to tooth movement is due to complete vascular occlusion in the compression area causing localized necrosis of bone and undermining resorption. When this happens the teeth start moving only after 12–15 days of bone remodeling. Therefore anchorage preparation is affected both by the magnitude of forces applied, the total root surface area of the teeth upon which the forces are applied, and the angulation of the teeth.

Increasing numbers of adults are seeking orthodontic treatment nowadays and in these cases anchorage becomes a critical concern. Extraoral anchorage appliances are not usually a feasible alternative for these individuals. Therefore the clinician must maximize all available resources such as the engagement and coligation of second molars (and third molars if present) into the dental anchorage unit, as well as the use of palatal anchorage devices such as the Nance acrylic button appliance. Also in multidisciplinary cases, implants and other fixed restorative devices can and should be incorporated into the treatment plan for use as anchorage units during orthodontics.

Histologic Responses

In general teeth can move through their investing tissues with or without histologic evidence of tissue injury. There is no evidence that the intra-alveolar phase of tooth movement during physiologic eruption, drift or relapse is mediated by pathologic processes.[15–17] However most studies on orthodontic tooth movement have described pathologic processes at sites of compression, including vascular collapse, compensatory hyperemia, and tissue necrosis. Hyperemic changes are not restricted to the periodontal tissues adjacent to compression, but have also been variously described in the adjacent marrow spaces and the dental pulp.

Tooth Movement Without Injury

The most obvious course of physiologic tooth movement is the intra-alveolar eruption of teeth. As the crown of a tooth completes mineralization and begins its process of migration through the alveolar bone, it becomes enclosed in a crypt. This crypt is translated bodily by a combined effort of osteoclastic bone resorption along the path of eruption and osteoblastic bone formation on the path that the crown has already taken. The rate-limiting factor of the earliest (intraosseous) stage of tooth eruption is bone resorption and eruption can be accelerated or retarded by the local delivery of factors that alter the rate of osteoclastic activity.[18] Certain hormones, such as parathyroid hormone-related protein (PTHrP), have been shown to be crucial in the normal tooth eruption processes and cementogenesis.[19,20] Pathologic systemic conditions with dysfunctional PTH/PTHrP or their cognate receptors can lead to the prevention of normal tooth eruption and inhibition of normal cementogenesis.

As the tooth erupts into the oral cavity, and even throughout life, there is a natural tendency for teeth to continue moving along the path of least resistance until they finally encounter an obstacle of resistance. Usually this barrier comes in the form of interproximal contact from an adjacent tooth or occlusal contact from a tooth in the opposing arch. In the absence of this resistance there will be continued mesiodistal tipping or supra-eruption, depending on the location of deficient contact. Studies have shown that mesial drifting of a tooth can have clinical significance on its morphologic composition. In the process of mesial migration, tensional forces on the distal root surfaces may account for the increased cementum thickness on the distal surfaces of mesially drifted teeth.[21] As for supra-eruption, in a mouse model where the opposing molar was extracted to induce occlusal hypofunction, histologic staining showed that after 15 days of hypofunction the PDL was significantly narrowed and the fibrous nature was very disorganized for a minimum of 30 days and for up to 3 months. There was concurrent deposition of disorganized woven bone at the top of the inter-radicular septa, at the bottom of the sockets, and along the modeling sides.[22] Thus it is evident that loading is an integral part of the maintenance of the supporting structures surrounding the tooth.

Tooth Movement With Injury

Necrotic lesions at compression sites in the PDL space have been described in the early literature documenting the histologic changes accompanying orthodontic tooth movement.[23] These areas are referred to as "hyalinization zones" because of their similarity in appearance to hyaline cartilage. Modern morphologic techniques have elucidated that these so-called "hyalinizations" are in fact areas of focal tissue necrosis.[24] As long as these lesions persist, orthodontic tooth movement does not occur. This period is coincident with the delay phase of the tooth movement cycle. Specialized phagocytic cells are recruited and migrate to the site to remove these necrotic lesions. These cells remove the injured tissue from the periphery, resulting in the resorption of not only the necrotic soft tissue lesion but also the adjacent alveolar bone and cementum.[25]

The tissue responses at sites of tension are consistent with those that have been described for other sites where soft tissue separates bone. In addition to the PDL, such sites can be found naturally in the craniofacial complex at sutures and artificially at sites of osteodistraction. Tensile forces are known to initiate an exuberant osteogenic response at these locations, with the first bone being deposited on the stretched soft tissue scaffold (Fig. 2-4). Through remodeling processes new compact bone is eventually deposited at these sites. This so-called consolidation process is slow to occur and therefore tends to lag behind the tissue removal activity that is simultaneously occurring at compression sites. The clinical result is the prevalence of increased mobility in teeth that are actively being treated orthodontically. This difference in timing between tissue removal and osteogenesis also accounts for the need to retain teeth that have recently been moved.

In addition to bone remodeling, histologic evidence has shown that initial root resorption occurs in the peripheries of the necrotic PDL following orthodontic treatment (Fig. 2-5). This is a result of mononucleated nonclast macrophage- and fibroblast-like cellular activity.[26,27] Minor resorptive lacunae created on the root surface by cemento-clasts can be repaired gradually over time. However heavy forces create extensive defects on the root surface, which exceed reparative capacity and lead to crater-like topography on the root surface and at the apex (Fig. 2-6).

Bone Turnover in Orthodontic Tooth Movement

Osteogenesis, and Bone Modeling and Remodeling

Bone structure can be changed in three principle ways: (1) osteogenesis; (2) bone modeling; and (3) bone remodeling. *Osteogenesis* is when bone is formed on soft tissue and generally occurs during embryonic development, the early stages of growth, and healing. There are two major subclassifications: intramembranous ossification and endochondral ossification, in which bone is formed on soft fibrous tissue and, usually, cartilage, respectively. Osteoblasts are a differentiation product from mesenchymal cells and act independently of osteoclasts, resulting in a large potential to create significant amounts of bone.

Modeling is characterized by bone formation on existing bone tissue over extended surface areas for significant periods of time. This type of bone turnover is prevalent

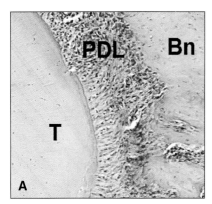
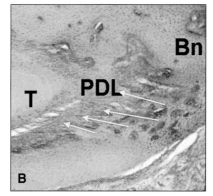
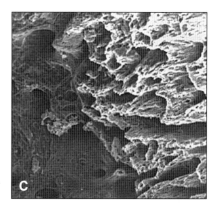

Fig. 2-4 Morphologic changes on the tension side during orthodontic tooth movement. **A** Initial changes are characterized by stretching of the principle periodontal ligament (PDL) fibers, seen here as linear orientation of cell nuclei adjacent to the tooth. **B** Later changes show deposition of bone on the stretched PDL fibers, oriented perpendicular to the tooth and socket wall (arrows). T = tooth root; Bn = alveolar bone. **C** The three-dimensional organization of these initial bony spicules can be appreciated with a scanning electron micrograph of the alveolar bone on the socket wall after removal of the tooth and PDL. The micrograph is looking into the socket with the tension socket wall on the right.

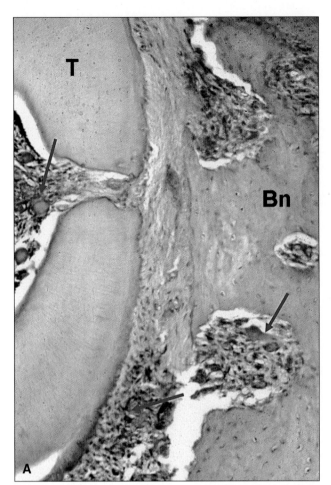 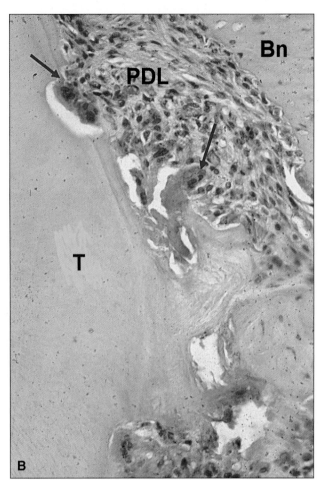

Fig. 2-5 Morphologic changes on the compression side showing tissue and cellular responses leading to root resorption during orthodontic tooth movement. **A** Initial changes are characterized by focal areas of periodontal ligament (PDL) necrosis, so-called hyalinization, seen as the clear area in the PDL running vertically down the center of this micrograph. Areas of vascular congestion can be seen adjacent (pulp, PDL, and marrow spaces) to the necrotic PDL (arrows). **B** Later changes show removal of the necrotic PDL and adjacent tissues, including the root cementum and dentin from the periphery by osteoclasts, cementoclasts, and macrophages (arrows). The remaining necrotic PDL is seen as the clear pink area in the lower middle of the micrograph. Vital adjacent PDL can be seen as the highly cellular areas above and below the necrosis. T = tooth root; Bn = alveolar bone.

during craniofacial growth and development, and leads to change in shape of the structure or translation of the surface. For example the mandibular alveolar process increases in length by resorptive modeling on the anterior surface of the ramus and by formative modeling on its posterior surface. From an orthodontics standpoint, modeling is important in normal growth of the craniofacial structure as well as changes in alveolar size and shape during tooth movement.

Remodeling is a reparative mechanism and involves a series of cellular events that occur cyclically throughout life (Fig. 2-7). It is the only physiologic mechanism for maintaining and repairing the structural integrity of bone. The bone remodeling cycle begins with a period referred to as activation that is characterized by the recruitment and activation of osteoclasts at the site to be remodeled. This is followed by a resorptive phase when a "packet" of bone is

removed. After a finite amount of time the resorptive process ceases. This phase is termed reversal. Reversal is followed be a formative phase characterized by the recruitment of bone formative cells to the site and the active repair of the defect created during the resorptive phase. Once the cycle is complete, the bone surface returns to a resting state. In healthy adults bone surfaces are primarily in a resting state, although a small fraction of the cell population can be seen to progress through the other phases. Remodeling is important in calcium homeostasis as well as in producing changes in bone matrices that modify the mechanical properties of the bone in response to altered loading. Remodeling and modeling of bone are differentiated by the fact that while osteoblast and osteoclast activities are found on the same site in remodeling, they occur on different sites in modeling, which enables morphologic changes in the bone.

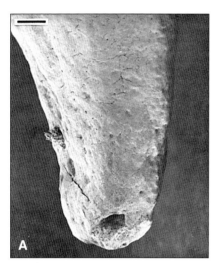 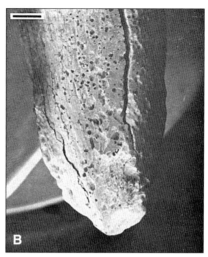 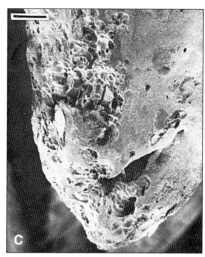

Fig. 2-6 Tooth injury resulting in root resorption following bone remodeling. **A** Apical third of the lingual root surface of the mandibular left bicuspid control tooth demonstrating the absence of resorption. **B** Apical resorption and loss of root length association with a multitude of resorption pits over the lingual root surface as a result of 2 weeks' application of a continuous 10 g intrusive force. Many of the resorption loci have coalesced to form extensive invasive lesions. **C** Lingual aspect of a maxillary right bicuspid showing early apical resorption caused by 14 days' intrusion with 50 g. Original magnifications for **A** and **B** are x 20 (bar = 300 μm) and for **C** is x 40 (bar = 200 μm). (Reproduced with permission from Harry MR, Sims MR. Root resorption in bicuspid intrusion. A scanning electron microscope study. Angle Orthod 1982;52:235–258).

Cellular and Molecular Mechanisms

Skeletal integrity is the result of a dynamic interaction between bone-forming osteoblasts and bone-resorbing osteoclasts. The rate of remodeling is defined primarily by cells of the osteoblast lineage which, in addition to bone formation, are also responsible for the activation and recruitment of osteoclast precursors.[28–30] However the basis of communication between osteoblasts and osteoclasts was unclear until several groups independently identified the presence of an intermediary factor on the surface of osteoblasts that was responsible for the induction of osteoclastogenesis. This factor is a member of the tumor necrosis factor (TNF) superfamily and was termed receptor activator of nuclear factor κB ligand (RANKL).[31,32] Binding of RANKL to its cognate receptor, receptor activator of nuclear factor κB (RANK), expressed on the surface of osteoclast progenitor cells, induces osteo-clastogenesis and activates osteoclasts (in the presence of macrophage-colony stimulating factor), resulting in increased bone resorption.[33,34] However RANKL also has the potential to bind to osteoprotegerin (OPG), a soluble decoy receptor protein that competitively binds to cell surface membrane-bound RANKL proteins and inhibits RANKL activation of osteoclastogenesis. RANKL–OPG interactions therefore decrease bone resorption (Fig. 2-8).[35] The ratio of RANKL/OPG expression by osteoblasts is believed to be a key determinant of the rate of recruitment and activation of immature osteoclasts. In dentistry these genes have already been strongly implicated as the causative factors of alveolar bone changes. RANKL and OPG protein production has been detected in human periodontal cells.[36] Pathological lymphocytes and macrophages in periodontitis tissues show correlations with RANKL protein production, and endothelial cells have associations with OPG production.[37] From an orthodontic perspective, it is very likely that pressure changes in the microenvironment of the tooth socket may cause up- and down-regulation of the RANKL and OPG genes as a means of modulating protein production and ultimately bone remodeling.

Besides the prominent role of the RANKL/OPG ratio in the regulation of osteoclasts by osteoblasts, the *rate* of bone remodeling is controlled by other local and systemic mechanisms. Local, or paracrine, mechanisms involve numerous inflammatory cytokines (e.g. interleukins, TNFs, and growth factors) that have biologic activities influencing individual phases of the cycle (Fig. 2-9).[38] In addition there is evidence that alterations in the genetic expression of bioactive agents can occur directly on bone cells. Systemic control of bone remodeling occurs through several endocrine mechanisms, including the calciotropic hormones (e.g. parathyroid hormone [PTH] and $1\alpha,25\text{-}(OH)_2$ vitamin D_3) and the sex steroids (e.g. estrogen).[39–41] These factors act on osteoblasts as an intermediary to regulate osteoblast/osteoclast equilibrium, and can either up- or down-regulate a cascade of downstream signaling pathways that ulti-mately affect the expression of specific genes necessary to synthesize proteins involved in bone remodeling. For example estrogen inhibits bone resorption, at least in part, by regulating the production of several cytokines, including

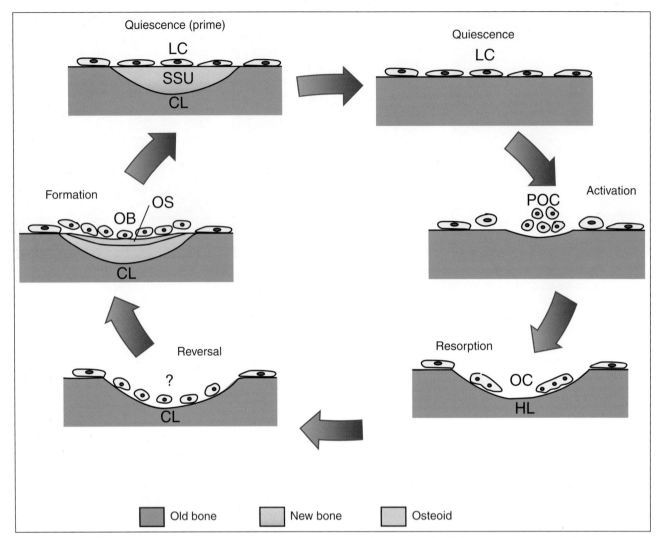

Fig. 2-7 Five phases of cellular activity in remodeling of trabecular bone. LC = lining cells; POC = osteoclast precursors; OC = osteoclasts; HL = Howship lacunae/resorption pit; OB = osteoblast; CL = closed lacunae; OS = osteoid; BSU = bone structural unit or newly formed bone structure.

interleukin-6 (IL-6), IL-1, RANKL, and OPG by cells of the osteoblastic lineage.[42] The potential implications of this knowledge to orthodontics are discussed at the end of this chapter.

The human bone remodeling cycle takes about 4 months and is characterized by a rapid period of resorption followed by a fairly slow period of formation. In a healthy adult bone resorption is coupled to formation so that there is no net loss or gain. However in certain disease conditions, this coupling can be lost, resulting in a net loss or gain of bone. Because it takes significantly more time to complete bone formation than it does resorption, stimulation of large amounts of remodeling often leads to a net bone loss. This can be a temporary condition if the level of remodeling activity returns to normal, permitting formation to "catch up" with resorption. This is characteristic of fracture healing. However if high levels of bone

remodeling persist, bone can be permanently lost, as in postmenopausal osteoporosis.

Conversely increased bone density resulting in osteopetrosis is a clinical manifestation of certain syndromes, such as Albers–Schonberg disease and Paget disease, where there is an excessive hyperactivity of the osteoclasts resulting in a concurrent compensatory excessive deposition of bone. Rates of bone remodeling may be increased up to 20-fold, but this coupling is imperfect. Since the newly formed bone is laid down so quickly, it is irregular and chaotic, resulting in a composite mixture of lamellar and woven bone which compromises the quality of the bone. The clinical consequences of this abnormal bone cell activity include diffuse sclerosis of the whole skeleton accompanied by pathologic bone fragility and delayed physical development, profound intractable myelophthisic anemia, neurologic deficits, and osteomyelitis, especially

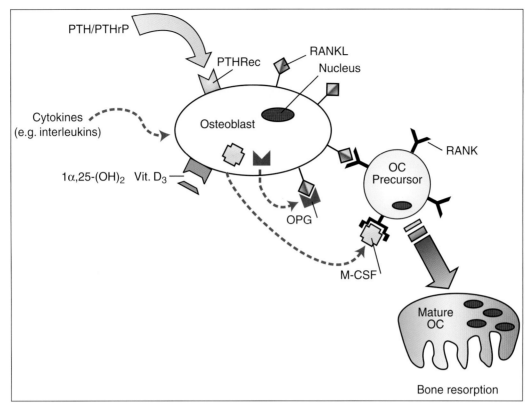

Fig. 2-8 Theoretical regulation of osteoclastogenesis by osteoblasts. Receptor activator of nuclear factor κB (RANKL) induces immature osteoclast (OC) precursors to differentiate into mature and functional osteoclasts, while osteoprotegrin (OPG) is a decoy receptor that acts as a competitive binding inhibitor of RANKL. Since RANKL is a cell-surface bound receptor protein, cell–cell interaction is required. Macrophage-colony stimulating factor (M-CSF) is also an essential co-factor. Vitamin D_3 and various cytokines have been demonstrated to have downregulatory effects on OPG gene expression and upregulatory effects on RANKL gene expression. PTH = parathyroid hormone; PTHrP = PTH-related protein.

of the jaws and skull. Eruption and development of the dentition can be impeded and delayed due to the irregular bone remodeling adjacent to the tooth bud and crown.

Biologic Responses in Clinical Treatment

In orthodontic tooth movement, sites of tension display osteogenesis over an extensive surface area, a framework consistent with modeling (Fig. 2-10A). However sites of compression undergo phases of a remodeling cycle (Fig. 2-10B).[43] Since large amounts of remodeling are initiated at these sites, there is a net loss of alveolar bone over the short term which subsequently returns to pretreatment levels over the course of orthodontic treatment. This ultimately leads to the clinical characterization of teeth being actively moved (i.e. radiographic evidence of widening of the PDL and clinical evidence of increased tooth mobility). This, along with the persistence of stretched ligament and gingival fibers, leads to rapid relapse of orthodontically moved teeth and necessitates stabilization,

at least until bone formation is able to return to pretreatment levels.[44]

There is a predictable relationship between mechanical strain and bone turnover. Increasing amounts of strain stimulate osteogenesis and conversely the lack of strain on bone (e.g. weightlessness during space flight) leads to osteopenia. Superficially this seems to contradict what happens in orthodontic tooth movement because sites of compression lose bone and sites of tension gain it. However it is important to realize that the PDL is loaded in tension sites and unloaded in compression sites. The latter also exhibit evidence of tissue damage and infiltration of inflammatory cells releasing cytokines, which can also stimulate large amounts of bone resorption. Recent studies show that alveolar bone at sites distant from the tooth socket wall contribute to the bone remodeling response, and this is consistent with what would be predicted by the bone literature (i.e. bony trabeculae adjacent to compression sites are osteogenic and those next to tension sites are not).[45] Evidence also indicates that tissues are directly sensitive to deformations and strains in their immediate environment in addition to pressure or tension.[46]

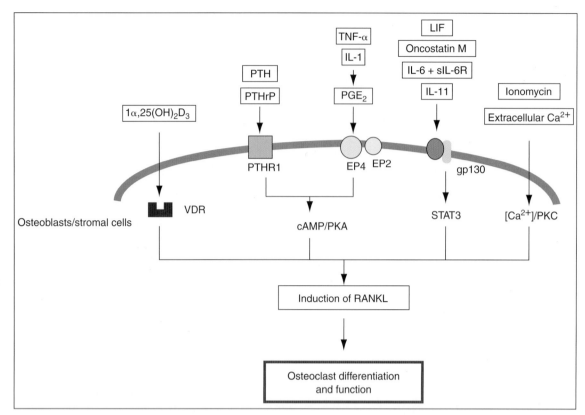

Fig. 2-9 Paracrine and endocrine regulation of receptor activator of nuclear factor κB (RANKL) in osteoblasts or stromal cells, which in turn induces osteoclastogenesis and results in the alteration of the osteoblast/osteoclast equilibrium. *Hormones and cytokine factors:* 1α, vitamin D (1α,25(OH)₂D₃) receptor; PTH/PTHrP = parathyroid hormone/TH-related protein receptor; PTHR1 = parathyroid hormone receptor type 1; TNF-α = tumor necrosis factor-α; IL-1, IL-6, sIL-6R = interleukin-1, interleukin-6, soluble IL-6 receptor; PGE₂ = progesterone; LIF = leukemia inhibitory factor. *Pathways:* VDR = vitamin D receptor; cAMP/PKA = cyclic adenosine monophosphate/protein kinase A pathway; STAT3 = signal transducer and activator of transcription 3 (important for the signal transduction of IL-6 and related cytokines); [Ca²⁺]/PKC = calcium concentration/protein kinase C pathway. (Reproduced with permission from Takahashi N, Udagawa N, Takami M, Suda T. Cells of bone: osteoclast generation. In: Bilezikian JP, Raisz LG, Rodan GA, eds. Principles of bone biology. San Diego: Academic Press, 2002:109–126.)

Biologic data are helpful in answering several clinically relevant questions in orthodontic tooth movement. How does bone density alter tooth movement? What is the relationship between force level and clinical response? How do intermittently applied forces compare to constant forces? What is the most effective rhythm for appliance reactivations? There is some controversy regarding the relationship between alveolar bone density and orthodontic tooth movement. Moreover the extent to which bone density impacts on root resorption is not fully understood. Some approaches to orthodontic treatment recommend taking advantage of the more dense cortical bone to enhance anchorage. This approach assumes that teeth would move more slowly through more dense alveolar bone. Although this appears to be a reasonable assumption, clinical studies have not been able to support the effectiveness of this approach. Some studies have found a relationship between root resorption and movement of teeth through dense cortical bone, while others have not. Orthodontic tooth movement in animal models has been

shown to be accelerated when alveolar bone density is experimentally reduced with less risk of root resorption.[47] Today bioactive agents show promise of being able to reduce localized bone density. The use of such agents in conjunction with conventional fixed appliances may provide more rapid tooth movement of individual teeth with less risk of root resorption.

The relationship between tooth movement and force magnitude is also controversial. Some data suggest that a force optimum exists, where there is a direct linear relationship at low force levels and an inverse one at high forces. Animal data have confirmed the direct linear relationship at low force levels, but seems to suggest there is a plateau at higher levels. Despite the persistence of biomechanic approaches to orthodontic treatment that assume the existence of an optimal force for orthodontic tooth movement, there is no direct evidence for it. Clinical studies aimed at addressing the concept are technically quite complex because of the difficulty of accurately measuring tooth movement, and force magnitude and

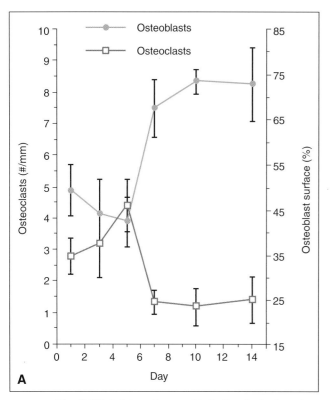

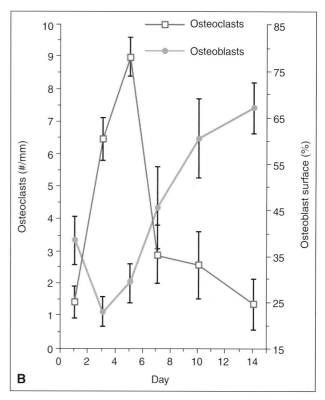

Fig. 2-10 Cell dynamics associated with orthodontic tooth movement. **A** Tension sites are characterized by an increase in osteoblasts and a reduction in resident osteoclasts in the latter part of the tooth movement. **B** Compression sites are characterized by an influx of osteoclasts in the early part of the tooth movement followed by their reversal to baseline levels, followed by an increase in osteoblasts in the latter part of the tooth movement.

distribution in a clinical environment. As technology develops, intraoral biomechanic sensors with data storage capacities should become available. These are currently in development for the headgear. Highly sensitive methods for measuring orthodontic tooth movement in three-dimensions using modern imaging instrumentation are also rapidly becoming a reality.[48] Together these two advances should make clinical studies of this relationship feasible in the near future.

Orthodontists realize that the biomechanics can be quite complex. Most appliances can be considered to be slowly dissipating. The goal of constant force may not be routinely achieved even with the use of superelastic wires. Clinicians also commonly use appliances with interrupted and intermittent durations of force application. Superimposed on the mechanics are the usual forces associated with oral physiology (e.g. chewing, deglutition, and speech). Most studies have attempted to model this complex mechanical environment by asking simple questions or creating simplified models about its component parts.

What does it take to initiate orthodontic tooth movement? The bone literature suggests that significant amounts of osteogenesis can be stimulated by short exposures to dynamic strains.[49] Orthodontists expect to see tooth movement in response to less than constant force application

(e.g. headgears and functional appliances). This is further supported by animal studies that have shown tooth movement with part-time exposure to mechanical signals.[50] A relevant question would be how long do the tissue changes stimulated during orthodontic tooth movement continue following appliance removal? Despite rapid relapse under these conditions, there is evidence that the cellular changes persist for a period of time, which would presumably be reflected in a more rapid response to a second appliance activation following a rest interval.[51] Some clinical studies have reported no difference in tooth movement when comparing constant and intermittent force protocols. Animal studies have suggested that the key factor may be the duration of force application with forces for about one-quarter of the time being effective, although other animals studies have shown that jiggling forces of extremely short duration can stimulate large numbers of osteoclasts and the tooth mobility characteristic of orthodontics.[52,53] This may be the case because intermittent protocols with short durations of force application provide long periods of time for significant amounts of relapse to occur.

Because most orthodontic appliances are slowly dissipating, clinical treatment can be viewed as a series of intermittent force applications. Experimental data from

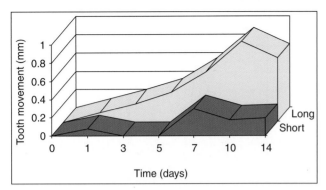

Fig. 2-11 Orthodontic tooth movement curves following short (1 day) and long (10 days) interval reactivation schedules. Note the greater overall tooth movement without a delay period.

animal models suggest that reactivating an orthodontic appliance over longer intervals stimulates more efficient tooth movement than reactivations over short intervals.[10] Biochemical analysis of known markers of active bone metabolism have demonstrated that significant amounts of alveolar bone turnover continue for an indeterminate period following appliance decay.[54] Studies of tooth movement and tissue responses following reactivations indicate that linear tooth movement and rapid recruitment of osteoclasts can be achieved if reactivation is timed to coincide with the latter part of the bone remodeling cycle initiated by the first activation.[55] Clinical data on reactivation rhythm are extremely important to improving the efficiency and safety of treatment. Again, in the absence of sensitive means to monitor biomechanics and tooth movement in three dimensions, these experiments will be difficult to accomplish (Fig. 2-11).

Related to the concept of reactivation timing is how the circadian rhythm factors into the biology of tooth movement. Since there is a decreased metabolism at night time during sleep, the question arises as to whether this becomes more favorable or less desirable for tooth movement. A research study was carried out on subjects divided into three groups: appliances were activated over a time frame of 21 days either continuously throughout the experimental period, only during the light (07:00–19:00 hours) period, or only during the dark (19:00–07:00 hours) period.[56] Results demonstrated that the tooth movement in the whole-day and light-period groups was about twice that in the dark-period group. Histologic evaluation of the periodontal tissues confirmed that there was greater new bone formation on the tension side in the whole-day and light-period groups and more osteoclastic activity on the pressure side compared to the dark-period group. Overall the light-period group exhibited decreased hyalinization of the PDL than the whole-day group. Therefore it is obvious that diurnal rhythms in bone metabolism and physiology have significant ramifications on orthodontic tooth movement.

Root Resorption

Root resorption is a relatively common sequel of orthodontic treatment. Consequences range from slight tooth mobility resulting from mild amounts of root resorption to complete loss of teeth due to excessive root resorption. The type and magnitude of root resorption vary substantially from mild apical root blunting in a large number of cases, to lateral root resorption, and infrequently, but unfortunately, to excessive root loss (Fig. 2-12). Because of the potential for significant clinical and legal implications of root resorption, assessment of the biologic and mechanical basis of root resorption has been the subject of extensive research and discussion for almost a century. Yet, because of the multiple factors contributing to this process, the research findings are inconclusive and remain a highly debated topic in the literature.[57,58] As early as 1914 clinical observers suggested a direct link between orthodontic treatment and root resorption.[59] In the late 1920s radiographic evidence demonstrating differences in root morphology before and after orthodontic treatment was presented.[60,61] Since then numerous potential causal relationships and contributory factors have been proposed and studied, but definitive explanations of why root resorption occurs, and what factors contribute to its occurrence, have remained controversial. A comprehensive understanding of this problem has remained elusive because of the difficulty in comparing the results and conclusions of various studies that have utilized different experimental designs, patient populations, treatment mechanics, and analyses. Additionally the variability in radiographic techniques and materials in different studies further contributes to the discrepant findings among studies. Finally because of inherent differences in both the characteristics of the patient and treatment, far too many potential etiologic factors have been considered in these studies, making it impossible to derive any meaningful conclusions. A better understanding of this important clinical problem requires controlled studies that are designed to examine the association between a limited set of variables and root resorption.

While the causative or contributory factors for orthodontic root resorption remain unknown, several studies have proposed a spectrum of factors that may predispose patients to root resorption. An hereditary component for orthodontic root resorption has been suggested by findings showing a significantly higher co-occurrence of root resorption among siblings than nonsiblings (Fig. 2-13).[62] In the context of genetic predisposition to root resorption, recent findings also support the notion of an association, albeit small, between IL-1α and TNF-α polymorphisms and root resorption.[63,64] Other studies have explored the relationship of force strength, as well as rate and direction of tooth movement, to root resorption with inconsistent findings.[65,66] A positive association between duration of treatment and root resorption has been demonstrated.[67,68] Root morphology, specifically abnormally shaped or

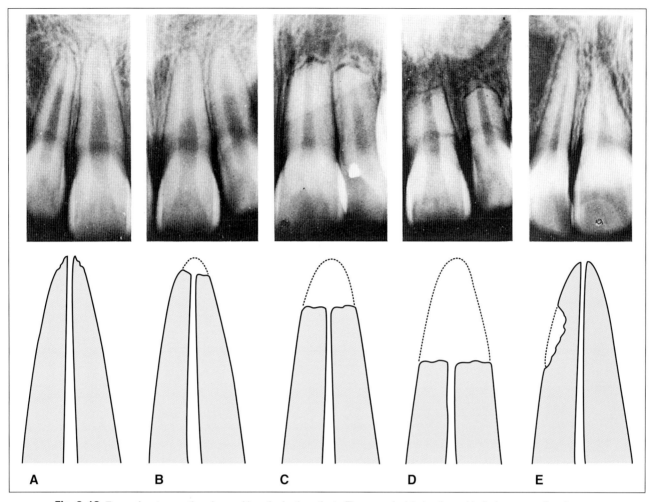

Fig. 2-12 Types of root resorption observed in orthodontic patients. These are depicted radiographically (upper panel) and diagrammatically (lower panel) and range from very mildly irregular apical root contours (**A**), mild apical root blunting (**B**), moderate apical root resorption (**C**), severe apical root resorption (**D**), and lateral root resorption (**E**). (Modified from Goldson L, Malmgren O. Orthodontic treatment of traumatized teeth. In: Andreasen JO, ed. Traumatic injuries of the teeth, 2nd edn. Philadelphia: WB Saunders, 1981:395).

dilacerated roots, also appear to influence the severity of root resorption.[69,70] Root resorption of varying degrees has been observed in all three planes of tooth movement (sagittal, transverse, and vertical).[71,72] Previous trauma to teeth treated orthodontically may also be a significant risk factor for root resorption.[73] However because of the low incidence of trauma to teeth, this factor possibly accounts for root resorption in relatively few patients.

In general much of the focus of previous studies has been on the mechanical variables, with little attention being paid to the potential contribution of biologic factors to orthodontic root resorption. One factor that may be associated with orthodontic root resorption is trabecular bone density. The hypothesis that trabecular bone density may be associated with orthodontic root resorption is based on the assumption that bone and roots with similar levels of calcification are likely to undergo comparable amounts of degradation when exogenous forces are applied. While

there is no conclusive evidence for this hypothesis, some studies have provided indirect evidence for a potential association between bone density and root resorption. For example it has been demonstrated that strong forces applied to teeth in less dense alveolar bone cause the same amount of root resorption as seen in roots in dense alveolar bone subjected to much weaker forces.[66] Additionally teeth being moved in close proximity to dense cortical bone undergo greater levels of root resorption than those in trabecular bone.[74] More appropriately, animal studies show that calcium-deficient rats exhibiting very low alveolar density have markedly low levels of root resorption following tooth movement (Fig. 2-14).[47] Similarly studies on hypocalcemic rats have also demonstrated a proportional relationship between bone density and magnitude of root resorption.[75] These studies provide important insights into the potential association between bone density and root resorption but require a more definitive validation.

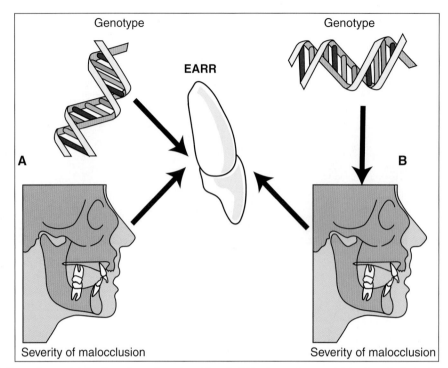

Fig. 2-13 Competing models for the pathway through which an individual's genotype modulates the extent of external apical root resorption (EARR) experienced during the course of orthodontic treatment. **A** The first paradigm suggests that the amount of EARR during treatment depends on an individual's genotype and, independently, on malocclusion. Genotype and malocclusion both have a modulating effect on the extent of EARR, but they operate along separate biologic and biomechanic pathways. With this model a patient's genotype would have a direct effect on the extent of EARR, and incorporating measures of severity of malocclusion into statistical design would not affect the estimate of heritability (h^2, the proportion of the total variance due to common genetic influences). **B** The alternative paradigm is that genotype has an *indirect* effect acting *through* malocclusion. This model acknowledges that craniometric studies show that facial size and shape have moderately high genetic components. Because siblings share similar craniofacial relationships, the genetic influence on EARR would be modulated through malocclusion. With this model, inclusion of skeletodental covariates would alter h^2 estimates—although it is not clear a priori that estimates should necessarily increase or decrease. (Reproduced from Harris EF, Kineret SE, Tolley EA. A heritable component for external apical root resorption in patients treated orthodontically. Am J Orthod Dentofacial Orthop 1997;111:301–309.)

Orthodontic Relapse

Many biologic and mechanical factors dictate the rate of tooth movement in orthodontics. Similarly this complex dynamic physiologic environment also dictates the amount of relapse which will occur following the completion of orthodontic treatment. Relapse can be defined as a natural tendency for a tooth or teeth to migrate back to their original pretreatment position and angulation in the dental arch. In general the amount of active tooth movement correlates strongly with the relapse potential (i.e. greater distances or greater rotations result in a greater tendency for relapse).[76] Factors involved in clinical orthodontic relapse include parameters of force duration, distance of tooth movement, and mechanical management to minimize relapse occurrence. The role of gingival and trans-septal fibers and the time period of bone remodeling following orthodontic tooth movement also play significant roles in the ultimate magnitude of the relapse that occurs.

The potential for relapse is great during a critical period of time immediately post orthodontic treatment when the teeth and roots have been moved into the desired final position (Fig. 2-15). In the process of tooth movement, bone resorption occurs in areas of pressure and bone deposition occurs in areas of tension, as defined by Wolff's law.[1] The type of bone that is deposited in the area of tension is a rather soft unorganized osteoid matrix. This bone is subsequently remodeled into organized lamellar bone architecture to provide a stronger alveolar support, a slow process which can take upwards of 6 months.[51] At the same time there are changes in the trans-septal fibers attached to the roots of the teeth. The tensile forces cause trans-septal fibers to adjust their length by rapid remodeling and this change continues to occur, as demonstrated by increased collagenous protein turnover within the middle third of the trans-septal fibers following release of orthodontic force.[77] In all cases it is apparent that the retention

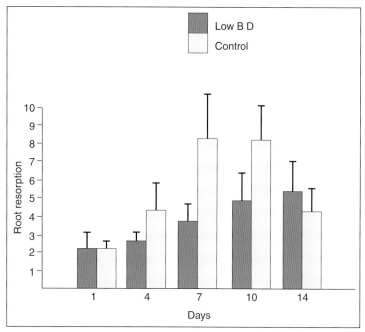

Fig. 2-14 Root resorption comparison between normal (control) and low bone density (low BD). Note that there is less root resorption in the low-density group. (Reproduced with permission from Goldie RS, King GJ. Root resorption and tooth movement in orthodontically treated, calcium-deficient, and lactating rats. Am J Orthod 1984;85:424–430.)

mechanism immediately post removal of the orthodontic appliances is a crucial component of the treatment plan.

Orthodontic relapse occurs when teeth are permitted to migrate out of position during this postorthodontic remodeling of the supporting structures. Histologic and electron micrograph studies have shown that rapid remodeling of the PDL and surrounding alveolar bones is the main cause of tooth relapse and that hyalinization formed subsequent to compression and/or mineralized tissues

subjected to compression are rapidly resorbed by osteoclasts, and macrophage- and fibroblast-like cells.[17] Biologic studies have provided evidence that teeth show a greater relapse tendency when continuous forces are used compared to intermittent forces.[78] This is because continuous forces are more effective in moving teeth and therefore the teeth are displaced farther from their original positions. The result of this is an increase in the potential of the teeth to revert back to their initial positions.

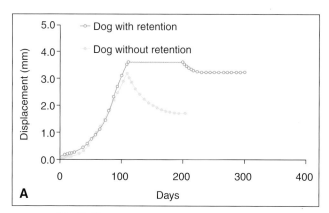
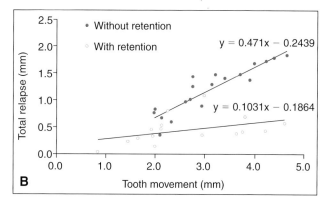

Fig. 2-15 Retention enhances stability following orthodontic tooth movement, and larger movements correlate with increased relapse, particularly in the absence of retention. **A** Time–displacement curves of two dog premolars, one with retention and one without. **B** Relation between active tooth movement and the total amount of relapse with or without retention. The plots represent linear regression lines for the two different conditions. (Reproduced with permission from van Leeuwen EJ, Maltha JC, Kuijpers-Jagtman AM, van't Hof MA. The effect of retention on orthodontic relapse after the use of small continuous or discontinuous forces. An experimental study in beagle dogs. Eur J Oral Sci 2003;111:111–116.)

This "relapse energy" phenomenon can also be observed in situations where teeth require rotational correction. As the tooth is rotated, the PDL is stretched (Fig. 2-16).[79] The greater the magnitude of rotation the further these fibers become elongated. In its new milieu the PDL is able to reorganize and invest its fibrils in alveolar bone and cementum during the deposition of new bone and cementum. However this process is slow and requires significant time.[80] Acceleration of this reorganization is facilitated by gingivectomy or supracrestal fiberotomies aimed at surgically releasing the stretched free gingival fibers and allowing reattachment of these fibers in a less stressed or less stretched configuration.[81,82] Scanning electron microscopy and histologic evaluation of post-fiberotomy teeth confirm that there is an eventual reparative reattachment of the collagen fibers of the PDL (Figs 2-17

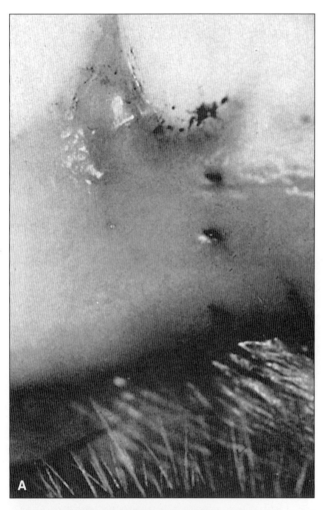

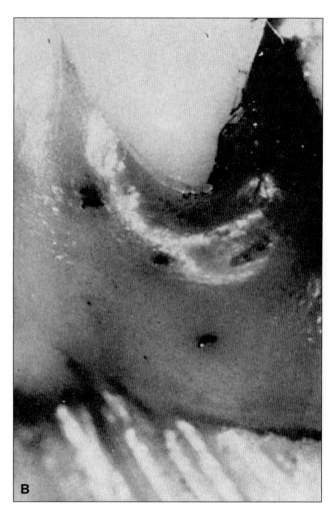

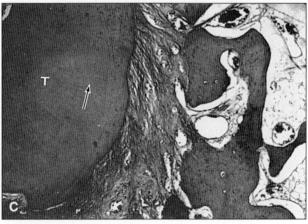

Fig. 2-16 Stretching of periodontal ligament (PDL) and gingival tissue by orthodontic rotation of teeth. **A** Tattoo marks on gingiva before rotation of the tooth. **B** Tattoo marks on gingiva show deviation in direction of rotational movement of the tooth. **C** PDL stretched and deviated (arrow) during rotation of the tooth (T). Magnification of original is × 64. (Reproduced from Edwards JG. A study of the periodontium during orthodontic rotation of teeth. Am J Orthod 1968;54:441–461.)

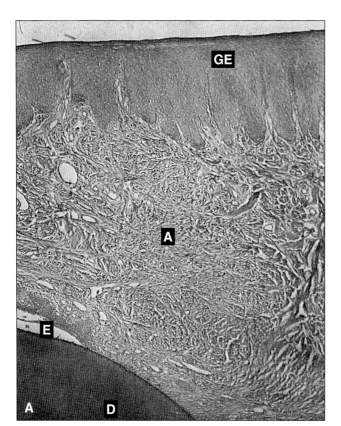
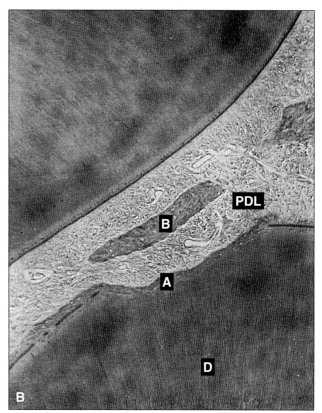

Fig. 2-17 Histologic changes of periodontal ligament (PDL) fiber adaptations in the presence and absence of surgical intervention. **A** Shows the PDL arrangement of an incisor with total repair 42 days following surgical intervention. Overall there was good orientation of the PDL ligaments as it slowly starts to reattach and reorganize into the more familiar parallel collagen bundles. The supragingival tissue showed a zone of healing where the fibers were much sparser than the adjacent fiber bundles. Fiber organization outside the area of healing was very similar to the fiber arrangement observed in comparable areas of unrotated incisors. **B** Histologic section of a nonsurgical control incisor with a similar degree of tooth rotation as in **A**. PDL showed areas of compression and damage on the distolingual aspect and a widening on the mesiolabial aspect. Observation of the supragingival tissues displayed a generalized discontinuity of the fiber pattern, areas of hemorrhage, and fiber disorganization. No evidence of any area of scarring or healing was observed. A = area of resorption undergoing healing; B = bone; D = dentin; GE = gingival epithelium. (Modified from Brain, 1969).

and 2-18). Longterm evaluation of 4–6 and 12–14 years after active treatment validate that circumferential supracrestal fiberotomies (CSF) are effective in improving retention of tooth position.[44] This study also validated that there was neither a clinically significant increase in the periodontal sulcus depth nor a decrease in the labially attached gingiva of the CSF teeth observed at 1 and 6 months following the surgical procedure. However recent biochemical studies propose that the rotational relapse of a tooth is not due to "stretched" collagen fibers but rather is a result of a change in the elastic properties of the whole gingival tissue.[83] Unlike bone and PDL, which regain their original structure after the removal of force, the gingival tissue does not regain its pretreatment structure and it may be this tension that contributes to orthodontic relapse.[84]

The factors noted above are considered intrinsic factors of orthodontic relapse related to the immediate supporting structures of PDL and alveolar bone surrounding the teeth. These relapse factors should be differentiated from extrinsic factors, such as continual craniofacial skeletal growth, external forces from facial muscles, and occlusal interdigitation. Despite the numerous studies over the years defining all the variables and contributory factors related to orthodontic relapse, to this day the degree of postretention anterior crowding is still both unpredictable and variable and no pretreatment variables, either from clinical findings, casts, or cephalometric radiographs before or after treatment, seem to be useful predictors.

Future Uses of Biologic Principles in Orthodontic Treatment

In future the principles gleaned from molecular biology and tissue engineering are expected to become part of the therapeutic regimen utilized during orthodontic treatment.

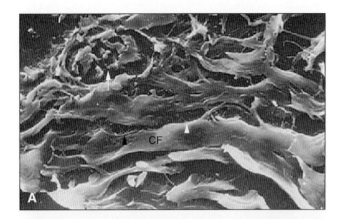

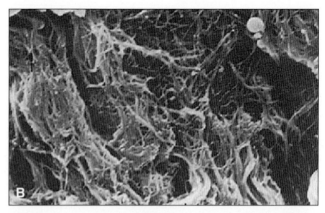

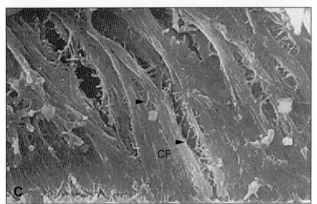

Fig. 2-18 Teeth that have undergone surgical release of the gingival fibers demonstrate a greater stability post orthodontic treatment. This is primarily due to the reattachment capability of the collagen fibers of the periodontal ligament (PDL). **A** Observations with scanning electron microscopy (SEM) of supra-alveolar fibers in palatal, buccal, and trans-septal gingival areas reveal well organized, parallel, and densely packed collagen fiber (CF) bundles with thin fibers connecting the large fiber bundles (arrowheads). **B** SEM analysis of the different gingival regions after rotation and retention reveal disorganized, torn, and ripped collagen fibers. **C** After gingival fiberotomy and release of retention the teeth remain stable in their rotated positions. SEM shows large, parallel, and densely packed collagen fibers. There is normalization of the longitudinally sectioned parallel and densely packed CF bundles interconnected with thinner fibers (arrowheads), resembling untreated controls. Bar in **A** is 0.1 mm and in **B** and **C** 10 μm. (Reproduced from Redlich M, Rahamin E, Gaft A, Shoshan S. The response of supraalveolar gingival collagen to orthodontic rotation movement in dogs. Am J Orthodont Dentofacial Orthop 1996;110:247–255.)

This paradigm of orthodontic treatment may involve the delivery of bioactive agents in combination with conventional biomechanics. Numerous agents already exist that have activities that should be of significance in accelerating or preventing tooth movement, and others are being reported monthly. For example localized application of calciotropic agents has significant effects on local bone remodeling dynamics and may be utilized to facilitate tooth movement, such as retraction of canines into extraction spaces, or impair tooth movement in cases with high anchorage needs where clinicians do not want molars to move forward. As more is learned about the biologic mechanisms in orthodontic tooth movement, methods of local pharmaceutical delivery will soon be developed. Data on efficacy and safety, as well as means of delivery in the context of orthodontic treatment, will likely be forthcoming.

Advances in technologic bioassays may also facilitate the biologic diagnostics and monitoring of bone turnover and metabolism. Medical researchers have already attempted to establish relationships between molecular biochemical markers of bone remodeling (e.g. osteocalcin, alkaline phosphatase, and procollagen I) and the metabolic rate of bone turnover in clinical subjects.[85] However the correlation and interpretation of results are complicated by numerous multifactorial variables, such as age, pubertal stage, growth velocity, mineral accrual, hormonal regulation, nutritional status, and circadian variation. Yet the rapid progression in developing more sensitive and specific assays, as well as recent discoveries of more specific metabolic bone markers, is making this potential assessment of bone turnover a likely reality in the near future.[86]

REFERENCES

1. Wolff J. The law of bone remodeling (trans). Berlin: Springer-Verlag, 1986:1–22.
2. Dorow C, Krstin N, Sander FG. Experiments to determine the material properties of the periodontal ligament. J Orofac Orthop 2002;63:94–104.
3. van Driel WD, van Leeuwen EJ, Von den Hoff JW, Maltha JC, Kuijpers-Jagtman AM. Time-dependent mechanical behaviour of the periodontal ligament. Proc Inst Mech Eng [H] 2000;214:497–504.
4. Tanne K, Nagataki T, Inoue Y, Sakuda M, Burstone CJ. Patterns of initial tooth displacements associated with various root lengths and alveolar bone heights. Am J Orthod Dentofacial Orthop 1991;100:66–71.
5. Yoshida N, Jost-Brinkmann PG, Koga Y, Mimaki N, Kobayashi K. Experimental evaluation of initial tooth displacement, center of resistance, and center of rotation under the influence of an orthodontic force. Am J Orthod Dentofacial Orthop 2001;120:190–197.
6. Tanne K, Yoshida S, Kawata T, Sasaki A, Knox J, Jones ML. An evaluation of the biomechanic response of the tooth and periodontium to orthodontic forces in adolescent and adult subjects. Br J Orthod 1998;25:109–115.
7. Tanne K, Inoue Y, Sakuda M. Biomechanic behavior of the periodontium before and after orthodontic tooth movement. Angle Orthod 1995;65:123–128.
8. Kyomen S, Tanne K. Influences of aging changes in proliferative rate of PDL cells during experimental tooth movement in rats. Angle Orthod 1997;67:67–72.
9. Ren Y, Maltha JC, van't Hof MA, Kuijpers-Jagtman AM. Age effect on orthodontic tooth movement in rats. J Dent Res 2003;82:38–42.
10. King GJ, Archer L, Zhou D. Later orthodontic appliance reactivation stimulates immediate appearance of osteoclasts and linear tooth movement. Am J Orthod Dentofacial Orthop 1998;114:692–677.
11. Iwasaki LR, Haack JE, Nickel JC, Morton J. Human tooth movement in response to continuous stress of low magnitude. Am J Orthod Dentofacial Orthop 2000;117:175–183.
12. van Leeuwen EJ, Maltha JC, Kuijpers-Jagtman AM. Tooth movement with light continuous and discontinuous forces in beagle dogs. Eur J Oral Sci 1999;107:468–474.
13. Andersson L, Malmgren B. The problem of dentoalveolar ankylosis and subsequent replacement resorption in the growing patient. Aust Endod J 1999;25:57–61.
14. Kurol J. Infraocclusion of primary molars. An epidemiological, familial, longitudinal, clinical and histological study. Swed Dent J 1984;21(Suppl):1–67.
15. King GJ, Keeling SD, McCoy EA, Ward TH. Measuring dental drift and orthodontic tooth movement in response to various initial forces in adult rats. Am J Orthod Dentofacial Orthop 1991;99:456–465.
16. Marks SC Jr, Schroeder HE. Tooth eruption: theories and facts. Anat Rec 1996;245:374–393.
17. Yoshida Y, Sasaki T, Yokoya K, Hiraide T, Shibasaki Y. Cellular roles in relapse processes of experimentally-moved rat molars. J Electron Microsc (Tokyo) 1999;48:147–157.
18. Marks SC Jr. The basic and applied biology of tooth eruption. Connect Tissue Res 1995;32:149–157.
19. Philbrick WM, Dreyer BE, Nakchbandi IA, Karaplis AC. Parathyroid hormone-related protein is required for tooth eruption. Proc Natl Acad Sci USA 1998;95:11846–11851.
20. Ouyang H, McCauley LK, Berry JE, Saygin NE, Tokiyasu Y, Somerman MJ. Parathyroid hormone-related protein regulates extracellular matrix gene expression in cementoblasts and inhibits cementoblast-mediated mineralization in vitro. J Bone Miner Res 2000;15:2140–2153.
21. Dastmalchi R, Polson A, Bouwsma O, Proskin H. Cementum thickness and mesial drift. J Clin Periodontol 1990;17:709–713.
22. Levy GG, Mailland ML. Histologic study of the effects of occlusal hypofunction following antagonist tooth extraction in the rat. J Periodontol 1980;51:393–399.
23. Rygh P. Ultrastructural changes in pressure zones of human periodontium incident to orthodontic tooth movement. Acta Odontol Scand 1973;31:109–122.
24. Rygh P. Hyalinization of the periodontal ligament incident to orthodontic tooth movement. Nor Tannlaegeforen Tid 1974;84:352–357.
25. Rygh P. Elimination of hyalinized periodontal tissues associated with orthodontic tooth movement. Scand J Dent Res 1974;82:57–73.
26. Brudvik P, Rygh P. The initial phase of orthodontic root resorption incident to local compression of the periodontal ligament. Eur J Orthod 1993;15:249–263.
27. Brudvik P, Rygh P. Non-clast cells start orthodontic root resorption in the periphery of hyalinized zones. Eur J Orthod 1993;15:467–480.
28. Suda T, Takahashi N, Martin TJ. Modulation of osteoclast differentiation. Endocrinol Rev 1992;13:66–80.
29. Takahashi N, Akatsu T, Udagawa N, et al. Osteoblastic cells are involved in osteoclast formation. Endocrinology 1998;123:2600–2602.
30. Udagawa N, Takahashi N, Akatsu T, et al. Origin of osteoclasts: mature monocytes and macrophages are capable of differentiating into osteoclasts under a suitable microenvironment prepared by bone marrow-derived stromal cells. Proc Natl Acad Sci USA 1990;87:7260–7264.
31. Anderson DM, Maraskovsky E, Billingsley WL, et al. A homologue of the TNF receptor and its ligand enhance T-cell growth and dendritic-cell function. Nature 1997;390:175–179.
32. ASBMR. Proposed standard nomenclature for new tumor necrosis factor family members involved in the regulation of bone resorption. American Society for Bone and Mineral Research President's Committee on Nomenclature. J Bone Miner Res 2000;15:2293–2296.
33. Hsu H, Lacey DL, Dunstan CR, et al. Tumor necrosis factor receptor family member RANK mediates osteoclast differentiation and activation induced by osteoprotegerin ligand. Proc Natl Acad Sci USA 1999;96:3540–3545.
34. Nakagawa N, Kinosaki M, Yamaguchi K, et al. RANK is the essential signaling receptor for osteoclast differentiation factor in osteoclastogenesis. Biochem Biophys Res Commun 1998;253:395–400.
35. Simonet WS, Lacey DL, Dunstan CR, et al. Osteoprotegerin: a novel secreted protein involved in the regulation of bone density. Cell 1997;89:309–319.

36. Hasegawa T, Yoshimura Y, Kikuiri T, et al. Expression of receptor activator of NF-kappa B ligand and osteoprotegerin in culture of human periodontal ligament cells. J Periodontal Res 2002;37:405–411.

37. Crotti T, Smith MD, Hirsch R, Soukoulis S, et al. Receptor activator NF kappaB ligand (RANKL) and osteoprotegerin (OPG) protein expression in periodontitis. J Periodontal Res 2003;38:380–387.

38. Takahashi N, Udagawa N, Takami M, Suda T. Cells of bone: osteoclast generation. In: Bilezikian JP, Raisz LG, Rodan GA, eds. Principles of bone biology. San Diego: Academic Press, 2002:109–126.

39. Huang JC, Sakata T, Pfleger LL, et al. PTH differentially regulates expression of RANKL and OPG during osteoblast development. J Bone Miner Res 2004;19:235–244.

40. Suda T, Ueno Y, Fujii K, Shinki T. Vitamin D and bone. J Cell Biochem 2003;88:259–266.

41. Bord S, Ireland DC, Beavan SR, Compston JE. The effects of estrogen on osteoprotegerin, RANKL, and estrogen receptor expression in human osteoblasts. Bone 2003;32:136–141.

42. Cheung J, Mak YT, Papaioannou S, Evans BA, Fogelman I, Hampson G. Interleukin-6 (IL-6), IL-1, receptor activator of nuclear factor kappaB ligand (RANKL) and osteoprotegerin production by human osteoblastic cells: comparison of the effects of 17-beta oestradiol and raloxifene. J Endocrinol 2003;177:423–433.

43. King GJ, Keeling SD, Wronski TJ. Histomorphometric study of alveolar bone turnover in orthodontic tooth movement. Bone 1991;12:401–409.

44. Edwards JG. A long-term prospective evaluation of the circumferential supracrestal fiberotomy in alleviating orthodontic relapse. Am J Orthod Dentofacial Orthop 1988;93:380–387.

45. Verna C, Zaffe D, Siciliani G. Histomorphometric study of bone reactions during orthodontic tooth movement in rats. Bone 1999;24:371–379.

46. Mundy GR. Cellular and molecular regulation of bone turnover. Bone 1999;24(5 Suppl):35S–38S.

47. Goldie RS, King GJ. Root resorption and tooth movement in orthodontically treated, calcium-deficient, and lactating rats. Am J Orthod 1984;85:424–430.

48. Ashmore JL, Kurland BF, King GJ, Wheeler TT, Ghafari J, Ramsay DS. A 3-dimensional analysis of molar movement during headgear treatment. Am J Orthod Dentofacial Orthop 2002;121:18–29; discussion 29–30.

49. Judex S, Boyd S, Qin YX, Turner S, Ye K, Muller R, Rubin C. Adaptations of trabecular bone to low magnitude vibrations result in more uniform stress and strain under load. Ann Biomed Eng 2003;31:12–20.

50. Gibson JM, King GJ, Keeling SD. Long-term orthodontic tooth movement response to short-term force in the rat. Angle Orthod 1992;62:211–215; discussion 216.

51. King GJ, Keeling SD. Orthodontic bone remodeling in relation to appliance decay. Angle Orthod 1995;65:129–140.

52. Proffit WR, Sellers KT. The effect of intermittent forces on eruption of the rabbit incisor. J Dent Res 1986;65:118–122.

53. Konoo T, Kim YJ, Gu GM, King GJ. Intermittent force in orthodontic tooth movement. J Dent Res 2001;80:457–460.

54. King G, Latta L, Rutenberg J, Ossi A, Keeling S. Alveolar bone turnover and tooth movement in male rats after removal of orthodontic appliances. Am J Orthodont Dentofacial Orthop 1997;111:266–275.

55. Gu G, Lemery SA, King GJ. Effect of appliance reactivation after decay of initial activation on osteoclasts, tooth movement, and root resorption. Angle Orthod 1999;69:515–522.

56. Miyoshi K, Igarashi K, Saeki S, Shinoda H, Mitani H. Tooth movement and changes in periodontal tissue in response to orthodontic force in rats vary depending on the time of day the force is applied. Eur J Orthod 2001;23:329–338.

57. Baumrind S, Korn EL, Boyd RL. Apical root resorption in orthodontically treated adults. Am J Orthod Dentofacial Orthop 1996;110:311–320.

58. Goldson L, Henrikson CO. Root resorption during Begg treatment; a longitudinal roentgenologic study. Am J Orthod 1975;68:55–66.

59. Ottolengui R. The physiological and pathological resorption of tooth roots. Items Interest 1914:36:332–362.

60. Ketcham AH. A preliminary report of an investigation of apical root resorption of vital permanent teeth. Int J Orthod 1927:13:97–127.

61. Ketcham AH. A progress report of an investigation of apical root resorption of vital permanent teeth. Int J Orthod 1929;15:310–328.

62. Harris EF, Kineret SE, Tolley EA. A heritable component for external apical root resorption in patients treated orthodontically. Am J Orthod Dentofacial Orthop 1997;111:301–309.

63. Al-Qawasmi RA, Hartsfield JK Jr, Everett ET, et al. Genetic predisposition to external apical root resorption. Am J Orthod Dentofacial Orthop 2003;123:242–252.

64. Al-Qawasmi RA, Hartsfield JK Jr, Everett ET, et al. Genetic predisposition to external apical root resorption in orthodontic patients: linkage of chromosome-18 marker. J Dent Res 2003;82:356–360.

65. McFadden WM, Engstrom C, Engstrom H, Anholm JM. A study of the relationship between incisor intrusion and root shortening. Am J Orthod Dentofacial Orthop 1989;6:390–396.

66. Reitan K. Initial tissue behavior during apical root resorption. Angle Orthod 1974;44:68–82.

67. Dermaut LR, De Munck A. Apical root resorption of upper incisors caused by intrusive tooth movement: a radiographic study. Am J Orthod Dentofacial Orthop 1986;90:321–326.

68. Taithongchai R, Sookkorn K, Killiany DM. Facial and dentoalveolar structure and the prediction of apical root shortening. Am J Orthod Dentofacial Orthop 1996;110:296–302.

69. Mirabella AD, Artun J. Risk factors for apical root resorption of maxillary anterior teeth in adult orthodontic patients. Am J Orthod Dentofacial Orthop 1995;108:48–55.

70. Newman WG. Possible etiologic factors in external root resorption. Am J Orthod 1975;67:522–539.

71. Harry MR, Sims MR. Root resorption in bicuspid intrusion. A scanning electron microscope study. Angle Orthod 1982;52:235–258.

72. Wainwright WM. Faciolingual tooth movement: its influence on the root and cortical plate. Am J Orthod 1973;64:278–302.

73. Linge L, Linge BO. Patient characteristics and treatment variables associated with apical root resorption during

orthodontic treatment. Am J Orthod Dentofacial Orthop 1991;99:35–43.

74. Horiuchi A, Hotokezaka H, Kobayashi K. Correlation between cortical plate proximity and apical root resorption. Am J Orthod Dentofacial Orthop 1998;114:311–318.

75. Engstrom C, Granstrom G, Thilander B. Effect of orthodontic force on periodontal tissue metabolism. A histologic and biochemical study in normal and hypocalcemic young rats. Am J Orthod Dentofacial Orthop 1988;93:486–495.

76. Reitan K. Principles of retention and avoidance of posttreatment relapse. Am J Orthod 1969;55:776–790.

77. Row KL, Johnson RB. Distribution of 3H-proline within transseptal fibers of the rat following release of orthodontic forces. Am J Anat 1990;189:179–188.

78. van Leeuwen EJ, Maltha JC, Kuijpers-Jagtman AM, van't Hof MA. The effect of retention on orthodontic relapse after the use of small continuous or discontinuous forces. An experimental study in beagle dogs. Eur J Oral Sci 2003;111:111–116.

79. Edwards JG. A study of the periodontium during orthodontic rotation of teeth. Am J Orthod 1968;54:441–461.

80. Reitan K. Tissue rearrangement during retention of orthodontically rotated teeth. Angle Orthod 1959;29:105–113.

81. Boese LR. Increased stability of orthodontically rotated teeth following gingivectomy in *Macaca nemestrina*. Am J Orthod 1969;56:273–290.

82. Brain WE. The effect of surgical transsection of free gingival fibers on the regression of orthodontically rotated teeth in the dog. Am J Orthod 1969;55:50–70.

83. Redlich M, Rahamim E, Gaft A, Shoshan S. The response of supraalveolar gingival collagen to orthodontic rotation movement in dogs. Am J Orthodont Dentofacial Orthop 1996;110:247–255.

84. Redlich M, Shoshan S, Palmon A. Gingival response to orthodontic force. Am J Orthod Dentofacial Orthop 1999;116:152–158.

85. Szulc P, Seeman E, Delmas PD. Biochemical measurements of bone turnover in children and adolescents. Osteoporos Int 2000;11:281–294.

86. Woitge HW, Seibel MJ. Biochemical markers to survey bone turnover. Rheum Dis Clin North Am 2001;27:49–80.

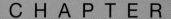

CHAPTER 3

Individualized Orthodontic Diagnosis

Flavio Uribe and Ravindra Nanda

The definition of diagnosis, according to Dorland's Medical Dictionary, is the determination of the nature of a case of disease.[1] In the case of orthodontics, the diseased or abnormal condition is the malocclusion, often linked to a facial disharmony. Although malocclusion is not a disease, it has esthetic and functional implications that may be categorized as handicapping. From the esthetic standpoint, there are psychologic implications to do with social acceptance and success,[2] and from the functional standpoint, mastication, speech, and protection of the structures in the whole stomathognathic system are important aspects to consider.

To define the abnormal or handicapping characteristics of the malocclusion, there needs to be an appreciation of what is normal. It is important to understand that in nature variation is the norm, and what is considered to be normal can be found within a wide range. Also, in the field of orthodontics esthetic perceptions vary through history and among individuals, races, and cultures. On the other hand, ideal occlusion and its functional implications are characterized by strict morphologic features. Thus, the definition of a normal occlusion is more objective than this.

Extensive research has determined the characteristics of normal functional occlusion. Concepts such as cusp-to-fossa or cusp-to-interproximal space occlusion, lateral and anterior guidance, and mutually protected occlusion are comprehensively described in other textbooks.[3] Needless to say, even though there is a certain leeway, the criteria for ideal occlusal function are better defined in comparison

to ideal esthetic values. Most of the occlusal concepts accepted today are derived from the assumed premise that good anatomy (good occlusal interdigitation) is analogous to proper function (Fig. 3-1).

From the esthetic viewpoint, orthodontists base their judgment on cephalometric norms obtained many decades ago from population samples with vaguely defined parameters of esthetics. In general, these studies assumed that good occlusion was directly related to good facial esthetics. Although these measurements provide some objective guidelines to start defining how each patient differs from the norm, there are some limitations to these analyses. Furthermore, it is not the absolute numeric amounts and their variation that dictate treatment, but the accurate interpretation of these and all the data obtained from the clinical examination and other patient records.

To properly diagnose a malocclusion, orthodontics has adopted the problem-based approach developed in medicine.[4] In this approach the patient is evaluated as a whole. Every factor that might be part of the etiology, might contribute to the abnormality, or might influence treatment, is evaluated. Information is gathered through a medical and dental history, clinical examination, and records that include models, photographs, and radiographic imaging. A problem list is generated from the analysis of the database that contains a network of interrelated factors influencing one another. The diagnosis is established after a continuous feedback between the problem recognition and the database. Ultimately, the diagnosis should provide some insight into the etiology of the maloclussion (Fig. 3-2).

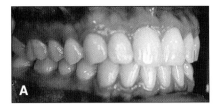 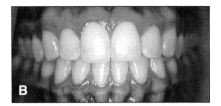 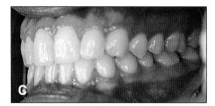

Fig. 3-1 A-C Frontal and lateral views of an ideal occlusion.

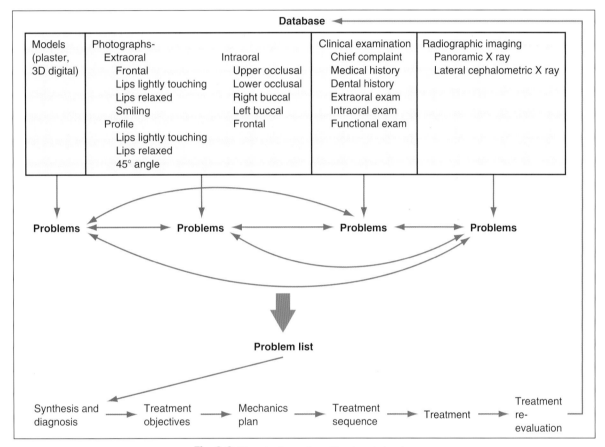

Fig. 3-2 Steps in diagnosis and treatment planning.

The diagnosis and problem list are the basis for the treatment objectives, and a subsequent treatment plan is tailored specifically to each patient's needs. An effort should be made to avoid solely classifying a patient into categories (Angle's classification) that tend to oversimplify the diagnosis and lead to certain standardized treatments being adopted.

From the treatment objectives perspective, one or various treatment plans can be determined that essentially help to organize the sequence of procedures and events needed to achieve the desired goals. The patient's informed consent, which includes the description of the advantages, disadvantages, and risks of each treatment plan, will ultimately determine the final treatment option. Finally, the treatment plan will dictate the mechanics plan designed to achieve the desired goals with the greatest efficiency and minimum side effects.

This chapter discusses some of the objective measures that define the range of normality both from an occlusal and a dentofacial standpoint. It is important to know that, although emphasis is placed on the whole dentofacial complex, there are limitations to the amount of correction that can be achieved with orthodontic treatment.

The clinician has to work within certain constraints and boundaries. The soft tissue envelope only allows a certain amount of correction. Major movements may involve other treatment options such as surgery, which although able to achieve a wider range of movements, is also limited by this soft tissue envelope. Overall, and given the limitations, the goal is to achieve the best possible facial balance and functional occlusion.

Finally, it is important to realize that the diagnosis and treatment plan are dynamic processes. As the plan is being executed, continuous monitoring and effective evaluation of the objectives is needed. Appropriate reassessment, adjustment, and corrective measures to the original plan are crucial if all the specific goals, and not only the occlusal goals, are to be achieved.

As described above, very precise collection of data is needed to achieve a proper diagnosis. This database should include a thorough medical and dental history, a set of models, the necessary radiographs, and a clinical examination accompanied by extra- and intra-oral photographs.

Clinical Examination

Medical and Dental History

The main question in any medical and dental interrogation is what is the chief complaint? This is the basis of the anamnesis and the treatment plan should at the minimum attempt to address these important patient's needs. It is the job of the experienced clinician to interpret this complaint, which may be vague in some cases. Good communication is the key to understanding a patient's expectations. In young patients, it is usually the parents who voice their complaint about their child's teeth. Commonly, the child is lacking in motivation or is too shy to express him/herself. The parents' concerns should be a major consideration but

the child should also be involved through a set of simple questions that will guide the clinician in finding out the child's motivation for treatment, if any.

The medical history gives pertinent information as to the physical well being of the patient. Numerous medical conditions can in some way or another affect treatment (Table 3-1).[5] For example, a history of a cardiac malformation or anomaly might be an indication for premedication before certain orthodontic procedures.[6] A history of rheumatoid arthritis can have direct implications on the temporomandibular joint (TMJ) and thus the occlusion. A patient with hemophilia may opt for a nonextraction treatment approach. All these conditions may affect the delivery of treatment in the various phases: pretreatment, treatment, and post-treatment.

Any metabolic disorder, such as diabetes, should be well controlled before and during treatment, as healing is greatly hindered in uncontrolled types of diabetes.[7]

Another common medical condition of concern, especially in young patients, is asthma, not only because of the respiratory implications, but also because there is some evidence that patients with asthma who undergo orthodontic treatment have an increased incidence of root resorption.[8]

The above are some of the more common medical conditions, but it is important that all medical conditions are

Table 3-1	Medical conditions to be considered in orthodontic treatment.	
Medical Condition	**Implications**	**Action**
Asthma	Root resorption	Monitor every 6 months for evidence of EARR
Allergies	Allergic reaction	Determine material causing allergy and substitute for a nonallergic material
Coagulation disorders	Bleeding risk	Avoid if possible treatment plans involving extractions
Diabetes	Periodontal disease	Monitor adequate control of diabetes. Manage with a periodontist
Epilepsy	Gingival hypertrophy (medications)	Monitor excellent plaque control. Manage with a periodontist for possible surgical intervention during treatment
Heart valve conditions	Endocarditis	Premedication when fitting bands
High blood pressure patient taking calcium-channel blockers	Gingival hyperplasia secondary to medications	Monitor oral hygiene. Complement brushing with chlorhexidine
HIV	Periodontal disease, opportunistic infections	Consult with physician about patient's general condition. Monitor oral hygiene and periodontal status
Leukemia	Mucositis, oral infections	Remove appliances until remission (consult physician)
Physical or mental handicap	Gingivitis, relapse (muscle hyper-/hypo-activity)	Electric toothbrushes may aid in oral hygiene. Consider mechanics plan where manual dexterity is not needed (noncompliance mechanics)
Rheumatoid arthritis	TMJ degeneration	Monitor TMJ. Manage with an oral surgeon if severe arthritic degeneration
Transplant patient	Gingival hyperplasia related to immunosuppressant drugs	Monitor oral hygiene. Consider chemical complement to brushing such as chlorhexidine.
Xerostomia (primary or secondary)	Caries	Monitor for loose appliances. Consider fluoride rinses as an oral hygiene supplement

EARR = external apical root resorption; TMJ = temporomandibular joint.

reviewed and further investigated (e.g. with a phone call to the patient's physician) if needed, as they may affect the treatment directly or indirectly. A more extensive review of these and other common medical disorders related to orthodontics may be found elsewhere.[5]

Another part of the medical history review, specific to female patients, is pregnancy. It is usually best to delay treatment until the pregnancy is over. The three basic reasons for postponing treatment are: radiographs are not usually recommended during pregnancy; there is an increased possibility of gingival hyperplasia due to hormonal influence; and in some instances the future mother's nutrition may be compromised as pain is elicited by tooth movement.

Other important information related to the medical history is the list of medications the patient might be taking and the existence of any allergies. Medications such as phenytoin (anticonvulsant), nifedepine (calcium channel blocker), and cyclosporine (immunosuppressive) need special attention as they have the potential to cause a hyperplastic gingival response.[9] Allergies that might be of importance are those related to the alloys used in orthodontics. Hypersensitivity to nickel has been reported with a prevalence of up to 28%.[10] Allergies to other metals used in orthodontics, such as chromium and cobalt alloys, have also been reported.[11] It is important to know the nature of the reaction to each allergen. Allergies related to the airway are also a significant finding as they impair normal nasal breathing, thus potentially affecting the growth and development of the jaws.[12]

Finally, the use of tobacco should be queried. It is not uncommon to encounter adolescent as well as adult patients who smoke. Smoking can have an adverse effect on the periodontal condition of patients,[13] is a risk factor for periodontal disease, and has been shown to delay wound healing.[14] Health providers also have an important duty to dissuade teenagers and adults from tobacco use.

Growth and Development

A specific section in the medical and dental interview should be dedicated to growth and development information. Most pediatricians keep a growth record of every child from birth (Fig. 3-3A and B). A growth chart classifies the child under a height and weight percentile for comparison to the established norms for gender and chronologic age. More importantly, this chart highlights any accelerations or peaks of growth that may have occurred. With this information the objective is to evaluate the skeletal maturational level of the patient. The underlying rationale for this information is to properly time orthodontic treatment to the period that would be most efficient and effective.[15] This implies that treatment will not only rely on tooth movement, but also on modifying growth to achieve a wider range of movement, thereby correcting larger dentofacial discrepancies.

The pubertal growth spurt is associated with a differential maxillomandibular growth that involves a more anterior positioning of the mandible (Fig. 3-4). The timing of this spurt has been of interest to orthodontists. During this period the orthodontist should be able to influence growth of the mandible and the midface by mechanically affecting the environment. Experiments in animal models have shown the possibility of mandibular growth enhancement during this period.[16] Unfortunately, there is no clear evidence that this additional mandibular growth enhancement is predictably achievable in humans.[17] Although clinical studies have shown impressive results at the occlusal level, the results may be the sum of a combination of small orthopedic and dental movements.[18,19] Some of the orthopedic movements involve remodeling within the temporal bone that is difficult to quantify with traditional research methods.[20]

Chronologic age, dental development, and eruption sequence are not good indicators of skeletal maturity. Biologic indicators, such as the menarche (females), voice change (males), hand–wrist ossification sequence, metacarpal ossification sequence, cervical vertebrae morphology, and statural growth curves, have been used to evaluate general skeletal craniofacial maturity.[15,21–23] Studies have shown a close correlation between peak height velocity and maximum acceleration in growth in the maxilla and mandible.[21,24]

Currently, there are no methods that can accurately predict the craniofacial size that a patient will achieve at the end of active growth. This predictive inability becomes a problem in young patients with moderate maxillomandibular discrepancies. In these patients a decision between a surgical or a growth modification approach is not simple. Moreover, both treatment strategies (surgery and growth modification) differ in timing, objectives, and often in the direction of tooth movement. Some studies suggest weak correlations can be drawn between final craniofacial form of growing children and their parents and other siblings.[25,26]

Although the absolute amount of growth cannot be predicted accurately, the direction of growth is more predictable. It has been shown that facial patterns are maintained.[27,28] Skieller et al also published findings related to the morphology of the mandible in the prediction of growth patterns.[29] Some controversy relates to their findings as their sample was made up of individuals with extreme patterns of vertical growth. Therefore, the applicability of these predictive methods to individuals with less severe aberrations in their growth pattern might be limited.[30]

Finally, the information regarding timing of active growth cessation is important for young patients needing maxillofacial surgery. Radiographic films can be used to evaluate this feature. If a hand–wrist radiograph shows fusion of the epiphysis and diaphysis of the radius, only further minimal growth can be expected, indicating the last stage of skeletal maturation.[21] The best method to confirm that no further growth will occur in the craniofacial region is to take two sequential lateral head films with a 6–12 month interval; the superimposition of these two radiographs should reveal no bony changes.[31]

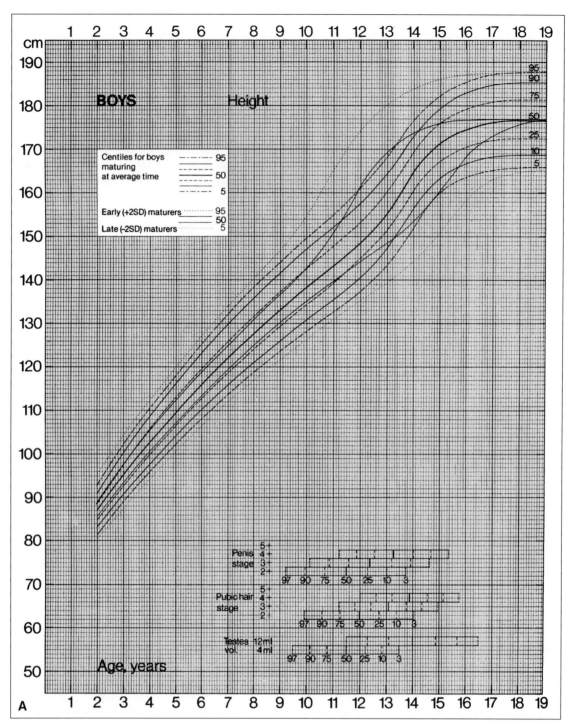

Fig. 3-3 Growth curves for **A** boys and **B** girls (height and weight). (Modified from Tanner JM, Davies PS. Clinical longitudinal standards for height and height velocity for North American children. J Pediatr 1985;107:317–329).

Continued

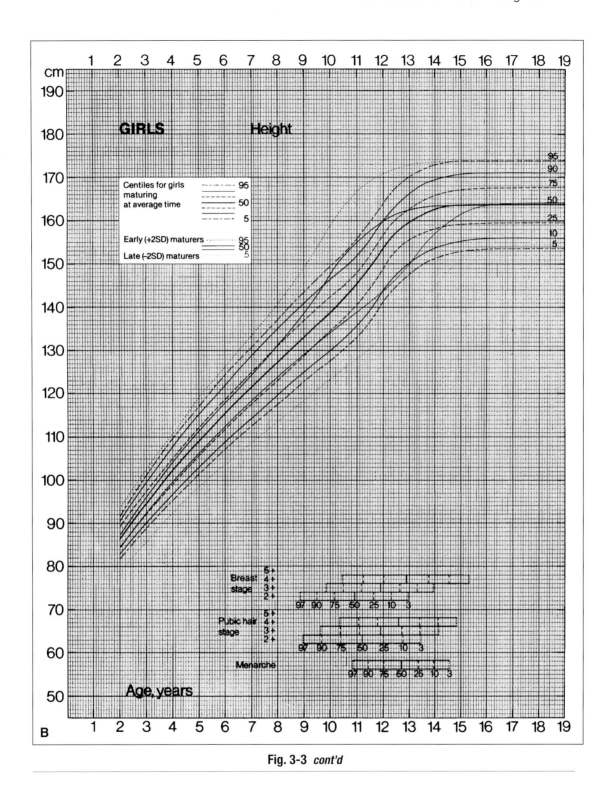

Fig. 3-3 *cont'd*

Factors Influencing Craniofacial Growth

It is well known that many conditions affect the growth and development of the craniofacial complex. Knowing the etiology of the malocclusion is of prime importance for the diagnosis and eventual success of treatment. The etiology of the malocclusion is often multifactorial. In general, the etiologic factors can be categorized into genetic factors, environmental factors, or a combination of the two. Genetic information can be gathered from the interview with the guardian of the child patient or from the adult patient. This information is of more importance in patients where syndromes or extensive craniofacial deviations are present. Also, as mentioned above, the parents' information may give some insight into the craniofacial form at the end

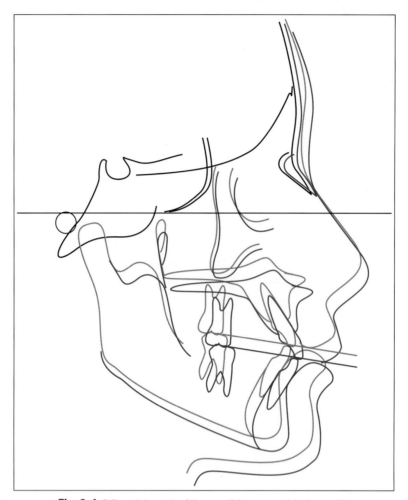

Fig. 3-4 Differential growth of the mandible compared to the maxilla.

of growth. The genetic component is also of further importance as it relates to abnormalities of tooth development and morphology, such as canine impaction, congenitally missing teeth, and abnormalities in tooth shape.[32,33]

Numerous environmental factors have been attributed to the etiology of the malocclusion. The classic example is the habit of thumb sucking. A longterm applied force (pressure) has been shown to affect all skeletal hard tissues. Muscle is a tissue that can apply this type of constant low force, and bone adapts to muscle force.[34] Muscular dysfunction either by hyper- or hypo-activity in certain diseases also may affect the normal growth and development of the jaws.[35] If the forces exerted by the muscles are not in equilibrium, the net effect will be reflected in the hard tissues in the form of displacement and eventually conditions leading to malocclusion and maxillomandibular skeletal discrepancy.[36,37]

Frontal Analysis

Traditionally, orthodontists have paid little attention to the facial analysis from the frontal view, and instead have focused mostly on the anteroposterior changes (i.e. Angle's classification). With the surge of three-dimensional (3-D) imaging technology more information from the frontal view will be available in the future, especially relating to the soft tissue analysis.[38]

When describing a patient from the frontal view, an overall assessment of the patient's symmetry is made. Attractiveness and pleasing facial esthetics have been linked to certain proportions and symmetry.[39,40] From the frontal view, the facial analysis is limited to the vertical and transverse dimensions.

Ideal facial proportions have been described since ancient times by Roman and Greek artists. Horizontal as well as vertical lines are used as reference planes to evaluate these proportions. The horizontal planes, such as the interpupillary, interauricular, alar base, and occlusal planes, should be parallel to each other and special attention should be paid to the presence of cants (Fig. 3-5). The proportions between these horizontal planes can also be evaluated on the profile view. From the frontal view the vertical reference lines are more important since it is only from this view that the transverse dimension can be evaluated (Fig. 3-6).

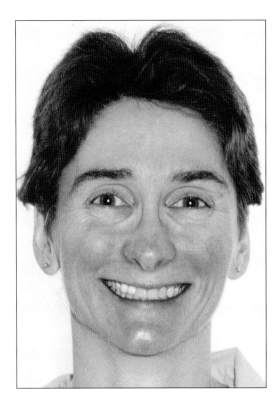

Fig. 3-5 Maxillary cant evidenced at smile. More gingival display is appreciated in the upper left buccal segment than in the right buccal segment.

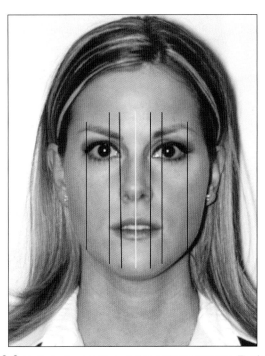

Fig. 3-6 Vertical reference lines used to evaluate symmetry. The face is divided into six portions in the transverse analysis. The yellow line is an estimate of the facial midline.

Midline

The frontal view is also helpful in the evaluation of the relationship between the facial and dental midline. It is important to note that the analysis of the facial midline can be difficult, especially in patients with deviated nasal septums (Fig. 3-7A). Thus, the commonly used technique of placing a piece of dental floss vertically through the facial midline to relate it to the dental midline can be deceiving. A better method is to assess the relationship between the cupid's bow and the dental midline (Fig. 3-7B).[41] Hence, the dental midline can be related to an adjacent well-defined midsagittal anatomic structure. A more detailed analysis of the dental midline is discussed later since many other factors need to be considered.

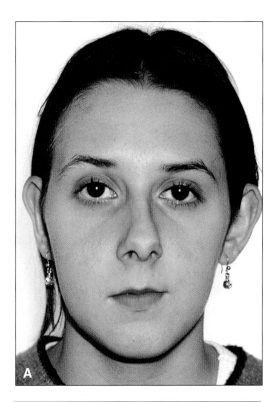

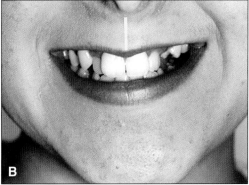

Fig. 3-7 A Patient exhibiting facial asymmetry, including a deviating septum. Estimating the facial midline using the nose as the reference structure may result in an inadequate reference line. **B** Same patient showing a coincident dental midline in relation to the philtrum.

Finally, the chin is evaluated for any deviation in relation to the facial midline (Fig. 3-8A). A view taken from above the patient (coronal) enhances the ability to detect any deviations (Fig. 3-8B). Similarly, observing the patient from the lower (ventral) aspect of the mandible can complement this analysis (Fig. 3-8C). This part of the clinical examination is very important as a large chin deviation is an indication for further analysis, perhaps with additional radiographic imaging.

Lips

A good analysis of the patient's lips is done at rest position and with the lips lightly touching each other (Fig. 3-9A and B). Indications of any muscle strain on lip closure should be noted. Upper and lower lip lengths can be assessed from the frontal as well as the profile view. Upper lip length when noted alone is not as important per se as its relationship to the upper incisors at rest and when smiling. The proper relationship between the upper lip and the amount of upper teeth exposure is a key factor in modern esthetic smile construction (Fig. 3-10A and B). Full display of the upper incisor crown upon smiling has been linked to youthful smiles.[42] A differential diagnosis between a short or long lip and a maxillary vertical excess or deficiency is

valuable in patients with an inadequate upper incisor display (Fig. 3-11).

Buccal Corridors and Smile Line

Other important relationships that can only be evaluated from the frontal view are the buccal corridors and the curvature of the smile line (relationship to lower lips). The buccal corridors and smile line concepts have been discussed extensively in the prosthetic literature.[43] The ideal esthetic parameter in smile design in the transverse dimension has been related to wide dental arches and narrow buccal corridors (Fig. 3-12). Some authors have described upper first molar display on a full smile as a feature of an attractive smile.[44] Although this does seem to be an attribute of beautiful smiles, its validity and applicability is doubtful. Anatomic structures limit the amount of transverse expansion needed in order to reduce the unattractive wide buccal corridors. The longterm periodontal health of teeth with expansion is not well understood. CT scans have shown that indiscriminate expansion of the maxillary arch results in buccal root dehiscences as these extend beyond the cortical plates.[45] Another important reason to avoid indiscriminate expansion relates to the longterm stability.[46] Skeletal tissues (bones and teeth) are

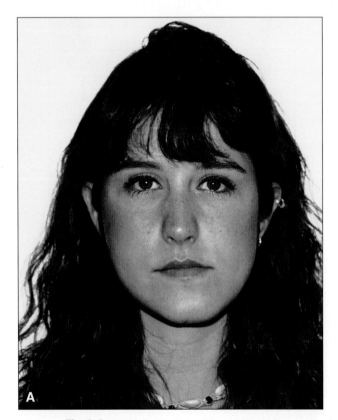

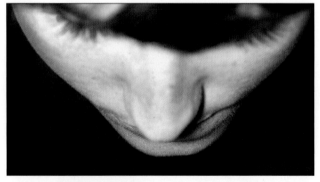

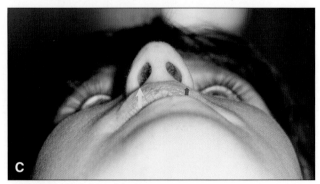

Fig. 3-8 **A** Patient with asymmetric mandible. **B** Coronal view to evaluate mandibular asymmetry during the clinical examination. **C** Ventral view complements the assessment for mandibular asymmetry. In this patient the ventral view provides better information about the asymmetry. Arrows show the asymmetry between the left and right sides in the lip region.

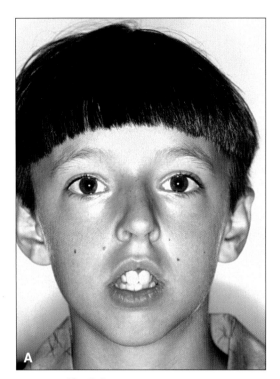 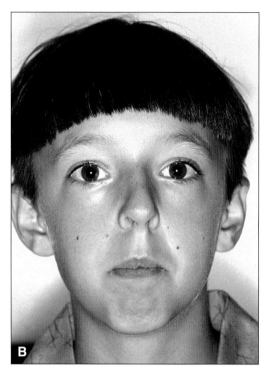

Fig. 3-9 **A** Patient showing incompetent lips at rest. **B** Upon lip contact the mentalis strain is noted.

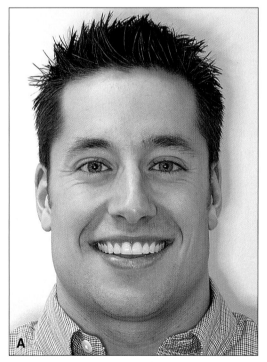 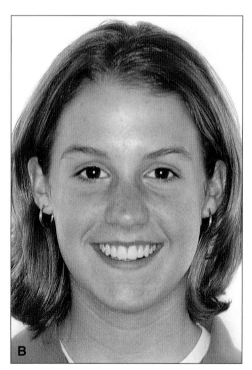

Fig. 3-10 Esthetic smiles in **A** a man and **B** a woman. Note the relationship of the upper lip to the gingival margins and the lower lip to the smile arc.

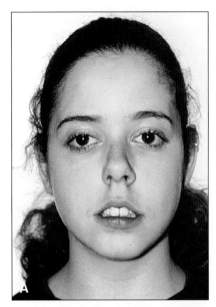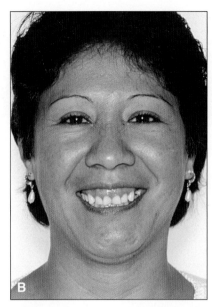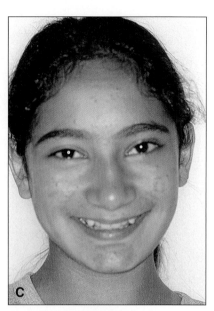

Fig. 3-11 Differential diagnosis for incisor display. **A** Patient with excessive incisor display due to a short upper lip. **B** Patient with excessive maxillary display due to a vertical maxillary excess. **C** Patient with an inadequate amount of incisor showing due to a short maxilla vertically.

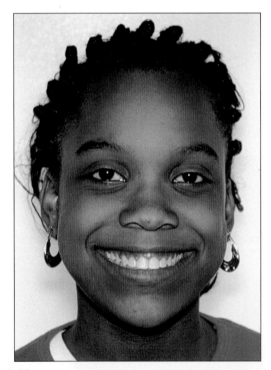

Fig. 3-12 Esthetically pleasing smile. Patient exhibits the upper first molars with very narrow buccal corridors and very wide dental arches.

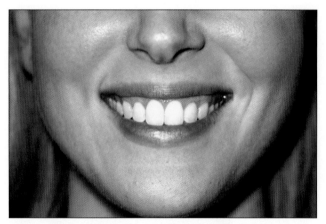

Fig. 3-13 Ideal parallelism between the incisal edges of the upper anterior teeth and the lower lip. The contact between the incisors and the lip is very slight.

usually in equilibrium with the surrounding musculature; the longterm stability might be compromised when teeth invade the neighboring muscle confinements.[36,37]

Another concept that has been related to esthetic smiles is the parallelism of the curve of the upper anterior teeth to the lower lip curvature on smiling (Fig. 3-13). Although this does seem to be an ideal objective, it should be noted that there are different types of smile and the lower lip posture varies accordingly.[47] Moreover, this smile arc is a resultant of the occlusal plane inclination and second-order crown angulations in the upper anterior teeth.[48] Thus, there are some limitations to the achievement of this ideal smile arc on every patient. A reasonable objective is to prevent a flat or reverse smile line (Fig. 3-14A) and to obtain some degree of curvature that resembles the one found in the lower lip (Fig. 3-14B).

Symmetry has always been linked to beauty. Not surprisingly, it has also been ascribed as one of the

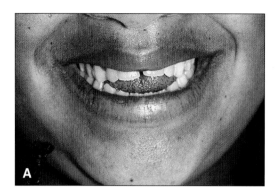

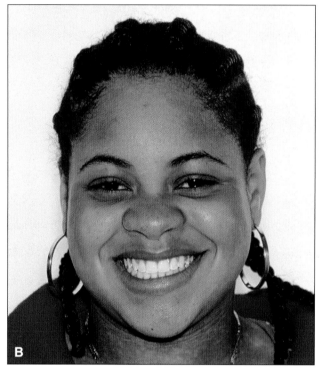

Fig. 3-14 A Reverse relationship between the upper incisors and the lower lips, which is frequently found in patients with a finger habit. **B** Correction of the reverse relationship after treatment. A better esthetic relationship to the lower lip was achieved.

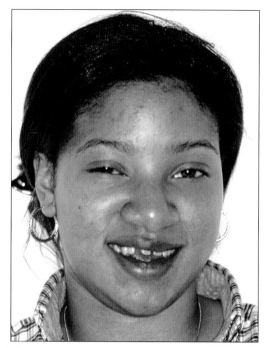

Fig. 3-15 Asymmetric smile with more tooth structure display on the right side. A reverse smile curve is also evident.

characteristics of a beautiful smile. This symmetry can be related to the size and shape of the teeth on both sides of each arch (see Fig. 3-10A). Also, it is related to the relationship of the intraoral tissues to the lips on both the right and left sides. Therefore, the same amount of gingival display should be seen upon smiling, on both sides of the arch. Reasons for any asymmetry include a cant in the maxillary skeletal base, different amounts of tooth eruption on the right and left sides, or asymmetric smiles. It is estimated that 8.7% of normal adults have asymmetric smiles (Fig. 3-15).[49]

The last feature related to symmetry in the smile is the dental midline. The ideal relationship of the dental midline to the facial midline was mentioned above. The upper dental midline has been considered more important than the lower dental midline in the esthetic smile design. It has been shown that a discrepancy of <2 mm (to the right or left) between the upper dental midline and the facial midline is not readily perceived (Fig. 3-16A).[50,51] However, any type of unparallel relationship between the interproximal contacts of the incisors related to the facial midline (incisal cant) is more easily perceived (Fig. 3-16B).[52]

Two further characteristics of an attractive smile are the gingival heights of the anterior teeth and the tooth shade. The gingival heights of the six upper anterior teeth are similar. The central incisors and the canines are at the same level, while the lateral incisors' free gingival level is approximately 0.5 mm incisal to the level of the canines and central incisors (Fig. 3-17). Moreover, the gingival heights of the premolars and molars should be approximately 1 and 1.5 mm less than the canines, respectively (Fig. 3-18A and B).[53] The significance of tooth shade in the esthetic smile has been reviewed extensively in the prosthodontic literature.[44] Light shades have always been considered one of the most important characteristics of an esthetic smile. Therefore, procedures such as tooth bleaching may be considered after orthodontic appliance removal. Tooth shade also becomes an important factor in patients where canine substitution for missing upper laterals is considered. Differences in the tone between the canines (dark yellow) and incisors may be an indication to opt to restore the laterals prosthetically instead of closing the edentulous space (canine substitution).

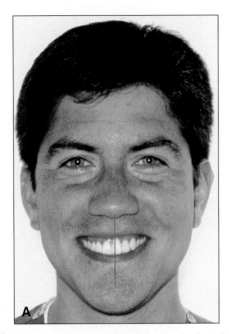 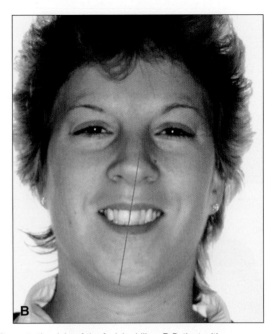

Fig. 3-16 **A** Patient with upper midline deviated approximately 2 mm to the right of the facial midline. **B** Patient with upper midline deviated approximately 1 mm from the facial midline. The inclination of the line described by the interproximal contact area accentuates the midline discrepancy.

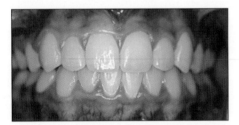

Fig. 3-17 Proper gingival heights. The upper central incisors and canines have the same gingival height; the lateral incisors' gingiva is 1 mm below the canines and central incisors.

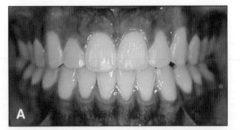

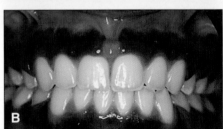

Fig. 3-18 **A** Gingival heights from the canines to the molars decrease gradually. **B** Abrupt change in gingival heights between the canine and the second premolar. This situation is commonly seen in upper first premolar extraction.

The last notable factor in the ideal smile is tooth shape. Incisors are the predominant teeth in the smile, especially the upper central incisor. The ideal proportion of this tooth is found when the width approximates 75–80% of the height (Fig. 3-19).[54] Similarly, lateral incisor size is often small in the mesiodistal dimension and should be considered in determining final occlusion and overall treatment outcome. Tooth shape will be discussed further later in this chapter.

Profile View

Orthodontists spend more time in evaluating patients from the profile view. Most of the literature is based on analysis from lateral cepahalometric films. The classification of malocclusions is also based on the anteroposterior dimension (i.e. Angle's classification). Even though the vertical dimension can be analyzed from this view, interest in this dimension has lagged. Later chapters describe the importance of the vertical dimension in the treatment

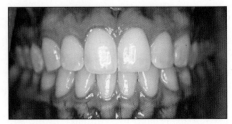

Fig. 3-19 Proper tooth proportions and shape, especially on the upper central incisors, is a key element in an esthetic smile.

of various malocclusions by an application of sound biomechanic principles.

Anteroposterior Dimension

The anteroposterior dimension is the backbone of most contemporary orthodontic analyses. In this dimension the soft tissue convexity is initially assessed by observing the spatial relationship between the forehead, maxilla, and mandible. These are separate, but interrelated, anatomic structures with independent timings in development. Each structure provides feedback to the others to maintain a normal facial growth pattern.[55] Normally, these three structures maintain a slight convexity that is reduced during puberty as a result of differential jaw growth.[28] During the pubertal growth spurt the mandible has a greater anterior displacement compared to the maxilla. It is important to note that at the end of growth there are also gender differences in the convexity of the profiles. On average the female profile is more convex due to a smaller chin projection.[56]

Once the magnitude of the facial profile convexity is assessed, the next step is to evaluate which of the three structures is contributing to the abnormality. With an increased angle of convexity or concavity, the question to be answered is which structure is causing the deformity (the mandible or maxilla). It has been reported that the majority of skeletal convexities exhibit a deficient mandible.[57] On the other hand, studies show that approximately half of skeletal concavities present with a deficient maxilla.[58]

To evaluate maxillary/mandibular position during the clinical examination, an adequate reference plane needs to be determined. During the clinical examination the easiest assessment can be done using the natural head position. This can be achieved when the extraoral photographs are taken. More detailed analysis of the soft tissue spatial relationships in the anteroposterior dimensions is obtained from the lateral cephalograms.

Nose

Although the nose is outside the limits of what can be affected by orthodontic treatment, it is important for facial balance. More importantly, the apparent nose projection can be affected by the anteroposterior position of the lips. During the clinical examination, the length and height of the nose are evaluated. Any morphologic variations in shape are noted (Fig. 3-20).

Lips

Lip response to orthodontic treatment is perhaps one of the most discussed topics in modern orthodontics. With the increased interest in esthetics, patients and practitioners are not only interested in the dental and skeletal changes, but also the response of the surrounding soft tissues to treatment. As teeth move, there is a direct effect on the lip support. Although this is a subject of perpetual research, no good predictor of the precise lip response to orthodontic movement has been identified.[59] The only predictable

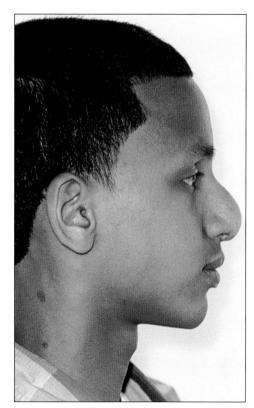

Fig. 3-20 Patient with an abnormal nose contour.

variable is the direction of lip response. It has been established that if any lip changes occur, these will be in the direction of the upper anterior tooth movement.[60,61]

During clinical examination an overall assessment of the lips at rest is necessary. Special attention should be given to lip posture and tonicity. The influence of lip pressure in the etiology of certain types of malocclusions has been suggested.[62] To evaluate lip posture, the anteroposterior and vertical relationship of the lips (rest position) to the incisors is examined (Fig. 3-21A and B).[63] In the anteroposterior dimension, a gap between the labial surface of the anterior teeth and the oral mucosa may be absent or present. In the vertical dimension the lip line may be high (middle of the incisor root) or low. If the lips and the incisors contact each other, the exact location (incisal, middle or apical third) of this junction is noted. The vertical and anteroposterior relationship of the lips to the incisors can aid in the prediction of upper lip movement in response to lingual incisor movement, and the longterm stability of the incisors to labial movement as well.[64]

The relationship between the upper and lower lip is another important feature that needs evaluation. When the lips are at rest, the normal interlabial gap ranges from 1 to 3 mm. As the patient closes his/her lips, any strain on the perioral musculature, such as mentalis strain, may be indicative of an excessive interlabial gap. Another very important dimension to note is the amount of incisor display with the lips maintained at this rest position.

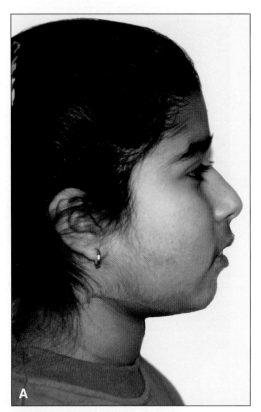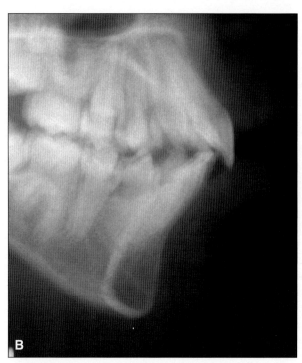

Fig. 3-21 A Patient with no contact between the crown of the upper incisors and the upper lip. The upper lip is not supported by the crowns of the upper central incisors. The effect on the upper lip after lingual tipping of the incisors would depend on the amount of movement of the coronal portion of the root. **B** Lateral cephalometric film showing the vertical and anteroposterior relationship of the lip to the incisors. Intimate contact is noticed with the alveolar process of the anterior teeth in the maxilla.

An excessive display of tooth or gum tissue may be the result of a single factor or combination of factors, such as vertical maxillary excess, short upper lip, or supra-erupted upper incisors. From the profile view, a general indication of a short upper lip is evident when an obtuse angle is found between a line drawn from the commissure of the mouth to the labrale superioris and the horizontal reference plane (Fig. 3-22). In general, the lower lip is almost parallel to the horizontal plane; therefore, these patients will present with an excessive interlabial gap.

Another important feature is lip thickness. It is well known that lip thickness varies between different races.[65–67] Moreover, the response to orthodontic tooth movement may be different between thin and thick lips. Some evidence suggests that thicker lips respond less and more variably to tooth movement than thinner lips (Fig. 3-23).[68]

The ideal anteroposterior position of the lips has been estimated by many studies using different reference lines. The definition of protrusive or retrusive lips varies with age, gender, and race. To define lip protrusion, different reference planes have been used. One of the most common reference planes used in clinical orthodontics is the E-line defined by Ricketts.[69] The limitation of this reference line is that it is influenced by the chin and nose. Any large deviation from normal of either the chin or the nose will

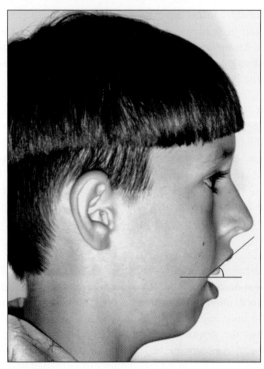

Fig. 3-22 Large interlabial gap. There is a large angle between the horizontal plane and a line from the angle of the mouth to the labrale superiore.

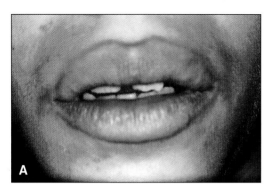
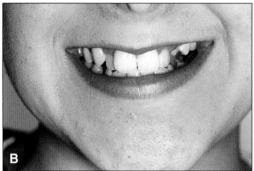

Fig. 3-23 **A** Patient with very thick lips. The response to incisor movement may be limited by the tissue mass. **B** Patient with very thin lips that may be more susceptible to lip changes with tooth movement.

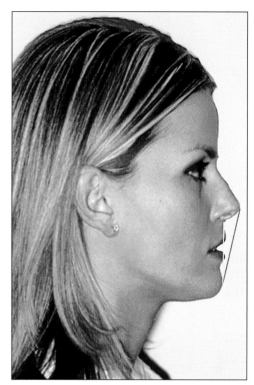

Fig. 3-24 Relationship of the lips to two commonly used reference lines: E-line (influenced by the nose, red) and Sn–Pg (yellow).

give a false impression of lip position. To control for the nose variability, Burstone proposed the Sn–Pg line (Fig. 3-24).[70,71] Others have used different angles using the chin and lips as reference points and not incorporating the nose (z angle, Steiner's S-line, and Holdaway angle).[72–74]

Another important measurement related to lip protrusion is the nasolabial angle. Although this angle is also influenced by the angulation of the nose (upturn or downturn of the nasal tip), it gives an indication of the upper lip inclination (Fig. 3-25).

Although numerically the soft tissue analysis can be better analyzed in a lateral cephalometric film, a general overview is achieved during the clinical examination. Using a combination of all these reference planes allows for a proper interpretation of lip position.

Another important structure that is analyzed from the lateral view is the chin projection. In adult patients the ratio of the chin-to-throat depth length compared to the lower facial height is 1.2:1.[75] It seems that not only the length of this line but the angulation to the true horizontal plane is an important feature in well balanced faces. Normally, a parallel relation or slightly negative angle (throat point above the menton) is found in esthetically pleasing faces (Fig. 3-26A and B).

Vertical Dimension

As stated above, this dimension can be analyzed from both the frontal and the profile view. Both these views

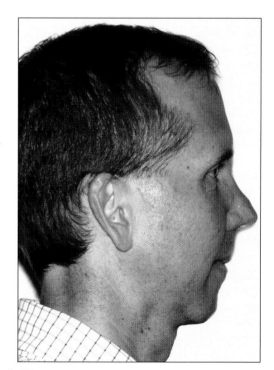

Fig. 3-25 Obtuse nasolabial angle. The upturned nasal tip and retrusive lip contribute to the obtuse angle.

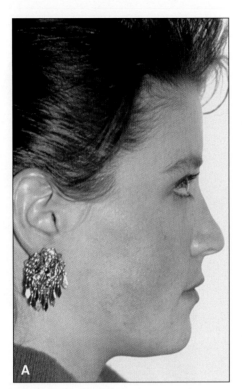 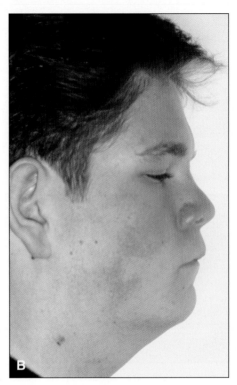

Fig. 3-26 **A** Parallel relationship of the chin–throat line to the horizontal plane. An adequate ratio between the lower facial height and throat depth is 1.2:1. **B** Inadequate ratio between the lower facial height and throat depth (no throat depth) gives an unesthetic inclination of the chin–throat line.

can be related through the vertical dimension to provide a composite 3-D analysis. The face can be divided into three equal thirds: upper, middle, and lower facial heights. The true upper facial height is seldom used as it is measured from the trichion to the glabella. More commonly the middle facial height is referred to as the upper facial height. The normal upper to lower facial height ratio is 1:1 (glabella to subnasale and subnasale to soft tissue menton) (Fig. 3-27A).

The lower facial third is very important since the effects of orthodontic treatment are most profound in this third. It is further subdivided into two proportional heights. One-third of the lower facial height normally corresponds to Sn to stomion and two-thirds from stomion to menton (Fig. 3-27B).

The vertical analysis is not limited to the anterior part of the face but also includes the posterior. The ratio between these two determines, to a degree, the steepness of the mandibular plane. The normal ratio of the lower facial height to the posterior facial height is 0.69.[76] An overall assessment of this relationship can be determined from the mandibular plane. Palpating and placing a flat object along the lower border of the mandible can give a general idea of the steepness of this plane.

In the vertical dimension from the profile view the face is generally categorized as convergent (short face) or divergent (long face). The general facial characteristics

of a long face are increased anterior facial height relative to the posterior facial height, steep mandibular plane angle, possible lip incompetence with large interlabial gap, and shallow mentolabial sulcus (Fig. 3-28A). At the other end of the spectrum, the short face is characterized by a flat mandibular plane angle with a similar posterior and anterior facial height, lip redundancy with deep mentolabial sulcus, and short lower facial height (Fig. 3-28B).

Most of the clinical analysis is static in nature; therefore, it is important during the examination to pay close attention to the animation of the facial soft tissues. During this time, an analysis of more natural lip function, including different smile heights, symmetry of the smile, and the amount of upper and lower incisor display during conversation, are more important than forced unnatural snap shots of animated features.

Photographs
Extraoral Photographs
Although the clinical examination provides an excellent opportunity for patient evaluation, it is important to document specific information (images, intraoral impressions). This information can be used later for data analysis (radiographs, photographs, and models), medicolegal reasons, and treatment progress and outcome evaluations.

Different photographic images from the profile and frontal views are recommended. Initially, a picture of the

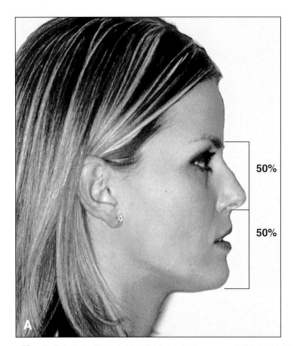
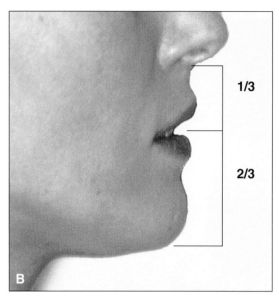

Fig. 3-27 A Facial heights divided into three equal thirds: trichion–glabella, glabella–subnasale, subnasale–menton. **B** Lower facial height is further divided into unequal thirds: subnasale–stomiom (1/3), stomiom–menton (2/3).

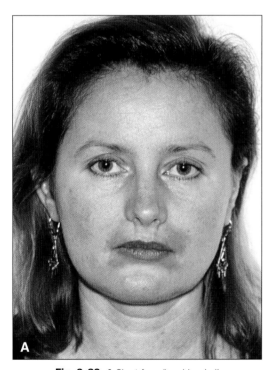
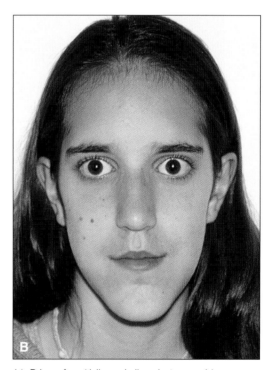

Fig. 3-28 A Short face (brachicephalic or mesoprosopic). **B** Long face (dolicocephalic or leptoprosopic).

patient with relaxed lips and lips lightly touching each other are taken from the frontal as well as the profile view (Fig. 3-29A-D). Frontal, and especially profile, view pictures are taken in the natural head position.

A 45° angle image between the profile and the frontal view provides information related to the amount of malar prominence and lower jaw shape (mandibular plane angle and gonial angle). This view usually confirms the findings of the analysis from the frontal and profile view (Fig. 3-29E).

Finally, a frontal photograph depicting a full smile should be taken. It is somewhat difficult to capture a natural,

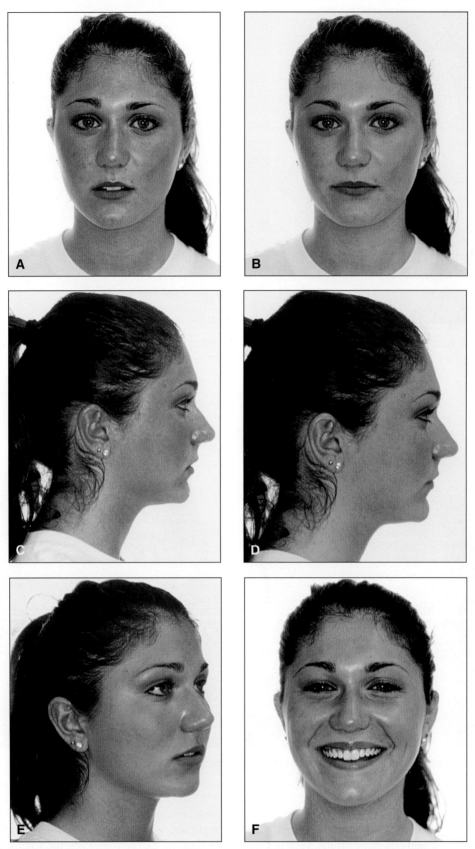

Fig. 3-29 Extraoral photographs for the records. **A** Frontal with lips at rest and **B** with lips lightly touching each other. **C** Profile with lips at rest and **D** with lips lightly touching each other. **E** 45° angle photograph. Assessment of the cheek projection and mandibular plane angle is obtained from this view. **F** Frontal smiling photograph.

unposed smile. Usually this photograph does not reflect the full extent of the smile. Thus, special attention is needed during the clinical examination to record important data such us the amount of tooth/gum display, the relationship of the upper teeth to the lower lip, and the width of buccal corridors (Fig. 3-29F). During the data analysis, this information can be correlated to the still images. As an alternative, a video image of the different animated facial features has recently been suggested to be used as part of the clinical record.[77]

Intraoral Photographs

A total of five views of the dentition and the occlusion are taken. These pictures include two buccal photos (left and right), two occlusal photos (upper and lower arch), and one frontal intraoral view. These photographs should be taken in maximum intercuspation (Fig. 3-30). Additionally, intraoral centric relation photographs are taken if a significant centric relation–centric occlusion (CR–CO) shift is present (mandibular shift).

Intraoral Examination

The intraoral examination for an orthodontic patient starts as any other dental examination. First, an overall inspection of the oral mucosa in search of any pathologic lesions is performed. Upon analyzing the soft tissue, special attention should be given to the gingival tissues. Periodontal status evaluation is of prime importance, especially in the adult. It is not uncommon to find active periodontal disease in adults around the molar areas. A random probing should be done around the first and second molars, and on some anterior teeth on every adult patient.

The quality of the attached gingiva is examined next. The thickness (gingivo-occlusal) and width of the attached gingiva is also very important. Many times this is overlooked and recession may occur as the teeth are displaced labially out of their alveolar housing. It should be noted that recession may also be present before starting treatment (Fig. 3-31).

Continuing with the intraoral soft tissue analysis, the labial frenum attachment is evaluated. A high insertion into the attached gingiva might contribute to a persisting diastema (Fig. 3-32).[78] Moreover, high frenum attachments have also been linked to recession of the labial surface of the lower incisors.[79]

Oral Hygiene

Good oral hygiene is very important during orthodontic treatment and should be stressed from the beginning. It only gets worse after the insertion of an appliance if proper education and motivation are not provided before the start of treatment. It is well established that orthodontic appliances hinder oral hygiene. Therefore, careful evaluation of the oral hygiene at the initial examination is needed, and treatment should be delayed until good plaque control is achieved by the patient.

Tongue

Initially, all the mucosa of the tongue should be screened for any signs of pathologic lesions. A general evaluation of the shape and size, and the relation to the lower dental arch, should be noted. Evidence of indentations on the lateral borders of the tongue, accompanied by generalized spacing between the teeth, may suggest macroglossia.

The tongue is a powerful muscle that applies constant pressure to the lingual surfaces of the teeth, counteracting the lip pressure on the buccal surfaces.[37] Functional evaluation of the tongue during speech and swallowing could give some insight as to etiology of the malocclusion. Finally, the lingual frenum is evaluated. Ankyloglossia or tongue

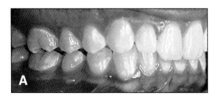 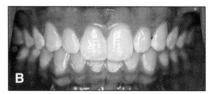 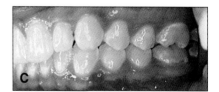

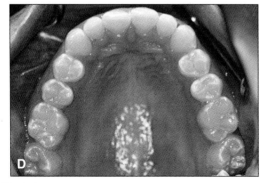 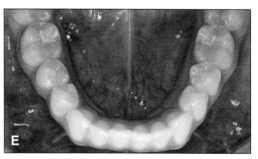

Fig. 3-30 Intraoral records. **A** Right buccal view. **B** Frontal view. **C** Left buccal view. **D** Upper occlusal view. **E** Lower occlusal view.

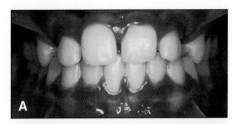

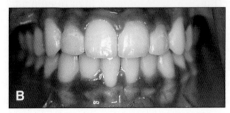

Fig. 3-31 A Preoperative photograph of the lower incisor gingival attachment. Incipient recession with a thin band of attached gingiva is seen. **B** Postoperative photograph shows no attached gingiva in the lower right central incisor and slight progression of gingival recession. Grafting of this area is indicated.

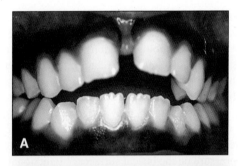

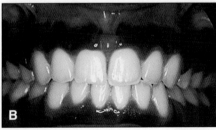

Fig 3-32 A Thick band of labial frenum possibly contributing to the diastema. **B** Diastema closure post treatment with the labial frenum still present. The patient rejected frenectomy. A bonded lingual retainer was placed between the incisors.

tie is found in some patients and may be a reason for impeded speech.[80]

Dentition

Before starting the dental examination per se, a thorough dental history is taken. First, the patient is asked if he/she is under regular dental care. Although an affirmative answer does not mean that there is no active disease, it can be assumed that the patient or guardian has an interest in maintaining good oral health. A patient's oral hygiene habits, i.e. brushing frequency, use of floss, etc, should also be noted.

History of previous orthodontic treatment is also important. It might give some insight into a patient's expectations, as well as relapse tendencies and sequelae (e.g. root resorption, decalcified lesions) after treatment. Additionally, the information can enable complications that may have occurred with previous orthodontic therapy to be anticipated.

Within the dental history, the patient is questioned about previous trauma to the jaws or teeth. A history of trauma to the jaws may explain asymmetries, abnormal growth or, in some cases, TMJ symptoms. A history of trauma and the nature of the trauma (i.e. avulsion, luxation, fractures, etc.) to the teeth should be noted. Certain types of dentoalveolar traumas have been related to external root resorption and ankylosis.[81] Orthodontic movement can be a precipitating factor to this resorption in severely traumatized teeth (Fig. 3-33).[82]

Finally, any history of deleterious habits, such as thumb/ finger sucking or a tongue posturing habit, might explain, in part, the etiology of the malocclusion. With regard to a habit, it is important to find out if this is an active or past habit. In the case of an active habit, the frequency and time during the day that the habit is performed are noted.

The dental examination starts by counting the number of teeth. The specific aim is to inspect for any supernumerary or missing teeth. Primary teeth should be distinguished from permanent teeth and any tooth transpositions should be noted. The panoramic film is a useful aid for corroborating the clinical examination findings.

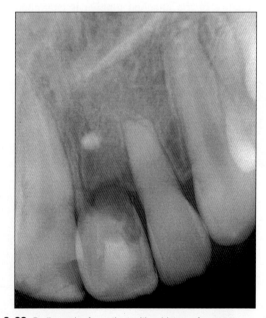

Fig. 3-33 Radiograph of a patient with a history of severe trauma to the upper central incisor taken after orthodontic treatment. Note the calcification of the pulp chamber in the lateral incisor and the severe resorption of the root of the central incisor.

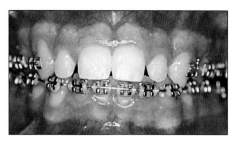

Fig. 3-34 Morphology of the peg laterals creates wide unesthetic incisal embrasures. Restoration of these teeth is generally recommended in the last stages of treatment if composites are the selected restorative material.

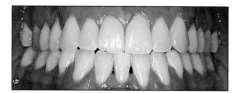

Fig. 3-36 Post-treatment black triangles after the extraction of a lower incisor.

The size and shape of the teeth are often overlooked. Attention to morphologic variation is especially important in the anterior segment. It is not unusual to find peg laterals, conical shaped teeth, or other dental anomalies in this esthetic zone. Peg laterals are unsightly teeth that usually generate a Bolton tooth size discrepancy (Fig. 3-34). Subtle discrepancies in tooth size and shape are often noticed at the end of treatment when the occlusal and esthetic goals are not met. Therefore, a careful evaluation of the tooth size is needed from the beginning of treatment. Different restorative alternatives will dictate the specific distribution of spaces and positioning of the teeth to facilitate and enhance the restorative result.[83]

Black triangles are a common unesthetic finding in adults. These black spaces are closely related to the tooth shape (Fig. 3-35) and are often a result of the papilla not filling the interproximal space. A study showed that if the interproximal contact of two adjacent teeth is 5 mm or less from the crestal bone, a papilla will be present almost 100% of the time.[84] Thus, triangular shaped teeth will have a low incisal contact that increases the distance to the crestal bone, resulting in a black triangle. At the initial examination the clinician should be aware that crowding between the upper incisors can displace the contact gingivally; therefore, as proper alignment is achieved in the initial phases of treatment, the contact may be displaced incisally, resulting in a black triangle. The black triangle frequently found with the extraction of a lower incisor is often related to the bone recession that occurs after a tooth extraction (Fig. 3-36).

Incisor crowns with a wider middle than incisal third may also result in excessive incisal embrasures (Fig. 3-37). Other abnormalities in tooth shape, such as irregularities in the borders of the incisors, may be related to a worn dentition or trauma to the incisors.

Tooth shape is not only related to the clinical crown but also to the root morphology and crown-to-root angulation. This is an important consideration in the straight wire technique as it is based on the coronal angulation to the occlusal plane in the three planes of space.[85] An acute angle between the root and the crown with a prescribed bracket may position the root outside the cortical bone in the third order or displace the root against the tooth adjacent to it in the second order (Fig. 3-38).

The tooth shade is the final factor to be evaluated. It has been shown that patients prefer lighter shades. More importantly, any white or brown spots should be noted in the initial examination, to distinguish them from the ones that

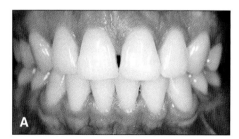
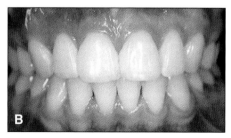

Fig. 3-35 A Black triangle as a result of the shape of the incisors. Contact between incisors was too low. **B** Good proportions between maximum height and width present in the incisal edge. Composite material was added to the mesial surfaces to alter the mesiodistal width in the middle and gingival thirds of the crowns.

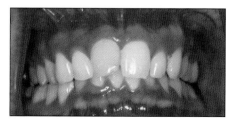

Fig. 3-37 Abnormal morphology of the central incisors. The mesiodistal width is larger in the middle third compared to the incisal third, resulting in large incisal embrasures.

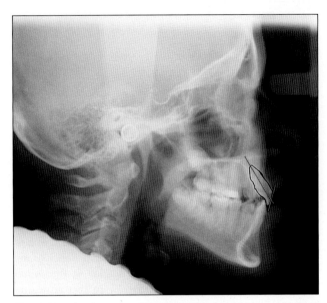

Fig. 3-38 Acute crown–root angulation. Caution should be used during root correction of the incisors as the lingual root portion may approximate the cortical plate of the palate.

can be caused by poor bacterial plaque control with fixed appliances.

The two most common dental diseases are caries and periodontal disease. Periodontal disease is more common in the adult population. Thus, molars in all adult patients should be probed on all surfaces. Any additional probing will depend on the degree of periodontal involvement of the posterior teeth or will be based on the radiographic evidence obtained.

The deleterious effects of traumatic forces to teeth with periodontal disease have been well reported (Fig. 3-39). Orthodontic forces have been shown to produce a similar breakdown effect on the tooth supporting structures in the presence of active periodontal disease. Therefore, prior to orthodontic treatment the clinician should ensure that no active disease is present and that suitable oral health conditions exist in the oral cavity.

Caries, the other common dental disease, is more prevalent in adolescents than in adults. Nevertheless, all patients should be screened for caries before and throughout orthodontic treatment. Any lesions present should be permanently restored and any pulpal involvement addressed before initiating treatment. It has been reported that infection within the confinement of the root canal can cause root resorption in response to an orthodontic force.[82] In addition, teeth with previous root canal treatment should be inspected for a good quality seal and no signs of periapical pathology. Referring the patient to a general or pediatric dentist for cleaning and check up before appliance placement is also recommended.

It is common for adults to present with missing teeth and heavily restored dentitions, i.e. crowns, bridges, and extensive amalgam or composite buildups. These patients should be checked for ill-fitting bridges and crowns. A good analysis of the tooth structure supporting the bridges should be done in collaboration with the restorative dentist.

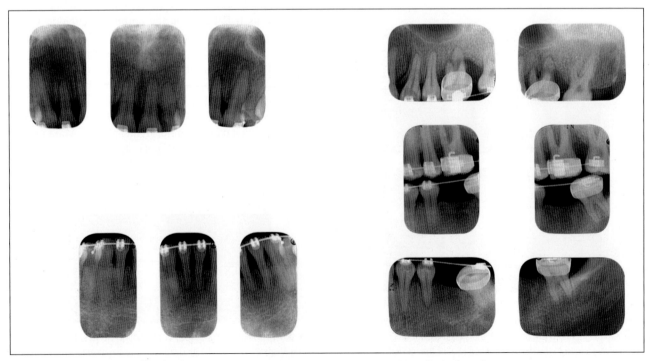

Fig. 3-39 Patient with severe localized bone loss exacerbated by orthodontic appliances.

A multidisciplinary approach is needed in these cases to carefully plan the orthodontic movement that will facilitate ideal subsequent crown and bridge work. Furthermore, it should be anticipated that appliance insertion in heavily restored dentition is complicated. Banding and bonding procedures in these patients are difficult due to irregular tooth shapes and variable surface characteristics of the restorative materials. Hence, appliance breakage during treatment is more common.

Orthodontics for the majority of patients is an elective procedure. Periodontal disease and caries affect many individuals seeking orthodontic treatment. Both dental diseases should be under control before orthodontic treatment is started. It should be stressed again that close communication with the general dentist is of key importance.

Tooth Eruption

As mentioned above, there is great variation in the timing of eruption of different teeth among individuals. Delayed eruption of teeth is not a problem per se. However, an abnormal eruption sequence has been considered to be one of the factors involved in the etiology of the malocclusion.[86] Other eruption disturbances, such as retained primary teeth, ankylosed teeth, and ectopic eruption are important etiologic factors in malocclusion (Fig. 3-40). It has been reported that there is a correlation between the abnormal eruption sequence and direction, abnormal shape of teeth, and congenitally missing teeth.[33]

Dental Arches

During the intra-arch analysis, a general appreciation of the arch shape, as well as an overall view of crowding or spacing, is achieved. Intra-arch evaluation of the tooth relationships also includes marginal ridge discrepancies. Severe marginal ridge discrepancies between adjacent teeth might be indicative of ankylosis. This condition is most often found between the permanent first molars and the lower second primary molars (Fig. 3-41).

A more thorough evaluation of the intra- as well inter-arch relationships can be achieved with the model analysis. Crowding, spacing, and problems with the angulations and orientation of teeth in the three dimensions of space can be analyzed more precisely in study models. Moreover, these models provide the unique possibility of analyzing the occlusion from the lingual aspect.

Extraoral Examination
Functional Analysis

One of the reasons that patients seek, or are referred, for orthodontic care is to achieve proper occlusal function. Therefore, the orthodontist must have a good understanding of the critical concepts in occlusion and how they relate to other structures such as the TMJ.

Much has been discussed about which type of occlusion provides the best function.[87] In general, it is accepted that ideal occlusal function relates to a mutually protected occlusion.[87,88] This means that the posterior teeth protect

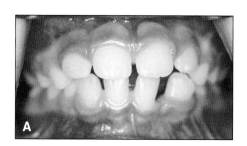
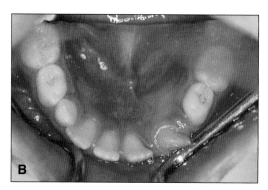
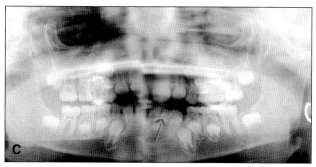

Fig. 3-40 Ectopic eruption of lower left lateral incisor. **A** Distal eruption of the lower lateral incisor exfoliated left primary canine instead of the lower lateral primary incisor. **B** Space for the left permanent canine is greatly reduced. **C** Panoramic radiograph shows the primary left lateral incisor is still present (arrow) mesial to the lower left permanent lateral incisor. Eruption of the lower left permanent canine is hampered.

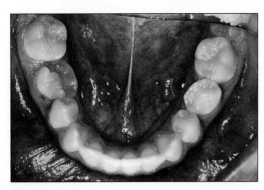

Fig. 3-41 13-year-old patient with the lower right second primary molar submerged below the occlusal plane. This clinical finding is highly suggestive of ankylosis of this primary tooth.

the anterior teeth in maximum intercuspation by receiving the majority of the occlusal load, and the anterior teeth protect the posterior teeth in the excursive movements. In lateral excursions, most clinicians agree that canine guidance is the ideal occlusal scheme. Yet, group function on lateral movements can also be an acceptable occlusal scheme. Overall, balancing occlusal contacts are considered deleterious for occlusal function.

Considerable controversy surrounds this area of occlusion and it is not within the scope of this chapter to discuss it. Needless to say, a good analysis of the different excursive movements is necessary in the initial clinical examination.

The different excursive movements to be analyzed are anterior protrusive, lateral, and lateral protrusive movements. As mentioned above, any contacts between the posterior teeth during the anterior protrusive movement should be noted. In the lateral movements, attention should be given to any posterior contacts in the working side, but most importantly on the balancing side. No anterior contacts should be present in lateral excursions. During all these excursive movements, close attention should be paid to wear facets and how these relate interocclusally in the different end movements.

Temporomandibular Disorders

Temporomandibular disorders (TMD) encompass certain conditions in and around the TMJ. These disorders have been subdivided into internal derangements (within the articulation) and myofacial pain dysfunction (masticatory and cervical muscles).[89] Internal derangements are classified according to the relationship of the articular disc to the condyle during jaw opening. Four distinct stages of condyle–disc relationships have been found that denote progressive degeneration. The first stage starts with initial incoordination between the condyle and the disc during opening. The second and third stages are characterized by anterior displacement of the disc, which is not recaptured in the third stage. The fourth stage involves damage to the retrodiscal tissue.

The four major characteristics of myofacial pain dysfunction (MPD) are pain of unilateral origin, limited jaw opening, masticatory muscle tenderness, and no radiographic or clinical evidence of joint degeneration.[90] Each patient should be examined for the presence of any of these symptoms. The masticatory muscles and the temporomandibular articulation are palpated in search of any areas or trigger points that elicit pain.

In general, the TMJ examination should focus on evaluating jaw movements and areas of pain in and around the joint upon palpation or function. Mandibular movements should be painless and within a normal range (50 mm approximately on maximum opening and 10 mm in lateral excursions).[88,91] The path followed during the opening movements of the mandible should be evaluated from the frontal view. This gives an indication of interferences, adhesions, or disc recapturing in the articulation. Although articular noises, such as clicking, popping, and crepitation, are important diagnostic findings, if any of these is the sole finding, it does not imply a diagnosis of TMD.[89]

In general, diagnosis and treatment of TMD is complex, as many other factors such as stress may be involved. In patients with a history of TMJ problems, a more advanced TMJ examination that may include the Helkimo index should be done.[92] All clinical examinations should be complemented with a very thorough medical and dental history that may include a psychostress analysis.[93]

CR-CO

A major area of controversy in orthodontics, and dentistry overall, is the relevance and importance of the centric relation.[94–97] Orthodontists should attempt to record the centric relation and detect if any major shifts to the centric occlusion are present. It is normal to find a shift of approximately 1.5 mm in most individuals. The correlation between these small shifts and temporomandibular adverse effects is marginal, but major shifts of 3–4 mm have been correlated with increased TMD.[98]

Some clinicians have recommended mounting every case in an articulator in order to treat an occlusion where CR–CO coincides. There is no evidence to support the need to mount every patient's models, less so if the potential source of error is considered in registering and transferring centric relation from the patient to an articulator.[99]

Radiographic Records

Several radiographic images can be used as diagnostic aids for orthodontic therapy. The most commonly used images are the panoramic and lateral cephalometric radiographic films.

Before concentrating on any measurement analysis, a careful screening of each radiograph for any signs of pathology is indicated. Pathologic images often pass undetected by clinicians as attention is usually centered on the orthodontic analysis instead of the anatomic structures.

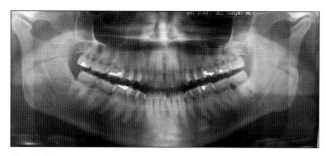

Fig. 3-42 Condylar shape on panoramic radiograph is indicative of osteoarthritic changes. Note also the radio-opaque structure between the root apices of the lower left premolars (compatible with idiopathic osteosclerosis).

Interestingly, it was found that 6% of orthodontic patients show some kind of anomalous or pathologic finding in orthodontic diagnostic radiographs (Fig. 3-42).[100,101]

Panoramic Radiograph

This radiograph provides a good general overview of the craniofacial anatomy, especially of the mandible, despite distortion of the image in some areas. Anatomy of the condyles should be carefully examined. Any asymmetry in length or width of the condyles, as well as in the shape of the articular surface, is noted. Ramus length and width symmetry should also be evaluated. Conditions such as hemimandibular hypo- or hyper-plasia can be also detected in this radiograph.[102] The most important information available in this radiograph includes the presence or absence of teeth, any variation in development or eruption timings, impaction of teeth, and variation in tooth anatomy.[103] The panoramic radiograph also provides general information on certain areas of interest that can be inspected closely with other more specific imaging.

The panoramic radiograph is also good for screening periodontal disease and caries. If an area looks suspicious for any of these diseases, a periapical or bite-wing radiograph should be taken.

With the advent of dental implants and their use in anchorage, the panoramic radiograph is also an important tool for inspection of the quality and quantity (height and width) of bone for possible implant sites.[104] It is also useful for evaluating the proximity of implant sites to vital structures such as the mandibular canal and the maxillary sinuses.

Lateral Cephalometric Radiograph

The lateral cephalogram is one of the oldest and still most often used radiographic images in orthodontics. Its limitation, as with any radiographs, is that it only displays a 2-D (vertical and anteroposterior) image of 3-D structures. Most orthodontic research and growth and development data are based on information obtained from this radiograph. It has been used for evaluation of the hard

tissue anatomy in the craniofacial structures, evaluation of growth, treatment planning, and treatment results.

Traditionally, angles and linear measurements have been used to evaluate the different anatomic structures in the craniofacial complex.[73,105] These measurements are compared to population means and the deviation from these norms is usually determined to be the problem. More recently, the development of numerous software programs enables an orthodontist to easily adopt his/her own relevant measurements from a plethora of cephalometric analyses. It should be emphasized that cephalometric analyses are only a diagnostic tool and are not diagnostic in themselves. Independent measures are meaningless if not interpreted properly; every deviation from the norm should be analyzed along with other measurements and within the whole context of the patient.

In the spatial analysis of an anatomic structure and its relation to others, three factors are important. The first is the size of the structure which can be measured, either in terms of height or width, and is usually defined by two points that determine a line. Second, the shape of the structure is usually defined by planes and angles and usually requires three or more points. Finally, the position of the structure is usually defined by angles and linear measurements to other reference structures.

The cephalometric analysis for orthognathic surgery (COGS) analysis developed at the University of Connecticut has been divided into five major craniofacial components in an attempt to define their size, shape, and position.[75] These components are: cranial base, maxilla, mandible, dentition, and soft tissue.

Before describing the specific spatial cephalometric analysis of these five components, a reference line or plane must be defined. This plane is important as it will determine the orientation of the cranium in space. Many of the angular and linear measurements that analyze facial morphology relate back to this plane.

The Frankfurt horizontal (FH) plane was defined by anthropologists in the 19th century and was adopted in cephalometry as the horizontal reference line. Although still used, there are inherent problems with this reference line as both porion and orbitale are difficult landmarks to locate. It is especially difficult to visualize porion since it is a bilateral landmark and is often not well defined on lateral head films. On the other hand, the sella–nasion (SN) line is composed of two easily visualized landmarks. At the University of Connecticut we have recommended an FH line located on average 7° lower than the SN line.[106] This constructed FH reference line is more reproducible and thus allows better evaluation of treatment progress and outcome.

For an accurate interpretation of the different structures in space, a reference line that was based on a physiologic posture instead of cranial anatomic landmarks has also been recommended. Studies have shown that variation in cranial base inclination may result in an unreliable impression of facial relationships.[107] A reference line that was made up of extracranial instead of intracranial points was recommended as being more reliable. This horizontal line should be parallel to the floor and represents the average head posture. The importance of this plane is that it not only reflects the normal position of the head in space, but also is a reproducible position not affected by intracranial landmarks. When a radiograph is taken in this natural head position (registered when a patient looks at a mirror in front of him/her at eye level), true vertical and horizontal reference lines can be traced.

Cranial Base

The cranial base is an important structure in the cephalometric analysis, particularly the anterior portion. Since growth of the anterior cranial base is nearly completed early in life, it can be used as a reference for the other structures. The anterior cranial base is also used to superimpose successive cephalograms in order to evaluate the overall changes related to growth and/or treatment. By knowing the length of the cranial base, size correlations to the other structures (maxilla and mandible) can be estimated (Fig. 3-43).

The saddle angle (N–S–Ar) (Fig. 3-43) and its influence on the craniofacial morphology has been evaluated in various studies. Its contribution to Class II and III malocclusions is somewhat controversial. It was proposed

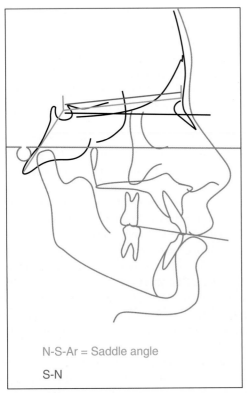

N-S-Ar = Saddle angle

S-N

Fig. 3-43 Commonly used measurements to evaluate the size and shape of the cranial base (first component in the cephalometric analysis).

that an obtuse angle related to the former and an acute angle to the latter,[108] but recent studies have not found a strong correlation between the two.[109]

Maxilla

The second component of the analysis is the maxilla. Initially a general idea of its size is obtained by measuring the posterior border to the anterior border (ANS–PNS). Thereafter the anteroposterior position is assessed. The distance from A point, which is related to a vertical reference line passing through N, provides good information relative to the position of the maxilla. It is important to remember that A point is affected by dentoalveolar movement. Another measurement used to assess the anteroposterior position of the maxilla is the perpendicular distance from PNS to a vertical line passing through PTM (Fig. 3-44).

To assess the vertical position of the maxilla, the distance from the anterior nasal spine (ANS) to the nasion (N) is measured. This is known as the upper facial height and its absolute measurement is not as important as the relationship to the lower facial height (ANS–Me): 45% for the upper to 55% for the lower facial height (Fig. 3-44).[106] Another important measurement indicating the vertical position or inclination of the maxilla is the angulation of the palatal plane (PNS–ANS) in relation to the horizontal line (Fig. 3-44). Usually in skeletal open bite patients this plane is tipped up anteriorly instead of being close to parallel, as is found in normal individuals.[110]

Mandible

The third major component of the cephalometric analysis is the mandible. The bulk of the cephalometric measurements relate to this craniofacial structure. All the mandibular anatomic structures, except for the condyles, are well visualized in the lateral cephalograms. For this reason, many of the mandibular length and angular measurements are taken from the constructed point articulare (Ar). This point may be confounding as mandibular positional or postural changes may give contradictory measurements.

To assess mandibular size, measurements such as Co–Gn, Co–Me, and Ar–Me are used (Fig. 3-45A). This can further be divided into ramus height and corpus length—Ar–Go and Go–Me, respectively (Fig. 3-45A). The anteroposterior position of the mandible is measured anteriorly by relating the distance of B point and the pogonion to a true vertical line (perpendicular to FH) passing through N (Fig. 3-45A). The difference between these two measurements gives an indication of the length of the hard tissue chin. Posteriorly, the anteroposterior position of the mandible can be evaluated from the angle formed by the ramus and the true horizontal (Fig. 3-45A). The shape of the mandible is defined by the gonial angle (Ar–Go–Me) (Fig. 3-45A).

The vertical measurement of the mandible anteriorly is done by evaluating the distance from ANS to Me (lower

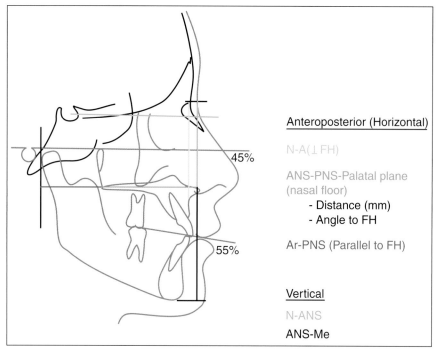

Anteroposterior (Horizontal)

N-A(⊥ FH)

ANS-PNS-Palatal plane
(nasal floor)
   - Distance (mm)
   - Angle to FH

Ar-PNS (Parallel to FH)

Vertical

N-ANS

ANS-Me

Fig. 3-44 Commonly used measurements to evaluate size and position of the maxilla (second component).

facial height). A ratio of the lower facial height to the posterior facial height (PNS–Go) can give an indication of the vertical pattern of the face (Fig. 3-45B). These measurements can be correlated to the mandibular plane angle (true horizontal Go–Me, Fig. 3-45B). Traditionally, these angular measurements have been used to describe vertical growth (high angle versus low angle) and facial patterns (long face versus short face).

Before starting the fourth major component (dental) of the analysis, a set of measurements that relate the maxilla and mandible to each other and the cranial base need to be mentioned. These measurements are A–B relative to the true horizontal and the occlusal plane, and the angle of convexity (N–A–Pg) (Fig. 3-46). Lastly, the S–Gn line is an isolated measurement that correlates directly with direction (angle with respect to the true horizontal) and magnitude (absolute length) of mandibular growth, and indirectly with the growth of the whole facial complex (Fig. 3-46).

Dental Measurements

The spatial relationship of the teeth is described in terms of their horizontal and vertical position within the bones. One of the reference planes for the dental measurements is the occlusal plane, which on average has a downward inclination anteriorly of approximately 12° related to the true horizontal or constructed FH plane.

Different types of occlusal planes have been described. Downs originally described the occlusal plane as a constructed line that bisects the upper and lower molars and the anterior teeth.[105] This plane does not take into consideration the axial inclinations of the posterior teeth. The inherent problem with this plane can be seen in patients who have no incisor overlap, such as is the case in anterior open bite patients.

A better method to define this plane is the anatomic or functional occlusal plane. This occlusal plane follows the occlusal contacts of the posterior teeth and is extended anteriorly. It can be determined easily as the longitudinal axis of the posterior teeth is almost perpendicular to this occlusal plane.

In the analysis of the dentition the inclination of the upper incisors is evaluated in relation to the maxillary palatal plane and the true horizontal plane (Fig. 3-47). In the lower arch, the ideal relationship of the incisors to the mandibular plane has been considered to be an angle close to 90° (Fig. 3-47). The interincisal angle should confirm the findings of the upper and lower incisor inclination to the palatal and mandibular plane respectively (Fig. 3-47).

Vertically, a measurement from ANS to 1 (ANS–upper incisor tip) determines the amount of eruption of the upper incisor. In the lower arch, the vertical height of the lower incisor is assessed by the measurement of Me to 1̄ (menton–lower incisor tip, Fig. 3-47).

Soft Tissue

Some of the reference lines used for cephalometric soft tissue analysis were introduced above in the description of the clinical examination. It is important to stress that

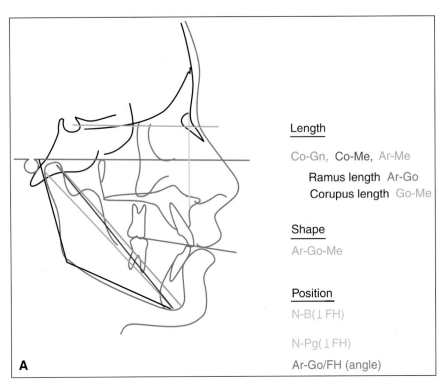

Length

Co-Gn, Co-Me, Ar-Me

Ramus length Ar-Go
Corupus length Go-Me

Shape

Ar-Go-Me

Position

N-B(⊥ FH)

N-Pg(⊥ FH)

Ar-Go/FH (angle)

A

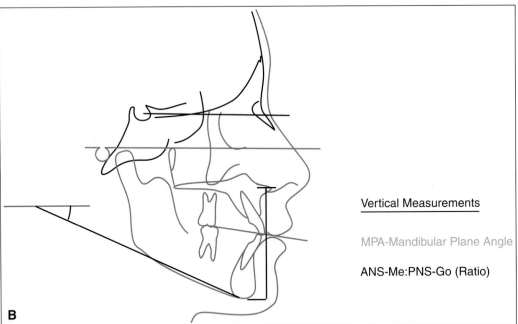

Vertical Measurements

MPA-Mandibular Plane Angle

ANS-Me:PNS-Go (Ratio)

B

Fig. 3-45 Commonly used measurements to evaluate size, shape and position of the mandible (third component). **A** Anteroposterior and **B** vertical images.

these lines are only guidelines based on averages and that esthetics is highly subjective and sometimes dependent on intangible aspects.

The soft tissue analysis should start by determining the general convexity of the profile (G–Sn–Pg, Fig. 3-48A). Thereafter, the anteroposterior position of the maxilla and the mandible can be analyzed separately by drawing a line perpendicular to the horizontal reference line passing either through the glabella, soft tissue nasion, subnasale, or any other anterior soft tissue landmark (depending on the analysis), and measuring the distance to the maxilla and the mandible (Fig. 3-48A). On average the mandible lies within this line (when a true vertical is drawn through the glabella) and the maxilla is 2–3 mm in front. It is important

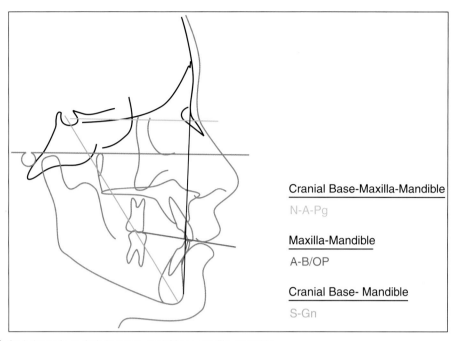

Fig. 3-46 Cephalometric analysis between cranial base–maxilla–mandible.

Cranial Base-Maxilla-Mandible
N-A-Pg

Maxilla-Mandible
A-B/OP

Cranial Base- Mandible
S-Gn

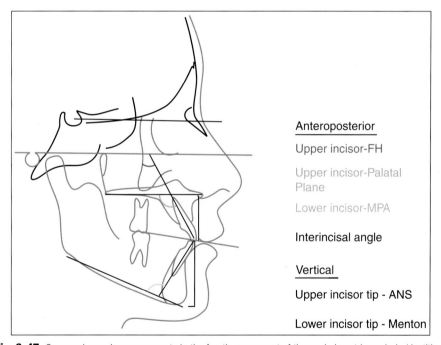

Fig. 3-47 Commonly used measurements in the fourth component of the cephalometric analysis (dentition).

Anteroposterior
Upper incisor-FH

Upper incisor-Palatal Plane

Lower incisor-MPA

Interincisal angle

Vertical
Upper incisor tip - ANS

Lower incisor tip - Menton

to determine the upper lip, lower lip, and soft tissue chin thickness since these elements might be compensating for a skeletal disharmony.

The next step in the soft tissue analysis is the evaluation of the lips. In general, measurements of the lip protrusion are made using Sn–Pg as the reference line (Fig. 3-48A). Other angles used to evaluate lip protrusion are the nasolabial angle for the upper lip, and the mentolabial angle for the lower lip (Fig. 3-48A). To eliminate the influence of the nose when measuring upper lip inclination, an angle is measured between the true horizontal and a line traced from Sn to the labrale superioris (Fig. 3-48B). A similar measurement to evaluate lower lip inclination has been used by connecting a line from the depth of the mentolabial sulcus to the labrale inferioris and measuring the angle to FH (Fig 3-48B).

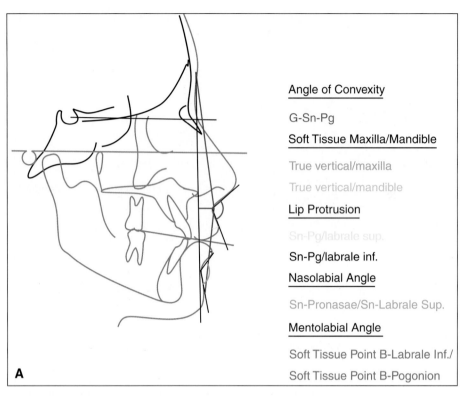

Angle of Convexity

G-Sn-Pg

Soft Tissue Maxilla/Mandible

True vertical/maxilla

True vertical/mandible

Lip Protrusion

Sn-Pg/labrale sup.

Sn-Pg/labrale inf.

Nasolabial Angle

Sn-Pronasae/Sn-Labrale Sup.

Mentolabial Angle

Soft Tissue Point B-Labrale Inf./
Soft Tissue Point B-Pogonion

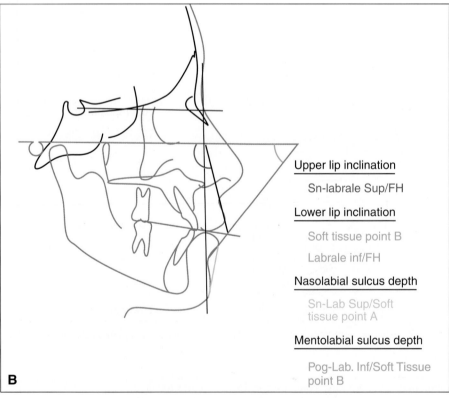

Upper lip inclination

Sn-labrale Sup/FH

Lower lip inclination

Soft tissue point B

Labrale inf/FH

Nasolabial sulcus depth

Sn-Lab Sup/Soft
tissue point A

Mentolabial sulcus depth

Pog-Lab. Inf/Soft Tissue
point B

Fig. 3-48 A and **B** Soft tissue analysis (fifth component).

To complement the lip analysis, the curl of both lips is evaluated. This is an important esthetic feature. The depth of the upper lip and the mentolabial sulcus is measured by drawing a line from the upper lip to Sn and the lower lip to Pg, respectively (Fig. 3-48B). Excessive depth in these measurements may indicate lip redundancy. Finally, a measurement of the chin to throat depth is important, especially in prospective surgery patients.

In general, when soft tissues are discussed, the tongue, soft tissue palate, and airway structures are rarely mentioned. It is important to evaluate the airway patency as well as the position of the hyoid bone. It has been reported that patients with obstructive sleep apnea have a low position of the hyoid bone.[111]

All the cephalometric measurements and their deviations from the norms are only guides to describe the problems. An explanation for each deviation from the norm is examined in conjunction with the other measurements to obtain a cephalometric summary. Attention should be paid to contradictory measurements and an explanation for these should be sought. Cephalometric analysis is a tool, and as such it is only one of the components in the database that needs to be complemented with the clinical examination, models, and other imaging.

Occlusal Radiograph

The occlusal radiograph has been used to locate supernumerary or impacted teeth. In conjunction with a panoramic radiograph, the occlusal X-ray has been reported to give a good indication of the location of the impacted/supernumerary tooth.[103] This radiograph is also indicated to evaluate the amount of suture distraction with rapid palatal expansion (Fig. 3-49).

Posteroanterio-Cephalometric Radiograph

The posteroanterio-cephalometric radiograph (posteroanterior cephalogram) is indicated in patients in whom a significant clinical asymmetry is noticed (Fig. 3-50). It

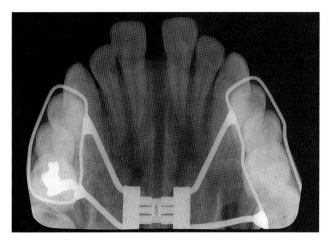

Fig. 3-49 Occlusal radiograph depicting an open palatal suture.

can be used for both skeletal and dental base asymmetry detection. Mandibular ramus heights as well as corpus lengths can be evaluated. A large discrepancy between the lower borders of the mandible observed in a lateral cephalometric radiograph is highly indicative of a skeletal asymmetry that can be better evaluated with a posteroanterior cephalogram.

This radiograph is also a good tool for evaluation of dental midline discrepancies. A method to obtain a differential diagnosis between an apical base midline problem and a dental midline problem has been described elsewhere.[112] In the transverse dimension, width measurements in the craniofacial region can be compared to recently published normative data obtained from a growth study.[113]

Submento-Vertical Radiograph

This is an excellent radiograph for evaluating mandibular asymmetry. An analysis of this radiographic image was developed for the evaluation of condylar position, as well as mandibular symmetry of the corpus and ramus.[114] Symmetry of the zygomaxillary complex can also be evaluated on this radiograph. The findings obtained from this X-ray can be correlated to those found on the posteroanterior cephalogram for a 3-D analysis of a skeletal asymmetry.

Other Imaging

Other imaging techniques can be used for a more detailed analysis of the TMD, including magnetic resonance imaging (MRI), especially for soft tissues, and computed tomography (CT). Although these imaging techniques show promise in orthodontics, especially in the area of 3-D analysis, most of their applications are limited by the cost/benefit ratio.

Hand–Wrist Films

This radiograph has been used to evaluate skeletal maturity. The stage of ossification of the wrist and phalanges in the hand correlates to skeletal maturity (Fig. 3-51). However, recent efforts to correlate skeletal maturation to the cervical vertebrae have diminished the need for a hand–wrist radiograph. It has been shown from a lateral cephalometric film that the peak of pubertal growth can be adequately estimated.[115] This new method eliminates the need for an additional radiograph since the lateral cephalometric radiograph is taken for almost every prospective orthodontic patient.

Diagnostic Models

One of the major advantages of models is the ability to inspect the malocclusion from the lingual side. Models also provide a more accurate and accessible way to evaluate arch shape, occlusion, and the 3-D position of each tooth in space (first, second, and third order) and how it relates to the other teeth. Also, arch symmetry can be analyzed from the deviation of the teeth from the midsagittal suture.

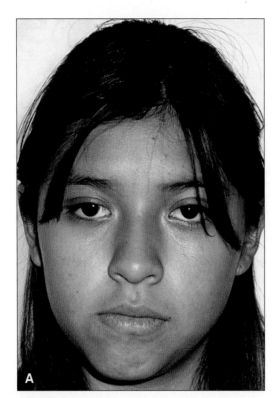 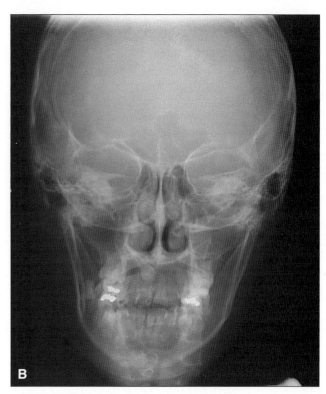

Fig. 3-50 **A** Significant mandibular asymmetry evidenced in the clinical examination and **B** on the posteroanterior cephalic radiograph.

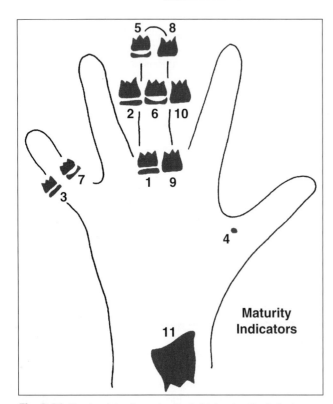

Fig. 3-51 Hand–wrist radiograph with skeletal maturation indicators. (Redrawn from Fishman LS. Radiographic evaluation of skeletal maturation. Angle Orthod 1982;52:88–112.)

Models can be used also for space analysis in the mixed dentition and as a template from which an occlusogram can be constructed. Recently, with the digital era and with the problem of storage space, new technologies have developed a digital model. Two methods are used to obtain a digital model from an alginate impression: one preserves the model and uses laser technology to recreate the complex topography of the poured model and transfer it to digital data. The second method destroys the model as it uses scanning technology to obtain the digital 3-D information. Once the model is digitalized there is also the possibility of creating a real model from the virtual one. The software allows a number of tests to be run, such as Bolton discrepancies, space analysis, and occlusograms.[116]

Summary

A synopsis of the most important components needed for the orthodontic diagnosis has been given. A detailed analysis of the clinical examination, radiographs, patient records, and additional imaging has been described. The basis for a good treatment outcome is heavily dependent on good data collection and analysis of the database. Ultimately, the diagnosis should answer the question why, so that later where are we going (objectives), how are we going to get there (treatment plan), and what is going to be used (mechanics plan), can be determined.

REFERENCES

1. Dorland's Illustrated Medical Dictionary, 30th edn. Philadelphia: WB Saunders, 2003.
2. Tobiasen JM. Social judgments of facial deformity. Cleft Palate J 1987;24:323–327.
3. Ash M, Ramfjord SR. Occlusion, 4th edn. Philadelphia: WB Saunders, 1995:472.
4. Barrows HS. Practice-based learning. Springfield, IL: Southern Illinois University School of Medicine, 1994:145.
5. Burden D, Mullally B, Sandler J. Orthodontic treatment of patients with medical disorders. Eur J Orthod 2001;23:363–372.
6. Epstein JB. Infective endocarditis: dental implications and new guidelines for antibiotic prophylaxis. American Heart Association. J Can Dent Assoc 1998;64:281–286, 289–292.
7. Devlin H, Garland H, Sloan P. Healing of tooth extraction sockets in experimental diabetes mellitus. J Oral Maxillofac Surg 1996;54:1087–1091.
8. McNab S, Battistulla D, Taverne A, Symons AL. External apical root resorption of posterior teeth in asthmatics after orthodontic treatment. Am J Orthod Dentofacial Orthop 1999;116:545–551.
9. Meraw SJ, Sheridan PJ. Medically induced gingival hyperplasia. Mayo Clin Proc 1998;73:1196–1199.
10. Janson GR, Dainsi EA, Consolaro A, Woodside DG, de Freitas MR. Nickel hypersensitivity reaction before, during, and after orthodontic therapy. Am J Orthod Dentofacial Orthop 1998;113:655–660.
11. Grimaudo NJ. Biocompatibility of nickel and cobalt dental alloys. Gen Dent 2001;49:498–503; quiz 504–505.
12. Smith RM, Gonzalez C. The relationship between nasal obstruction and craniofacial growth. Pediatr Clin North Am 1989;36:1423–1434.
13. Bergstrom J, Preber H. Tobacco use as a risk factor. J Periodontol 1994;65 (Suppl):545–550.
14. Scabbia A, Cho KS, Sigurdsson TJ, Kim CK, Trombelli L. Cigarette smoking negatively affects healing response following flap debridement surgery. J Periodontol 2001;72:43–49.
15. Franchi L, Baccetti T, McNamara JA Jr. Mandibular growth as related to cervical vertebral maturation and body height. Am J Orthod Dentofacial Orthop 2000;118: 335–340.
16. Oudet C, Petrovic A, Stutzmann J. Time-dependent effects of a 'functional'-type orthopedic appliance on the rat mandible growth. Chronobiol Int 1984;1:51–57.
17. Chen JY, Will LA, Niederman R. Analysis of efficacy of functional appliances on mandibular growth. Am J Orthod Dentofacial Orthop 2002;122:470–476.
18. Woodside DG. Do functional appliances have an orthopedic effect? Am J Orthod Dentofacial Orthop 1998;113:11–14.
19. Baccetti T, Franchi L, Toth LR, McNamara JA Jr. Treatment timing for twin-block therapy. Am J Orthod Dentofacial Orthop 2000;118:159–170.
20. Voudouris JC, Woodside DG, Altuna G, et al. Condyle-fossa modifications and muscle interactions during Herbst treatment, part 1. New technological methods. Am J Orthod Dentofacial Orthop 2003;123:604–613.
21. Fishman LS. Radiographic evaluation of skeletal maturation. A clinically oriented method based on hand–wrist films. Angle Orthod 1982;52:88–112.
22. Hagg U, Taranger J. Menarche and voice change as indicators of the pubertal growth spurt. Acta Odontol Scand 1980;38:179–186.
23. Hagg U, Taranger J. Skeletal stages of the hand and wrist as indicators of the pubertal growth spurt. Acta Odontol Scand 1980;38:187–200.
24. Silveira AM, Fishman LS, Subtelny JD, et al. Facial growth during adolescence in early, average and late maturers. Angle Orthod 1992;62:185–190.
25. Saunders SR, Popovich F, Thompson GW. A family study of craniofacial dimensions in the Burlington Growth Centre sample. Am J Orthod 1980;78:394–403.
26. Suzuki A, Takahama Y. Parental data used to predict growth of craniofacial form. Am J Orthod Dentofacial Orthop 1991;99:107–121.
27. Bishara SE. Facial and dental changes in adolescents and their clinical implications. Angle Orthod 2000;70:471–483.
28. Nanda RS. The rate of growth of different facial components. Am J Orthod 1955;41:658–673.
29. Skieller V, Bjork A, Linde-Hansen T. Prediction of mandibular growth rotation evaluated from a longitudinal implant sample. Am J Orthod 1984;86:359–370.
30. Leslie LR, Southard TE, Southard KA et al. Prediction of mandibular growth rotation: assessment of the Skieller, Bjork, and Linde-Hansen method. Am J Orthod Dentofacial Orthop 1998;114:659–667.
31. Kokich VG. Managing complex orthodontic problems: the use of implants for anchorage. Semin Orthod 1996;2:153–160.
32. Peck S, Peck L, Kataja M. Concomitant occurrence of canine malposition and tooth agenesis: evidence of orofacial genetic fields. Am J Orthod Dentofacial Orthop 2002;122:657–660.
33. Baccetti T. A controlled study of associated dental anomalies. Angle Orthod 1998;68:267–274.
34. Katz JL. The structure and biomechanics of bone. Symp Soc Exp Biol 1980;34:137–168.
35. Kiliaridis S. Masticatory muscle influence on craniofacial growth. Acta Odontol Scand 1995;53:196–202.
36. Proffit WR. Equilibrium theory revisited: factors influencing position of the teeth. Angle Orthod 1978;48:175–186.
37. Weinstein S, et al. On an equilibrium theory of tooth position. Angle Orthod 1963;33:1–26.
38. Mah J, Bumann A. Technology to create the three-dimensional patient record. Semin Orthod 2001;7:251–257.
39. Thornhill R, Gangestad SW. Facial attractiveness. Trends Cogn Sci 1999;3:452–460.
40. Scheib JE, Gangestad SW, Thornhill R. Facial attractiveness, symmetry and cues of good genes. Proc R Soc Lond B Biol Sci 1999;266:1913–1917.
41. Arnett GW, Bergman RT. Facial keys to orthodontic diagnosis and treatment planning. Part I. Am J Orthod Dentofacial Orthop 1993;103:299–312.
42. Vig RG, Brundo GC. The kinetics of anterior tooth display. J Prosthet Dent 1978; 39:502–504.
43. Frush JO, Fisher RD. The dysesthetic interpretation in the dentogenic concept. J Prosthetic Dent 1958;8:55–58.
44. Dunn WJ, Murchison DF, Broome JC. Esthetics: patients' perceptions of dental attractiveness. J Prosthodont 1996;5:166–171.

45. Fuhrmann RAW. Three-dimensional evaluation of periodontal remodeling during orthodontic treatment. Semin Orthod 2002;8:23–28.

46. Schiffman PH, Tuncay OC. Maxillary expansion: a meta analysis. Clin Orthod Res 2001;4:86–96.

47. Sarver DM, Ackerman JL. Evaluation of facial soft tissues. In: Proffit WR, ed. Contemporary treatment of facial deformity. St Louis: Mosby, 2003:92–126.

48. Burstone C. 2003. Personal communication.

49. Benson KJ, Laskin DM. Upper lip asymmetry in adults during smiling. J Oral Maxillofac Surg 2001;59:396–398.

50. Cardash HS, Ormanier Z, Laufer BZ. Observable deviation of the facial and anterior tooth midlines. J Prosthet Dent 2003;89:282–285.

51. Beyer JW, Lindauer SJ. Evaluation of dental midline position. Semin Orthod 1998;4:146–152.

52. Kokich VO Jr, Kiyak HA, Shapiro PA. Comparing the perception of dentists and lay people to altered dental esthetics. J Esthet Dent 1999;11:311–324.

53. Caudill R, Chiche GJ. Establishing an esthetic gingival appearance. In: Chiche G, ed. Esthetics of anterior fixed prosthodontics. Chicago: Quintessence Publishing Co, 1994:177–198.

54. Chiche G, Pinault A. Replacement of deficient crowns. In: Chiche G, ed. Esthetics of anterior fixed prosthodontics. Chicago: Quintessence Publishing Co, 1994:53–73.

55. Petrovic A, Stutzmann J. (Growth hormone: mode of action on different varieties of cartilage [author's transl]). Pathol Biol (Paris) 1980;28:43–58.

56. Nanda RS, Meng H, Kapila S, Goorhuis J. Growth changes in the soft tissue facial profile. Angle Orthod 1990;60:177–190.

57. McNamara JA Jr. Components of class II malocclusion in children 8–10 years of age. Angle Orthod 1981;51:177–202.

58. Guyer EC, Ellis EE 3rd, McNamara JA Jr, Behrents RG. Components of class III malocclusion in juveniles and adolescents. Angle Orthod 1986;56:7–30.

59. Lai J, Ghosh J, Nanda R. Effects of orthodontic therapy on the facial profile in long and short vertical facial patterns. Am J Orthod Dentofacial Orthoped 2000;118:505–513.

60. Kocadereli I. Changes in soft tissue profile after orthodontic treatment with and without extractions. Am J Orthodont Dentofacial Orthoped 2002;122:67–72.

61. Rains M, Nanda R. Soft-tissue changes associated with maxillary incisor retraction. Am J Orthod 1982;81:481–488.

62. Thuer U, Ingervall B. Pressure from the lips on the teeth and malocclusion. Am J Orthod Dentofacial Orthop 1986;90:234–242.

63. Lapatki BG, Mager AS, Schulter-Moenting J, James IE. The importance of the level of the lip line and resting lip pressure in Class II, division 2 malocclusion. J Dent Res 2002;81:323–328.

64. Burstone C. Arch form and dimension: anteroposterior positioning of the incisors. In: Burstone C, ed. Problem solving in orthodontics: goal-oriented treatment strategies. Chicago: Quintessence Publishing Co, 2000: 87–144.

65. Lew KK, Ho KK, Kong SB, Ho KH. Soft-tissue cephalometric norms in Chinese adults with esthetic facial profiles. J Oral Maxillofac Surg 1992;50:1184–1189; discussion 1189–1190.

66. Flynn TR, Ambrogio RI, Zeichner SJ. Cephalometric norms for orthognathic surgery in black American adults. J Oral Maxillofac Surg 1989;47:30–39.

67. Rhine JS, Campbell HR. Thickness of facial tissues in American blacks. J Forensic Sci 1980;25:847–858.

68. Oliver BM. The influence of lip thickness and strain on upper lip response to incisor retraction. Am J Orthod 1982;82:141–149.

69. Ricketts R. Planning treatment on the basis of the facial pattern and an estimate of its growth. Angle Orthod 1957;27:14–37.

70. Burstone C. The integumental profile. Am J Orthod 1958;44:1–25.

71. Burstone CJ. Lip posture and its significance in treatment planning. Am J Orthod 1967;53:262–284.

72. Merrifield L. The profile line as an aid in critically evaluating facial esthetics. Am J Orthod 1966;52:804–822.

73. Steiner C. The use of cephalometrics as an aid to planning and assessing orthodontic treatment. Am J Orthod 1960;46:721–735.

74. Holdaway R. A soft tissue cephalometric analysis and its use in orthodontic treatment planning. Part I. Am J Orthod 1983;84:1–28.

75. Legan H, Burstone CJ. Soft tissue cephalometric analysis for orthognathic surgery. J Oral Surg 1980;38:744–751.

76. Horn A. Facial height index. Am J Orthod 1992;102:180.

77. Sarver DM, Ackerman MB. Dynamic smile visualization and quantification: part 1. Evolution of the concept and dynamic records for smile capture. Am J Orthod Dentofacial Orthop 2003;124:4–12.

78. Edwards J. The diastema, the frenum, the frenectomy: a clinical study. Am J Orthod 1977;71:489–508.

79. Kopczyk R, Saxe SR. Clinical signs of gingival inadequacy: the tension test. J Dent Child 1974;41:352–355.

80. Fletcher SG, Meldrum JR. Lingual function and relative length of the lingual frenulum. J Speech Hearing Res 1968;11:382–390.

81. Andreasen J, Andreasen FM. Textbook and color atlas of traumatic injuries to the teeth. Copenhagen: Munksgaard, 1994.

82. Hamilton RS, Gutmann JL. Endodontic–orthodontic relationships: a review of integrated treatment planning challenges. Int Endodont J 1999;32:343–360.

83. Kokich VG, Spear FM. Guidelines for managing the orthodontic-restorative patient. Semin Orthod 1997;3:3–20.

84. Tarnow DP, Magner AW, Fletcher P. The effect of the distance from the contact point to the crest of bone on the presence or absence of the interproximal dental papilla. J Periodontol 1992;63:995–996.

85. Andrews L. Straight wire: the concept and appliance. San Diego: K-W Publications, 1989.

86. Dale J, Dale HC. Interceptive guidance of occlusion with emphasis on diagnosis. In: Graber T, ed. Orthodontics: Current principles and techniques. St Louis: Mosby, 2000:375–469.

87. Clark JR, Evans RD. Functional occlusion: I. A review. J Orthod 2001;28:76–81.

88. Ash M, Ramfjord SP. Occlusion. Philadelphia: WB Saunders, 1994.

89. Laskin DM. The clinical diagnosis of temporomandibular

disorders in the orthodontic patient. Semin Orthod 1995;1:197–206.

90. Greene C, Lerman MD, et al. The TMJ pain-dysfunction syndrome: Heterogenicity of the patient population. J Am Dent Asocc 1969;79:1168–1172.

91. Cox S, Walker DM. Establishing a normal range for mouth opening: its use for oral submucous fibrosis. Br J Oral Maxillofac Surg 1997;35:40–42.

92. Helkimo M. Studies on function and dysfunction of the masticatory system. II. Index for anamnestic and clinical dysfunction and occlusal state. Swedish Dent J 1974;67:101–121.

93. Fricton JR. Management of masticatory myofascial pain. Semin Orthod 1995;1:229–243.

94. Roth RH. Occlusion and condylar position. Am J Orthod Dentofacial Orthop 1995;107:315–318.

95. Rinchuse DJ. A three-dimensional comparison of condylar change between centric relation and centric occlusion using the mandibular position indicator. Am J Orthod Dentofacial Orthop 1995;107:319–328.

96. Hew SK. Comment on the Roth/Rinchuse responses. Am J Orthod Dentofacial Orthop 1996;109:15A–16A.

97. Chhatwani B. More comments on Rinchuse Counterpoint. Am J Orthod Dentofacial Orthop 1995;108:13A.

98. McNamara JA Jr, Seligman DA, Okeson JP. Occlusion, orthodontic treatment, and temporomandibular disorders: a review. J Orofac Pain 1995;9:73–90.

99. Clark JR, Hutchinson I, Sandy JR. Functional occlusion: II. The role of articulators in orthodontics. J Orthod 2001;28:173–177.

100. Kuhlberg AJ, Norton LA. Pathologic findings in orthodontic radiographic images. Am J Orthod Dentofacial Orthop 2003;123:182–184.

101. Kuhlberg A, Norton LA. Finding pathology on cephalometric radiographs. In: Athanasiou AE, ed. Orthodontic cephalometry. London: Mosby-Wolfe, 1995:175–180.

102. Obwegeser HL, Makek MS. Hemimandibular hyperplasia—hemimandibular elongation. J Maxillofac Surg 1986;14:183–208.

103. Jacobs SG. Radiographic localization of unerupted teeth: further findings about the vertical tube shift method and other localization techniques. Am J Orthod Dentofacial Orthop 2000;118:439–447.

104. Tyndall D, Brooks S. Selection criteria for dental implant site imaging: A position paper of the American Academy of Oral and Maxillofacial Radiology. Oral Surg Oral Med Oral Pathol Oral Radiol Endodont 2000;89:630–637.

105. Downs W. Variations in facial relationships: their significance in treatment and prognosis. Am J Orthod 1948;34:812.

106. Burstone CJ, James RB, Logan H, Murphy GA, Norton LA. Cephalometrics for orthognathic surgery. J Oral Surg 1978;36:269–277.

107. Moorrees C. Natural head position: The key to dephalometry. In: Jacobsen A, ed. Radiographic cephalometry. Chicago: Quintessence Publishing Co, 1995:175–184.

108. Bjork A. Cranial base development. Am J Orthod 1955;41:198–225.

109. Dhopatkar A, Bhatia S, Rock P. An investigation into the relationship between the cranial base angle and malocclusion. Angle Orthod 2002;72:456–463.

110. Cangialosi TJ. Skeletal morphologic features of anterior open bite. Am J Orthod 1984;85:28–36.

111. Tangugsorn V, Krogstad O, Espeland L, Lyberg T. Obstructive sleep apnea: a principal component analysis. Int J Adult Orthod Orthognath Surg 1999;14:215–228.

112. Torres M. Treatment objectives and treatment planning. Dental Clin North Am 1981;25:27–41.

113. Basyouni AA, Nanda SK. An atlas of the transverse dimensions of the face. In: McNamara JA Jr, ed. Craniofacial Growth Series, vol 37. Ann Arbor: 2001, University of Michigan Center for Human Growth and Development.

114. Forsberg CT, Burstone CJ, Hanley KJ. Diagnosis and treatment planning of skeletal asymmetry with the submental-vertical radiograph. Am J Orthod 1984;85:224–237.

115. Baccetti T, Franchi L, McNamara JA Jr. An improved version of the cervical vertebral maturation (CVM) method for the assessment of mandibular growth. Angle Orthod 2002;72:316–323.

116. Tomassetti JJ, Taloumis LJ, Denny JM, Fischer JR Jr. A comparison of 3 computerized Bolton tooth-size analyses with a commonly used method. Angle Orthod 2001;71:351–357.

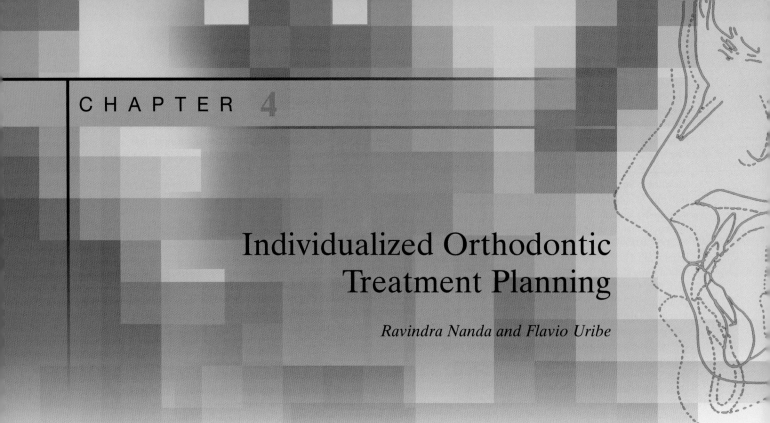

CHAPTER 4

Individualized Orthodontic Treatment Planning

Ravindra Nanda and Flavio Uribe

A well executed, individualized treatment plan is one of the most important aspects of orthodontic treatment. Treatment planning starts with optimal diagnosis and sequential categorization of the identified problems in order of importance. From the problem list, specific treatment objectives are set. Greater priority is given to problems that appear more severe, or for which the timing of orthodontic intervention is an issue. Also, a patient's chief complaint should be given high priority.

The treatment planning sequence should closely follow diagnostic findings (see Ch. 3) in the anteroposterior, transverse, and vertical dimensions. Although all these dimensions have direct and indirect relationships to each other, each is analyzed separately in the problem list. In addition to problems in these three dimensions, any remarkable dental and medical findings, and alignment issues are also listed.

The most common remarkable medical and dental findings to be considered during orthodontic treatment are discussed in Chapter 3. In summary, any important systemic disease or medical condition that may have an impact on the treatment plan should be included in the problem list. Not only may these conditions affect the course of orthodontic treatment, but orthodontic treatment may have an adverse effect on any existing medical and dental problems. Furthermore, the effect of some medications on orthodontic treatment should also be explored.[1,2]

Significant dental problems may have a direct impact on treatment planning. An example can be seen in a patient with extensive decay in the first molars. A decision between extracting and restoring these teeth has to be made not only from a purely orthodontic perspective, but also in conjunction with other factors such as cost–benefit and longterm prognosis.

Treatment Objectives

The cornerstone of treatment planning is the treatment objectives. These can easily be visualized in the three dimensions by means of a visualized treatment objective (VTO) and an occlusogram.[3] It is important to note that there are general and specific treatment objectives, which are related, but distinct as far as determination of treatment goals is concerned. General treatment objectives are those that can be applied to any orthodontic patient regardless of his/her malocclusion. These objectives include most of the characteristics of an ideal occlusion, such as: Class I occlusion (canine), normal overjet and overbite, coincident midlines, slight curve of Spee, arch width coordination, and absence of crowding, spacing, rotations and marginal ridge discrepancies.[4] These objectives do not provide the clinician with any information on how specifically they are to be achieved. For example, an ideal overjet can be obtained in a Class II patient by retracting the upper incisors, flaring the lower incisors, or a combination of the two. Moreover, the nature of the incisor movement can be translation, controlled tipping, or uncontrolled tipping. If the specific objectives are not known then any appliance (Herbst, headgear, pendex, twin force bite corrector, elastics, bionator) or any therapy (extraction, nonextraction, surgery, implants) for Class II correction can be used since the general objective is overjet reduction. A very wise phrase applies here: "If you don't know where you are going, it doesn't matter which road you take."[5]

To provide an individualized treatment plan, specific treatment objectives must be determined.[6] It is worth emphasizing that general treatment objectives allow the orthodontist to communicate with the patient and/or his/her guardian, while specific objectives act as a template (blueprint) for the desired treatment outcome.

Specific Treatment Objectives

Seven specific treatment objectives will guide the clinician to achieve the desired outcome in the three planes of space: skeletofacial, soft tissue, occlusal plane, arch width, midlines, anteroposterior position of the incisors and molars, and vertical position of the incisors and molars.[4]

Skeletofacial Objectives

This objective relies on understanding the growth status of the patient and often on the ability to predict the amount, direction, and rate of remaining growth. Due to the great variability in growth, it is difficult to define specific skeletofacial objectives. Perhaps this inability to accurately predict growth is the reason why many clinicians do not believe specific objectives can be set in treatment planning for growing patients. This is not an issue in the adult patient for whom skeletal objectives can be defined adequately, although for them a similar problem is encountered in determining the soft tissue objectives (see below).

Even though there is great variability in predicting growth, this objective is important and can not be disregarded. A good approach is to underestimate future growth in skeletal Class II patients and overestimate growth in Class III patients. In this manner, any additional growth in the former and any normal or decrease in growth in the latter, in relation to the prediction, would be favorable. Of course this is not always easy, especially in patients with moderate-to-severe dentofacial deformities, since growth can be the deciding factor between a surgical and nonsurgical approach to treatment.

Useful growth information is best obtained with a series of lateral cephalometric radiographs taken at 6 month to 1 year intervals. These radiographs provide important information since growth patterns are usually maintained in the majority of patients.[7] Unfortunately serial cephalograms are often unavailable. Therefore, an assessment of growth potential (amount of growth left in relation to puberty) and evaluation of craniofacial morphology (Bjork indicators)[8] may aid in the prediction.

It is important to note, however, that even if growth can not be extensively modified at the level of the apical bases, significant skeletofacial changes can be achieved by affecting the dentoalveolar apparatus. This is especially evident in the vertical control of the molar, where favorable skeletofacial vertical and anteroposterior changes can be obtained with carefully selected mechanics.

Soft Tissue Objectives

Soft tissue objectives are very much related to the skeletofacial objectives. The only aspect not covered in the skeletofacial objectives is the soft tissue changes due to dentoalveolar movement. The most remarkable changes in this area relate to the lips: reduction of interlabial gap, and lip protrusion or retrusion. Direct effects on the soft tissue drape are seen with dentoalveolar movement in the vertical dimension at the molar level, and in the anteroposterior dimension at the incisor level.

Anteroposterior incisor movement can result in changes at the lip level, at least to some degree.[9-11] Accurate prediction of soft tissue response to incisor movement is difficult. Therefore, the objectives should be set in terms of direction (more predictable) rather than the magnitude of change.

Occlusal Plane Objectives

Occlusal plane objectives are often overlooked in treatment planning. Occlusal plane goals should be considered from a frontal and lateral perspective and in conjunction with skeletal and soft tissue objectives.[12] In the lateral view, anterior and posterior occlusal planes should be coincident. For example, in openbite and deep overbite patients, the anterior and posterior occlusal planes are often at different levels. When determining specific objectives for a patient, it is a good idea to predetermine the level of the occlusal plane in order to apply proper mechanics during treatment. In deep overbite patients it may be desirable to intrude anterior teeth to the level of the posterior teeth or vice versa. A straight wire ligated into all the brackets has no ability to selectively intrude or extrude teeth. These mechanics are not optimal; the wire ends up controlling the occlusal plane objectives rather than the clinician. Similarly in open bite patients, placement of a straight wire can have very undesirable results. The best option in this situation may be to treat the posterior and anterior segments separately.

Specific occlusal plane objectives in the frontal view should also be determined carefully. Often a cant in the anterior occlusal plane is associated with a midline deviation. This can be effectively treated by selective ligation of an intrusion arch or use of a cantilever to rotate the anterior teeth as a whole.[13]

Treatment objectives should outline not only the level of the occlusal plane, but also the cant. Level is an almost parallel vertical movement, whereas cant refers to angular movement of the occlusal plane. A level change can be achieved, for example, by using an anterior bite plane which allows eruption of posterior teeth. In addition, the application of box elastics to the posterior teeth aids in the occlusal plane leveling of the buccal segments by extrusion.[14] Indiscriminate use of Class II elastics for a prolonged period of time will invariably cant (steepen) the occlusal plane, whether or not this is a desired part of the treatment plan.

Arch Width Objectives

Arch width objectives relate mainly to the intercanine and intermolar width. The lower intercanine width has been considered to be almost unalterable as changes in this distance yield unstable results.[15] Any significant increase in lower intercanine width should be followed by a longterm fixed retention.[16] More leeway has been given to the alteration of the upper canine and molar width. Increasing the arch width depends largely on the occlusal and esthetic objectives.

For occlusal correction, a definite indication for expanding the upper arch width is the presence of a skeletal crossbite. With regard to esthetics, the objective of filling the buccal corridors is the justification given by some clinicians for a nonextraction expansion treatment plan.

Midline Objectives

The midline is an important occlusal and esthetic objective. This topic is discussed extensively in numerous chapters in this book. Needless to say, the facial and dental midlines should coincide. The planning of this objective becomes more elaborate when a surgical correction due to apical base midline problems is considered. In these patients the desired dental movement has to be determined in conjunction with the apical base movement.[17]

Anteroposterior Objectives

Incisor Objectives. The incisor anteroposterior objectives should be planned with consideration given to the skeletofacial and soft tissue (lips) objectives.[18] The final anteroposterior position is decided after taking into consideration the nasolabial angle, facial convexity, size of nose, and ethnicity.[19] Anteroposterior objectives that can not be obtained skeletally are obtained through dental compensations (camouflage). Usually the anteroposterior incisor objective is described in terms of the incisal edge (flare, maintain, or retract). The nature of the tooth movement should be described further (controlled tipping, uncontrolled tipping, or translation). If the incisor edge is to be maintained, root correction (controlled root movement) is the other type of incisor movement in this plane.

The anteroposterior movement of the incisor depends largely on occlusion and esthetics. Arch crowding, protrusion, overbite, and overjet are some of the occlusal factors to consider. Esthetic considerations relate to lip changes (which greatly vary in magnitude) and third-order inclination of the upper incisors.[20] The final position of the upper incisors, due to their esthetic importance, must be decided during treatment planning.[21] This is especially the case in surgical patients, where the incisor is positioned ideally in space and the orthodontic and surgical movements are planned from it. In adolescent patients, the final upper incisor position also needs to be considered relative to the desired lower incisor position, the overjet, and the potential differential jaw growth.

Proper lower incisor inclination has been considered essential and tied to a cephalometric norm (90°) by various techniques. Labial movement beyond this norm in patients with an ideal mandibular plane to the Frankfort horizontal plane (25°) has been related to instability and gingival recession. Although some evidence does not completely support the predisposition of recession after labial flaring,[22] this movement has traditionally been considered undesirable.

Molar Objectives

The anteroposterior position of the molar greatly depends on the final position of the incisors. Once the incisor anteroposterior position is established, the molars will either need to be protracted, maintained, or distalized, depending on the arch width and amount of crowding present. Incorporating growth into the planning of the anteroposterior molar position becomes somewhat challenging if growth modification is planned.

Vertical Incisor and Molar Objectives

As mentioned above, the final vertical position of the upper and lower incisors is influenced by the occlusion (overbite) and esthetics (incisor display). The incisor vertical position, together with the anteroposterior position, are good starting reference points for treatment planning. The vertical position of the incisors can be easily defined by boundaries determined by the incisor display and overbite. Chapter 15 discusses the different considerations for final vertical incisor position when significant dental attrition is present in adults.

The influence of the molar vertical position on the skeletofacial objective makes this tooth a key factor in the vertical and anteroposterior dimensions. The molars can be held against growth (relative intrusion) or absolutely intruded with the use of implants. They can also be extruded for overbite correction, although the longterm stability of this type of extrusion in adults is questionable.[23] Furthermore, extrusion of molars should be carefully considered due to the resultant clockwise rotation of the mandible, which may negate any positive changes occurring during adolescent mandibular growth.

Dynamics of Treatment Planning

It must be emphasized that treatment plans and specific objectives are not static.[3] Due to the difficulty in accurate prediction of remaining growth, an undesirable outcome may be encountered during orthodontic treatment. Moreover, the biologic response to the mechanic stimulus may also be unfavorable. It should be determined whether the undesirable outcome resulted from poor mechanics and/or unfavorable growth. Ultimately, the treatment objectives should be adjusted after a reanalysis of the new clinical situation.

Occlusogram and Visualized Treatment Objective

Two powerful tools for visualizing the treatment plan are the occlusogram and the VTO.[3] With the advent of computers, these two procedures have become less cumbersome to perform.[24] The occlusogram is a two-dimensional analysis of what would be considered a diagnostic wax setup.[25] Since it is done either on a piece of paper or a screen, it allows visualization of the original problem in comparison to the desired dental and skeletofacial corrections. Through the anteroposterior dimension, the occlusogram and VTO are related to each other, generating the three-dimensional visual goals of treatment.[26]

To obtain a consensus between the wishes of the patient and the clinician, more than one treatment plan is often developed. Different treatment plans give the patient options that may be helpful when difficult choices have to be made due to issues with finance, compliance, or other personal circumstances. Therefore, in instances where treatment plans are developed, the pros and cons of each option should be evaluated. An evaluation of the different options will help the clinician successfully present the treatment plan to the patient as well as to obtain informed consent.

Once the treatment plan has been defined with specific goals, the appliance or group of appliances needed to achieve these goals are selected. Although the mechanics plan is done after the treatment objectives have been set, many seasoned clinicians tend to be biased by their own experience as to what can be achieved with the tools (appliances) they traditionally use. It is important to understand the biomechanics and potential side effects of all the appliances chosen for treatment in order to achieve the desired treatment goals. A solid understanding of the effects of each appliance, when applied to specific populations, is essential as well. Knowledge of scientific controlled trials that look at various orthodontic appliances in different populations will help achieve this goal.[27] Overall, it is important to remember that evidence-based orthodontics in conjunction with sound biomechanic knowledge allows the clinician to develop individualized mechanics with predictable results.

Case Reports

Three patients are presented from a diagnosis and treatment plan perspective.

CASE REPORT 1

Patient Profile (Fig. 4-1)

- 16.2-year-old postpubertal, female
- Chief complaint: "Bottom teeth crowded and top front teeth stick out".

Medical History

- Noncontributory
- No allergies; no medications.

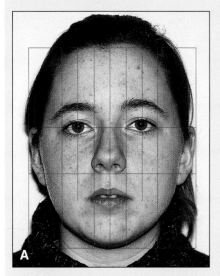 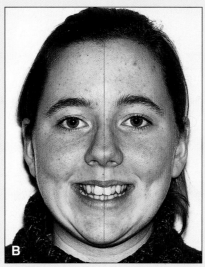 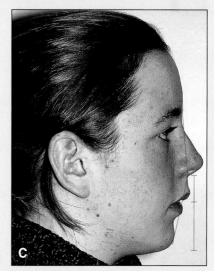

Fig. 4-1 Case 1. **A** Extraoral frontal view. Ovoid facial form; slight mentalis strain upon closure; no apparent pathology; interlabial gap 3.0 mm; incisor display at rest 6.0 mm; midline—no major asymmetries; transverse fifths—narrow intercommissural width at rest; vertical thirds—short middle facial height relative to upper and lower facial height; long upper lip and philtrum. **B** Extraoral smile. Incisor display on smile 90%; excessive mandibular incisor show; midlines: maxillary—1.0 mm right of facial, mandibular—2.0 mm left of facial, 3.0 mm midline discrepancy; narrow smile; excessive buccal space/corridor. **C** Extraoral profile. Convex soft tissue profile; protrusive upper lip; nasolabial angle is within normal limits (WNL); lower facial height: throat depth WNL; long upper lip. *Continued*

CASE REPORT 1—cont'd

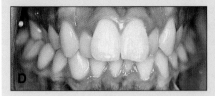 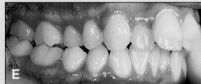 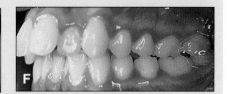

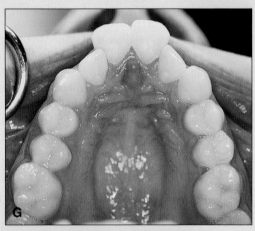 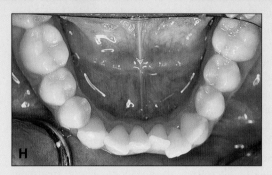

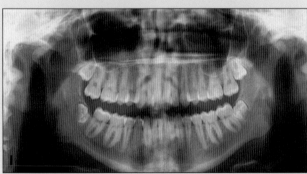

Fig. 4-1 *Cont'd.* **D** Intraoral frontal view. Bilateral maxillary (skeletal) constriction and posterior crossbite (no shift noted); maxillary midline: 1 mm right of facial; mandibular midline: 2 mm left of facial; 50% overbite; good oral hygiene; attached/keratinized tissue levels WNL. **E** Intraoral right and **F** left buccal views. Class II molar and cuspid (more severe on left); posterior crossbite bilaterally; 11 mm overjet; protrusive maxillary incisors; retroclined mandibular incisors. **G** Intraoral occlusal view. 7–7 present; V-shaped arch; mild (3 mm) crowding in anterior segment; no caries present; high palatal vault. **H** Intraoral occlusal view. 7–7 present; U-shaped arch; moderate (5 mm) crowding in anterior; no caries present. **I** Panoramic X-ray.

Dental History

- Patient has received routine dental care
- Presents in permanent dentition: 7-7/7-7 present
- No history of trauma or decay
- History of bruxing.

Psychosocial Profile

Enthusiastic about receiving orthodontic treatment.

Cephalometric Summary

Mild Class II skeletal with convex skeletal profile (Fig. 4-2, Tables 4-1–4.4) due to:
- Mildly retrognathic mandible
- Protrusive maxillary incisors and retroclined mandibular incisors
- Convex soft tissue profile
- Tipped-up palatal plane.

Overall Summary

- Convex/Class II skeletal profile
- Bilateral posterior crossbite
- Class II, Division 1 subdivision
- 11 mm overjet; 50% overbite.

Problem List

1. *Medical/dental findings of significance:*
   - Asymptomatic, bilateral click of temporo-mandibular joint (TMJ) on maximum opening (dislocation with reduction)
   - Potential impaction of mandibular 8s
   - Poor oral hygiene.

2. *Anteroposterior:*
   - Skeletal: mild Class II/convex skeletal profile due to mildly retrognathic mandible

CASE REPORT 1-cont'd

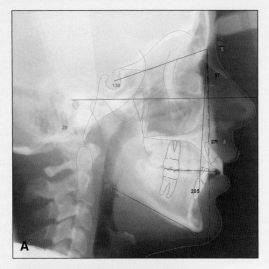

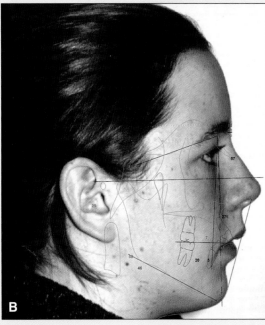

Fig. 4-2 Case 1. **A** Lateral cephalometric tracing. **B** Lateral cephalometric superimposition.

Table 4-2 Case 1: Cranial base—maxilla and mandible

Measurement	Value	Norm	SD	Dev. norm
PNS-ANS (mm)	52.9	52.6	3.5	0.1
Ar-PTM (HP) (mm)	28.8	32.8	1.9	−2.1**
y axis (mm)	127.9	131.0	6.0	−0.5
y axis (degrees)	78.4	67.0	5.5	2.1**
Ramus height (Ar–Go) (mm)	47.4	46.8	2.5	0.2
Body length (Go–Pg) (mm)	71.5	74.3	5.8	−0.5
Gonial < (Ar–Go–Me) (degrees)	124.5	122.3	4.0	−0.9
MPA (MP–HP) (degrees)	28.6	26.0	5.0	0.5
SNA (degrees)	73.0	82.0	3.5	−2.6**
SNB (degrees)	67.9	80.0	3.4	−3.8***
ANB (degrees)	5.1	1.6	1.5	2.3**
N–A (HP) (mm)	1.0	−2.0	3.7	0.8
N–B (HP) (mm)	−8.7	−4.3	4.1	−1.1*
N–A–Pg (degrees)	−4.2	−6.5	5.1	−0.5
N–ANS (mm)	55.8	50.0	2.4	2.4**
ANS–Gn (mm)	69.2	61.3	3.0	2.4**
Ratio		45:55	45:55	

Table 4-1 Case 1: Cranial base analysis.

Measurement	Value	Norm	SD	Dev. norm
Ant CB SN (mm)	71.7	75.3	3.0	−1.2*
Post CB SN (mm)	31.4	35.0	4.0	−0.9
Saddle Angle	130.4	124.0	5.0	1.3

Each asterisk means one standard deviation from the mean.

Table 4-3 Case 1: Dentition

Measurement	Value	Norm	SD	Dev. norm
IMPA (L1–MP) (degrees)	85.4	95.0	7.0	−1.4*
U1–HP (degrees)	117.1	116.0	5.5	0.1
Witts (mm) (A–B/OP)	7.0	−0.4	2.5	2.9**
Interincisal angle (degrees)	128.6	127.0	9.0	0.2

CASE REPORT 1—cont'd

Table 4-4 Case 1: Soft tissue.

Measurement	Value	Norm	SD	Dev. norm
ST convexity (G1–SN–Pg') (degrees)	16.7	12.0	2.0	2.4**
NLA (Col–Sn–UL) (degrees)	104.1	102.0	8.0	0.3
UL–(SN–Pg') (mm)	7.0	3.0	1.0	4.0**
LL–(SN–Pg') (mm)	2.0	2.0	1.0	0.0

- Dental: (1) Class II, Division 1 subdivision; (2) severe Class II denture base discrepancy; (3) protrusive maxillary incisors and retroclined mandibular incisors; (4) 11 mm overjet.
3. *Transverse*:
   - Skeletal: constricted maxilla
   - Dental: (1) posterior teeth in crossbite bilaterally; (2) maxillary midline 1 mm right of facial; mandibular midline 2 mm left of facial (due to mandibular asymmetry), resulting in 3 mm dental midline discrepancy.

4. *Vertical*:
   - Skeletal: within normal limits
   - Dental: (1) 50% overbite; (2) 3 mm interlabial gap, 6 mm incisor display at rest, 90% incisor display at smile; (3) lip incompetent.

5. *Alignment*:
   - Maxillary arch: mild (3 mm) crowding
   - Mandibular arch: moderate (5 mm) crowding.

Treatment Objectives (Fig. 4-3 and Table 4-5)

1. *Significant medical and dental objectives*:
   - Monitor development of 8s (especially mandibular)
   - Educate patient about TMJ (dislocation with reduction)
   - Oral hygiene instructions.

2. *Skeletofacial*: reduce convexity of profile (camouflage).

3. *Anteroposterior*:
   - Incisors: (1) retract maxilla; (2) flare mandible
   - Molars: (1) protract maxilla bilaterally to establish Class I relationship on right and Class II relationship on left; (2) hold mandible left and protract right to Class I.

4. *Vertical*:
   - Incisors: (1) maintain maxilla; (2) intrude mandible 1 mm
   - Molars: (1) maintain maxilla; (2) maintain mandible.

5. *Arch width/transverse*: expand maxilla to eliminate crossbite.

6. *Midlines*:
   - Maxilla: move 1 mm to left
   - Mandible: move 2 mm to right (using asymmetric extraction space on right side).

7. *Occlusal plane*: Maintain natural occlusal plane.

8. *Soft tissue*: Decrease convexity.

General Treatment Plan

- Expand maxilla (rapid palatal expansion [RPE])—one turn/day for first week, then two turns/day if diastema is visible
- Re-evaluate postexpansion
- If dentition is truly asymmetric/subdivision, extract maxillary 4s and mandibular right 5
- Finish Class I molar on right; Class II molar on left.

Table 4-5 Case 1: Orthodontic treatment sequence.

Maxilla	Mandible
Consultation; place separators	Consultation
Pick up impression for RPE	
Insert RPE; expand	
Re-evaluate	
Extract first bicuspids	Extract right second bicuspid
Align and retract cuspids separately	Level and align
Space closure (group C right, group A left)	Space closure (group C right)
Retract four anteriors	
Finish	Finish
Retention	Retention

RPE = rapid palatal expansion.

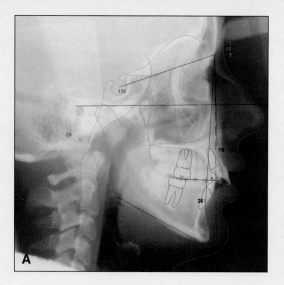

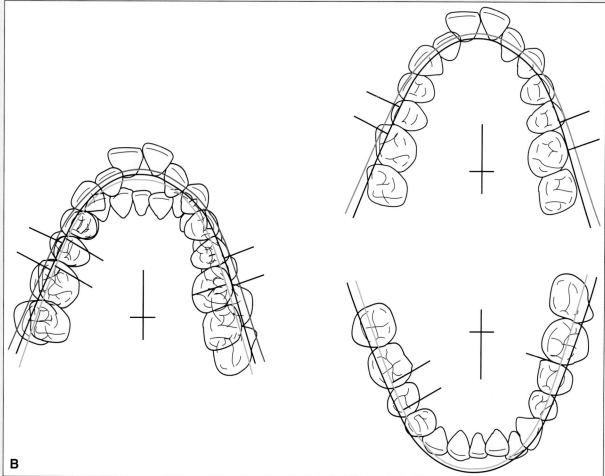

Fig. 4-3 Case 1. **A** Visualized treatment objective (black is initial and blue VTO; black Md-6 = left side; blue Md-6 = right side). **B** Occlusogram.

CASE REPORT 2

Patient Profile (Fig. 4-4)

- 16.7-year-old, postpubertal male
- Chief complaint: "I just want my teeth a little more straight".

Medical History

- Asthma: albuterol—cold weather-induced
- Tumor removed behind left ear (2001)
- Tumor removed from right leg tibial region (2001).

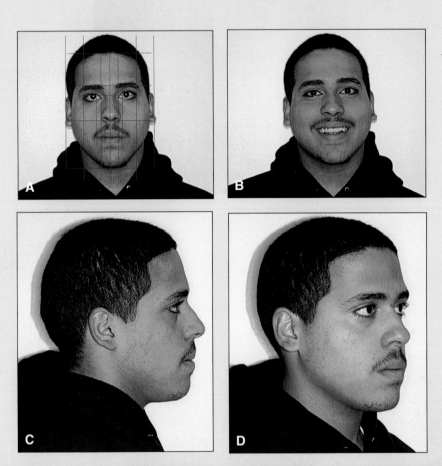

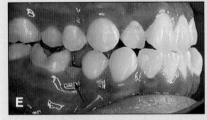
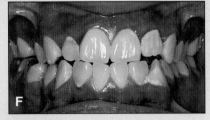
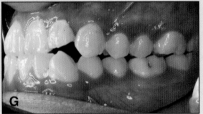

Fig. 4-4 Case 2. **A** Extraoral frontal view. Normofacial with trapezoidal facial form; lip competent; interlabial gap at rest is 1 mm; incisor show at rest 0 mm; long lower facial height (LFH); asymmetries: right eye slightly lower than left eye, chin deviates to left. **B** Extraoral smile. Incisor show 70%; no buccal corridors; thick lips; upper midline on with face and Cupid's bow; incisal plane does not follow lower lip (reverse smile line); no mandibular incisor show. **C** Extraoral profile. Straight to slightly bimaxillary protrusive soft tissue profile; nasolabial angle is within normal limits (WNL); slightly larger LFH; mildly retrusive upper lip to E-plane; UL:LL ~1:2; LFH: throat depth ~1.4:1; mentolabial fold is WNL. **D** Extraoral 45° view. Weak malar prominence; normal mandibular plane angle; moderate lip protrusion. **E–G** Intraoral buccal and frontal views. **F** Intraoral frontal view: maxillary and mandibular midlines coincident with facial midline; 0% open bite (anterior open bite tendency); fair/poor oral hygiene (plaque accumulation, numerous white spot lesions present and localized gingival erythema); good attached keratinized tissue; tight transversely (dental crossbite UR5–LR6). **E** and **G** Intraoral buccal views: Class III molars and canine—1 mm overjet; crossbite UR5 and LR6; LR5 impacted (arrow); LR6 tipped mesially.

Continued

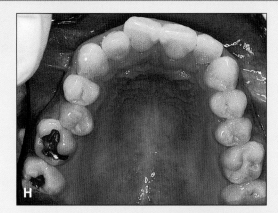
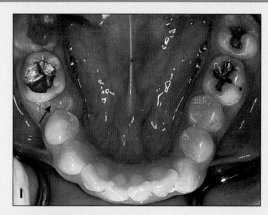

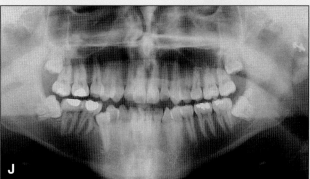

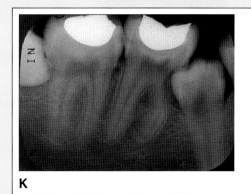
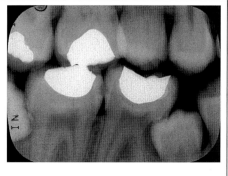

Fig. 4-4 *Cont'd.* **H** Intraoral occlusal view. 7–7 present; U-shaped arch; occlusal restorations on 6s and UR7; mild crowding (3–4 mm). **I** Intraoral occlusal view. 7–7 present; U-shaped arch; occlusal restorations on 6s and 7s (deep on LR6); impacted LR5 (arrow); mesially impacted LR8; severe crowding ~11 mm. **J** Panoramic X-ray. **K** Periapicals of LR5 area.

Dental History

- Extensive dental care, large posterior amalgams
- Lost lower right primary second molar prematurely.

Psychosocial Profile

Extremely quiet and shy.

Cephalometric Summary (Fig. 4-5, Tables 4-6–4.9)

- Moderately concave skeletal profile due to prognathic mandible
- Slightly larger lower facial height (LFH)
- Class III denture base relationship

CASE REPORT 2–cont'd

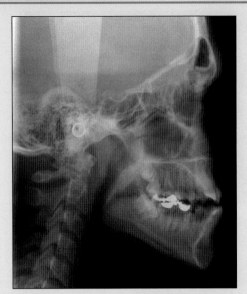

Fig. 4-5 Case 2. Cephalometric X-ray.

Table 4-6 Case 2: Cranial base analysis.

Measurement	Value	Norm	SD	Dev. norm
Ant CB (SN) (mm)	72.2	70.9	3.0	0.5
Post CB (S–Ar) (mm)	44.2	39.1	4.0	1.3*
Saddle angle (degrees)	121.8	124.0	5.0	–0.4

Table 4-7 Case 2: Cranial base—maxilla and mandible.

Measurement	Value	Norm	SD	Dev. norm
SNA (degrees)	85.5	82.0	3.5	1.0*
SNB (degrees)	85.5	82.0	3.5	1.0*
ANB (degrees)	–1.8	1.6	1.5	2.3**
N–A (HP) (mm)	2.8	0.0	3.7	0.8
N–B (HP) (mm)	8.7	–5.3	6.7	2.1**
N–A–Pg (degrees)	–3.5	4.4	3.0	–2.7**
PNS–ANS (mm)	55.8	57.7	2.5	–0.7
Ar–PTM (HP) (mm)	33.1	37.1	2.8	–1.4*
y axis (mm)	163.9	132.5	6.0	5.2*****
y axis (degrees)	66.6	67.0	5.5	–0.1
Ramus height (Ar–Go) (mm)	51.9	50.9	4.5	0.2
Body length (Go–Pg) (mm)	100.1	83.7	4.6	3.6***
Gonial angle (Ar–Go–Me) (degrees)	122.2	113.4	6.7	1.3*
MPA (MP–HP) (degrees)	27	23	5.9	0.7
N–ANS (mm)	57.0	65.4	3.0	–3.8***
ANS–Gn (mm)	87.8	57.4	3.5	8.7********
Ratio		39:61	45:55	

Table 4-8 Case 2: Dentition.

Measurement	Value	Norm	SD	Dev. norm
IMPA (L1–MP) (degrees)	91.9	95.0	7.0	–0.4
U1–HP (degrees)	122.6	117.0	5.5	1.0*
Witts (mm) (A–B/OP)	–8.1	–1.0	1.0	–7.1*******
Interincisal angle (degrees)	118.3	127.0	9.0	–1.0*

Table 4-9 Case 2: Soft tissue.

Measurement	Value	Norm	SD	Dev. norm
ST convexity (G1–SN–Pg') (degrees)	177.5	154.0	5.6	4.2****
NLA (Col–Sn–UL) (degrees)	98.3	102.0	8.0	0.3
UL–(SN–Pg') (mm)	3.0	0.0	1.0	3.8***
LL–(SN–Pg') (mm)	7.7	0.0	1.0	7.7*****

- Slightly flared upper centrals, inclination of lower incisors is within normal limits (WNL)
- Flat occlusal plane
- Slightly steep mandibular plane angle.

Overall Summary

- Skeletal Class III with long LFH

- –1 mm overjet and 0 mm overbite
- UR-5 and LR-6 in crossbite
- LR-5 impacted
- LR-6 tipped mesially with mesial root resorption and very poor prognosis
- Large restoration on LL6.

CASE REPORT 2—cont'd

Problem List

1. *Medical/dental findings of significance*:
   - See medical history above
   - Caries LR-6^D, LR-7^M
   - Fair/poor oral hygiene
   - LR-5 impacted resorbing mesial root of LR-6
   - Radiopacity distal to LL8
   - Lower third molars horizontally impacted.

2. Anteroposterior:
   - Skeletal: (1) moderately concave profile due to a prognathic mandible; (2) soft tissue profile is straight to bimaxillary protrusive
   - Dental: (1) Class III; (2) –1 mm overjet; (3) slightly flared maxillary incisors.

3. *Vertical*:
   - Skeletal: long LFH

- Dental: (1) no incisor show at rest; (2) 0% deepbite (openbite tendency).

4. *Transverse*:
   - Skeletal: chin deviates slightly to left
   - Dental: (1) UR-5 in crossbite with LR-6; (2) tight transversely.

5. *Alignment*:
   - Maxillary arch: mild (3–4 mm) crowding
   - Mandibular arch: (1) severe (10 mm) crowding; (2) Bolton discrepancy (mandibular excess 3–4 mm).

Treatment Objectives (Fig. 4-6 and Table 4-10)

1. *Significant medical and dental objectives*:
   - Improve oral hygiene
   - Restore caries along with full oral examination by general dentist

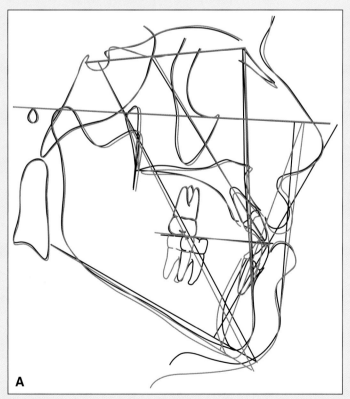

Fig. 4-6 Case 2. **A** Visualized treatment objective (black is initial and blue is growth and treatment [blue is LR-7^M]). **B** Occlusogram. Extract lower 6s. *Continued*

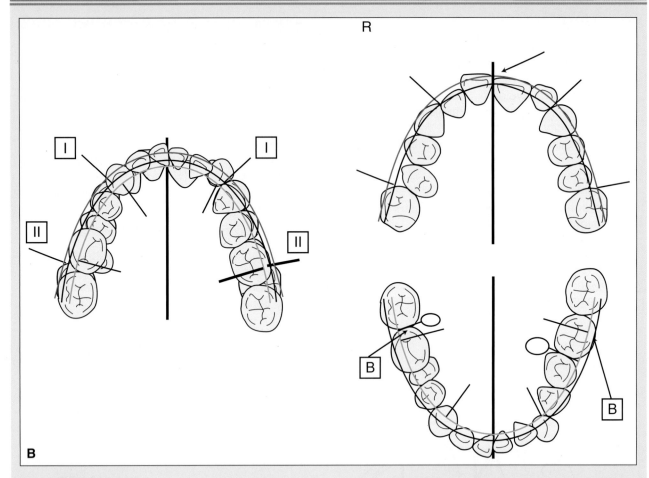

B

Fig. 4-6 *Cont'd*

- Extract LR-6 (root resorption)
- Extract 8s at end of orthodontic treatment and diagnose radiopacity distal to LL8 when extracted (biopsy)
- Monitor radiographs for possible signs of pathology (tumors).

2. *Skeletofacial*: maintain.

3. *Anteroposterior*:
   - Incisors: (1) maintain maxilla; (2) retract mandible 2–3 mm
   - Molars: (1) maintain maxilla; (2) mandible–protract second molars.

4. *Arch width/transverse*: maintain.

5. *Vertical*:
   - Incisors: (1) extrude maxilla 1–2 mm; (2) maintain mandible

Table 4-10 Case 2: Orthodontic treatment sequence.

Maxilla	Mandible
	Extract lower 6s
Spacers, bond 7–7, band 6s	Spacers, bond 5–5, band 7s
Align buccal segments and anterior segments separately	Align and maintain lower curve of Spee
Upper extrusion arch	Group B space closure
Finish	Slenderize 3–3 (Bolton discrepancy)
Retention (bond bar 6–7)	Finish
	Retention

CASE REPORT 2–cont'd

- Molars: (1) maintain maxilla (avoid extrusive mechanics); (2) maintain mandible (avoid extrusive mechanics).

6. *Midlines*:
  - Maintain maxilla
  - Maintain mandible.

7. Occlusal plane: maintain.

8. Soft tissue: maintain.

General Treatment Plan

- Nonsurgical
- Extract mandibular first molars
- Retract mandibular incisors to create positive overjet and overbite
- Extrusion of maxillary incisors to increase incisor display and create positive overbite.

CASE REPORT 3

Patient Profile (Fig. 4-7)

- 16.10-year-old postpubertal female presents in permanent dentition
- Chief complaint: "My teeth are really crooked".

Medical History

Noncontributory.

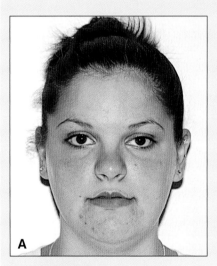
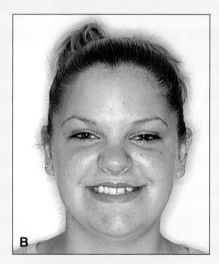
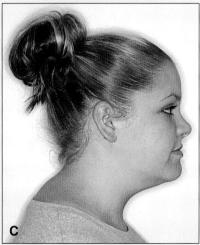
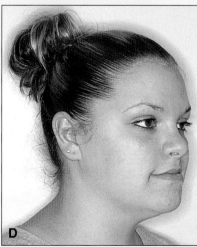

Fig. 4-7 Case 3. **A** Extraoral frontal view. Normofacial with ovoid facial form; interpupillary plane cants slightly down to patient's left; chin point on with facial midline; interlabial gap at rest: 1–2 mm; incisor show at rest: 1–2 mm. **B** Extraoral smile. Incisor show ~80% (determined clinically); distinct cupid's bow; maxillary midline 2 mm left of facial midline; mandibular midline on with facial midline. **C** Extraoral profile. Straight soft tissue profile; nasolabial angle within normal limits; upper facial height to lower facial height ~50:50; upper lip mildly retrusive to E-plane; lower facial height to throat depth ~1:1.3; upper lip to lower lip = 1:2.5. **D** Extraoral 45° view. Malar prominences within normal limits; flat mandibular plane; lip competent; thin lateral aspects of upper lip. *Continued*

CASE REPORT 3-cont'd

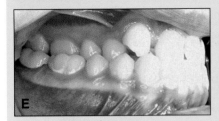
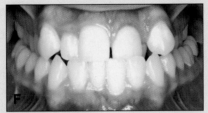
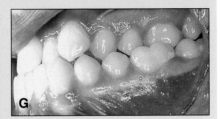

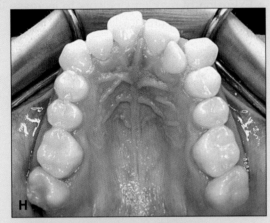
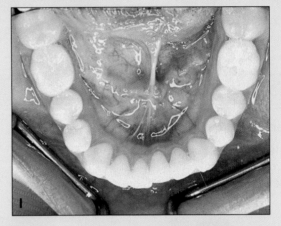

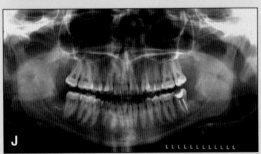

Fig. 4-7 *Cont'd.* **E–G** Intraoral frontal, and right and left buccal views. **F** Intraoral frontal view: Maxillary midline 2 mm left of facial; mandibular midline on with facial; bilateral skeletal crossbite including anterior crossbite; minimal overbite ~5–10%; 1 mm diastema between upper centrals; mild gingival inflammation; good thickness of keratinized/attached gingiva; white spot lesions localized to maxillary anteriors and several posterior locations. **E** and **G** Intraoral right and left buccal views: super Class I cuspids and molars on right; Class I molars and cuspids on left; bilateral buccal crossbite; –2 to +1 mm overjet. **H** Intraoral occlusal view—maxilla. 7–7 present; U-shaped arch; UL two blocked out palatally; severe crowding (~8 mm) localized to anterior; 6s rotated mesial-in. **I** Intraoral occlusal view—mandible. 7–7 present; U-shaped arch; mild crowding (~1–2 mm); rotated LL-5; PFM crown LL7. **J** Panoramic X-ray.

Dental History

- 1/2003: root canal therapy (RCT) in lower left 7 (LL7) due to severe caries
- 3/2003: all four 8s removed
- 5/2003: porcelain fused to metal (PFM) crown LL7
- Regular visits to general practitioner every 6 months.

Psychosocial Profile

- Patient very motivated to receive treatment. Has wanted braces for a long time
- Patient has family problems at home. Moves around between grandmother's and stepmother's homes (important for future compliance issues and maintaining appointments).

Cephalometric Summary (Fig. 4-8 and Tables 4-11–4-14)

- Straight skeletal profile due to a mildly prognathic mandible
- Mildly flat mandibular plane angle
- Mildly long lower skeletal facial height
- Mildly flared maxillary incisors
- Mildly upright mandibular incisors
- Large soft tissue chin.

Overall Summary

- Straight skeletal profile
- Super Class I molars and canines on right

CASE REPORT 3—cont'd

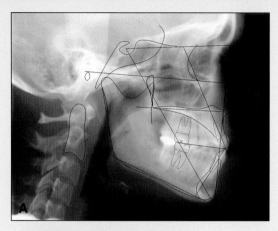

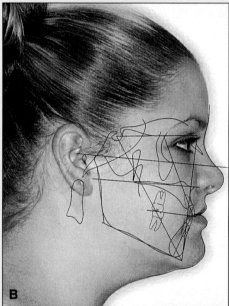

Fig. 4-8 Case 3. **A** Cephalometric X-ray. **B** Lateral cephalometric superimposition.

Table 4-12 Case 3: Cranial base—maxilla and mandible.

Measurement	Value	Norm	SD	Dev. norm
SNA (degrees)	82.5	82.0	3.5	0.2
SNB (degrees)	83.0	80.9	3.4	0.6
ANB (degrees)	−0.4	1.6	1.5	−1.4*
N–A (HP) (mm)	−0.5	−2.0	3.7	0.4
N–B (HP) (mm)	−0.1	−4.3	8.5	0.5**
N–A–Pg (degrees)	0.3	4.9	3.0	−1.5*
PNS–ANS (mm)	52.8	52.6	3.5	0.1
Ar–PTM (HP) (mm)	33.1	32.8	1.9	0.2
y axis (mm)	130.7	131.0	6.0	−0.1
y axis (degrees)	62.4	67.0	5.5	−0.8
Ramus height (Ar–Go) (mm)	53.7	48.5	4.5	1.2*
Body length (Go–Pg) (mm)	79.0	74.3	5.8	0.8
Gonial angle (Ar–Go–Me) (degrees)	122.7	122.9	6.7	−0.0
MPA (MP–HP) (degrees)	18.7	24.2	5.0	−1.1*
N–ANS (mm)	47.8	50.0	2.4	−0.9
ANS–Gn (mm)	66.1	60.6	3.5	1.6*
Ratio	42.1:57.9	45:55	1.0	

Table 4-11 Case 3: Cranial base analysis.

Measurement	Value	Norm	SD	Dev. norm
Ant CB (SN) (mm)	76.1	75.3	3.0	0.3
Post CB (S–Ar) (mm)	33.2	35.0	4.0	−0.4
Saddle angle	125.2	124.0	5.0	0.2

Table 4-13 Case 3: Dentition.

Measurement	Value	Norm	SD	Dev. norm
IMPA (L1–MP) (degrees)	89.9	95.0	7.0	−0.7
U1–HP (degrees)	116.9	116.0	5.5	0.2
Witts (mm) (A–B/OP)	−1.2	−1.0	1.0	−0.2
Interincisal angle (degrees)	134.6	127.0	9.0	−0.8

CASE REPORT 3–cont'd

Table 4-14 Case 3: Soft tissue.

Measurement	Value	Norm	SD	Dev. norm
ST convexity (G1–SN–Pg') (degrees)	0.9	12.0	2.0	–5.6*****
NLA (Col–Sn–UL) (degrees)	101.6	102.0	8.0	–0.1
UL–(SN–Pg') (mm)	3.7	2.8	2.0	0.5
LL–(SN–Pg') (mm)	4.2	2.3	2.0	1.0

- Class I molars and canines on left
- Bilateral posterior crossbite
- Severe maxillary crowding
- –2 mm to +1 mm overjet
- 5–10% overbite.

Problem List

1. *Medical/dental findings of significance*:
   - RCT/PFM crown LL 7
   - Recently extracted 8s
   - White spot lesions localized to maxillary anteriors and several posterior locations.

2. *Anteroposterior*:
   - Skeletal: straight skeletal profile with a mildly prognathic mandible; anterior skeletal crossbite (UR2 and UL 1,2)
   - Dental: (1) super Class I molars and canines on right; (2) weak Class I molars and canines on right; (3) Maxillary 6s rotated mesial-in.

3. *Transverse*:
   - Skeletal: bilateral posterior crossbite due to skeletally constricted maxilla
   - Dental: upper midline 2 mm left of facial midline.

4. *Alignment*:
   - Maxillary arch: severe (~8 mm) crowding localized to anterior segment
   - Mandibular arch: mild (1–2 mm) crowding.

5. *Vertical*:
   - Skeletal: (1) mildly flat mandibular plane angle; (2) mildly long lower facial height
   - Dental: (1) minimal overbite (~5–10%); (2) 80% incisor display upon full smile.

Treatment Objectives (Fig. 4-9 and Table 4-15)

1. *Pathology/other*:
   - Monitor apical area of LL 7 with periapical radiographs
   - Monitor bony fill of extraction sites (8s)

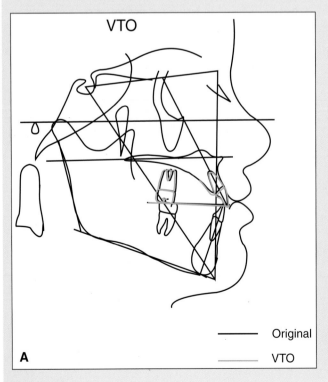

VTO

——— Original

——— VTO

A

Fig. 4-9 Case 3. **A** Visualized treatment objective (VTO) (black is initial and pink VTO). **B** Occlusogram. *Continued*

CASE REPORT 3—cont'd

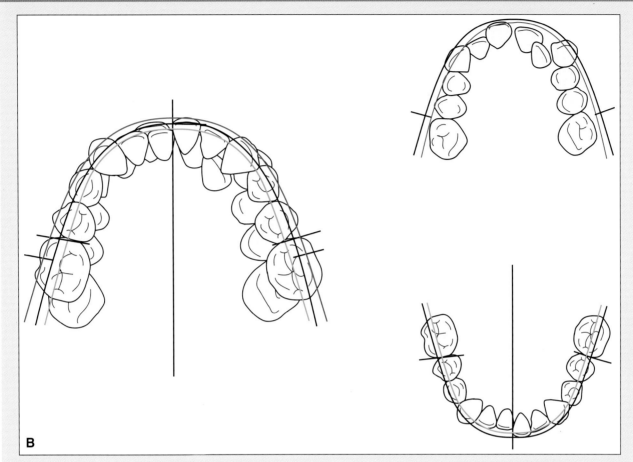

B

Fig. 4-9 *Cont'd*

- Discuss white spot lesions and proper oral hygiene.

2. *Skeletofacial*: maintain.

3. Anteroposterior:
   - Incisors: (1) maintain maxilla (UR 1); (2) maintain mandible (LL 1)
   - Molars: (1) maintain maxilla; (2) maintain mandible.

4. *Arch width/transverse*: skeletally expand maxillary arch.

5. *Vertical*:
   - Incisors: (1) extrude maxilla ~1.5 mm; (2) maintain mandible
   - Molars: (1) maintain maxilla (avoid extrusive mechanics); (2) maintain mandible (avoid extrusive mechanics).

6. *Midlines*:
   - Shift maxilla midline 2 mm right
   - Maintain mandible.

7. *Occlusal plane*: maintain.

8. *Soft tissue*: maintain.

General Treatment Plan

- Nonsurgical, nonextraction
- Expand maxilla (RPE) one turn/day until achieving proper overexpansion
- Re-evaluate vertical dimension after removal of expander
- Use auxiliary torquing/extrusion arch 2–2 to obtain positive overbite if needed
- Finish Class I molars and canines.

CASE REPORT 3—cont'd

Table 4-15 Case 3: Orthodontic treatment

Maxilla	Mandible
Spacers 4s and 6s	
Band 4s and 6s; pick up impression of bands; replace spacers	
Cement RPE; activate two turns/day; patient to wear vertical pull chin cap at night with 200 g force for 1 month; patient to return in 5 days for evaluation	
Retain RPE for 6–9 months	
Bond 5–5	Bond 5–5/spacers 6s
	Band 6s
Align	Level and alignment; strip mandibular anteriors as necessary
Remove expander 6–9 months later and re-evaluate vertical dimension; use auxillary torquing arch 2–2 (stiff segment 4–6) to obtain positive overbite	
Finishing/root correction	Finishing/root correction
Retention	Retention

RPE = rapid palatal expansion.

Summary

This chapter describes a systematic way to diagnose an orthodontic patient, devise a list of treatment objectives, and based on that develop a treatment plan. Specific treatment objectives provide the blueprint for desired outcome. The importance of the specific objectives is highlighted when a decision among the myriad of orthodontic appliances for correction of any maloclussion is needed.

REFERENCES

1. van Venrooy JR, Proffit WR. Orthodontic care for medically compromised patients: possibilities and limitations. J Am Dent Assoc 1985;111:262–266.
2. Roberts WE, Hohlt WF, Baldwin JJ. Adjunctive orthodontic therapy in adults: Biologic, medical, and treatment considerations. In: Bishara SE, ed. Textbook of orthodontics. Philadelphia: WB Saunders, 2001: 494–531.
3. Lindauer S. Orthodontic treatment planning. In: Nanda R, ed. Biomechanics in clinical orthodontics. Philadelphia: WB Saunders, 1997:23–47.
4. Kuhlberg AJ, Glynn E. Treatment planning considerations for adult patients. Dent Clin North Am 1997;41:17–27.
5. Proffit WR, Sarver DM. Treatment planning: Optimizing benefit to the patient. In: Proffit WR, Sarver DM, White RP, eds. Contemporary treatment of dentofacial deformity. St Louis: Mosby, 2003:172–244.
6. Kuhlberg AJ. Steps in orthodontic treatment. In: Bishara SE, ed. Textbook of orthodontics. Philadelphia: WB Saunders, 2001.
7. Bishara SE. Facial and dental changes in adolescents and their clinical implications. Angle Orthod 2000;70:471–483.
8. Bjork A. Prediction of mandibular growth rotation. Am J Orthod 1969;55:585–599.
9. Burstone C. The integumental profile. Am J Orthod 1958;44:1–25.
10. Rains MD, Nanda R. Soft-tissue changes associated with maxillary incisor retraction. Am J Orthod 1982;81:481–488.
11. Kocadereli I. Changes in soft tissue profile after orthodontic treatment with and without extractions. Am J Orthod Dentofacial Orthop 2002;122:67–72.
12. Lamarque S. The importance of occlusal plane control during orthodontic mechanotherapy. Am J Orthod Dentofacial Orthop 1995;107:548–558.

13. Nanda R, Margolis MJ. Treatment strategies for midline discrepancies. Semin Orthod 1996;2:84–89.

14. Nanda R. The differential diagnosis and treatment of excessive overbite. Dent Clin North Am 1981;25:69–84.

15. Rossouw P, Preston CB, Lombard CJ, Truter JW. A longitudinal evaluation of the anterior border of the dentition. Am J Orthod Dentofacial Orthop 1993;104:146–152.

16. Little RM. Stability and relapse of dental arch alignment. In: Burstone C, Nanda R, eds. Retention and stability in orthodontics. Philadelphia: WB Saunders, 1993:97–106.

17. Torres M. Treatment objectives and treatment planning. Dental Clin North Am 1981;25:27–41.

18. Sarver DM. The importance of incisor positioning in the esthetic smile: the smile arc. Am J Orthod Dentofacial Orthop 2001;120:98–111.

19. Nanda R. Biomechanic basis of edgewise orthodontics and craniofacial orthopedics. Monograph, IOK Center for Continuing Education in Orthodontics. Munich: 1988:27–54.

20. Peluso C, Kuhlberg A. The axial inclination of central incisors and its effects on the perception of the facial profile.

Annual American Dental Association Meeting, Scientific Program, Memphis, 2002.

21. Arnett GW, Jelic KS, Kim J, et al. Soft tissue cephalometric analysis: diagnosis and treatment planning of dentofacial deformity. Am J Orthod Dentofacial Orthop 1999;116:239–253.

22. Allais D, Melsen B. Does labial movement of lower incisors influence the level of the gingival margin? A case–control study of adult orthodontic patients. Eur J Orthod 2003;25:343–352.

23. Burzin J, Nanda R. The stability of deep bite correction. In: Nanda R, Burstone, C, eds. Retention and stability in orthodontics. Philadelphia: WB Saunders, 1993. 61-80.

24. Fiorelli G, Melsen B. The "3-D occlusogram" software. Am J Orthod Dentofacial Orthop 1999;116:363–368.

25. Marcotte MR. The use of the occlusogram in planning orthodontic treatment. Am J Orthod 1976;69:655–667.

26. Braun S. The extraction–nonextraction decision revisited. Am J Orthod Dentofacial Orthop 1999;116:21A–22A.

27. Huang GJ. Making the case for evidence-based orthodontics. Am J Orthod Dentofacial Orthop 2004;125:405–406.

CHAPTER 5

Social Psychology of Facial Appearance

Jill Bennett Nevin and Robert Keim

"At first glance, the disciplines of social psychology and clinical orthodontics would seem to be as separate as any two disciplines one could find. It has been stated that 'One is mental, the other is dental'. Indeed, it is difficult to bring these two sciences together. One involves clinical treatment; the other is a social science. The clinician measures physical characteristics with direct precision in terms of millimeters and degrees; the psychologist measures less specific entities, such as verbal social actions and attitudes. Yet while these two sciences appear to be dichotomous, there are areas of overlap where interdisciplinary considerations are both useful and necessary."[1]

"Social psychology: The scientific study of the way in which people's thoughts, feelings and behaviors are influenced by the real or imagined presence of other people."[2]

According to Hassebrauk,[3] the smile is the second facial feature, after eyes, that people tend to view when evaluating another's attractiveness.[3] A person's facial appearance and its degree of attractiveness can significantly impact diverse aspects of his/her personal, professional, and social life. Orthodontists by definition are involved with clinical procedures that alter, and hopefully improve, a patient's facial appearance. While, as Dr Graber notes above, "one field is mental and the other is dental,"[1] considering the impact that alterations in facial appearance

can have on a patient's overall wellbeing in life, it is imperative that the practicing orthodontist has an understanding of the social psychological underpinnings of facial attractiveness theory. This chapter provides the practitioner with a research-based introduction to postulated components of perceived facial attractiveness, and an understanding of selected social and psychological outcomes associated with facial appearance. The science of social psychology not only provides a context for that understanding, but the basis for a deeper appreciation of the contribution clinical orthodontists make to patients' lives.

Social Psychology

Social psychology is that branch of psychology that examines human cognition, affect, and behavior in the context of social factors. It emphasizes information processing mechanisms shared by most people. As such, it shares with cognitive psychology an interest in cognitive processing, particularly of situational and social influences on cognition, emotion, and action. Enquiry into the origins of human perception and behavior can lead social psychologists into explorations of evolutionary psychology and neurobiology and, like personality psychology, the focus may shift to the psychological status of individuals, i.e., "individual differences" that influence thoughts, feelings, and behavior. Finally, like sociology, social psychology sometimes considers the impact of macro-level factors, such as culture or intergroup relations, on topics of interest.[2] Situated at a rich intersection of scientific and theoretic traditions, it is well suited to examine the socially-embedded topic of facial appearance.

Appearance-Based Inferences and Attributions

From a very early age we are admonished not to "judge a book by its cover," and taught that "beauty is more than skin deep." Judging others' personalities and character based on superficial qualities of facial appearance over which they have little control violates our cultural value of fairness. Beyond making trait inferences or behavioral attributions based on "looks," discriminating against or rewarding others on this basis may seem even more offensive to our moral sensibilities. Shouldn't distribution of social rewards be based on merit? Yet research overwhelmingly shows that facial appearance has a pervasive and nontrivial influence on how individuals are viewed and treated in every major social domain of life. For example, studies suggest that on the basis of facial appearance, parents treat infants better or worse, teachers make flattering or pejorative inferences about their students, social support is proffered or withheld, work opportunities are gained or lost, potential mates are pursued or shunned, and juries even find defendants innocent or guilty.[4,5] As the sections below will show, social psychological research demonstrates that facial appearance tends to have a significant impact on quality of life.

Social psychology recognizes that people are "naïve scientists" in their everyday lives, regularly making inferences about both themselves and others. In the social realm, individuals make inferences about their own and others' personality traits, as well as formulating causal attributions for behavior. Facial appearance often plays a strong role in impression formation of others, especially in the initial stages of acquaintance.[6] Why?

In face-to-face interactions with others, a social perceiver generally engages in shortcuts in reasoning in order to quickly understand and categorize the other. Cognitive processing shortcuts, generally termed *heuristics*, are time and/or effort saving, albeit potentially inaccurate ways of reasoning to conclusions. During initial impression formation of others, people tend to use cues that are readily available (*availability heuristic*), and whatever cues are first available (*primacy heuristic*). Perceivers' initial impressions generally prime and provide categories for an ongoing understanding of the other. Subsequent information received about the target will tend to be subjected to *selective perception* biases, as the perceiver attends to data that confirms initial judgments, and discounts or fails to notice evidence that is at odds with his/her initial assessment. Selective perception is thought to take place partly because people have an innate need for consistency in their sense making, seeking to avoid (whether consciously or subconsciously) the discomfort (*cognitive dissonance*) of

inferences that are internally contradictory.[6] For all of these reasons, initial impressions based on the often first available cue of facial appearance tend to be extra influential on the outcomes of social interactions.

Stereotypes and Facial Appearance

A stereotype is "a generalization about a group of people in which identical characteristics are assigned to virtually all members of the group, regardless of actual variation among the members."[2] Studies suggest that people have a tendency to engage in a kind of stereotyping based on facial appearance, whether intentionally or unintentionally, and whether consciously or unconsciously. Specific stereotypes corresponding to certain facial types (e.g., "babyfaceness," see below) have been identified.[4]

More generally, there is much evidence for a human tendency to negative attitudes and discriminatory behavior toward those perceived as unattractive, and on the other hand, for more positive impressions and treatment of people with attractive faces.[5] The preferential reaction to and treatment of people with attractive faces has been termed the "attractiveness halo."[4] The tendency to make more positive trait inferences and behavioral attributions to those who are more attractive has been posited as reflecting a rather pervasive, underlying "What is beautiful is good" mindset.[7] For example, attractive individuals are judged as having more social appeal, and as being more interpersonally, academically, and occupationally competent.[5] While there are rare circumstances in which attractiveness appears to be a possible liability, e.g., potentially eliciting inferences of vanity,[8] those with attractive faces frequently experience beneficial halo effects from "cradle to grave," reaping more positive social outcomes throughout the lifespan in areas such as parent–child interactions, teacher–student interactions, and occupational success, as demonstrated below.

Social Psychological Impact of Facial Appearance

Parent–Child Interactions

Beginning in infancy, unattractive children tend to be perceived more negatively even by their own mothers. In a study of maternal behaviors and attitudes, Langlois et al[9] showed that mothers of newborns with attractive faces were more affectionate and playful with their babies than were mothers of less attractive infants. In contrast, mothers of less attractive babies tended to engage in comparatively perfunctory caregiving and to attend to others in the environment, rather than to their own infants. In addition to differential treatment, mothers of less attractive newborns expressed relatively more negative attitudes about infants being a burdensome interference in parents' lives. A subsequent assessment at the age of 3 months revealed a gender-specific effect, with attractive boys still being treated to more affectionate play than their less attractive male counterparts, though differential treatment of girls had dissipated. At the age of 3 months, the differential attitudes of burdensomeness did not remain—unless an infant had become less attractive over time. In such cases a mother's attitude that her infant was interfering with her life tended to increase, corresponding with her infant's increased unattractiveness.

Additional studies have revealed similarly discrepant maternal behavior toward babies with craniofacial abnormalities (e.g., cleft lip/palate) compared to maternal behavior toward normal infants. Field and Vega-Lahr[10] found that mothers of infants with craniofacial abnormalities tended to behave less positively toward them, e.g., smiling at and vocalizing less to them. Fathers' participation in caregiving has also been significantly and positively correlated with their infants' attractiveness according to a study by Parke et al.[11]

Likewise, in childhood, attractive children continue to experience the effects of the presence or absence of the "attractiveness halo" in relation to their parents. For example, Elder et al's study[12] examining relationships between fathers and their adolescents during the Great Depression found that fathers were more punitive and harsh toward their less attractive daughters than the more attractive ones, pursuant to family income loss. Regarding these findings, Langlois et al[9] surmise, "apparently, the girls' attractiveness provided some buffer or protection against irritable parenting." Indeed, a variety of laboratory experiments have examined the influence of attractiveness on punishment severity, revealing a propensity to inflict harsher sanctions on less attractive children.[4] For example, college women playing the role of mother to a 10-year old in a laboratory setting administered more severe punishments (louder noises) to a less attractive child for erring during a learning process.[13]

Teacher–Student Interactions

The attractiveness halo extends from the home to school. It can affect both teacher–student and student–peer relations, and academic outcomes. In an early study of the impact of facial attractiveness in the classroom, Clifford and Walster[14] studied how school children's facial attractiveness affected teachers' expectations. Teachers were asked to estimate a child's IQ based on a photograph, report card information, and attendance records. Independent of alternate diagnostic information, a child's attractiveness was found to have a medium-sized effect on estimates of IQ, and a large effect on teachers' expectations of his/her eventual educational attainment.[14] Additional studies report similar findings for teachers' judgments of their own students' academic potential. Further, identical essays have been shown to be rated higher if attributed to more attractive rather than less attractive students.[4]

Considering decades of well-documented evidence for the powerful impact of teacher expectancies in the schoolroom, teachers' attractiveness-based academic expectations may have far from trivial effects. *Interpersonal expectancy effects* occur when one person's expectations of another bring about a *self-fulfilling prophecy*, in which the target person's behavior is influenced—often very subtly, but powerfully—to confirm the other's expectations.[15] A seminal classroom study exploring such a phenomenon, which came to be popularly known as the "Pygmalion effect," demonstrated that teachers' expectations can influence students' actual IQ gains. In this study, teachers were informed that certain students had been determined to have unusual potential for a spurt in intellectual growth. In reality, the designated "bloomers" had been selected randomly. During the school year, the unfounded prophecy of enhanced performance somehow resulted in significant intellectual (IQ) gains by the designated "bloomers" compared to the control group.[16]

The link between teacher expectations and student performance is proposed to be mediated in large part by teacher behavior. Prominent facial attractiveness scholar, Leslie Zebrowitz, reported that a synthesis of findings from over 100 studies revealed that teachers' positive expectancies for given students' performance generally correlate with a host of supportive teacher behaviors toward those students. These behaviors include "more interaction with the student, presentation of more material or more difficult material, more praise of the student, more smiling and eye contact, staying closer to the student, and providing more encouragement."[4] Zebrowitz notes that while evidence for differential attractiveness-based expectations is strong, the evidence for related differential treatment of students is thus far less consistent.[4] However, the combined evidence for teachers' attractiveness-based expectations, and evidence for teachers' expectations generally leading to different treatment which in turn impacts student achievement, raises a red flag of concern that less attractive children may be unfairly disadvantaged in the classroom.

Teachers' attitudes and behavior toward students have also been shown to be influential in the opinions that students form of their peers. Specifically, research reveals that teachers' negative or positive expectancies and public classroom feedback about students can directly influence student peers to have similar attitudes and beliefs. In one study of this phenomenon, White et al[17] found that negative teacher feedback caused students to view a hypothetical student in a video to be less liked, perceived as less deserving of reward, and rated as more likely to engage in inappropriate behavior. Given the influential role teachers can play in influencing peer-to-peer attitudes—which if negative can be linked to bullying—it is clearly important for an instructor to guard against differential treatment of students based on facial attractiveness. Providing reason for optimism, there is some evidence that the effects of attractiveness-based bias on teacher expectations can be outweighed by providing teachers with additional personalized information about a student's conduct, work habits, and attitudes.[17]

In an ironic turnabout, it has been shown that teacher attractiveness influences students' preferences and evaluations relative to teachers. For example, in one study, teachers rated as either attractive or unattractive read a story to groups of first graders. Children were asked which teacher they would prefer as a substitute. They tended to choose the teacher with the more attractive face, with many of the children explaining that they liked the teacher better because she was pretty, and that prettier teachers are smarter.[18]

Occupational Outcomes

The benefits of attractiveness extend to the workplace. Meta-analyses reveal that attractive individuals fare better than their less attractive counterparts with regard to perceived job qualifications, hiring decisions, predicted job success, and compensation. Both men and women are subject to these biases, and the magnitude of effects is sizeable.[19]

Research exploring the outcome of attractiveness and employment discrimination has often utilized simulation studies. In such experimental settings, attractiveness can be isolated from other potential confounds, e.g., actual performance, occurring in natural work settings. Typically, identical résumés are paired with photographs of individuals rated as either attractive or unattractive. Findings reveal that attractive candidates are generally perceived more positively and are recommended for better treatment.[4] For example, in an experiment on the effect of facial disfigurement (in this case a portwine stain) on personnel decisions, a combination of 59 students and 57 professional recruiters made decisions based on a mock job application. Despite identical résumés, the hypothetical applicant was disadvantaged in the disfigured condition compared to the nondisfigured condition. In the disfigured condition, she received lower ratings on personal qualities and job skills by both groups, and was less likely to be hired by the student group.[20] Despite the professional recruiters' reported willingness to hire in either condition, it seems reasonable to surmise that in a real-world setting, recruiters' demonstrated tendency to give lower competency ratings due to facial disfigurement might eventually translate into differential hiring practices in a competitive job market.

Indeed, the association of attractiveness and biased treatment has been shown to occur in actual practice in the workplace. For instance, a large scale study by Frieze et al[21] of male and female MBA graduates from a large Middle Atlantic university found facial attractiveness correlated with—among other fiscal benefits—higher starting salaries for the males. Attractiveness was also positively correlated with subsequent salaries for both men and women, followed for 10 years after completing their MBAs. For women, each point on a five-point attractiveness scale was associated with a $2150 per year (1983) salary difference. For men, each point was worth an average of $2600. Over time, the difference in salary for someone in the highest attractiveness category compared to someone in the lowest was approximately $10,000 per year.

As researchers have noted, the real-world implications of differential workplace practices based on attractiveness can be consequential. Not surprisingly, legal actions have been brought on the grounds of appearance-based discrimination.[4] Reflecting legitimate societal concern about the injustice of "lookism" in the workplace, the Rehabilitation Act of 1973 has been interpreted as protecting people against employment discrimination on the basis of (fundamentally immutable aspects of) physical appearance.[4,22]

Orthodontics and the Social Psychological Impact of Facial Appearance*

In the 1990s there was an evolution in the understanding of the interplay of psychological factors and dentofacial disharmony. Contemporary researchers have continued to pursue a deeper understanding of the critical interplay of a patient's psychological profile, orthodontic treatment objectives, and psychological outcomes.

Shaw et al[23] evaluated the risk–benefit appraisal for orthodontic treatment. They discussed the benefit of "social psychological wellbeing" in terms of three subgroups. First they looked at "nicknames and teasing" and stated that the contribution of orthodontic treatment should not be underestimated where conspicuous dentofacial deviation has attracted the hurtful mockery of peers. Second they evaluated "dental appearance and social attractiveness" and found that faces displaying a range of dental conditions affected the perception of social characteristics, such as perceived friendliness, social class, popularity, and intelligence. Third they discussed "self-esteem and popularity" and found an association between dental attractiveness and self-esteem and other factors. They concluded, "when personal dissatisfaction with dental appearance is felt in childhood, it might well remain for a lifetime."

It is taken for granted by many practitioners that improved dentofacial appearance brought about by orthodontic treatment enhances self-esteem but the literature in support of that assumption is equivocal. Graber[1] suggested that there is a complex interaction between dentofacial form and overall self-esteem. He suggests that the first variable to be considered is the level of overall self-esteem of the subject. When self-esteem is low before treatment, alterations in

---

*Reproduced in part with permission from Rahbar F. Changes in self-esteem and self-concept as a result of orthodontic treatment. Master's thesis, University of Southern California, 2001.

facial esthetics are more likely to have an important psychological impact than when self-esteem is already high before the treatment begins. The second variable to look at is the location and degree of deformity. Alterations that are proximal to the dental region and cause distortion of balanced facial form close to the communicative zones are more likely to result in changes in self-esteem than those that are more distant from the mouth and have less effect on the soft tissue facial contours. Major facial form deformities, e.g. cleft lip, are likely to evoke special coping mechanisms that protect self-esteem, while more minor, self-perceived facial form disproportion, e.g., malocclusion, may produce anxieties with resultant changes in self-esteem. The final variable of import is the differential importance of esthetics between males and females, i.e., the sex factor. Females tend to value good facial esthetics more highly in their self-esteem constructs than do males. Hence, most dentofacial disproportion is more significant to the overall self-esteem of females than of males.

In a study by Rahbar,[24] findings suggest that the patient's view of his/her own physical sense improved by virtue of simply going into braces, as the psychological benefits were achieved prior to the actual facial changes from treatment. The author administered the Tennessee self-concept scale (TSCS) to a sample of 330 subjects selected at random from the active patient pool of the Graduate Orthodontic Clinic at the University of Southern California. The sample was stratified according to the stage of treatment: Group 1 consisted of preorthodontic patients, group 2 of mid-treatment, and group 3 of post-treatment/retention. The patients' view of their own physical appearance was found to be within normal limits initially and improved with orthodontic treatment. These results indicate that the patients' self-identity scores were within normal limits for all groups initially and improved upon beginning orthodontic treatment. These results underscore the beneficial nature of orthodontic treatment in the psychological wellbeing of adolescents. The interpretation of these findings is twofold. First there was a significant improvement in the patients' perception of their own physical sense pre- and post-orthodontic treatment. This suggests that the resolution of malocclusion or facial disharmony resulted in improvement of the individual's satisfaction with his/her body and physical sense. Second the significant difference between the pre- and mid-treatment groups (groups 1 and 2) suggests that the mere initiation of treatment has a positive effect on the individual's view of his/her body, state of health, physical appearance, skills, and sexuality. The improved feelings of self-esteem and self-concept may be attributable to the patients' perception of embarking on a path of self-improvement. The findings of this investigation are similar to those reported by Dennington[25] who stated that the mere placement of orthodontic appliances resulted in improved self-esteem.

More recently, O'Brien et al[26] conducted a multicenter randomized clinical trial to investigate early treatment of Class II malocclusions. In addition to the anatomic changes found with early treatment, findings indicated improvement in patient self-esteem as a result of orthodontic treatment. While many studies have addressed the pros and cons of early Class II correction from a structural and functional point of view, this study directly addressed the psychological benefits of early Class II correction with functional appliances. The sample of 174 children aged 8–10 years with Class II, Division 1 malocclusions was randomly allocated to a treatment group receiving twin-block appliances or to an untreated control group. They found that Class II correction resulted in an increase in self-concept and a "reduction of negative social experiences."

Is There Universal Agreement on Facial Attractiveness?

"I know not what beauty is, but I know that it touches many things." (Albrecht Dürer c. 1500)

If improving facial attractiveness does indeed tend to enhance self-esteem and overall psychosocial wellbeing, just what constitutes "facial attractiveness?" Does the old adage "beauty lies in the eye of the beholder" represent the fact that perceptions of beauty are based on idiosyncratic individual preferences? Or, on the contrary, is there evidence for agreement between human beings as to what constitutes facial attractiveness? A substantial body of research literature has examined this question.

Intracultural and Cross-Cultural Agreement on Attractiveness

Current research indicates that there is significant within and cross-cultural agreement about who and what is attractive. Langlois et al[5] conducted a large scale quantitative meta-analysis examining attractiveness ratings which assessed the amount of agreement about facial attractiveness between thousands of people representing diverse ages (children to adults) and ethnic and cultural groups. Inter-rater reliability about attractiveness was very high (effective reliability ranging from $r = 0.85$ to $r = 0.94$) both within and across ethnicities and cultures.[5]

Agreement on Attractiveness in Infancy

Remarkably, evidence suggests that even young infants respond to attractiveness, apparently displaying preferences that coincide with those of adults. Multiple methodologies have been used to ascertain infants' facial esthetic preferences, with results pointing to infant–adult agreement.[27] One method of estimating infant esthetic preference is

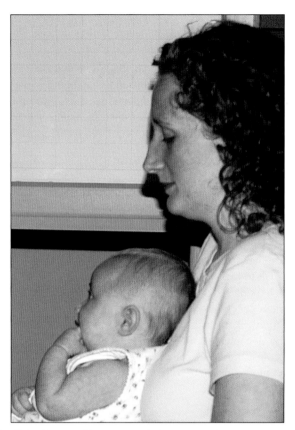

Fig. 5-1 "Gaze time" is one method of estimating infant esthetic preference.

"gaze time" (Fig. 5-1). Under controlled conditions, when infants (newborns [several days old] to 25 months) are presented simultaneously with two facial photographs—one rated more attractive by adults—they tend to gaze significantly longer at the face previously rated more attractive. While this methodology relies on the speculative assumption that longer gaze time equals preference, it is suggestive of agreement between infants and adults on attractiveness.[27] Subsequent studies employing different methodologies have provided additional support for this conclusion.

In an ingenious experiment, Langlois et al[28] observed 60, 1-year-old infants interacting with a stranger acting as caretaker. The caretaker wore a thin, lifelike mask which was either attractive or unattractive. Rigorous procedures included blinding the caretaker as to the mask she was wearing, having her follow a strict interaction script, and blinding raters to the mask she was wearing (by having them observe her from behind). Raters coded her behavior toward the infants as having no significant differences between mask conditions, yet infants exposed to the un-attractive mask displayed more avoidance behavior toward the caretaker and more distress and negative emotion. In another study, Langlois et al[28] provided 12-month olds with dolls which were identical except for unattractive

versus attractive faces. Infants played with the attractive dolls for a significantly longer duration.

A gradual socialization model of attractiveness preference development suggests that preferences are gradually developed through exposure to and enculturation by parents, peers, and the media. However the above studies challenge such a model by suggesting either an innate schema (a cognitive representation present at birth) of facial attractiveness, or a cognitive predisposition for very early acquisition (via environmental exposure to faces) of a preference for attractive faces.[27] While not discounting possible later influences of enculturation, and regardless of the specific mechanism underlying infants' early preferences, research demonstrates a remarkable preference for attractive faces—beginning in early infancy.

What is Attractive and Why?

"Tis not a lip, or eye, we beauty call, but the joint force and full result of all."

(Alexander Pope 1711)

While there is good overall agreement between observers about which faces are attractive, identifying those properties responsible for perceived attractiveness is more complex. Facial attractiveness has been postulated to consist of the following, either in combination or primarily alone: "averageness," symmetry, neonate-like features or "babyfaceness", secondary-sexual characteristics (sexual dimorphism), youthfulness, familiarity, straight profiles, and facial expression (particularly smiling). Aspects of these postulated components will be explored in the following sections.

Averageness

In the late 1800s, Sir Francis Galton, criminologist and pioneer of statistical regression, was studying whether or not different groups of people had distinctive facial morphologies. His methodology involved the creation of composite faces by overlying multiple images of faces onto a photographic plate. The multiple images that contributed to each composite included individuals from the different groups defined by Galton. Two of the groups included "criminals" and "vegetarians." Galton asked if there was a typical "criminal" face or a typical "vegetarian" face. His hypothesis about intragroup facial similarity was not supported; rather his most significant finding was that the composites were more attractive than individual faces taken singly. Thus was born the "averageness hypothesis" of facial beauty.[27]

Since Galton's serendipitous observation of the association of "averaged" faces and attractiveness, formal evidence has accrued for the averageness hypothesis of attractiveness. For example, Langlois and Roggman[29] found that facial composites formed through computerized averaging of multiple faces were, with very rare exception, rated more attractive than the individual faces which comprised them. A strong linear trend was also noted in which faces were judged more attractive as more faces were combined (e.g., a 32-face composite was rated higher than a 16-face composite, which was rated higher than an 8-face composite). Challenging the critique that such findings may be influenced by methodological artifacts which might enhance attractiveness (e.g., blurring of skin blemishes), a number of studies in which the faces under consideration were not generated by artificial means have linked high facial typicality with attractiveness. However, some studies suggest that the most attractive faces may have one or a few aspects which deviate slightly from the norm (e.g., larger than average eyes), thereby optimizing appeal.[30,31]

It is important to make clear that the term "averageness" as used here does not indicate a rating of mid-level attractiveness, but rather indicates a representation of facial features that is closer to the population mean. Orthodontists have utilized cephalometric population norms and analyses for this very purpose for the better part of a century. Witness the plethora of cephalometric analyses in the orthodontic literature. Attempts to correct patients' dental and skeletal relationships to published cephalometric standards reflect a clinical predilection to accept averageness as attractive.

To the extent that an individual has a mental representation of an average face, he/she has a *prototype* in mind. "Cognitive representations, called prototypes, may be defined as a central exemplar or 'average' of a category... prototypes are perceived as 'typical' and are 'good' examples of a category of stimuli."[27] Faces which typify an average of faces within the population are proposed to have features which coincide more closely with the mathematical mean of the population.

Why is Averageness Attractive?

Preference for Prototypes. First there may be an innate cognitive preference for prototypic members of categories, including human faces.[32] Also prototypes may be useful components for engaging in cognitive "heuristics," i.e., making decisions more quickly on less information, sometimes called "*frugal heuristics.*" Some researchers have posited that on an evolutionary scale, a face that is closer to representing the population average could be quickly recognized as a member of the same species as the observer.[33] An early capacity to quickly identify and be attracted to a prototypical human face could have constituted an evolutionary advantage. Miller and Fishkin[34] hypothesized that if, indeed, the human infant—who has an unusually long period of utter dependency on caretakers—is "hard-wired" to identify human faces, this "design element" could be adaptive for survival, helping the infant (and later toddler) to identify and maintain proximity to its human caregivers.[34]

Averageness Appears Familiar. Another possible explanation for part of the appeal of averageness is that it makes faces appear more *familiar*, even if never seen before, and facial familiarity is associated with perceived attractiveness.[35] Mita et al[36] found that people like the look of their own face better when viewed as it would look in a mirror (as they are accustomed to seeing it), while their friends prefer the photographic (non-mirror) image, in keeping with a familiar view of them.

Mate Selection: Theory that Averageness Equates with "Good Genes". Thornhill and Gangestad[37] proposed that preference for facial averageness could represent an evolved advantage in mate selection, by virtue of average faces being an accurate advertisement of better genes. They theorized that those with more average faces have a more heterozygous (diverse) set of genes which are more resistant to parasites. Propounding a complementary theory, they hypothesized that potential mates representing non-average genotypes (and hence, having less-average faces) are more likely to be genetically homozygous for potentially detrimental alleles—presumably rendering them more susceptible to parasites which are typically adapted to exploit common vulnerabilities of a specific host population.

Symmetry

Averageness Versus Symmetry

A potential critique of the "averageness hypothesis" is grounded on the fact that "average faces are typically more symmetrical than individual ones."[38] This raises the question as to whether the real attractiveness factor underlying averageness is symmetry, as some researchers have theorized.[39] However, faces composed of perfectly symmetrical features which are nonetheless unattractive can easily be imagined.

Faces naturally have a (greater or lesser) degree of bilateral asymmetry. Some studies designed to ascertain the potential contribution of symmetry to attractiveness use computer-created symmetric facial photos called "chimeras," which subjects typically rate for attractiveness in comparison to less symmetric versions (Fig. 5-2).

Current research suggests that both averageness and symmetry contribute to attractiveness. Rhodes et al[40] found that symmetry impacts attractiveness independent of averageness, but averageness appears more robust. Rubenstein et al[27] concluded that "averageness is the only characteristic discovered to date that is both necessary and sufficient to ensure facial attractiveness—without a facial configuration close to the average of the population, a face will not be attractive...no matter how symmetrical. Averageness is fundamental."

The essential role of averageness in attractiveness notwithstanding, symmetry has been found to correlate positively with attractiveness, and asymmetry has been found to have a negative correlation with assessments of

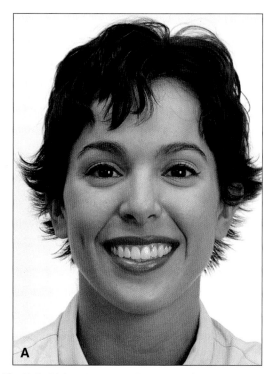 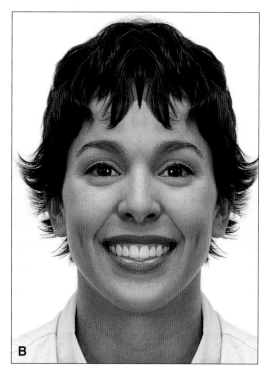

Fig. 5-2 **A** Initial photograph of a model. **B** Chimeric photograph created from the original photograph of the same model in which the right facial hemisphere has been mirrored on the left to create a symmetric image.

attractiveness.[41,42] In one novel experiment designed to see if symmetry was an independent predictor of attractiveness, Mealy et al[43] studied sets of monozygotic twins. While genetically identical, phenotypic expression differs due to developmental differences—and hence, so does the amount of symmetry between members of the identical-twin dyad. The more facially-symmetric twin within each of the 34 pairs was consistently rated as the more attractive of the two.

Why is Symmetry an Important Aspect of Attractiveness?

Symmetry May Signal Genetic Fitness and/or Good Health. It is hypothesized that facial symmetry may be a marker of good health and/or good genes and developmental stability. Environmental stressors such as parasites and pollutants are postulated to cause asymmetry, i.e., fluctuating asymmetry (FA), unless an organism is strong enough, e.g., via good-enough genes, to withstand the disturbances without impact on its symmetry. On an evolutionary analysis, selecting a mate with good genes facilitates passing on good genes to offspring, thereby improving the offspring's viability and consequently propagating that gene set. It is hypothesized that the predilection for symmetry to add to perceived attractiveness is an evolved tendency to avoid mates with physical cues connoting poor genes and/or health.[44] But does symmetry correlate with good genes or good health?

A number of physical and psychological abnormalities correlate with minor physical anomalies, including those of the head and face. Thornhill and Moller[45] have found correlations between minor physical anomalies and genetic or mental impairments: Down syndrome, schizophrenia, autism, and learning disabilities. Zebrowitz[4] specifies several other links: cretinism (due to thyroid deficiency) characterized by, for example, atypical ears; impaired brain development associated with a receding chin and forehead; fetal alcohol syndrome with characteristic atypical facial features signifying mild mental deficiency; and schizophrenia, which may be associated with crooked smiles.

Given the variety of psychological and physical abnormalities associated with facial anomalies, any potential psychological cue, such as facial asymmetry, may be perceived as less attractive due to some (hypothetically, hard-wired and usually subconscious) perception of lesser fitness. It is possible that the majority of small deviations from the population norm or from symmetry may not be indicative of lesser fitness in given individuals, if at all. However cognitive processing heuristics may result in a "sickness similarity" *over*generalization from facial anomalies truly indicative of lesser fitness to similar facial stimuli, signaling potential mates—potentially without cause—to stay away.[4]

So far there is mixed evidence for the link between a person's physiological health status and attractiveness. On the one hand, some studies fail to find a correlation.

For example, Kalick et al,[46] using photographs from late adolescence for a group of 164 males and 169 females, failed to find attractiveness ratings predictive of health data gathered from adolescence through later adulthood. However, a meta-analysis of the literature by Langlois et al[5] revealed at least a tentative connection. As they note, some measures used thus far in studies are questionable (e.g. blood pressure, which could arguably be adversely affected by the discriminatory treatment that unattractive individuals tend to face, rather than signifying underlying genetic weakness). Given the importance of the proposed link between health and attractiveness posited by evolutionary fitness theories, the subject warrants further investigation.[5]

Babyfaceness or Facial Neoteny

An infant's face characteristically has features which distinguish it from a mature face. Picturing a baby's face, a layperson can probably readily call to mind a number of the aspects which have been identified by researchers as typical of infants. These "neotenous" characteristics include a large forehead with lower set eyes, nose and mouth; a smaller, shorter, more recessive chin; fuller lips; larger eyes; a smaller nose; higher, thinner eyebrows; and a rounder, less angular face.[4] The presence of babyface features has been correlated with attractiveness for both females and males, although the effect is more consistent and larger for females, and is curvilinear (increasing, and then at a point, reducing attractiveness) for males.[47,48] Adult females tend to retain more neoteny than male faces and as such babyfaceness is to a degree definitional of facial feminity.[49] However, adult male and female faces rated most attractive also exhibit some mature components constituting secondary sexual characteristics, e.g., high cheekbones in women and larger chins in males[47,48] (Box 5-1).

Why is Babyfaceness Attractive?

Studies have shown that babyfaceness tends to have a natural appeal to human adults, eliciting sympathy and care, and deterring aggression. On an evolutionary analysis, infants and children who were better able to elicit more caretaking by displaying such "cute" and appealing features as large eyes may have had a better survival rate, producing similarly babyfaced children. In a complementary selection process, those parents who responded to neotenous characteristics with heightened caretaking behavior are posited to have raised more surviving offspring.[51]

Neotenous features may also have been adaptive for mate selection for several reasons. In female adults, youthfulness is associated with fertility and lengthier reproductive prospects.[51] Also the same neotenous features that elicit care and deter aggression toward children are proposed to do so for adults, and so may have helped to produce a secure and nurturing bond between mates, particularly by deterring male aggression.[52] As noted above, female faces generally retain more neoteny, and so neoteny is in part definitional of facial femininity. Male faces which are to an extent "feminized" have been found to be associated with raters' attributions of being a "good parent" and correlate with higher ratings by females as desirable longterm mate prospects than wholly masculinized faces. A review of the literature reveals that women tend to find some combined balance of masculine and feminine (alternately fairly neotenous) features in men most attractive, with preferences shifting toward the masculine (e.g. larger chin and brow ridge) during the phase of their menstrual cycle when most likely to conceive[53] (Box 5-2).

Babyface Stereotype

An abundance of research has identified a "babyface" stereotype in which observers have a tendency to view individuals whose features are neotenous as having certain traits typically ascribed to children. Studies have found

---

Box 5-1	Sexual dimorphism and mate selection

It is hypothesized that certain exaggerated secondary sex characteristics may advertise "good genes" to prospective mates because the sex hormones (especially testosterone) required to produce them during pubescence places a handicap on the immune system. Therefore only the more immunocompetent individuals can reach adulthood having been able to "afford" these costly sexual displays.[44,50] Also certain facial features associated with estrogen during development are found particularly attractive in females, e.g., fuller lips, and are postulated as possible honest "advertisements" of female fertility.[50] In addition, secondary sex characteristics help to indicate that a prospective mate has reached the age of reproductive capacity.

Box 5-2	Opposite sex attractiveness: multiple theories

The fact that women tend to find a blend of masculine and feminine features attractive in men has been hypothesized to be a function of desiring a combination of qualities, e.g., the "good genes" signaled by masculine features, and the perceived propensity for caretaking (and consequent investment in offspring) stereotypically attributed to feminized faces.[53] One hypothesis regarding female shift in desire for more masculine faces during the high-risk conception phase is that as a short-term mating strategy, women may seek copulation with men likely to provide "good genes,"[54] represented by exaggerated masculine features.[55] Alternately there are compelling evolutionary arguments for the highly adaptive value of pair-bonding and longterm mating strategies,[34,56] as well as adaptation to cooperative group-level social environments.[34,57] Also, it is important to bear in mind that in the overall picture, while attractiveness is generally valued in prospective life mates, research reveals that other personal qualities such as provision of social support, acceptance, and honesty are ranked above attractiveness. Cunningham et al found attractiveness ranked fifth in level of importance by men, and seventh by women.[58]

babyfaced adults to be perceived as more honest, warm, approachable, friendly, dependent, intellectually naïve, physically weak, and submissive than their mature-faced peers.[4,59]

This babyface stereotype, based on an overgeneralization of childlike traits to bearers of childlike faces, can be attended by benefits. For example, in employment simulation studies, babyfaced job applicants were favored over those with mature-looking faces for jobs involving warmth and social sensitivity.[52] Babyfaceness can also be advantageous in the courtroom. In a study of over 500 small claims court cases, there was a robust finding that babyfaced defendants were judged less guilty of intentional crimes when they plead innocence than mature-faced defendants, perhaps due to the attribution of greater honesty and social appeal.[60] Research also shows that individuals with neotenous faces tend to elicit more help from others.[52] In one such study, Keating et al[61] left fictitious identical "lost" job résumés in public areas (e.g., indoor malls and outdoor sidewalks) with attached photographs which had been computer manipulated to look either more mature faced or more babyfaced. This was achieved by either decreasing lip and eye size, or enlarging them, respectively. A self-addressed, stamped envelope was attached to the packet. In order to elicit sympathy from whoever found the "lost" résumé, the application indicated that the applicant sought "to obtain a job…that will allow me to relocate near my family." The hypothesis that the babyfaced photograph would elicit more helping behavior was supported overall, with a generally higher return rate of such résumés, compared to those with less neotenous photographs.

In terms of persuasive ability, being babyfaced tends to confer credibility based on attributions of honesty and sincerity. However, those with more mature features tend to be perceived as higher in expertise and knowledgeability. Zebrowitz[4] observed that advertisers exploit the different persuasive strengths of mature versus babyfaced individuals by strategically type-casting them in commercials according to whether credibility, e.g., as in personal testimonials, or expertise is most likely to influence the target audience.

Profile Considerations

Orthodontists from Angle[62] to McLaughlin[63] have emphasized the importance of profile analysis in the assessment of facial esthetics. Angle's classification of malocclusion, originally applied strictly to dental occlusal relationships, has been extended to include sagittal anteroposterior relationships of the facial skeleton and the soft tissue profile as well. Thus orthodontists commonly speak of "skeletal class IIs" or "Class I profiles". Even prior to Angle, Woolnoth[64] noted "The straight face is considered the handsomest…The profile falls vertical down the brow and again from upper lip to point of chin." Clearly the esthetic preference for a straight profile dominates the profile literature of orthodontics. Charles Tweed enthusiastically expounded the esthetic preference for a Class I profile.[65]

While social psychological research on facial attractiveness has predominantly focused on frontal assessments, several studies provide support for the hypothesis that the straight profile is more appealing. For example, in a study on dentofacial appearance, Lucker et al[66] explored which occlusal characteristics, both frontal and profile, contribute to a child's facial esthetic evaluations of peer-aged children. Provided with frontal and profile photographs of children ranging from 10 to 14 years old, peers (children aged 10–13) were more likely to say that a face had "nothing wrong" with it if a Class I profile was evident in the assessment photographs. Conversely, children were more likely to identify photographs of children with a retrognathic or prognathic profile as having "something wrong with it" than a "straight profile" (Fig. 5-3).

Why is the Straight Profile Attractive?

The evolutionary advantage of a straight profile preference has been hypothesized as connoting appropriate masticatory function to potential mates. This attribute may have conferred enhanced survival and subsequent reproductive success to individuals possessing it and as such, may have been a selective psychological cue in mate selection.[30]

Expressiveness

Facial "expressiveness" is comprised of features which cue perceivers to infer responsiveness, friendliness, openness, interest in the perceiver, and/or approachability, e.g., low dominance. For example, dilated pupils may be interpreted (likely subconsciously) by a perceiver as showing interest in him/her. Raised eyebrows may convey openness, non-dominance, interest, happiness and/or flirtatious attention. Fuller lips convey babyfaceness (and hence, e.g., approachability), tend to be associated with higher levels of estrogen during development (hence femininity), and fuller, redder lips are associated with sexual excitement in both sexes.[4] Smiling, a dynamic expressive feature, can convey a variety of prosocial states, such as friendliness, agreeableness, and social supportiveness.[51]

Cunningham et al[51] suggested that research trends reveal expressive features to be particularly attractive in women. The presence of some of the above expressive features in males, such as smiling, has heightened attractiveness ratings by contemporary women—when balanced by mature, masculine features, such as thick eyebrows and a large chin.[47] Some researchers[67] have noted that across primates and humans raised brows (one aspect of "expressiveness") can connote receptivity or submission, while lowered brow expressions are associated with dominance. They also found that non-smiling poses were rated as slightly higher in dominance.[67] The extent to which preferences regarding expressivity features are enculturated versus biologically driven/selected remains open to specula-tion. However, according to an evolutionary "multiple fitness model" of mate selection, female preference for a seemingly paradoxical blend of facial

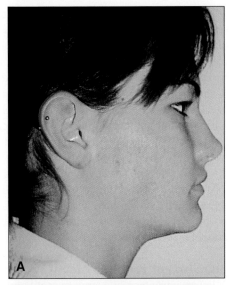

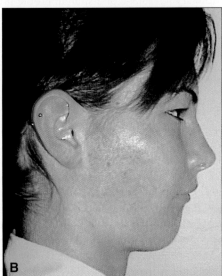

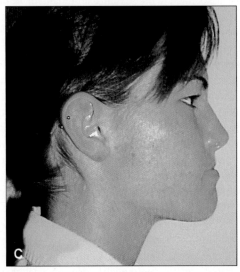

Fig. 5-3 A "Straight", **B** retrognathic, and **C** prognathic profile.

qualities may represent an evolved attraction to a complementary balance of expressiveness connoting social warmth, and dominance cues signaling a male's propensity to be protective and to compete for mate/offspring-beneficial resources.[47]

Expressiveness: The Smile

The orthodontic literature is rife with descriptions of what constitutes an attractive smile: appropriate tip and torque of incisors, down–up–down vertical configuration of the central–lateral–cuspid incisal edges, appropriate gingival display, minimal buccal corridors with cuspids just inside the labial commissures, and phi ratios of crown length/width as well as central width/lateral width. It is not the purpose of this section to reiterate well-known dogma with respect to appropriate tooth positioning within the labial arcade of the smile, but rather to focus on several social psychological findings regarding the smile.

Ekman and colleagues' early pioneering studies[68] of universal emotions and the pancultural facial configurations which convey them revealed at least five universally recognizable combinations (for happiness, fear, surprise, anger, disgust, and sadness). Disgust, for example, is universally expressed by certain facial movements, central to which is a scrunched-up nose gesture. Happiness or enjoyment is universally expressed by upturned lips and corners of the mouth: the smile.

Some smiles are voluntarily enacted social displays used primarily as means to accomplishing social goals, while others (albeit potentially socially beneficial) arise spontaneously out of inner contentment or pleasure. There is evidence that the former type of smile tends to involve the mouth only, while the most genuine smiles—truly representing subjective enjoyment—involve muscles around both the mouth and the eyes. Darwin expressed his indebtedness to Duchenne de Boulogne, a French anatomist, for making this early, keen observation. In 1862, Duchenne wrote: "The emotion of frank joy is expressed on the face by the combined contraction of the zygomaticus major muscle and the orbicularis oculi. The first obeys the will but the second is only put in play by the sweet emotions of the soul…"[69]

Accordingly, Ekman et al[70] suggested that this kind of "felt smile" be called the "Duchenne smile." Scientific research has confirmed Duchenne's discovery. For example, Ekman et al[70] had raters observe and code subjects' expressions as they watched films which were likely to produce genuine amusement versus films which were not. While there was no difference between the overall amount of smiling in film conditions, there was a significant interaction between film type and smile type: there were more Duchenne smiles during the amusing films, and "D-smiles" also correlated with higher self-reported enjoyment.

Display rules are learned social rules governing regulation of facial expression. While smiling is usually socially positive, there are cases when it is deemed appropriate to refrain from smiling, e.g., when hiding enjoyment of others' misfortune.[71] In other cases, smiling is socially sanctioned, whether genuine or not. A meta-analysis derived from 162 research reports found that women and girls smile more than their male counterparts, and a study of potential moderators supported the authors' hypothesis that females smile more according to whether "gender-appropriate" behavioral rules and roles are conspicuous in a given situation.[72] For example, under conditions of social tension, women tended to smile more than men. This is compatible with the theory that management of emotions in a social situation or "emotion work" is often "gendered work." In short, the fact that females smile significantly more than men within socially tense situations may be due to their being socially conditioned to mitigate or diffuse negative emotions and to take care of the emotional needs of others, while concealing their own.

Smiling is generally a very important and positive social behavior for human beings. It is a common and reciprocated greeting, can induce positive mood, build relational rapport, and can serve as a positive reinforcer for behavior change. Infants' moods and responses to the environment can be influenced by parents' smiles.[73]

Indeed, infants can be greatly influenced by the absence of smiling or expressionlessness on an adult face. So-called "still-face" experiments involve play between an infant and parent in which the parent maintains an unresponsive and expressionless face while interacting with the infant. Studies reveal that infants consistently show increased grimacing, distress, and crying, and decreased smiling and gazing at the parent.[74] From infancy, people appear to crave and expect facial responsiveness, and to be distressed when that expectation is frustrated when interacting with nonexpressive faces.

Positive facial expression, conveyed by smiling, has been found to generally increase ratings of attractiveness. For example, studies have shown that women and men find the expressive feature of a big smile attractive in the opposite sex.[47,48] Moreover, smiling can elicit more positive person perceptions, e.g., of sociability, kindness, and sincerity.[4,75]

Attractive and Smiling Faces Make Us Feel Good

Recent research utilizing event-related functional magnetic resonance imaging (fMRI) technology suggests that adults actually respond neurologically to an attractive and happy face as if it were a reward stimulus. O'Doherty et al[76] hypothesized that facial attractiveness and smiling would evoke fMRI-measurable responses in regions of the brain typically activated by reward stimuli. Their hypothesis was supported by a study in which subjects viewed attractive and unattractive faces while monitored by fMRI. Based on their findings, the researchers concluded that viewing attractive faces is experienced as a reward stimulus, and

viewing *smiling* attractive faces further increases reward-associated brain activity.

Indeed, the positive affect (emotion) thought to be induced by attractive/pleasant faces has been used to help explain the attractiveness "halo effect," wherein attractiveness is associated with stereotypically positive evaluations.[4,77] Research has demonstrated that in general, when people are in a good mood, they tend to render more positive judgments of others.[6] Coupled with evidence that facial attractiveness tends to invoke pleasant emotions,[76,77] perceivers may be predisposed by mood to render more positive trait and behavioral inferences about an attractive target.

The fact that smiling can enhance attractiveness reveals one of the possible ways that individuals can be empowered to help "level the playing field" with respect to the attractiveness halo. To the extent that smiling enhances a person's perceived attractiveness and induces positive emotion in the perceiver, a less attractive individual may be able to mitigate negative attributions or increase positive attributions made about him/herself by smiling in social situations. Not infrequently, orthodontists hear of patients' reluctance to smile due to self-consciousness about their teeth. Gently encouraging patients to overcome such inhibitions and to smile whenever they feel inclined (depending on their goals/appropriate display rules) may help them to benefit from the attractiveness halo—regardless of stage of treatment.

Conclusion: Functionalist and Soft Tissue Paradigms

Throughout the 20th century, the functionalist paradigm prevailed as the major philosophy of dentistry. Functional considerations were deemed the ultimate indications for dental and orthodontic treatment. Heavy emphasis was placed in dental school curricula on functional occlusion: tripod centric stops with cuspid rise and anterior guidance on Posselt excursions. Treatment rendered in the name of curing, preventing, or restoring the effects of disease was deemed of paramount importance. As a result of this paradigm, procedures done to improve a patient's appearance were deemed cosmetic and of lesser importance than dentistry rendered to deal with disease and its sequelae. The tenets of the functionalist paradigm were so restrictive that procedures performed with the specific goal of improving facial appearance were deemed "elective" and not really necessary. This hierarchy of priorities held so much sway that funding provided by third parties for dental treatment frequently denied or placed extreme restrictions on what would be covered for "cosmetic" purposes. As a result, many dental insurers either denied coverage for orthodontic care or imposed ridiculously low "lifetime maximums" for orthodontic coverage.

Fortunately, the functionalist paradigm is on the wane. It is crystal clear from the evidence presented from over a half century of social psychology literature that facial esthetics can affect every aspect of a patient's life. As shown above, facial attractiveness can influence social success from infancy to geronition. It can affect the quality and quantity of nurturing an infant receives. It can influence academic expectations and outcomes of students from elementary school through college. It can influence whether or not a job applicant is hired for a particular position and what level of income he/she can eventually expect. The powerful effect of facial attractiveness can influence the process of mate selection. It can even influence whether a person is found guilty or innocent in a court of law.

Historically, diagnostic emphasis has been placed on the skeletal and dental relationships as determined by two-dimensional cephalometric and plaster dental casts. Current diagnostic trends, as illustrated by the Arnett analysis (Fig. 5-4), still consider skeletal and occlusal relationships but place appropriate emphasis on soft tissue relationships and facial esthetics. It is hard to imagine any other aspect of dentistry that is more important or even more functional—to use an obsolete buzzword—than facial esthetics. Various authors have described a new paradigm, the *soft tissue paradigm*, that recognizes the influential importance of facial esthetics on the quality of a patient's life, and places functional and esthetic considerations in an appropriate relationship—on a par—in the hierarchy of necessities.

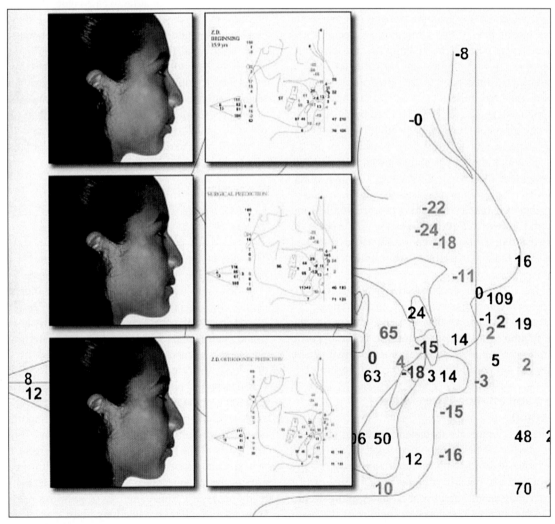

Fig. 5-4 Example of the Arnett analysis, which emphasizes soft tissue relationships and facial esthetics. (From Keim RG: JCO Interviews Dr. Richard McLaughlin. Journal of Clinical Orthondontics 38(4), 199–210, April 2004).

REFERENCES

1. Graber T. In: Lucker GW, Ribbens KA, McNamara JA, eds. Psychological aspects of facial form. Craniofacial Growth Series. Michigan: Ann Arbor, 1980.
2. Aronson E, Wilson TD, Akert RM. Social psychology, 3rd edn. New York: Longman, 1988.
3. Hassebrauck M. The visual process method: A new method to study physical attractiveness. Evolution Hum Behav 1998;19:111–123.
4. Zebrowitz LA. Reading faces: Window to the soul? Boulder: Westview Press, 1988.
5. Langlois JH, Kalakanis LE, Rubenstein AJ, Larson AD, Hallam MJ, Smoot MT. Maxims or myths of beauty: A meta-analytic and theoretical overview. Psychol Bull 2000;126:390–423.
6. Fiske ST, Taylor SE. Social cognition, 2nd edn. New York: McGraw-Hill, 1991.
7. Eagley AH, Ashmore RD, Makhijani MG, Longo LC. What is beautiful is good, but…: A meta-analytic review of research on the physical attractiveness stereotype. Psychol Bull 1991;110:109–128.
8. Dermer M, Thiel DL. When beauty may fail. J Personality Soc Psychol 1975;31:1168–1176.
9. Langlois JH, Ritter JM, Casey RJ, Sawin DB. Infant attractiveness predicts maternal behaviors and attitudes. Dev Psychol 1995;31:466–472.
10. Field TM, Vega-Lahr N. Early interactions between infants with cranio-facial anomalies and their mothers. Infant Behav Dev 1984;7:527–530.
11. Parke RD, Hymel S, Power T, Tinsley B. Fathers and risk: A hospital based model of intervention. In: Sawin DB, chair. Symposium on psychosocial risks during infancy, University of Texas, Austin, November 1977. As cited in Langlois JH, Ritter JM, Casey RJ, Sawin DB. Infant attractiveness predicts maternal behaviors and attitudes. Dev Psychol 1995;31:466–472.
12. Elder GH, Van Nguyen T, Caspi A. Linking family hardship to children's lives. Child Dev 1985;56:361–375.
13. Berkowitz L, Frodi L. Reactions to a child's mistakes as affected by her/his looks or speech. Soc Psychol Q 1979;42:420–425.
14. Clifford M, Walster E. The effects of physical attractiveness on teacher expectation. Sociol Educ 1973;46:248.
15. Rosenthal R. Covert communication in classrooms, clinics, courtrooms, and cubicles. Am Psychol 2002;57:839–849.
16. Rosenthal R. Teachers' expectancies: Determinants of pupils' IQ gains. Psychol Rep 1966;19:115–118.
17. White KJ, Jones K, Sherman MD. Reputation information and teacher feedback: their influences on children's perceptions of behavior problem peers. J Soc Clin Psychol 1998;17:11–37.
18. Klein J, producer. The value of beauty, 20/20, ABC News. As cited in Zebrowitz LA. Reading faces: window to the Soul? Boulder: Westview Press, 1998.
19. Hosoda M, Stone-Romero EF, Coats G. The effects of physical attractiveness on job-related outcomes: A meta-analysis of experimental studies. Personnel Psychol 2003;56:431–462.
20. Stevenage SV, McKay Y. Model applicants: The effect of facial appearance on recruitment decisions. Br J Psychol 1999;90:221–234.

21. Frieze IH, Olson JE, Russell J. Attractiveness and income for men and women in management. J Applied Soc Psychol 1991;21:1039–1057.
22. Harvard Law Review 1987:2035. As cited in Zebrowitz LA. Reading faces: window to the soul? Boulder: Westview Press, 1998.
23. Shaw WC, O'Brien KD, Richmond S, Brook P. Quality control in orthodontics: Risk/benefit considerations. Br Dental J 1991;170:33–37.
24. Rahbar F. Changes in self-esteem and self-concept as a result of orthodontic treatment: Master's thesis, University of Southern California, 2001.
25. Dennington RJ. The self-concept of seventy-seven orthodontic patients treated at St. Louis University. Master's thesis, St Louis University, 1975.
26. O'Brien K, Wright J, Conboy F, et al. Effectiveness of early orthodontic treatment with the twin-block appliance: A multicenter, randomized, controlled trial. Part 2: Psychosocial effects: Am J Orthod Dental Orthop 2003;124:5.
27. Rubenstein AJ, Langlois JH, Roggman LA. What makes a face attractive and why: The role of averageness in defining facial beauty. In: Rhodes G, Zebrowitz LA, eds. Facial attractiveness: Evolutionary, cognitive, and social perspectives. Advances in Visual Cognition. Westport: Ablex, 2002.
28. Langlois JH, Roggman LA, Rieser-Danner LA. Infants' differential social responses to attractive and unattractive faces. Dev Psychol 1990;26:153–159.
29. Langlois JH, Roggman LA. Attractive faces are only average. Psychol Sci 1990;1:115–121.
30. Rhodes G, Harwood K, Yoshikawa S, Nishitani M, McLean I. The attractiveness of average faces: cross-cultural evidence and possible biological basis. In: Rhodes G, Zebrowitz LA, eds. Facial attractiveness: evolutionary, cognitive, and social perspectives. Westport: Ablex, 2002.
31. Geldart S, Maurer D, Carney K. Effects of eye size on adults' aesthetic ratings of faces and 5-month-old's looking times. Perception 1999;28:361–374.
32. Whitfield TW, Slatter PE. The effects of categorization and prototypicality on aesthetic choice in a furniture selection task. Br J Psychol 1979;70:65–75.
33. Penton-Voak I, Perrett D. Consistency and individual differences in facial attractiveness judgements: An evolutionary perspective. Soc Res 2000;67:219–242.
34. Miller LC, Fishkin SA. On the dynamics of human bonding and reproductive success: Seeking windows on the adapted-for human-environmental interface. In: Simpson JA, Kenrick DT, eds. Evolutionary social psychology. Mahwah, NJ: Lawrence Erlbaum Associates, 1997.
35. Monin B. The warm glow heuristic: When liking leads to familiarity. J Personality Soc Psychol 2003;85:1035–1048.
36. Mita TH, Dermer M, Knight J. Reversed facial images and the mere-exposure hypothesis. J Personality Soc Psychol 1977;5:597–601.
37. Thornhill R, Gangestad SW. Human facial beauty: Averageness, symmetry, and parasite resistance. Hum Nature 1993;4:237–269.
38. Enquist E, Ghirlanda S, Lundqvist D, Wachtmeister C. An ethological theory of attractiveness. In: Rhodes G, Zebrowitz LA, eds. Facial attractiveness: Evolutionary,

cognitive, and social perspectives. Westport: Ablex, 2002:136.

39. Alley TR, Cunningham MR. Averaged faces are attractive, but very attractive faces are not average. Psychol Sci 1991;2:123–125.

40. Rhodes G, Sumich A, Byatt G. Are average facial configurations attractive only because of their symmetry? Psychol Sci 1999;10:52–58.

41. Grammer K, Thornhill R. Human (Homo sapiens) facial attractiveness and sexual selection: The role of symmetry and averageness. J Comparative Psychol 1994;108:233–242.

42. Jones BC, Little AC, Penton-Voak IS, Tiddeman BP, Burt DM, Perrett DI. Facial symmetry and judgements of apparent health: Support for a "good genes" explanation of the attractiveness-symmetry relationship. Evolution Hum Behav 2001;22:417–429.

43. Mealy L, Bridgstock R, Townsend GC. Symmetry and perceived facial attractiveness: A monozygotic co-twin comparison. J Personality Soc Psychol 1999;76:151–158.

44. Thornhill R, Gangestad S. Human facial beauty: Averageness, symmetry, and parasite resistance. Hum Nature 1993;4:237–269.

45. Thornhill R, Møller AP. Developmental stability, disease and medicine. Biol Rev 1997;72:497–548.

46. Kalick SM, Zebrowitz LA, Langlois JH, Johnson RM. Does human facial attractiveness honestly advertise health? Longitudinal data on an evolutionary question. Psychol Sci 1998;9:8–13.

47. Cunningham MR, Barbee AP, Pike CL. What do women want? Facialmetric assessment of multiple motives in the perception of male facial physical attractiveness. J Personality Soc Psychol 1990;59:61–72.

48. Cunningham MR. Measuring the physical in physical attractiveness: Quasi-experiments on the sociobiology of female facial beauty: Interpersonal relations and group processes. J Personality Soc Psychol 1986;50:925–935.

49. Zebrowitz LA. Stability of babyfaceness and attractiveness across the life span. J Personality Soc Psychol 1993;64:453–466.

50. Grammer K, Fink B, Juette A, Ronzal G, Thornhill R. Female faces and bodies: N-Dimensional feature space and attractiveness. In: Rhodes G, Zebrowitz LA, eds. Facial attractiveness: evolutionary, cognitive, and social perspectives. Westport: Ablex, 2002:91–125.

51. Cunningham MR, Barbee AP, Philhower CL. Dimensions of facial physical attractiveness: The intersection of biology and culture. In: Rhodes G, Zebrowtiz LA, eds. Facial attractiveness: evolutionary, cognitive, and social perspectives. Westport: Ablex, 2002:193–238.

52. Keating CF. Charasmatic faces. Social status cues put face appeal in context. In: Rhodes G, Zebrowitz LA, eds. Facial attractiveness: Evolutionary, cognitive, and social perspectives. Westport: Ablex, 2002:153–192.

53. Little AC, Penton-Voak IS, Burt DM, Perrett DI. Evolution and individual differences in the perception of attractiveness: How cyclic hormonal changes and self-perceived attractiveness influence female preferences for male faces. In: Rhodes G, Zebrowitz LA, eds. Facial attractiveness: Evolutionary, cognitive, and social perspectives. Westport: Ablex, 2002:59–192.

54. Buss DM, Schmitt DP. Sexual strategies theory: An evolutionary perspective on human mating. Psychol Rev 1993;100:204–232.

55. Penton-Voak IS, Little AC, Jones BC, Burt DM, Tiddeman BP, Perrett DI. Female condition influences preferences for sexual dimorphism in faces of male humans (Homo sapiens). J Comparative Psychol 2003;117:264–271.

56. Miller LC, Putcha-Bhagavatula A, Pedersen WC. Men's and women's mating preferences: distinct evolutionary mechanisms? Curr Directions Psychol Sci 2002;11:88–93.

57. Caporeal LR, Brewer MB. Hierarchical evolutionary theory: there is an alternative and it's not creationism. Psychol Inquiry 1995;6:31–80.

58. Cunningham MR, Rowatt TJ, Shamblen S, et al. Men and women are from earth: Life-trajectory dynamics in mate choices. University of Louisville. As cited in Cunningham MR, Barbee AP, Philhower CL. Dimensions of facial physical attractiveness: The intersection of biology and culture. In: Rhodes G, Zebrowitz LA, eds. Facial attractiveness: evolutionary, cognitive, and social perspectives. Westport: Ablex, 2002:193-238.

59. Zebrowitz LA, Montepare JM. Impressions of babyfaced individuals across the life span. Dev Psychol 1992;28:1143–1152.

60. Zebrowitz LA, McDonald SM. The impact of litigants' babyfacedness and attractiveness on adjudications in small claims courts. Law Hum Behav 1991;15:603–623.

61. Keating CF, Randall DW, Kendrick T, Gutshall K. Do babyfaced adults receive more help? The (cross-cultural) case of the lost résumé. J Nonverbal Behav 2003;27:89-109.

62. Angle EH. Treatment of malocclusion of the teeth and fractures of the maxillae. Angle's system, 6th edn. Philadelphia, SS White Dental Mfg Co, 1990.

63. Arnett GA, McLaughlin RP. Facial and dental planning for orthodontists and oral surgeons. St Louis: Mosby, 2004.

64. Woolnoth T. The study of the human face. London: Tweedie:1865:181–244. Cited in Peck H, Peck S. A concept of facial esthetics. Angle Orthod 1970;40:289.

65. Tweed CH. Clinical orthodontics. St Louis: Mosby, 1966.

66. Lucker GW, Graber LW, Pietromonaco P. The importance of dentofacial appearance in facial esthetics: A signal detection approach. Basic Appl Soc Psychol 1981;2:261–274.

67. Keating CF, Mazur A, Segall MH, et al. Culture and the perception of social dominance from facial expression. J Personality Soc Psychol 1981;40:615–626.

68. Fridlund AJ, Ekman P, Oster H. Facial expressions of emotion: Review of the literature, 1970–1983. In: Siegman AW, Feldstein S, eds. Nonverbal behavior and communication, 2nd edn. Hillsdale: Erlbaum, 1987.

69. Duchenne B. The mechanism of human facial expression or an electro-physiological analysis of the expression of emotions. (A Cutherbertson, translator). New York: Cambridge University Press, 1990. (Original work published 1862).

70. Ekman P, Friesen WV, Davidson RJ. The Duchenne smile: Emotional expression and brain physiology II. J Personality Soc Psychol 1990;58:342–353.

71. Salem JE. Development and validation of a self-report measure of adherence to display rules for the facial expression of emotion. Dissertation Abstracts Int: Section B: Sci Eng 1999;9:3712.

72. LaFrance M, Paluck EL, Hecht MA. The contingent smile: A meta-analysis of sex differences in smiling. Psychol Bull 2003;129:305–334.

73. Knapp ML, Hall JA. Nonverbal communication in human interaction, 4th edn. Fort Worth, Harcourt Brace Publishers, 1997.

74. Delgado CEF, Messinger DS, Yale ME. Infant responses to direction of parental gaze: A comparison of two still-face conditions. Infant Behav Dev 2002;25:311–318.

75. Otta E, Abrosio FFE, Hoshino RL. Reading a smiling face: Messages conveyed by various forms of smiling. Perceptual Motor Skills 1996;82:1111–1121.

76. O'Doherty JO, Winston J, Critchley H, Perrett D, Burt DM, Dolan RJ. Beauty in a smile: the role of medial orbitofrontal cortex in facial attractiveness. Neuropsychologia 2003;41:147–155.

77. Mehrabian A, Blum JS. Physical appearance, attractiveness, and the mediating role of emotions. Curr Psychol Dev Learning Personality Soc 1997;16:20–42.

78. Sarver DM. Esthetic orthodontics and orthognathic surgery. St Louis: Mosby, 1998.

79. Proffit WR. The soft tissue paradigm. Annual Cecil Steiner Memorial Lecture, University of Southern California, February, 2004.

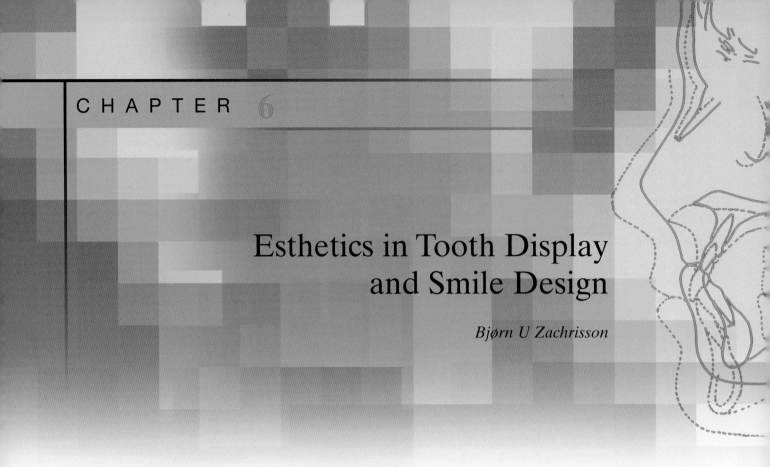

CHAPTER 6

Esthetics in Tooth Display and Smile Design

Bjørn U Zachrisson

The orthodontic profession has always been in pursuit of the ideal dentition. The profession is now on the threshold of a paradigm shift that apparently will change the fundamental conceptual basis of orthodontics and the traditional emphasis in diagnosis and treatment planning.[1,2] The former emphasis on dental and skeletal components is still valid, but greater attention to the soft tissue aspects of orthodontics is now required. In an effort to create natural esthetics, the orthodontist must give careful consideration to the patient in his/her entirety. Individual attributes of a tooth or segment of teeth may represent only part of the story, because teeth do not exist individually and separate from the patient to whom they belong. Combinations of tooth positions can create an effect that is greater than, equal to, or less than the sum of the parts.[3] The discipline of esthetics in orthodontics can be broken down into at least four parts: microesthetics (the elements that make teeth look like teeth); gingival esthetics; macroesthetics (the principles that apply when groupings of individual teeth are considered); and facial esthetics.[3] The focus of this chapter will be the principles of macro-esthetics in orthodontics and how to apply them clinically. The dynamic relationship between the teeth and the surrounding soft tissues during and after orthodontic corrections, and the patient's facial characteristics will be emphasized. The display (amount and shape of crown structure that shows in various views and lip positions) will be related to age, sex, and facial characteristics. The purpose is to provide guidelines for orthodontists on how to analyze esthetic factors by viewing the patient from the front, and to discuss some new concepts on how to achieve the desirable characteristics of tooth display in the vertical and transverse dimensions during normal social interaction.

Evaluating Esthetics in the Dentist's Chair

Esthetics, which is derived from the Greek word for "perception", deals with beauty and the beautiful. It may be divided into two dimensions: objective (admirable) and subjective (enjoyable) beauty.[4] Objective beauty implies that the object possesses properties that make it unmistakably praiseworthy. Subjective beauty is value laden, and is related to the tastes of the person contemplating it. Contemporary techniques in orthodontics should lend objective esthetics to the entire orofacial complex, involving unity, form, structure, balance, color, function, and display of the dentition. In addition, the creation of subjective beauty according to an individual orthodontist's preferences may enhance the cosmetic value of the treatment given to each patient.

In discusssing the principles of visual perception and its clinical application to dentofacial esthetics, Lombardi[5] remarked that detailed esthetic judgments can only be made by viewing patients from the front, in conversation, using facial expressions, and smiling. The traditional dentist's view from above and behind the patient is skewed, differing markedly from the "true" perception of the patient in a mirror or by other persons during normal social interaction.

For example, it is not possible to gain adequate information on details such as midline alignment (maxillary and mandibular relative to facial) and right–left symmetry of canine and premolar crown torque unless the patient is observed directly from the front. A direct "eye-to-eye" view of the dentition can, in fact, be obtained when the patient is sitting in the dentist's chair,[6] and the trick is to move the patient's head to the side of the head rest (Fig. 6-1). By this means, it is possible to analyze important esthetic factors, like:

- Crown lengths of the upper and lower incisors
- Incisal edge contours (before and after recontouring by grinding)
- Position and symmetry of gingival margin levels on the upper and lower anterior teeth
- Axial inclinations of all anterior teeth
- Midlines (maxillary to mandibular and facial)
- Connector areas (the zone in which two adjacent teeth appear to touch)
- Symmetry and degree of crown torque of the canines and premolars
- Harmony of the front-to-back tooth display curve.

After carefully studying these features, the orthodontist can make the required finishing archwire bends and perform any other esthetic procedures needed. For analysis of tooth display when speaking and smiling, and viewing of the buccal corridors on smiling, a better impression is obtained with the patient sitting up or standing in front of the dentist than when sitting in the dentist's chair.[5,6]

Standards of Normality

It is useful for esthetic oral rehabilitation to describe some average desirable smile features. These normative standards may serve as a guideline for enhancement of esthetics for the anterior component of the dentition.

Smile Type – Incisor and Gingival Display

Lip coverage of the maxillary incisors in full smiles can be distinguished into three types: low, average, and high smiles.[7] The most frequent type (about 70% of the young adult population) is the *average* smile that reveals 75–100% of the upper incisors. The *low* smile displays <75% of the maxillary incisors in the full smile and may be found in about 20% of a population, whereas the *high* smile ("gummy smile"), revealing the complete cervicoincisal length of the upper incisors and a contiguous band of gingiva, occurs in about 10% of the US population.[7]

Upper lip coverage tends to increase with age, and therefore the percentage of "gummy smiles" may be greater among younger age groups,[8,9] and smaller among older adults.[10] There is also a sexual dimorphism in that low smile lines are a predominantly male characteristic, and high smiles are predominantly female.[7]

It is noteworthy that some marginal gingival display in smiling is not as objectionable to lay people as orthodontists may imagine.[9,11] A moderately gummy smile should

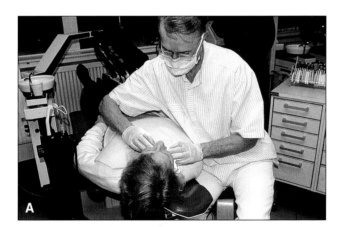

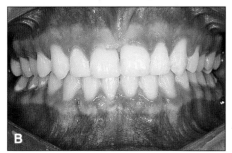

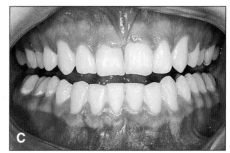

Fig. 6-1 Moving a patient's head to the side of the head rest (**A**) allows a direct frontal view of the dentition (**B**) and a realistic impression of the esthetic features. **C** Incisal edge contours can be examined on slight mouth opening.

therefore be viewed as an acceptable anatomic variation well within the usual range of lip–tooth–jaw relationships, especially for women.[8,9]

Smile Curve (Smile Arc[12])

The relationship of the maxillary incisal curve to the inner contour of the lower lip also can be divided into three types: parallel, straight, and reverse. In a survey of young adults in the Los Angeles area, Tjan et al[7] found that a great majority (85%) had a maxillary incisal smile curve *parallel* to the inner contour of the lower lip, 14% showed a *straight* rather than a curved line, and only 1% had a *reverse* smile curve. Since parallelism is the normal finding in untreated persons, it is the optimal goal for objective beauty in esthetic oral rehabilitations,[13,14] including orthodontic (Figs 6-2 and 6-3) and orthodontic–prosthetic treatment (Fig. 6-4). A straight or reverse smile curve may contribute

to a less attractive facial appearance.[5,13] The reverse curve is frequently associated with marked abrasive wear of the upper incisors.

Number of Teeth Displayed in the Smile

The Los Angeles survey[7] also revealed that in a typical or average smile in young adults, the six maxillary anterior teeth and the first or second premolars are displayed. The number of teeth displayed in the full smiles of 454 students were: six anteriors only, 7%; six anteriors and first premolars, 48.5%; six anteriors and first and second premolars, 40.5%; six anteriors, first and second premolars, and first molars, 4%.

Vertical Position of the Incisors

Normal Age Changes in Lip–Incisor Relationship

There are progressive changes with age in upper and lower lip positions that are caused by the effects of gravity. Some normative studies for the optimal vertical incisor positions in the faces of persons in different age groups have been reported. Peck et al[8] showed that the normal display of maxillary incisors with relaxed lips at 15 years of age is 4.7 mm (SD 2.0 mm) for boys and 5.3 mm (SD 1.8 mm) for girls. The sexual dimorphism is evident at all ages. Vig and Brundo[10] have provided normative mean values for different adult age groups (Table 6-1). Dong et al[15] compared the age changes in maxillary and mandibular incisor display at rest and when smiling (Fig. 6-5) and confirmed the observations that the age changes with relaxed lips were dramatic (Fig. 6-6). Mandibular incisor display shows a corresponding increase with age. The amount of mandibular incisor display after age 60 is approximately equal to the amount of maxillary incisor display before age 30 (Fig. 6-6D). There is a close correlation between

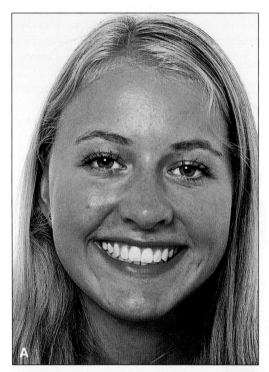

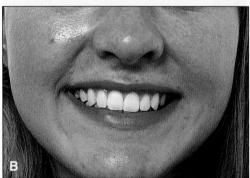

Fig. 6-2 A and **B** Esthetic smile curve (arc) with parallelity between the maxillary teeth and the inner contour of the lower lip. Upright canine and premolar crowns contribute to fullness of smile.

Table 6-1	Maxillary and mandibular incisor display with lips gently parted (in mm). (Modified from Vig RG, Brundo GC. The kinetics of anterior tooth display. J Prosthet Dent 1978;39:502–504).	
Age group (years)	Mandibular central incisor	Maxillary central incisor
Up to 30	3.5	0.5
30–40	1.5	1.0
40–50	1.0	2.0
50–60	0.5	2.5
Over 60	0.0	3.0

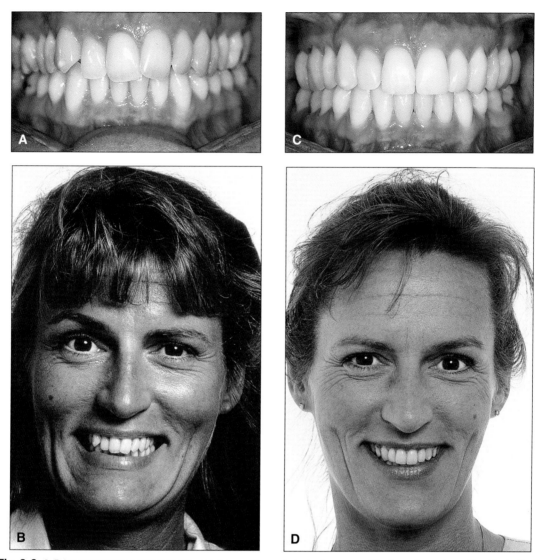

Fig. 6-3 A-D Improvement in parallelism between the maxillary anterior tooth curve and the lower lip contour with orthodontic treatment in an adult female case of bimaxillary crowding. The cant of maxillary central incisor midline is corrected.

the incisor exposure at rest and during normal speech. The tooth display in speaking may be every bit as important as the tooth display in smiling to express personality and age.

The most important esthetic information in treatment planning is obtained when the patient is observed during normal conversation. The tooth display in smiling will not provide the same information, since when a person is smiling the upper lip is raised actively by three different muscle groups.[16] For this reason, nearly everyone, irrespective of age, will display the maxillary incisors nicely in the full smile, even if only the mandibular incisors are visible during speech. In other words, the age changes in incisor display are much more pronounced and apparent when the patient is speaking or with the lips relaxed, than when he or she is smiling (Fig. 6-7).[15]

Sagging of the perioral soft tissue is partly due to the natural flattening, stretching, and decreasing elasticity of the skin with age.[17] The upper lip becomes longer and hides more and more of the maxillary incisors, whereas the drooping of the lower lip will expose gradually more of the mandibular incisors. As a consequence, show of maxillary incisors with relaxed lips signifies youth and beauty, whereas display of mandibular incisors is a characteristic of the elderly (see Fig. 6-6). The importance of the vertical dimension in tooth display has been demonstrated in prosthetic dentistry[13,14] and in orthognathic surgery involving maxillary repositioning.[18,19]

Sex Differences

The sexual dimorphism in anterior tooth display implies that females have significantly more maxillary and less mandibular tooth exposure than males at all ages. In a group of adults, Vig and Brundo[10] found almost twice as much maxillary anterior tooth display with the lips at rest

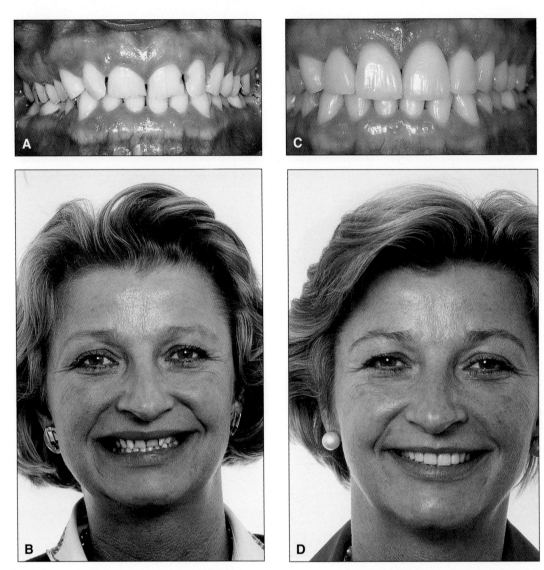

Fig. 6-4 A-D Orthodontic–prosthetic interdisciplinary approach to improve parallelism between the maxillary incisor curve and the lower lip contour in an adult female case of Class II, Division 2 malocclusion with worn central incisors. Four porcelain laminate veneers (courtesy of Dr S Toreskog, Göteborg, Sweden) were used to restore and elongate the maxillary incisors.

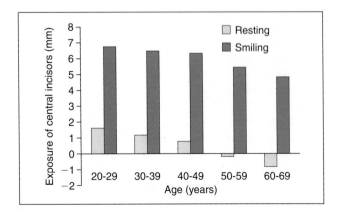

Fig. 6-5 Comparison of maxillary incisor display by age with lips at rest and on smiling. (Reproduced with permission from Dong JK, Jin TH, Cho HW, Oh SC. The esthetics of the smile. A review of some recent studies. Int J Prosthodont 1999;12:9–19.)

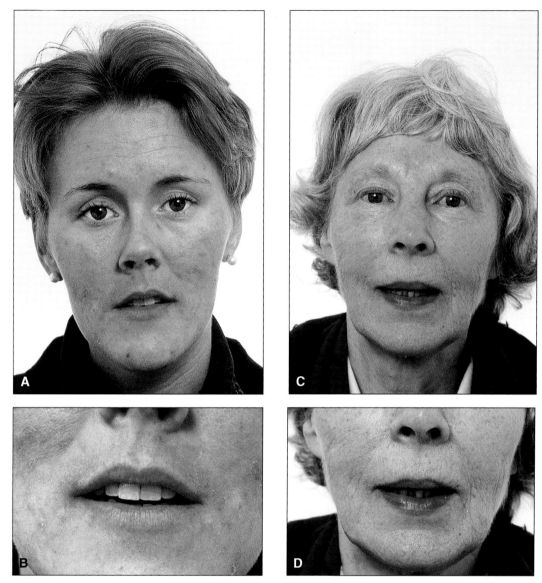

Fig. 6-6 Age changes in vertical incisor display with relaxed lips, demonstrated by female patients aged 25 (**A** and **B**) and 65 (**C** and **D**). Note that the younger woman shows only maxillary incisors, whereas the older woman shows only mandibular incisors.

in women (3.4 mm) as in men (1.9 mm). Men displayed much more of the mandibular incisors (0.5–1.2 mm).

Standardized Extraoral Records

A standardized procedure for recording the incisor display in (1) the rest position (see Fig. 6-6) and (2) a posed smile (see Fig. 6-2) before and after orthodontic treatment is recommended and will help the clinician avoid undesirable treatment effects on the maxillary incisor reveal. Each patient should be coached and asked to achieve the same lip position at least twice in succession before a photograph is taken. A short video sequence is very helpful in demonstrating the rest position, normal conversation, and smiling.[20,21] But most people are able to attain reasonably reproducible lip positions,[8,9] and still photographs can provide important clinical information. In the rest position (instruct the patient to say "Emma" or "Mississippi"),[6,22] the teeth should be slightly apart, and the perioral soft tissue and mandibular posture must both be unstrained. At the posed smile (instruct the patient to bite together, smile and say "cheese"),[6] the teeth should be lightly closed.

Clinical Implications for Deep Overbite Correction

Average and Low Smile Types

Correction of deep anterior overbite can be made with various combinations of incisor intrusion and molar

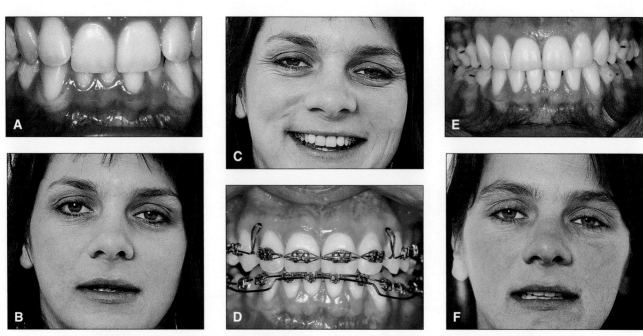

Fig. 6-7 Deep anterior overbite in a 30-year-old female patient before (**A-C**), during (**D**), and after orthodontic treatment (**E** and **F**). The initial maxillary incisor display with lips at rest (**B**) corresponds to a much older person. For this reason, the maxillary central incisors were extruded with stepdown bends in the archwire and the mandibular incisors were intruded using an overlay base arch (**D**). Final result shows overbite correction (**E**) and a maxillary incisor display more relevant to the patient's age (**F**).

extrusion.[23] The treatment concepts for cases of deep overbite have changed significantly during the past 10 years due to the increasing emphasis given to the esthetic importance of the vertical display of the *maxillary* incisors during normal speech and with relaxed lips. While active intrusion of maxillary incisors with intrusion arches, utility arches, overlay base arches, and similar approaches, has previously been considered a cornerstone of deep bite correction, the risk of too much intrusion (so-called "overintrusion") with such approaches is apparent. Overintrusion tends to hide the maxillary incisors behind the upper lip when the patient is speaking. Such a mistake can go undetected by the orthodontist unless the incisor display on speaking and smiling is analyzed from the front. With increasing age of the patient and concomitant drooping of the upper lip, an unesthetic incisor display at adolescence will predictably worsen with time.

The optimal vertical reference position for the *maxillary incisal edge* in orthodontic treatment planning is with *relaxed* lips (see Fig. 6-6). The clinical guideline should be that the maxillary incisors should be moved in the vertical direction that improves their relationship to the resting lip position relative to the patient's age (see Fig. 6-5). In a young adult between 20 and 30 years of age, there should be at least 3 mm of maxillary incisors showing. For an adult 30–40 years of age, approximately 1.5 mm of the maxillary incisors should show with the lips in their rest position, and at age 40–50 years, about 1 mm. In patients over 50–60 years of age, the maxillary incisors normally should

not show at all when the lips are relaxed. According to Frush and Fischer,[24] an optimal incisor position for adults occurs when the maxillary lateral incisors show "when the patient is speaking seriously". The degree to which the tips of the lateral incisors should show will depend on the sex and age of the patient. The tooth-to-lip position at rest should be monitored constantly throughout the orthodontic treatment. Since no orthodontist would wish to make his/her patients look older than they really are, it is important to carefully analyze each patient's tooth display on speaking before deciding whether or not maxillary intrusion mechanics should be used. In some cases of deep overbite, extrusion rather than intrusion of the maxillary incisors may be indicated (see Fig. 6-7), or a combination of orthodontics and prosthetic crown lengthening with porcelain laminate veneers will be the method of choice (see Fig. 6-4).

From an esthetic point of view, the best treatment strategy in the majority of cases of deep overbite is to actively intrude the *mandibular* rather than the maxillary incisors. This is particularly true when the curve of Spee is marked, and when the six mandibular anterior teeth are above the functional occlusal plane at the start of treatment. Mandibular incisor intrusion can be achieved with segmented intrusion arches, utility arches, overlay base arches, etc. The rate of intrusion can be controlled by recording the position of the maxillary central incisal edges relative to fixed points on the mandibular appliances. Using overlay base arches (Fig. 6-8) the mandibular incisor intrusion

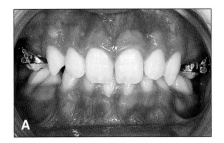

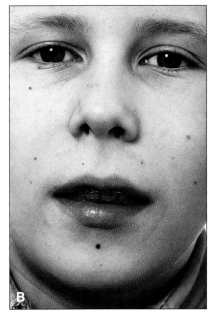

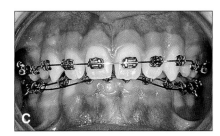

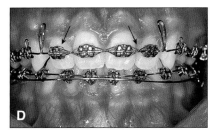

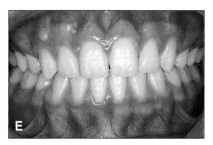

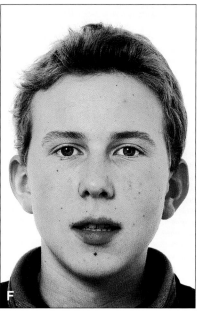

Fig. 6-8 A Young male patient with deep anterior overbite. **B** Rest position photograph indicates that maxillary incisors should not be intruded. **C** and **D** Mandibular incisor intrusion using overlay base arches from double tubes on the mandibular first molars. Final result demonstrates **E** overbite correction and **F** optimal maxillary incisor display with lips at rest.

usually occurs at a rate of 0.5 mm per month. It should be emphasized that it is not possible to effectively intrude mandibular incisors with one continuous archwire. Compared to a conventional continuous archwire, segmented mechanics (Burstone) will produce overbite correction by (1) more incisor intrusion and (2) less molar extrusion and subsequent posterior rotation of the mandible.[25,26]

Another situation that calls for the use of segmented archwires is children with reduced anterior overbite and maxillary canines erupting in a high position.[22] If a continuous leveling archwire is used, the intrusive counterforce on the incisors may overintrude them into functionally and esthetically unacceptable positions. In such instances, the first molars should be connected with a solid transpalatal bar to yield a reliable posterior anchorage unit, and a cantilever wire from the extramolar tube used to bring down the canines and secure an optimal vertical incisor display after treatment.

An alternative to incisor intrusion for deep overbite correction may be active molar extrusion. Such effects can be obtained with functional appliances, bite planes, headgears, etc.[27] Molar extrusion may be of merit in a growing child with normal or low-angle face type and vertical growth pattern,[28] but it would be calamitous in a high-angle case, and generally cannot be recommended in adults because of stability concerns.[28,29]

The second most common mistake in orthodontic treatment and finishing in the vertical plane is to create a straight smile line rather than an incisal smile curve.[12,21,22,30,31] Undesirable arc flattening is probably underestimated in orthodontics. Ackerman et al[31] reported that the smile arc of as many as 32% of their patients was flattened during orthodontic treatment. One reason why such changes may remain unnoticed by orthodontists is that they are only observed when patients are examined from the front.

It may seem difficult to achieve the desired parallelism between the maxillary incisors and the lower lip in smiling. In clinical practice, however, this appearance can readily be achieved if the maxillary central incisors are symmetrically positioned 0.5–1.5 mm longer than the lateral incisors[32] (Fig. 6-9). If the lower lip shows a marked curvature in smiling, the distoincisal edges of the maxillary central incisors can be ground slightly with a diamond instrument,

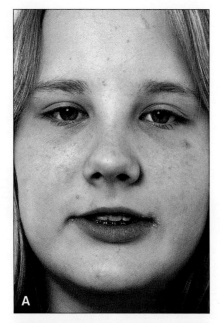
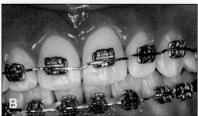
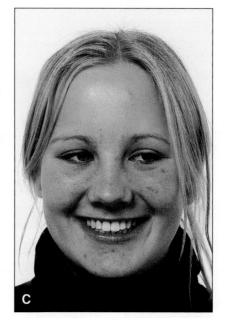

Fig. 6-9 When the smile curve is flattened during treatment (**A**), the central incisors may be extruded with stepdown bends (**B**) to improve the curve and the parallelism to the lower lip contour (**C**).

as this procedure will not affect the functional occlusion[33] (Fig. 6-9).

It is particularly undesirable to combine maxillary incisor overintrusion with a straight rather than a curved arrangement of these teeth. This display gives the impression of a typical static denture that results in the so-called "denture mouth".[22,24]

High Smile Types – "Gummy" Smiles

The "gummy" smile, which can be defined as 2 mm or more of maxillary gingival exposure in full smiling, has provoked considerable interest and concern among orthodontists. Its biologic mechanism appears to involve the combined effects of anterior vertical excess, an increased muscular capacity to raise the upper lip in smiling, and associated factors such as excessive interlabial gap at rest and excessive overjet and overbite.[14] Surprisingly, upper lip length, clinical crown length of the incisors, and mandibular and palatal plane angles do not appear to relate to the "gummy" smile line.[9]

A different treatment strategy may be needed for patients with high lip lines than for those with average or low smile types. Treatment alternatives include various combinations of orthodontic, periodontal, and surgical

therapy. The differential diagnosis should take into consideration both the amount of maxillary incisor display with the lips in their rest position and the amount of gingiva shown on smiling. If the maxillary incisor show at rest is optimal, active upper incisor intrusion should not be initiated. Instead, surgical crown lengthening with removal of crestal alveolar bone[34–36] should be made. Such procedures are particularly indicated in cases with altered passive eruption, excessive marginal gingivae, and short clinical crowns, since they will expose more of the anatomic crowns. When crestal alveolar bone is removed during surgical crown lengthening, the gingival margin will stabilize within 6 months at about 3 mm from the new bone level.[36]

Treatment of the most severe "gummy" smiles may require maxillary superior repositioning surgery (LeFort I osteotomy), along with reduction of the associated vertical maxillary excess.[9]

Midlines

Dental to Facial Midline Positions

As mentioned above, it is virtually impossible to check the relationship of the upper and lower midlines to the facial midline from the normal dentist–patient positions, since it only allows a view from the side (see Fig. 6-1). However, moving the patient's head to the side of the headrest[6] will allow direct frontal observation.

Midline Guides

The most practical guide to locate the facial midline is an imaginary vertical line extending through the soft tissue nasion and the midpoint of the Cupid's bow in the upper lip.[3,37] A line between these landmarks not only locates the position of the facial midline but also determines the direction of the midline. Whenever possible, the maxillary dental midline should be coincident with the facial midline (see Fig. 6-2). If this is not possible, the midline between the maxillary central incisors should be strictly vertical and parallel to the facial midline.[3,38–40]

Esthetically Acceptable Midline Deviations

Kokich et al[11] recently reported an interesting interaction between the maxillary central incisor midline deviation and crown angulation. As long as the dental midline was parallel to the facial midline, even a 4 mm maxillary midline deviation was not detected by dentists and lay people. However, all evaluators rated a 2 mm deviation in incisor angulation (canted midline) as noticeably unattractive. A significantly slanted dental midline is displeasing and will be easily noticed. This data demonstrates that a precise dental midline is not necessary for optimal esthetics, as long as the incisal crown angulation is not canted (see Figs 6-3, 6-4, and 6-7–6-9). On the other hand, if the mid axis between the right and left maxillary central incisors is markedly canted, it will look unacceptably skewed even if the incisor contact point is located in the middle of the face.

While alignment of the maxillary and mandibular dental midlines is desirable in orthodontic treatment for occlusion reasons, the mandibular midline becomes a lesser issue in esthetics. The narrowness and uniform sizes of the mandibular incisors make visualization of their midpoint more difficult.

Connector Area Versus Contact Point

Morley and Eubank[3] recently introduced the term *connector area* as a useful tool and a visual goal to optimize smile esthetics in dental patients. Connector areas are larger, broader areas than the contact points between teeth, and can be defined as the zone in which two adjacent teeth appear to touch. The most esthetic relationship between the maxillary anterior teeth is referred to as the 50–40–30 rule. This rule defines the ideal connector area between the two maxillary central incisors as 50% of their clinical crown length (see Figs 6-2 and 6-9–6-11). The ideal connector area between a maxillary lateral incisor and a central incisor is 40% of the central incisor's clinical crown length, and between a lateral incisor and a canine it is 30% of the clinical crown length of the central incisors.[3]

The most important connector area is the one between the two maxillary central incisors. Since it should be quite long in orthodontically well-treated cases, it is clinically important to carefully check the clinical mid axis between the mesial surfaces of the central incisors before appliance removal. In cases of pretreatment crowding, it is almost always necessary to recontour these mesial surfaces by grinding (see Figs 6-1, 6-3, and 6-12). This will relocate the contact point in an apical direction to reduce or avoid interdental gingival recession (dark triangles between the teeth due to loss of the gingival papillae)[41] and result in an optimally long and vertical connector area (see Figs 6-2 and 6-9–6-11). If the connector area is canted undesirably, it can be improved in the finishing stages of treatment using small artistic archwire bends. A prerequisite for detecting the need for such corrections is that the patient's dentition is studied from the front.

Transverse Dimension

Most orthodontists are familiar with the fact that too little lingual root torque of the maxillary central incisors during treatment will have a negative esthetic effect in most patients. Partly due to a different reflection of the incoming light, patients with optimal incisor crown inclination are considered to look more attractive than patients who finish orthodontic treatment with large interincisal angles. The evidence base with regard to what is the most desirable esthetic labiolingual crown inclination of the maxillary canines, premolars, and molars is limited. Thus, any discussion on what constitutes the most esthetic positions of the upper canines and posterior teeth in different patients will be subjective.

As discussed and illustrated elsewhere,[42,43] our working hypothesis is that fullness of the smile should be sought through adjustment of the clinical crown torque of the maxillary canines and premolars to their most esthetic appearance in different face types, rather than through nonextraction heroics or unnecessary lateral expansion and labial tipping of the maxillary dentition. Some important elements for the transverse dimension in orthodontics are:

- Labiolingual crown inclination of the terminal tooth in each quadrant that shows in smiling
- Crown inclination symmetry of the contralateral teeth
- Harmony of the front-to-back tooth display curve
- Relationship between the size of the maxillary apical base and the labiolingual crown inclination of the maxillary teeth
- Occurrence of buccal corridors (negative space).

Terminal Tooth on Smiling

Generally speaking, about 90% of people show either the first or the second premolar as the last tooth when they are smiling.[7,20] To create the illusion of smile fullness, the last premolar displayed should be positioned relatively

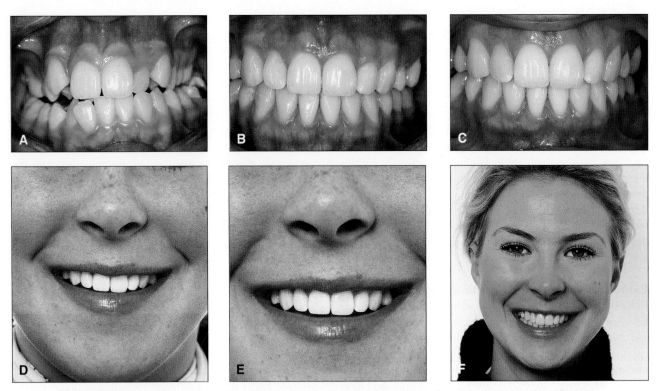

Fig. 6-10 Which maxillary canine provides optimal esthetics to the smile? Comparisons of crown torque before (**A** and **D**), at the end of (**B** and **E**), and 10 years after orthodontic treatment (**C** and **F**). Note the right–left side asymmetry of canine torque at all stages. The smile is broader on the patient's right side with a more upright canine position.

upright[42,43] (see Figs 6-2, 6-10, and 6-11). It is particularly important to avoid a lingual inclination of the maxillary premolars in patients with a relatively small maxillary apical base (Fig. 6-13) and in premolar extraction cases (see Figs 6-2 and 6-11).[42,43] When there is crown inclination asymmetry between the right and left last premolar on smiling, the smile invariably appears narrower on the side where the premolar has more tilt.[43]

The torque prescriptions for most preadjusted appliance systems tend to create too much lingual crown inclination of maxillary and mandibular canines and posterior teeth.[44] The view that the canines and premolars should have considerable lingual crown inclination (Fig. 6-14) in an optimally treated orthodontic case,[45] irrespective of tooth size, jaw size, face type, and facial expressivity is disputed from an esthetic perspective.

The normative crown inclination values proposed by Andrews[45] (Fig. 6-14), which have influenced available preadjusted appliance systems, were based on careful study of 120 nonorthodontic patients with normal occlusion and teeth that were "straight and pleasing in appearance", and 1150 successfully treated orthodontic cases. Although this information has been of great value, well-finished orthodontic cases may not be the optimal basis for optimal crown torque estimations from an esthetic perspective.

Crown Inclination Symmetry on Contralateral Teeth

Crown inclination symmetry of the contralateral teeth on the right and left sides of the maxilla and mandible will contribute to an optimally esthetic appearance (see Figs 6-2 and 6-11–6-13). It is generally easier said than done to obtain bilateral crown inclination symmetry (see Figs 6-10, 6-15, and 6-16). A prerequisite to detect asymmetries is to view the patient directly from the front at the start of orthodontic therapy (see Figs 6-10, 6-13, and 6-15), so that the necessary correction bends can be made in the archwires.

Front-to-Back Progression

The front-to-back progression of the maxillary canine, premolars, and molars is a critical factor for the display of the dentition when the patient is speaking and smiling. The principles of gradation and smoothness must be observed, so the decrease in size and detail occurs gradually.[5] Lombardi[5] noted that the teeth should have a harmonious perspective from the dominant central incisors transitioning posteriorly, with each tooth in harmonious proportion to those adjacent to it. The apparent widths may, or may not, be in "golden proportions"[46–48] to one another. Analyzing

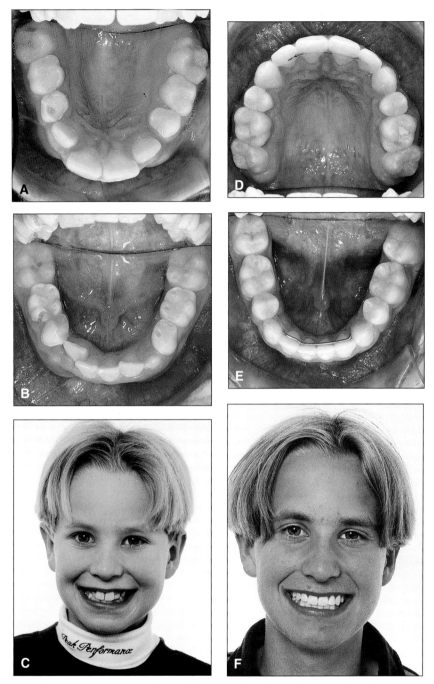

Fig. 6-11 Four premolar extraction case with full and radiant smile after orthodontic treatment. Note the upright canines and premolars (**F**). The original mandibular arch form is maintained (**B** and **E**), whereas the maxillary arch is moderately expanded and rounded (**A** and **D**).

students in California, Preston[48] found the golden proportion between the perceived width of the maxillary central and lateral incisors in only 17% of cases, and not between any perceived lateral incisor and canine widths. He claimed that there is nothing mystical or exclusively correct about the use of the golden proportion. Its use may well provide a pleasing outcome, as might many other approaches (see Figs 6-2, 6-11, 6-13, and 6-17). From a clinical point of view, it may be more important to avoid any interruption of the harmony and gradual smoothness. This implies that a canine or premolar with excessive lingual tipping (Figs 6-15 and 6-16), or a premolar placed too far buccally,[5] will lessen the harmony of the tooth display curve laterally and reduce the esthetic impression.

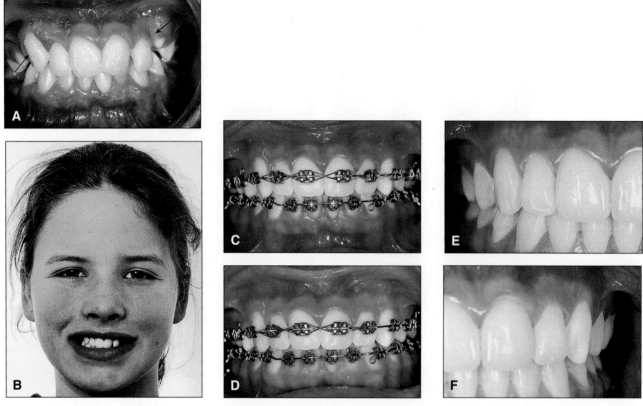

Fig. 6-12 A markedly different clinical crown inclination between the maxillary right and left canines in a young female patient (**A** and **B**). Due to the individualized torque with intentional lingual root torque bends in the archwire, the right canine improved its inclination at 9 (**C**) and 12 months (**D**) until it was upright and symmetric with the left canine at the end (**E** and **F**). Also note the uprighted positions of the maxillary and mandibular posterior teeth (**A-F**).

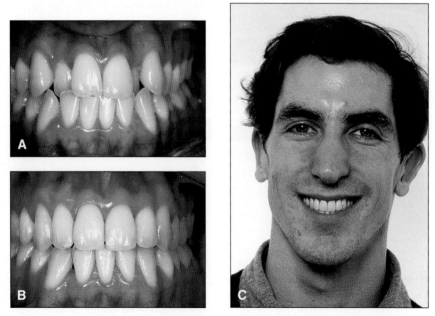

Fig. 6-13 Nature's way of compensating for a small maxillary apical base is to tilt the maxillary posterior teeth (canines through molars) labially (**A**). This position was respected during the treatment with outcome showing slight labial inclination of the crowns (**B**) to provide a full and pleasing smile (**C**).

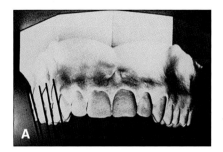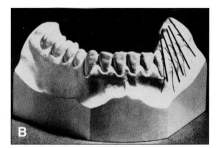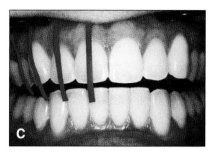

Fig. 6-14 The optimal lingual crown inclination in normally occluded upper (**A**) and lower posterior crowns (**B**) according to Andrews.[45] (**C**) Progressive medial tipping of the axial inclinations of the teeth according to Morley and Eubank.[3]

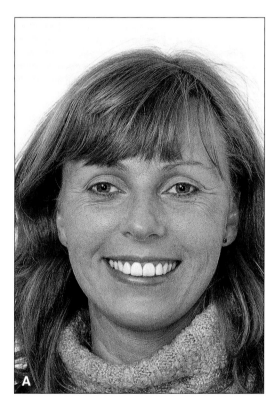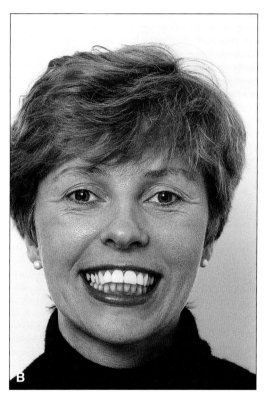

Fig. 6-15 A Excessive lingual tipping of the maxillary right canine at the end of orthodontic treatment disturbs the harmony and smoothness of the front-to-back tooth display curve. **B** Note that right–left comparison from the front also identifies canine crown inclination asymmetry before treatment, but this was not noticed and was not properly corrected.

Apical Base Size and Crown Inclination Variations

With regard to jaw size, it appears to be a general rule for obtaining optimal esthetics that the smaller the maxillary apical base, the more labial tilt may be given to the canines and premolars to allow a broader smile (see Fig. 6-13). This will copy nature's way of compensating for different sizes of maxillae. For most patients, optimal esthetics will be achieved with upright canines or a very mild lingual crown inclination (see Figs 6-2, 6-10, 6-11–6.13, and 6-17). Too much lingual crown inclination of the canines will generally disrupt the harmony of the front-to-back tooth display curve (see Figs 6-10, 6-15, and 6-16).

Buccal Corridors ("Negative Space")

Several studies have reported lay people's perception of and reaction to the buccal corridors.[20,24,30,31,49] None found a relationship between this trait and smile esthetics. Frush and Fischer[24] considered the buccal corridor to be a normal feature of a dentition that prevents the "60 tooth smile" that is often characteristic of a denture. Apparently, the labiolingual inclination of the maxillary canine and

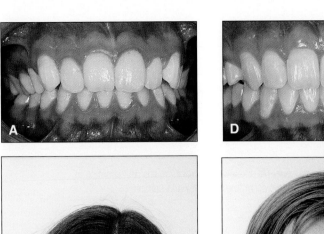

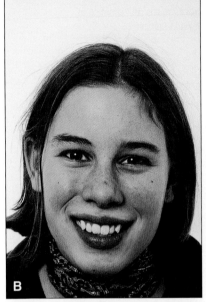

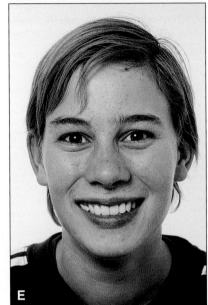

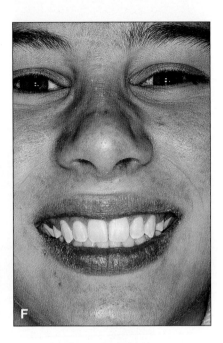

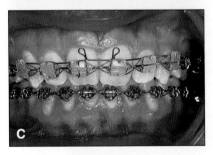

Fig. 6-16 Asymmetry in crown inclination of posterior teeth in a young female patient, with excessive lingual tipping on the right side (**A** and **B**). The discrepancy remained undiagnosed and was not corrected during treatment (**C** and **D**). The post-treatment lingual canine inclination is esthetically undesirable, particularly on the patient's right side (**E** and **F**).

premolars are equally as or more important than the presence or absence of dark buccal corridors for reflection of dental arch fullness. It should be emphasized that dark shadows between the buccal surfaces of the dentition and the corners of the mouth are more apparent on frontal photographs than in real life, as they are generally due to inadequate flash lightning of the posterior areas of the mouth in routine photography.[20,31] If the pretreatment maxillary dental arch is acceptable with regard to shape and width, it may seem preferable from a longterm stability point of view to obtain smile fullness by intentionally adding buccal crown torque to lingually inclined canines and premolars during treatment (see Figs 6-2, 6-11, 6-12, and 6-17). Maxillary lateral expansion is indicated whenever the maxillary and mandibular dental arches are

notably constricted in the beginning, whether or not posterior crossbite is present. Excessive intentional lateral expansion of the dental arches is likely to introduce a disequilibrium and longterm relapse.[42]

The above principles and considerations may be supplemented with a discussion of the optimal crown torque from an esthetic perspective for individual teeth.

Maxillary Canine

There is a very large variation in labiolingual inclination of the maxillary canines and premolars between patients (Fig. 6-18). The patient in Figure 6-18A and B has a broad maxilla and marked lingual tipping of all teeth. In marked contrast, the patient in Figure 6-18C and D has a narrow

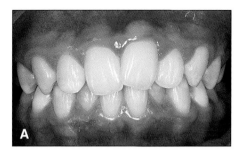
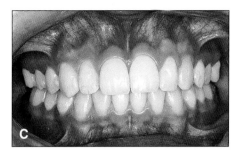
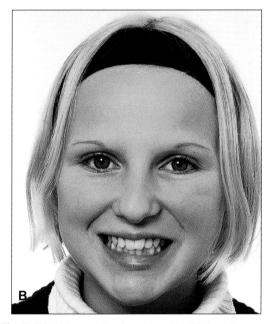
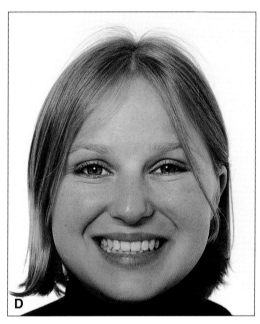

Fig. 6-17 Adolescent female patient with mild bimaxillary crowding (**A** and **B**) treated without extraction and without lateral expansion and/or incisor proclination. Space along the dental arches was provided by stripping oval premolars and triangular incisors toward their ideal shapes. The improved fullness of the smile (compare **B** and **D**) is due primarily to intentional uprighting (lingual root torque placed in the archwires) of the canines and posterior teeth.

maxillary apical base and a pronounced labial tilt of all clinical crowns. The crown torque discrepancies between these two patients demonstrates why it is unrealistic to try and produce the same orthodontic treatment result for both of them, and it is also obvious that they cannot be treated to optimum esthetics by the same preadjusted bracket prescription system without archwire bending. An individualized esthetic goal should be set for each patient before the orthodontic treatment is started.

The question of what is the optimal esthetic labiolingual inclination for the maxillary canines in different patients is examined using photographs of a young female patient before and after orthodontic therapy, and at 10-year follow-up (see Fig. 6-10). When studying the treatment result from the front, the crown inclination is different between the right and left maxillary canines. Thus, two questions arise: (1) which of the canines is esthetically most preferable? and (2) why is the treatment result asymmetric with regard to crown inclination? Since subjective beauty is dependent on the person observing an object, each orthodontist may make his/her judgment in this regard. In our opinion, the maxillary right canine has a more esthetic inclination than the left canine, since the lingual tipping of the left canine makes the smile narrower on that side (see Fig. 6-10). The asymmetry of the finished case is explained by the fact that the crown inclination was different between the right and left canine at the start of treatment. The same bracket prescription was used on both sides, and no torquing bends were made in the archwires. Since no intentional attempt was made to correct the asymmetry, this outcome was logical. The longterm follow-up records showed that the canine crown inclination asymmetry was not self-correcting. To achieve symmetry of labiolingual crown inclination between the teeth on the right and left sides of the mouth, intentional individualization is needed (see Fig. 6-12). The easiest and most practical way to achieve symmetry is to carefully study each case from the front, and make the necessary archwire bends early in treatment (see Fig. 6-12).

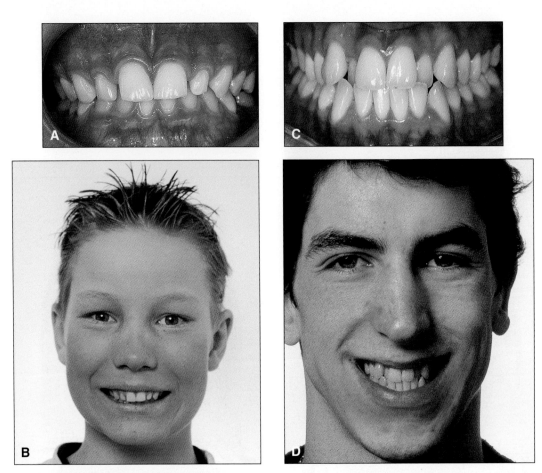

Fig. 6-18 Two male patients demonstrating the wide range of individual variation in crown inclination of posterior teeth (canines through molars). The young boy (**A** and **B**) has a large maxillary apical base with marked lingual tilt of the teeth. The older patient (**C** and **D**) has a small maxilla, a large mandible, and a labial tilt of the teeth.

Excessive lingual tipping of the maxillary canine is undesirable for esthetic reasons, whether it occurs uni- or bilaterally (see Figs 6-15 and 6-16).

It is apparent from these and other cases that (1) the *preferred labiolingual crown inclination* of the maxillary canine from an *esthetic* viewpoint in the majority of cases is *relatively upright*; and (2) that *pretreatment asymmetries in crown inclination between right and left canines will remain* after orthodontic therapy if no intentional measures are taken to correct it. Such adjustments may involve the use of individual archwire bends at different time periods during treatment, or possibly by the use of custom-made appliances specifically engineered for the individual needs of every patient.

Maxillary First and Second Premolars

Premolars with an upright position will produce a broader smile than premolars that are tipped lingually. Particularly when orthodontic treatment results in some lingual tipping of the maxillary premolars behind the upright canines, the smile becomes undesirably narrow in the posterior segments, and does not reach an optimal fullness (Fig. 6-19).

For this reason, the esthetically preferable first and second premolar crown torque for most patients is around 0°. For patients with a wide maxillary apical base, a few degrees of lingual crown torque may be desirable. For patients with a small apical base, upright premolar crowns or even some labial crown inclination may produce a nice display of their dentitions (see Fig. 6-13).

Maxillary First Molar

Only a small percentage of the population will show the maxillary first molars when smiling.[7] For these patients, the molars should be relatively straight in order to contribute to a full smile (Fig. 6-20).

Mandibular Canine

The optimal outcome of orthodontic treatment with regard to the mandibular canines is to achieve: (1) relatively upright positions when viewed from the front (see Figs 6-10, 6-12, 6-16, and 6-17); and (2) bilateral crown inclination symmetry (see Figs 6-10, 6-16, and 6-17). Upright rather than lingually tipped mandibular canines allow more labial crown torque of the maxillary canines,

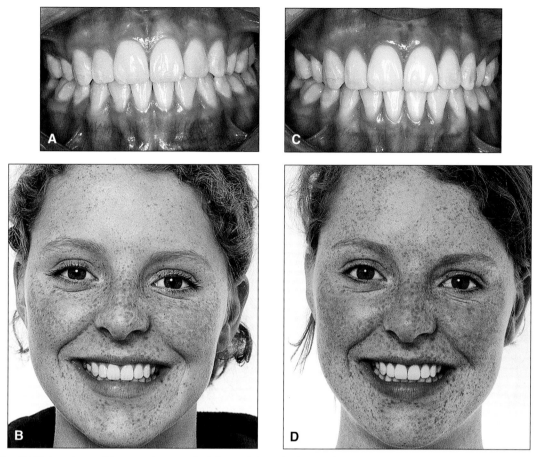

Fig. 6-19 Importance of the premolar crown for fullness of the smile. A young female patient at the end of orthodontic treatment (**A** and **B**) and 5 years later (**C** and **D**). The post-treatment intraoral result may appear optimal according to the prevailing concepts (compare with Fig. 6-12**A** and **C**). However, the smile photograph displays that the lingually tilted premolars are almost hidden behind the upright canines. The smile is much narrower than for the patient in Fig. 6-17**D** with upright premolars.

producing a broader smile (see Figs 6-11, 6-12, 6-17, and 6-20). Many preadjusted prescription appliances place lingual crown torque in the mandibular canines, which appears undesirable from both esthetic and functional viewpoints. Particularly when the mandibular canines are tipped lingually before orthodontic treatment is started, appliances with built-in lingual crown torque will tend to produce an excessive lingual tipping of the canines (Fig. 6-21). The correction of such lingual tippings is time consuming and difficult, and may remain unnoticed at the end of treatment (Figs 6-3, 6-13, and 6-21). A mandibular canine torque prescription that induces some labial crown torque (lingual root torque) will counteract such side effects.

Mandibular Premolars and Molars

A common side effect of routine orthodontic treatment with both preadjusted and standard edgewise appliances is that the crowns of the mandibular posterior teeth tend to tip lingually.[44] This is undesirable not only from an esthetic point of view, but also for functional reasons. If the mandibular premolars and molars receive marked lingual crown torque, the maxillary posterior teeth may erupt into

occlusion with their lingual cusps hanging down. This arrangement may cause balancing side interferences in side movements of the mandible. This side effect can be avoided by careful clinical observation and archwire bending and/or by using nontorqued attachments for the mandibular posterior teeth, including the second molars (see Figs 6-10, 6-12, 6-17, and 6-20).

How to Achieve Both an Optimal Smile and Dental Stability

The available research evidence with regard to longterm stability of orthodontic treatment results implies that the patient's pretreatment mandibular intercanine width and mandibular arch form may be the optimal guide to future dental and arch form stability.[50–55]

If these measures are within a normal range, which implies that the intercanine width is around 25–26 mm, the mandibular incisors are in front of the A–pogonion line, and the arch form is symmetric, with no need for transverse uprighting (buccal crown torque) of the premolars and

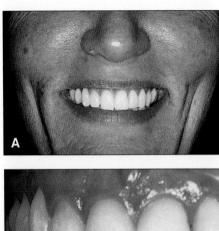

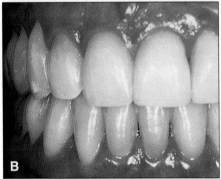

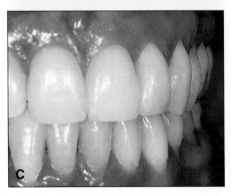

Fig. 6-20 A-C When the terminal teeth displayed in the smile are the maxillary first molars, their position should be upright in order to produce fullness of smile (same patient as in Fig. 6-3).

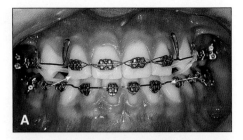

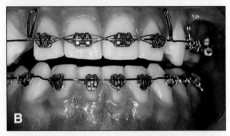

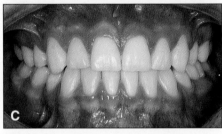

Fig. 6-21 Unintentional excessive lingual tipping of mandibular canines (and premolars) during orthodontic treatment (**A** and **B**) is difficult and time consuming to correct, and may remain undercorrected at the end of treatment (**C**). Note the right–left side asymmetry of the canine crown inclination throughout treatment.

molars, then the mandible should be treated orthodontically without incisor proclination and lateral expansion (see Figs 6-11 and 6-17). Mild-to-moderate dental crowding is managed by mesiodistal enamel reduction (stripping).

The maxillary dental arch is placed on top of and coordinated with the mandible. The original maxillary arch form is respected, but frequently has to be rounded and slightly expanded posteriorly (see Fig. 6-11A and D) to occlude properly with the mandibular teeth.[42,43] With this approach, smile fullness is sought not through lateral expansion or tipping of the maxillary dentition, but rather through intentional adjustment of the labiolingual crown inclination of the maxillary canines and premolars to their most esthetic appearance (see Fig. 6-17).[42] Maxillary lateral expansion is indicated, however, whenever the maxillary and mandibular arches are notably constricted

in the beginning, whether or not a posterior crossbite is present.

Clinical Guidelines

Vertical Dimension

The following guidelines are recommended for the purpose of obtaining an optimally esthetic tooth display in normal conversation and on smiling:

- Study the patient's dentition directly from the front to make a reliable esthetic evaluation. In the dentist's chair, move the patient's head to the side of the head rest, which allows an "eye-to-eye" perspective.
- Routinely take extraoral photographs before and after treatment to record the maxillary incisor display with the lips at rest. A short video with the patient speaking is very helpful.
- Provide a curve of the maxillary incisors that is parallel to the inner contour of the lower lip on smiling. This is generally achieved by making the maxillary central incisors 0.5–1.5 mm longer than the lateral incisors.
- Be careful not to actively intrude the maxillary incisors when their pretreatment vertical position is normal for

the patient's age. Do not overintrude and hide away the maxillary incisors behind the upper lip!

- Establish an age-appropriate vertical incisor display in the rest position and normal conversation for each orthodontic patient.

Midlines

The following guidelines may be clinically useful for optimal smile design in orthodontic patients:

- A vertical line from the nasion to the base of the philtrum may be the most practical guide to locate the facial midline.
- A precise dental midline coincident with the facial midline is not necessary for optimal esthetics.
- Moderate maxillary midline deviation is acceptable to most individuals, as long as the central incisor crown angulation is not significantly canted.
- Securing optimal connector areas between the maxillary anterior teeth according to the 50–40–30 rule is useful for esthetic smile design.
- The connector area between the two maxillary central incisors should be long (approximately half their clinical crown lengths), vertical, and parallel to the facial midline.
- The mandibular midline is less important for esthetics.

Transverse Dimension

What constitutes the most desirable and esthetic crown inclinations is not evidence based, but the following clinical recommendations are useful:

- Provide an individualized, esthetic, symmetric labiolingual crown inclination of canines and premolars for each patient.

- Crown inclination asymmetries between contralateral canines and premolars in the right and left side of the mouth are common. They must be (1) recognized early in treatment by studying the dentition from the front; and (2) intentionally corrected by archwire torquing (or possibly by custom-made bracket torque prescriptions). Otherwise, the finished result will be asymmetric with regard to clinical crown inclination.
- The terminal teeth shown on smiling should be straight to provide smile fullness. In about 90% of cases, this will be the maxillary first or second premolar.
- A smooth, gradual front-to-back tooth display curve laterally provides harmony and beauty to the treatment result. Any disruption will reduce the esthetic outcome.
- Avoid tipping the mandibular canines, premolars, and molars lingually during the orthodontic treatment.
- The secret to excellence in orthodontics is to learn to see important details in the dentition as they occur before, during, and after treatment.

Summary

This chapter has discussed some esthetic elements of tooth display and smile design associated with orthodontic treatment. Normative standards of the lip–incisor relationships are provided. The importance of a patient's display of his/her dentition during speech and on smiling was evaluated (1) in the vertical dimension; (2) with regard to midlines; and (3) in the transverse dimension. Clinical guidelines were provided. Together, these should help to improve the esthetic outcome of contemporary orthodontic treatment results.

REFERENCES

1. Ackerman JL, Proffit WR, Sarver DM. The emerging soft tissue paradigm in orthodontic diagnosis and treatment planning. Clin Orth Res 1999;2:49–52.
2. Proffit WR. The soft tissue paradigm in orthodontic diagnosis and treatment planning: A new view for a new century. J Esthet Dent 2000;12:46–49.
3. Morley J, Eubank J. Macroesthetic elements of smile design. J Am Dent Assoc 2001;132:39–45.
4. Nash DA. Professional ethics and esthetic dentistry. J Am Dent Assoc 1988;115:7E–9E.
5. Lombardi RE. The principles of visual perception and their clinical application to denture esthetics. J Prosthet Dent 1973;29:358–382.
6. Zachrisson BU. Esthetic factors involved in anterior tooth display and the smile: Vertical dimension. J Clin Orthod 1998;32:432–445.
7. Tjan AHL, Miller GD, The JPG. Some esthetic factors in a smile. J Prosthet Dent 1984;51:24–28.
8. Peck S, Peck L, Kataja M. Some vertical lineaments of lip position. Am J Orthod Dentofacial Orthop 1992;101:519–524.
9. Peck S, Peck L, Kataja M. The gingival smile line. Angle Orthod 1992;62:91–100.
10. Vig RG, Brundo GC. The kinetics of anterior tooth display. J Prosthet Dent 1978;39:502–504.
11. Kokich VO Jr, Kiyak HA, Shapiro PA. Comparing the perception of dentists and lay people to altered dental esthetics. J Esthet Dent 1999;11:311–324.
12. Sarver DM. The importance of incisor positioning in the esthetic smile: The smile arc. Am J Orthod Dentofac Orthop 2001;120:98–111.
13. Mack MR. Vertical dimension: A dynamic concept based on facial form and oropharyngeal function. J Prosthet Dent 1991;66:478–485.
14. Mack MR. Perspective of facial esthetics in dental treatment planning. J Prosthet Dent 1996;75:169–176.
15. Dong JK, Jin TH, Cho HW, Oh SC. The esthetics of the smile. A review of some recent studies. Int J Prosthodont 1999;12:9–19.
16. Rubin LR. The anatomy of a smile: Its importance in the treatment of facial paralysis. Plast Reconstr Surg 1974;53:384–387.
17. Peck S, Peck H. The aesthetically pleasing face: An orthodontic myth. Trans Eur Orthod Soc 1971;47:175–185.
18. Rosen HM, Ackerman JL. Porous block hydroxyapatite in orthognathic surgery. Angle Orthod 1991;61:185–191.

19. Turley PK. Orthodontic management of the short face patient. Semin Orthod 1996;2:138–152.
20. Ackerman MB, Ackerman JL. Smile analysis and design in the digital era. J Clin Orthod 2002;36:221–236.
21. Mah J, Korrodi Ritto A. Imaging in orthodontics: Present and future. J Clin Orthod 2002;36:619–625.
22. Zachrisson BU. Mechanical intrusion of maxillary incisors: A treatment strategy to be abandoned? World J Orthod 2002;3:358–364.
23. Nanda R. Differential diagnosis and treatment of excessive overbite. In: Nanda R, ed. Symposium on orthodontics. Dental Clinics of North America. Philadelphia: WB Saunders, 1981:195–202.
24. Frush JP, Fisher RD. The dynesthetic interpretation of the dentogenic concept. J Prosthet Dent 1958;8:558–581.
25. Weiland FJ, Bantleon HP, Droschl H. Evaluation of continuous arch and segmented arch leveling techniques in adult patients—A clinical study. Am J Orthod Dentofac Orthop 1996;110:647–652.
26. AlQabandi A, Sadowsky C, Sellke T. A comparison of continuous archwire and utility archwires for leveling the curve of Spee. World J Orthod 2002;3:159–165.
27. Dolce C, Babb LK, McGorray SP, Taylor MG, King GJ, Wheeler TT. Vertical skeletal and dental changes in early treatment of Class II malocclusion. Semin Orthod 2002;8:141–148.
28. Simons ME, Joondeph DR. Change in overbite: A ten-year postretention study. Am J Orthod 1973;64:349–367.
29. Braun S. Biomechanic considerations in the management of the vertical dimension. Semin Orthod 2002;8:149–154.
30. Hulsey CM. An esthetic evaluation of lip-teeth relationships present in the smile. Am J Orthod 1970;57:132–144.
31. Ackerman JL, Ackerman MB, Brensinger CM, Landis JR. A morphometric analysis of the posed smile. Clin Orth Res 1998;1:2–11.
32. Brisman AS. Esthetics: a comparison of dentists' and patients' concepts. J Am Dent Ass 1991;100:345–352.
33. Kokich VG, Spear FM. Guidelines for managing the orthodontic–restorative patient. Semin Orthod 1997;3:3–20.
34. Kokich VG. Esthetics: The orthodontic–periodontic–restorative connection. Semin Orthod 1996;2:21–30.
35. Garber DA, Salama MA. The aesthetic smile: Diagnosis and treatment. Periodontology 1996;11:18–28.
36. Brägger U, Lauchenauer D, Lang NP. Surgical lengthening of the clinical crown. J Clin Periodontol 1992;19:58–63.
37. Zachrisson BU. Dental to facial midline positions. World J Orthod 2001;2:266–269.
38. Miller EL, Bodden WR Jr, Jamison HC. A study of the relationship of the dental midline to facial median line. J Prosthet Dent 1979;41:657–660.
39. Beyer JW, Lindauer SJ. Evaluation of dental midline position. Semin Orthod 1998;4:146–152.
40. Johnston CD, Burden DJ, Stevenson MR. The influence of dental to facial midline discrepancies on dental attractiveness ratings. Eur J Orthod 1999;21:517–522.
41. Tarnow DP, Magner AW, Fletcher P. The effect of the distance from the contact point to the crest of bone on the presence or absence of the interproximal dental papilla. J Periodontol 1992;63:995–996.
42. Zachrisson BU. Making the premolar extraction smile full and radiant. World J Orthod 2002;3:260–265.
43. Zachrisson BU. Maxillary expansion: Long-term stability and smile esthetics. World J Orthod 2001;2:266–272.
44. Ugur T, Yukay F. Normal faciolingual inclinations of tooth crowns compared with treatment groups of standard and pretorqued brackets. Am J Orthod Dentofacial Orthop 1997;112:50–57.
45. Andrews LF. The six keys to normal occlusion. Am J Orthod 1972;62:296–309.
46. Levin EL. Dental esthetics and the golden proportion. J Prosthet Dent 1978;40:244–252.
47. Ricketts RE. The biologic significance of the divine proportion. Am J Orthod 1982;81:351–370.
48. Preston JD. The golden proportion revisited. J Esthet Dent 1993;5:247–251.
49. Rigsbee OH III, Sperry TP, BeGole EA. The influence of facial animation on smile characteristics. Int J Adult Orthod Orthogn Surg 1988;3:233–239.
50. Little RM, Wallen TR, Riedel RA. Stability and relapse of mandibular anterior alignment—first premolar extraction cases treated by traditional edgewise orthodontics. Am J Orthod 1981;80:349–365.
51. Little RM, Riedel RA, Årtun J. An evaluation of changes in mandibular anterior alignment from 10 to 20 years postretention. Am J Orthod Dentofacial Orthop 1988;93:423–428.
52. Felton JM, Sinclair PM, Jones DL, Alexander RG. A computerized analysis of the shape and stability of mandibular arch form. Am J Orthod Dentofacial Orthop 1987;92:478–483.
53. Franklin GS, Rossouw PE, Woodside DG. A longitudinal study of dental and skeletal parameters associated with stability of orthodontic treatment. Am J Orthod Dentofacial Orthop 1996;109:109 (thesis abstract).
54. Vaden JL, Harris EF, Ziegler Gardner RL. Relapse revisited. Am J Orthod Dentofacial Orthop 1997;111:543–553.
55. Boley JC. Class I extraction treatment: A case report at 20 years postretention. World J Orthod 2002;3:50–56.

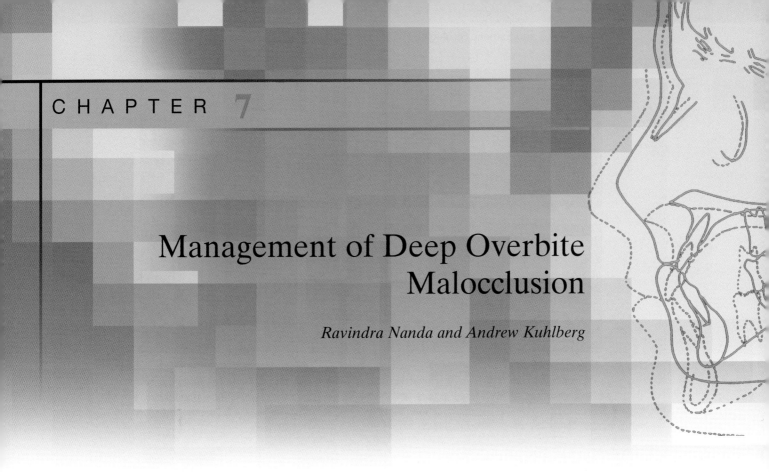

CHAPTER 7

Management of Deep Overbite Malocclusion

Ravindra Nanda and Andrew Kuhlberg

Overbite, the vertical overlap of incisors, is often expressed as the percentage of the lower incisor crown length that is covered by the upper incisors. An excessively deep overbite may be associated with incisor wear, palatal impingement, and compromised esthetics. Figure 7-1 shows four variations of malocclusions with deep overbite. The prevalence of severe deep overbite is about 8% in the US,[1] with the average overbite ranging from 36.5 to 39.2% in children between the ages of 5 and 6 years, and from 37.9 to 40.7% in adults.[2–4] While an anterior deep overbite may be associated with nearly any other dimension of malocclusion, it is frequently associated with Class II malocclusions. In Class II, Division 1 patients, with an excess overjet and proclined maxillary incisors, a deep overbite is associated with overeruption of the mandibular incisors (Fig. 7-1C). Alternatively, Class II, Division 2 patients present with a short lower vertical dimension, flat mandibular plane, retroclined maxillary incisors and deep overbite.

The history of orthodontics reveals the wide variety of methods developed to correct deep overbite. Clinically successful results have been obtained with many techniques; no single approach is best. Each manner of deep overbite correction has advantages and disadvantages, and must be carefully selected in light of the specific etiology of the individual's malocclusion and the desired treatment outcomes. This chapter will present the classic mechanisms on which most approaches to deep overbite correction are based, with an emphasis on selecting the appropriate method for the specific clinical presentation of the indivi-

dual. Optimal correction of deep overbite requires proper diagnosis, individualized treatment planning, and efficient execution of treatment mechanics.[5] A careful combination of treatment planning and mechanics to correct deep overbite can help to achieve a desirable esthetic result and to minimize relapse during the postretention phase.

The three fundamental orthodontic treatment strategies for deep bite correction (not including the surgical option) are: extrusion of posterior teeth; flaring of anterior teeth; and intrusion of upper and/or lower incisors. These effects are most often achieved biomechanically via bite plates, reverse curve archwires, step bends in archwires, and intrusion arches (Table 7-1).

Treatment Strategies for Correction of Deep Bite

Extrusion of Posterior Teeth

Extrusion of posterior teeth is one of the most common methods to correct deep overbite (Fig. 7-2).[6] This can be an efficacious method of bite opening. One millimeter of upper or lower molar extrusion effectively reduces the incisor overlap by 1.5–2.5 mm. A very common method to extrude posterior teeth in patients with a deep curve of Spee is to level the arches with the sequential use of straight continuous archwires.[7] A close variation of this technique is to use mandibular reverse curve of Spee and/or maxillary exaggerated curve of Spee wires. Progressively increasing step bends in an archwire (or purposely altering bracket

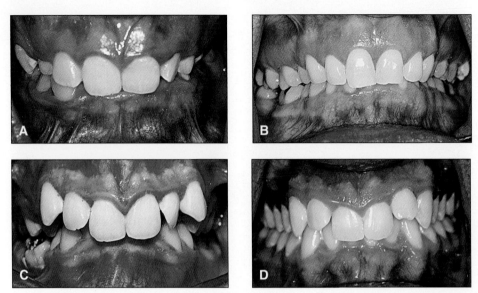

Fig. 7-1 Frontal view showing 100% deep bite in four different patients. Lingual crown inclination of central incisors with labial prominence of roots in **A** a young patient and **B** an adult. This type of deep bite correction may need flaring of the incisors to correct axial inclinations and intrusion of lower incisors. Note the gingival margins have minimal problems. **C** and **D** Deep bite with lingually inclined incisors as well as discrepancy between the gingival heights of the upper anterior teeth. This type of deep bite needs intrusion of maxillary with or without mandibular incisors to correct gingival heights.

Table 7-1	**Popular approaches to deep overbite correction.**			
	Bite plate	**Reverse curve archwire**	**Step-bend archwire**	**Intrusion arch**
Molar/posterior extrusion	****	***	***	Variable effect
Incisor flaring	(–)	***	**	Variable effect
Incisor/anterior intrusion	(–)	**	**	****
Indications	Short lower facial height Deep overbite correction in lower Excessive lower curve of Spee	Moderate-to-minimal upper incisor display Class I occlusion	Step between anterior and posterior occlusal planes (lower) Moderate-to-minimal upper incisor display Class I occlusion	Excessive gingival display on smiling Excessive incisor display Short upper lip Incisor hyper-eruption Simultaneous Class II molar correction
Special concerns	Comfort and compliance Questionable stability in nongrowing patients Increases lower facial height	Protrusive incisors/ excessive IMPA[†] Questionable stability in nongrowing patients Increases lower facial height	Indiscriminate posterior extrusion versus anterior intrusion	Segmental spring Canine-to-incisor levels Minimal upper incisor display

*Less effect
**Medium effect
***Moderately high effect
****High effect
(–) Negligible effect
[†]Incisor Mandibular Plane Angle

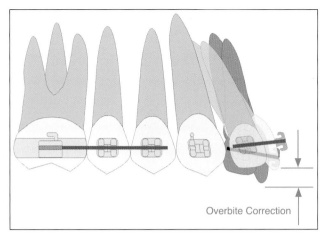

Fig. 7-6 Vertical incisal edge change associated with incisor flaring and resulting in a reduction of the overbite.

of proclined incisors because of the possible disturbance of the perioral neuromuscular balance.[17] In nonextraction patients with anterior crowding, arch expansion and alignment takes place by proclination of the incisors as well as widening of the arch circumference.

Intrusion of Incisors

Intrusion of upper and/or lower incisors is a desirable method to correct deep bite in many adolescent and adult patients (Figure 7-7).[18–20] Intrusion of incisors is most

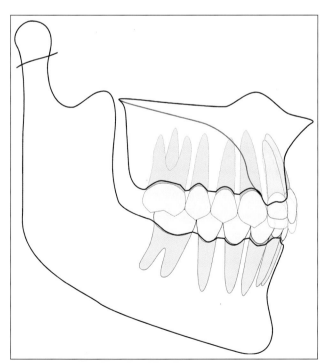

Fig. 7-7 Objectives of deep overbite correction by anterior intrusion. The goal of incisor intrusion is overbite correction without affecting the jaw position.

reliably accomplished if a pure intrusive force is applied to the incisors. Intrusion is particularly indicated in deep bite patients with a large vertical dimension, excessive incision–stomion distance, and a large interlabial gap.

The four most common methods to facilitate intrusion of the upper incisors have been described by Burstone,[8] Begg and Keeling,[21] Ricketts,[22] and Greig.[23] All four designs apply tipback bands at the molars to provide an intrusive force at the incisors. The wire size, material, method of attachment to the brackets, and the application of torque in these four techniques are diverse, but all recognize the need for a light and continuous force application. This chapter describes the mechanics of incisor intrusion and how side effects can either be controlled or used advantageously to correct various components of a malocclusion, such as a Class II molar relationship and discrepancies in the occlusal planes, midlines, and axial inclination of incisors.

Treatment Plan Considerations

Individualized treatment planning requires selecting an optimal strategy for management and correction of a patient's dentofacial problems. Setting specific objectives provides a blueprint for treatment and allows the clinician to determine an effective mechanics plan. The following factors contribute to the development of the treatment and mechanics plans for deep overbite correction.

Soft Tissue Considerations

A careful clinical examination of a patient's soft tissue facial features (Fig. 7-8) can help in strategy selection between extrusion of molars and intrusion of upper and/or lower incisors. The face is evaluated in frontal (Fig. 7-8B) and profile views (Fig. 7-8A, C, and D), both with relaxed lips and lips closed. Facial evaluation should include an assessment of the interlabial gap, incision–stomion distance (incisor display), and lip support with the upper and lower lips in their relaxed position. Observation of the patient during an unforced smile is also important to determine the relationship of the upper lip to the gingival line, as well as the smile line.[24]

Interlabial Gap

In a relaxed lip position, an interlabial gap of 3–4 mm is considered esthetically acceptable. The interlabial gap is increased in children with a long vertical dimension (see Fig. 7-8A and B) and/or respiratory obstruction. Maintaining an acceptable interlabial gap should be considered when selecting a strategy for deep overbite correction. If a patient exhibits an excessive interlabial gap, the objective should be to help reduce the discrepancy, if possible, or at least to avoid worsening the problem. Class II, Division 1 patients with deep overbite, normal-to-long lower facial heights, and increased anterior vertical dimension, frequently present with these associated concerns. An important

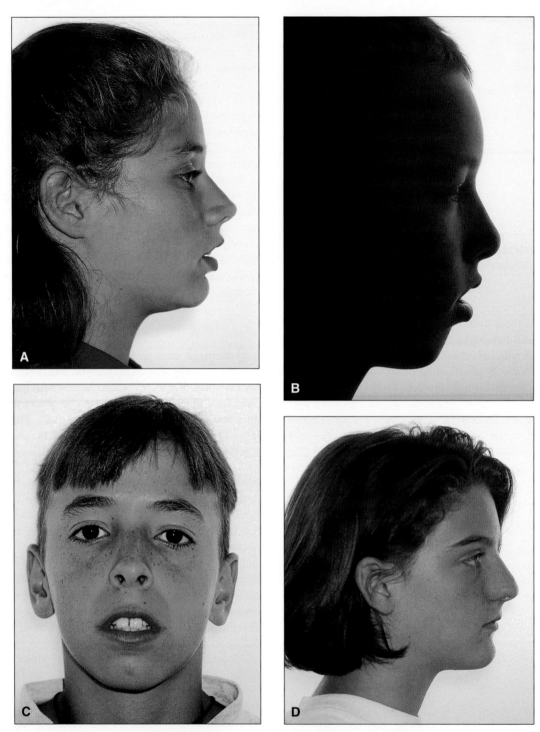

Fig. 7-8 Interlabial gap is an important determinant of the type of mechanics plan to correct deep bite. **A-C** These patients can be corrected by intrusion of maxillary incisors. **D** This patient has no interlabial gap in the relaxed lip position, and may need intrusion of the lower incisors and/or extrusion of posterior teeth to correct deep bite.

consideration in treatment planning in these cases is the effect of posterior extrusion. Extrusion of the posterior teeth increases the lower vertical dimension by rotating the mandible downward and backward (see Fig. 7-2), thereby worsening an already excessive interlabial gap.

Upper Incisor Display

Burstone was among the first orthodontists to emphasize the importance of describing the relationship of the upper incisors to the upper lip and the interlabial gap (see Fig. 7-8C).[8] Upper incisor display has been shown to decrease with maturity in the 40s and 50s as lip musculature gradually loses its tonicity (see Ch. 6).[25] The selection of alternative treatment options should take into account the patient's age. While the effects of aging cannot be discounted, targeting treatment goals to address less predictable longterm aging of the face may be questioned. Rather, the clinician should set treatment objectives for a balanced and harmonious appearance at the end of treatment for each stage of maturity.

In a clinical situation where a patient's incisor display at rest (the distance of the upper incisal edge to the lower lip, or the incision–stomion distance) measures 3–4 mm, with a deep overbite and a normal-to-long vertical dimension, the treatment of choice may be intrusion of the lower incisors. In adult patients, intrusion of the upper incisors should only be planned if the incision–stomion distance is >3 mm. A vast number of these patients with deep overbite often benefit from lower incisor intrusion, as its display increases with age.

Both adolescent and adult Class II, Division 2 patients demand a very careful evaluation of the interlabial gap and incisor display. Some patients may exhibit a minimal interlabial gap, a redundant lip length, and an inverted lower lip. Careful consideration should be given when planning to increase the vertical dimension by extrusion of the posterior teeth with or without intrusion of the lower incisors. In adolescent patients, this treatment approach is often successful in part due to the overall growth and adaptation by the neuromuscular complex of the patient. In adults, this approach may be less successful without growth and the potentially reduced neuromuscular adaptive capacity.

Smile Line

Evaluating a natural smile provides valuable information for planning deep overbite correction. The upper lip, upper incisors, gingival levels, and lower lip contour interrelate in an esthetic smile (see Ch. 2). The arc of the upper teeth should follow the curvature of the lower lip and the upper lip should be at or slightly above the upper gingival line.[26] Females frequently show more gingiva on smiling than males. Planning deep overbite correction with these important esthetic considerations aids in determining appropriate individualized treatment goals.

Lip Length

Upper lip length can also contribute to the overall dental esthetics of the patient at rest or smiling. A short upper lip may play a role in an excessive interlabial gap, the appearance of excessively long maxillary anterior crown lengths, or a gummy smile. Upper incisor intrusion is a valuable alternative for patients with deep overbite and a short upper lip.

Crown–Gingival Relationships

The most favorable crown–gingival relationship is for the central incisors and canine gingival margins to be higher than the lateral incisor margins. The canine and central incisors should be at similar levels. This idealized "high–low–high" appearance of the gingival line of the maxillary incisors improves the harmony of a smile. Kokich et al have detailed important considerations in analyzing these esthetic factors.[24] Class II, Division 2 malocclusions commonly show severe discrepancies in this relationship. As shown in Figure 7-1D, the central incisor gingival margins are far more occlusal than the canine margins. This relationship can be corrected efficiently by anterior intrusion of the four incisors. In patients with a larger discrepancy, the central incisors can be intruded first to the level of the lateral incisors. Further deep overbite correction with intrusion of all four incisors may follow to obtain the proper gingival relationship with the canine. In select cases, gingivectomy may further enhance this appearance.

Occlusal Plane Considerations

The occlusal plane essentially describes the dentition relative to the facial skeleton. The level and cant of the occlusal plane can be identified from a lateral cephalometric analysis (see Ch. 3). The level of the occlusal plane describes its vertical position and the cant describes its angle, usually relative to the horizontal reference (i.e. Frankfort horizontal) (Fig. 7-9). Additionally, there may be steps between the anterior and posterior teeth within the occlusal plane (Fig. 7-10). These considerations may impact on treatment planning for deep overbite correction.

Figures 7-10 and 7-11 illustrate the interrelationships between deep overbite correction and occlusal plane changes. Selecting consistent treatment objectives for both the occlusal plane and vertical tooth movements (anterior intrusion versus posterior extrusion) directs the orthodontist toward alternative approaches to deep overbite correction.

One common presentation of deep overbite malocclusions is an excessive curve of Spee. The upper and lower occlusal planes are parallel and a step or exaggerated curve exists between the canine and first premolar. Indiscriminate leveling of these arches may result in the undesirable effect of creating upper and lower occlusal planes that converge toward the anterior without adequate overbite correction. These convergent occlusal planes may be more difficult to correct than the original problem. It can be more effective

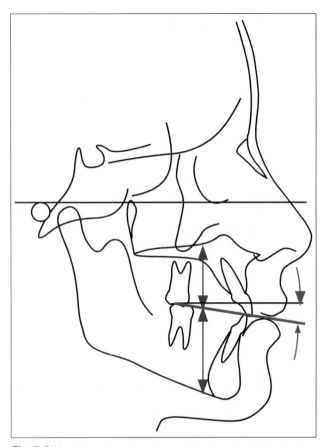

Fig. 7-9 Cephalometric tracing diagramming the occlusal plane level (blue) and cant (red).

to direct the vertical tooth movements and overbite correction to specific occlusal plane objectives.

Skeletal Considerations

Three skeletal considerations can significantly affect the outcome of overbite correction in patients: vertical dimension; anteroposterior relationship of the maxilla to the mandible; and in younger patients, the amount of growth remaining and its direction.

As described above, extrusion of the posterior teeth can affect the skeletal vertical dimension and soft tissue appearance. The approximate average of the anterior upper facial height ratio (nasion–anterior nasal spine [N–ANS])/ lower facial height (anterior nasal spine–menton [ANS–Me]) is 45–55%. Extrusion is contraindicated in patients with excessive lower facial heights. The increased tooth eruption tends to promote downward and backward mandibular rotation.[27] Pure intrusion of the anterior teeth allows a correction of the malocclusion without detrimental skeletofacial side effects.

In brachyfacial (short face) patients with deep overbite malocclusions, increasing the vertical dimension through posterior extrusion may be advised. It is important to consider function in these patients as a strong musculature increases the risk of post-treatment relapse. Slow correction during growth may allow the masticatory muscles to adapt to the treatment changes.

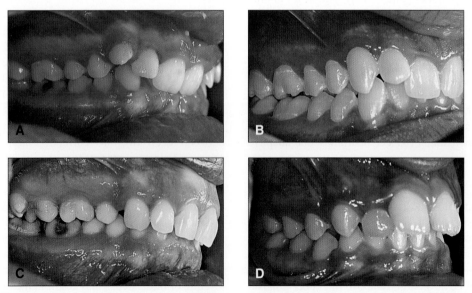

Fig. 7-10 Lateral view of deep bite showing the importance of the occlusal plane. **A-C** In these examples, the posterior occlusal plane needs to be maintained and the anterior occlusal plane (incisors) needs intrusion of the upper incisors. Placement of a straight wire before the incisor intrusion and axial inclination correction should be avoided as this would only steepen the occlusal plane by changing the axial inclinations of the posterior teeth. **D** Deep bite correction may need retraction of maxillary incisors without any extrusion to maintain the occlusal plane.

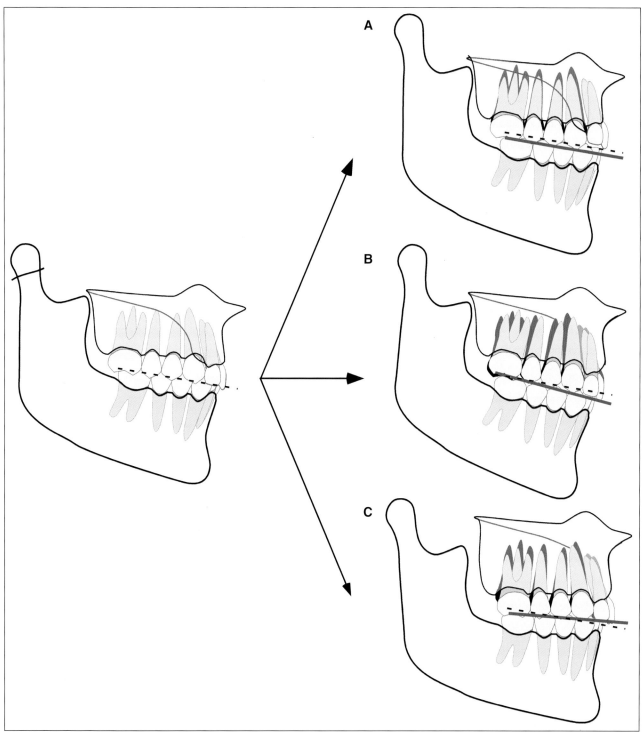

Fig. 7-11 Interrelationships between occlusal plane changes and deep overbite correction. **A** Posterior eruption and changing the level of the occlusal plane results in overbite correction by extrusion and the concurrent mandibular rotation. **B** Steepening the occlusal plane (rotation of the occlusal plane in a clockwise direction) also requires mandibular movement. **C** Flattening the occlusal plane (rotation of the occlusal plane in a counterclockwise direction) reduces the mandibular response.

Intrusion Arch Biomechanics

Burstone first described intrusion arch mechanics as part of the segmented arch technique.[8,28–30] Until 1980, intrusion arches were made of stainless steel wires with helical springs in front of the molars to reduce the load deflection rate. In 1980, beta-titanium alloys replaced stainless steel, eliminating the need for a helical spring due to the titanium wire's lower stiffness. Preformed nickel–titanium wires (Connecticut Intrusion Arch*) were introduced in 1998.[18] These preactivated and precalibrated wires deliver a force of 35–45 g (the force depends on the distance between the molars and incisors).[31] Each alloy remains an alternative for the fabrication of intrusion arches.

A major objective of using auxiliary springs, such as an intrusion arch, is the improved control of the applied forces, both relative to the qualitative and quantitative force systems. The design of the intrusion arch allows accurate prediction of the directions of the forces that the springs exert on the teeth. Springs of this design are statically determinant, i.e. it is possible to measure the magnitude of all the forces produced by their activation. The vertical intrusive force on the incisors is balanced by an equal but opposite extrusive force at the molar tube. These two forces produce an "interbracket" couple which is opposed by an "intrabracket" couple of equal magnitude but in an opposite direction at the molar tube. The following biomechanic factors are important in understanding intrusive mechanics:
1. Magnitude of force
2. Force constancy/load deflection rate
3. Point of force application
4. Molar tipback moment.

Magnitude of Force

Intrusive tooth movements appear to occur most effectively with low force magnitudes. This may be due to both the nature of the stresses acting on the periodontal ligament as well as the concentration of the stresses at the apices of the teeth. Lower force magnitudes also reduce the strength of the tipback moment acting on the molar or posterior segment. Clinical experience and experimental studies indicate that the force values listed in Table 7-2 are effective for the intrusion of anterior teeth.

Generally, it is recommended that canines are intruded separately. Including canines into a maxillary anterior segment requires an increase in the applied intrusion force. The reciprocal extrusive force on the molars and the increased tipback moment may result in undesirable side effects. Separate canine intrusion may be readily achieved with the use of cantilever springs.

Force Constancy/Load Deflection Rate

Compared to conventional/continuous wire activations, segmented springs exert forces in a range greater than the

*Ortho Organizers Inc, San Marcos, CA

Table 7-2	Force values for the intrusion of anterior teeth.[31]	
Teeth	**Force value (g)**
Maxillary central incisor	12–15
Maxillary lateral incisor	8–10
Maxillary cuspid incisor	25
Mandibular central incisor	8–10
Mandibular lateral incisor	8–10
Mandibular cuspid incisor	25
Maxillary four incisors	35–50
Mandibular four incisors	30–40

intended tooth movement (Fig. 7-12). The deflection of the spring engaging it to the incisors exceeds the amount of overbite correction. This feature both reduces the magnitude of the applied force and improves its constancy. A more continuous, low force allows increased time intervals between adjustments and may be gentler on the responding tissues.

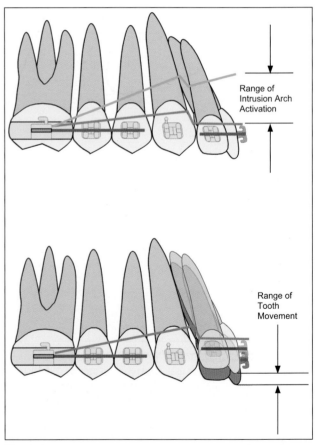

Fig. 7-12 A and **B** Range of spring activation for intrusion arches exceeds the desired tooth movement. The increased range of activation allows more force constancy through the reduction in load/deflection rate and reduced force magnitudes.

Point of Force Application

An essential feature of an intrusion arch is that it applies force via a point in contact with the incisors. Therefore, the expected clinical actions may be understood by assessing the applied force vector. Force magnitude, line of action, and origin are three key features of vectors. Each feature is important in understanding the clinical effects.

The point of force application and the direction of the line of action determine the tendency for the force to produce rotational movement. An applied force with a line of action passing through the center of resistance of the tooth produces pure bodily movement (Fig. 7-13A).[32] The point of force application for intrusion is most often at the central incisor brackets. A pure vertical force vector passes anterior to the center of resistance of the incisors (Fig. 7-13B). The effect of this force vector on the incisor is both an upward movement and a crown–labial/root apex–lingual rotation due to the moment of this force. Although there is no "applied torque," the expected tooth movement has a rotational component.

Figure 7-14 illustrates four clinical scenarios of intrusion arches, demonstrating the importance of the point of force application and its line of action. The expected movements are shown by the shadowed tooth in each figure. In Figure 7-14A, the incisors have an average axial inclination with a vertical, intrusive force applied at the central bracket. The force is placed more distally in Figure 7-14B; the intrusion arch is attached at the lateral incisor bracket. Figure 7-14C has a similar intrusion activation as Figure 7-14A, except that the incisors are excessively flared. Figure 7-14D depicts excessively upright central incisors, as may occur in an extreme Class II, Division 2 malocclusion.

In Figure 7-14A the intrusion force would be expected to move the incisor gingivally and to simultaneously

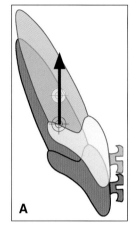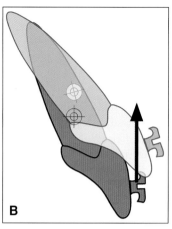

Fig. 7-13 Effect of point of force application and the line of action on movement. **A** Force line of force action passes through the tooth's center of resistance resulting in bodily movement. **B** Point of force application at the bracket with the line of force anterior to the tooth's center of resistance results in a combination of bodily movement and rotation due to the moment of the force.

flare it. Flaring is a result of the moment of the force. The amount of flaring depends on the magnitude of the moment, which is the product of the force magnitude times the distance of the line of action to the tooth's center of resistance. In contrast, the intrusive force passes through the center of resistance in Figure 7-14B. In this case the moment of the force is zero. With no moment, there would be a vertical movement without any change in the axial inclination of the tooth. Figure 7-14C shows that when incisors are severely flared, the large distance between the line of force and the center of resistance causes a much larger moment on the incisors, causing further undesirable

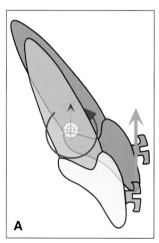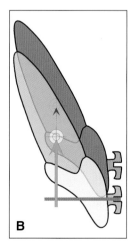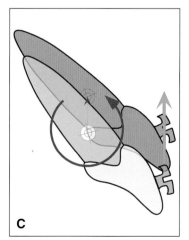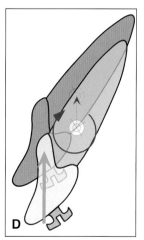

Fig. 7-14 Four scenarios for point of force application. **A** Force applied at the bracket produces a vertical movement and rotation. **B** Force applied acting through the center of resistance produces bodily movement. **C** Force applied at the bracket on a flared tooth increases the rotational effect due to the increased moment of the force. **D** Intrusive force on an incisor with an extreme lingual axial inclination will increase the lingual tilt because of the direction of the moment of the force.

flaring. At the other end of the spectrum is the severely upright incisor (Fig. 7-14D). The intrusive force passes lingual to the center of resistance, producing a small moment with a crown–lingual/root–labial direction. Rather than flaring the incisors, the force would tend to increase their uprightness.

These figures illustrate the ways that the same spring produces different clinical effects depending on the specific circumstances of its use. The point of force application is determined by selecting the appropriate tie-in point. The line of action of the intrusive force is a function of the spring's activation. To vary the line of force, applying additional force(s) is necessary. In most cases, this is a distally directed force. Combining a distal component of force to the intrusion arch alters the force by producing a resultant force. Figure 7-15A shows the resultant force vector from the addition of an intrusive and distal force. Clinically, the distal force can be produced in several ways. A small distal force may be applied by cinchback of the intrusion arch in the molar tube. The cinchback minimizes the potential for the overjet to increase by fixing the point of rotation of the intrusion arch spring (Fig. 7-15A). Without the cinchback, the intrusion arch is free to slide forward, with the potential for increased expression of the incisor flaring (Fig. 7-15B).

A greater level of control of the force vector can be obtained with the addition of an even greater distal force. In Figure 7-15C, an additional distal force is applied to the incisors, producing a resultant force vector that follows the long axis of the tooth. It is important to note that the distal force magnitude is smaller than the intrusive force (as mentioned above the intrusive force for the four incisors may be as little as 40 g). This light distal force redirects the line of action and results in an intrusive effect along the long axis of the incisor. A combination of deep overbite correction and overjet reduction can be achieved at the same time.

Molar Tipback Moment

An intrusion arch also applies forces to the molars. An extrusive force on the molar balances the intrusive incisor force. Additionally, the spring delivers a tipback moment on the molar. The magnitude of this moment is calculated by multiplying the distance between the molar tube and the point of attachment at the incisors. The span between these points varies based on the clinical situation, but frequently ranges between 25 and 40 mm. With an intrusive force of 40 g, the tipback moment acting on the molars may range from 1000 to 1600 g-mm. The moment magnitude is sufficient to produce a significant amount of distal molar movement (Figs 7-16 and 7.17).

This tipback moment aids in the correction of Class II molar relationships. Following tipback, molar uprighting and distal root movement can be achieved with the use of a high-pull headgear. Another approach is to use successively stiffer archwires for molar uprighting; however, this

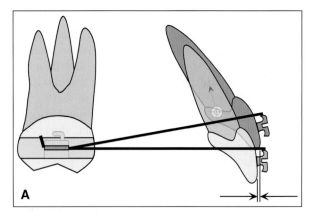

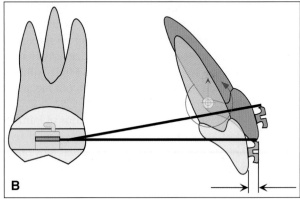

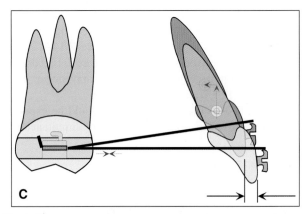

Fig. 7-15 Effect of intrusion arch cinchback. **A** Distal cinchback of the intrusion arch fixes the length of the spring and restricts the amount of incisor flaring. **B** Without the cinchback, the spring may slide anteriorly with the incisor movement resulting in flaring. **C** Combining a slight distal force with the intrusion force prevents incisor flaring and alters the direction of the resultant force vector, allowing simultaneous intrusion and retraction along the long axis of the incisor.

approach may be less predictable in maintaining the Class I molar relationships.

In Class I deep overbite problems, molar tipback is usually unnecessary and unwanted. Increasing the number of teeth in the posterior anchorage unit (first molar to first premolar) with passive heavy segments helps reduce the posterior effects of the intrusion arch (Fig. 7-18). In

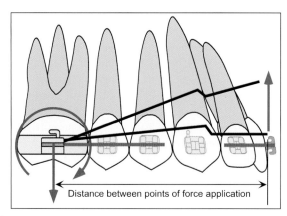

Fig. 7-16 Determining the magnitude of the tipback moment. The moment of magnitude is the product of the force magnitude times the perpendicular distance between the two forces.

Distance between points of force application

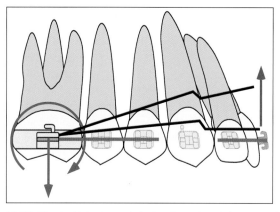

Fig. 7-17 Standard intrusion arch design. Separate anterior segments (four incisors) and posterior segments (first molar, second molar, premolar, first premolar) along with the active intrusion arch spring.

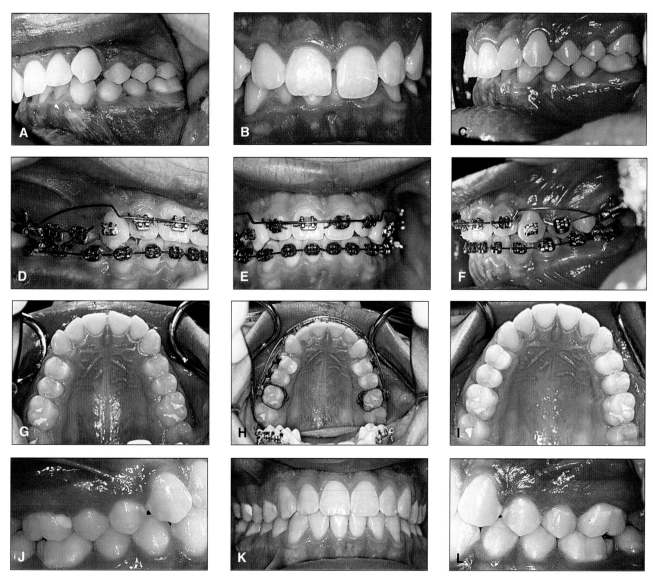

Fig. 7-18 Patient DM is a good example of intrusion arch use to correct deep bite, unilateral Class II occlusion and dental midline discrepancy (**A-C**). The intrusion arch (CIA) is ligated at three places on the anterior segment (**D-F**). A buccal segment is placed once the molars and bicuspids achieve a Class I relationship (**D, F**). The time lapse between **B** and **E** is 5 months. **G-I** show occlusal views before and during the intrusion (**G, H**) and during the retention phase (**I**). **J-L** Buccal occlusion and frontal intraoral view during the retention phase.

the mixed dentition, it may be advisable to use lighter force magnitudes to limit the amount of molar movement.

It should be noted here that distal movement of the upper molar is accomplished by the use of a vertical intrusive force in the anterior region. This is significantly different from various methods of molar distalization, which deliver reciprocal horizontal forces, thereby exacerbating the severity of the Class II relation in the canine region.

For intrusion of mandibular incisors, lower force values are recommended; therefore, the moments on the molar are much smaller. In the lower arch, buccal segments are valuable in enhancing the posterior anchorage during incisor intrusion.

Appliance Design

The primary characteristics of intrusion arches are similar regardless of the material from which they are made. This chapter discusses two versions: nickel–titanium intrusion (CIA*) arches and beta-titanium intrusion arches (CNA*). The basic form of the intrusion arch is shown in Figures 7-12 and 7-16–7.18.

Nickel–Titanium Intrusion Arches

These intrusion arches are fabricated from nickel–titanium wire, providing the advantages of low force magnitude and force constancy from the memory and springback characteristics of the material. Because nickel–titanium is not deformable under regular clinical circumstances due to its material properties, these springs are preformed. Comfort steps allow the wire to bypass the canine and premolar brackets with insertion into the molar auxiliary tube. Once inserted, the preactivation bend is located anterior to the molar tube.

The CIA* wires are available in two dimensions (0.016 × 0.022 and 0.017 × 0.025). For the same spring activations and interbracket distances, the smaller cross-section wires provide a reduced force magnitude compared to the larger sizes. Wires are also available in long and short sizes for both maxillary and mandibular arches. Long and short CIA* wires are based on moment bends placed in front of the molars. Longer arches are for nonextraction patients, and short wires are common for extraction patients.

Beta-Titanium Intrusion Arches

CNA* wires are advantageous due to their lower elastic modulus compared to stainless steel while retaining formability, which is not possible with the nickel–titanium wires. For equivalent spring activations (the vertical distance between the passive intrusion arch and the tie-in point at the incisors), a beta-titanium spring has a higher force magnitude compared to nickel–titanium.[33,34] Adjusting the preactivation bends allows the clinician to control the magnitude of force.

Preparation of the Patient for Intrusive Mechanics

Since intrusion arches are most commonly used as auxiliary or accessory springs, triple tube molar attachments are recommended. This allows use of the auxiliary tube (0.018 × 0.025) for the active intrusion spring and the main slot of the tube can be used for primary archwires or buccal segments. Additionally, the headgear tube permits the use of extraoral anchorage control.

Typically, the four incisors are bracketed for intrusive mechanics. A rigid anterior segment joining the incisors is ideal for intrusion as it minimizes the interincisor movement (see Fig. 7-18D). At the same time, four incisors can move as one multirooted tooth. However, if the incisors are crowded, rotated, or spaced, lighter wires can be used initially to align the anterior segment. During the aligning stage, intrusion mechanics can proceed.

The use of buccal segments (see Fig. 7-18C) on posterior teeth depends on the occlusion, stage of dental development (i.e. the eruption of premolars), and the anchorage needs of the individual treatment. Buccal segments redistribute the reactive extrusive and molar tipback effects to several teeth, limiting their expression. For simultaneous correction of deep bite and Class II molar correction (Figs 7-19 and 7-20) no buccal segment is needed, which allows a greater amount of molar correction.

While buccal segments may reduce the expression of the molar tipback and extrusion, they may not always eliminate them. Within the buccal segment, there is greater risk of extrusive tooth movement of the teeth anterior to molar (Fig. 7-21). The combination of the tipback rotation and extrusion is magnified in teeth more mesial to the molar tube. This effect could be especially problematic with respect to the canines. Excluding the canines from buccal segments prevents this untoward reaction. Figures 7-22–7-26 show patients with deep bite and flared incisors, deep bite treated with mandibular intrusion, deep bite with anterior occlusal plane, and smile problems, respectively. The patients were treated either with CIA* or CNA* intrusion arches.

Controlling Anchorage and Molar Correction with Headgear

The intrusive force on the incisors expressed by an intrusion arch is balanced by an equal and opposite extrusion force and a crown–distal tipback moment on the molars. When indicated, efforts to control or eliminate these potential effects may be necessary. Two methods of boosting anchorage with the use of intrusion arches are high-pull headgear and increasing the number of teeth in the anchor unit.

*Ortho Organizers Inc, San Marcos, CA

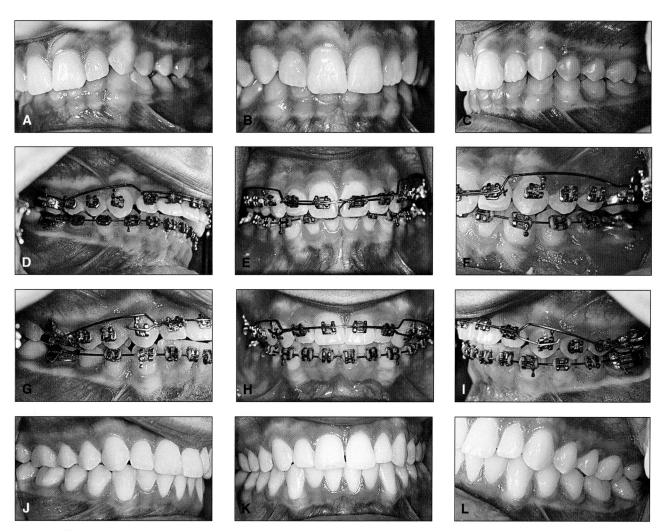

Fig. 7-19 Patient JK shows deep bite with a significant step between the maxillary anterior and posterior occlusal planes (**A-C**). A CIA intrusion arch is first ligated to the anterior segment only between the maxillary incisors to flare them and then the wire is ligated at three places (**D-F**). No buccal segment is placed to allow the molar tipback. At the third visit, a high-pull headgear is given. Note that the occlusal plane of the maxillary molar cusps shows that headgear wear was good. If the overbite is corrected before the molar correction, an anterior segment is placed to include the cuspids (**G-I**). This effectively stops intrusion as upper six anterior teeth need almost twice the force needed for incisors. The moment intrusion arch now only will move the molars distally into a Class I occlusion. **J-L** Patient at the retention stage with good overbite correction and Class I molar occlusion. *Continued*

High-pull headgear can effectively minimize or prevent unwanted posterior tooth movements during intrusion. The headgear opposes the extrusive force and generates a moment countering the tipback moment of the intrusion spring. The moment of the force produced by the headgear depends on the distance between the line of action of the headgear force vector and the center of resistance of the molar. The center of resistance of the upper first molars is approximately at the bifurcation of roots, or about 10 mm superior to the molar tube.[35] The force can be adjusted based on the distance of the point of attachment at the outer bow to the center of resistance of the upper first molar. For example, an outer bow 10 mm above the molar center of resistance with a force of 200 g will deliver 2000 g-mm of distal root moment. If the outer bow is closer to the molar center of resistance, the force can be increased to achieve the desired moment. The moment delivered by the headgear should be higher than the intrusion arch moment as the latter is active all the time, while headgear use is intermittent (10–12 h per night). In Class II correction,

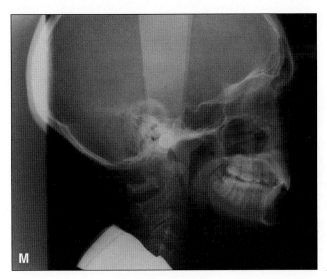

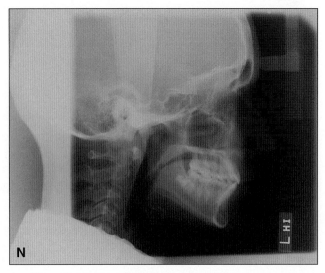

Fig. 7-19 *cont'd.* **M** and **N** Cephalometric radiographs of the patient before and after the treatment.

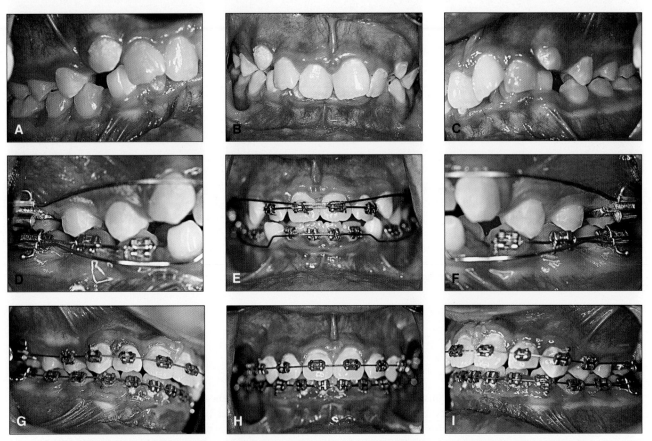

Fig. 7-20 Patient LC shows a >100% deep bite and edge-to-edge molar relationship, cuspids erupting in a Class II relationship, maxillary incisor crowding and problems with gingival height of maxillary incisors (**A-C**). **D-F** Correction of deep bite. The intrusion arch at this time is only ligated at a single point between the central incisors to slightly flare them. Maxillary bicuspids are not ligated yet as the molars are being allowed to achieve Class I occlusion. The patient at this stage also wears high-pull headgear. Note the minimal tipping of the maxillary molars. The lower incisors were also intruded 3 mm and, following intrusion, the CIA wire is ligated into the brackets. Buccal segments are placed in the mandibular posterior teeth to prevent any tipback. Once intrusion is complete and satisfactory buccal occlusion is achieved with the intrusion arch, finishing wires can be placed (**G-I**). *Continued*

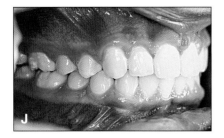
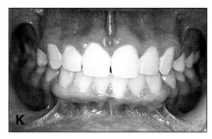
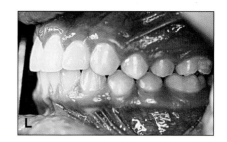

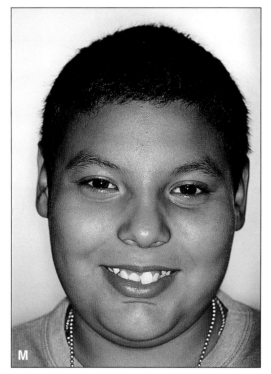
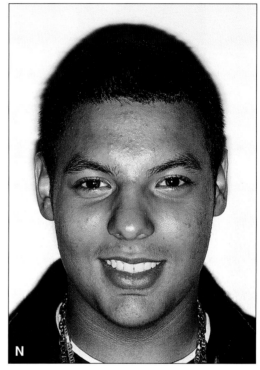

Fig. 7-20 *cont'd.* Finished intraoral views (**J-L**) show correction of deep bite and posterior occlusion. Maxillary incisal edges at this stage need restorative build up due to their shape. **M** and **N** Frontal smile views of the patient before and after treatment.

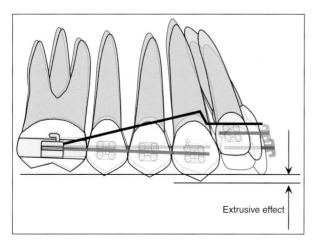

Fig. 7-21 Incorporating the canine into the buccal segment risks extrusive movement of the canine secondary to posterior segment tipback.

combining high-pull headgear with maxillary incisor intrusion provides an efficient approach to move molars distally. Generally, a 3–4 month period of headgear wear during the night only is sufficient to upright molars.

In Class I patients with deep bite, posterior anchorage can be maintained by using as many teeth as possible in the buccal segment. Distributing the extrusive and tipback forces over a large unit of teeth tends to lessen the amount of anchor movement and other unwanted side effects. A passive CNA* palatal arch further enhances the anchorage control.

*Ortho Organizers Inc, San Marcos, CA

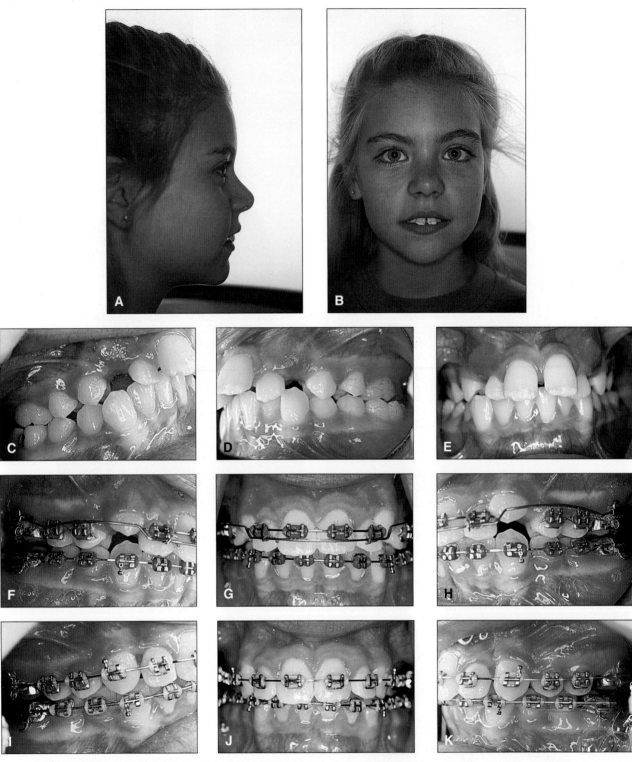

Fig. 7-22 Patient KM shows a large interlabial gap and a very large incision–stomion distance (**A, B**). Lateral intraoral views show a full cusp Class II molar relationship and molar crossbite (**C, D**). Frontal view (**E**) shows flared incisors camouflaging deep bite and midline discrepancy. **F-H** show that the intrusion arch is only ligated distal to the lateral incisors which has resulted in retraction of incisors and correction of deep bite. Buccal views (**F, H**) show partial correction of the posterior Class II relationship. The patient is also using a high-pull headgear at this stage. Note the ligation of the bicuspids with the molars and the flat occlusal plane of the molars, indicating patient cooperation in headgear wear. **I-K** show correction of deep bite and Class I buccal occlusion.

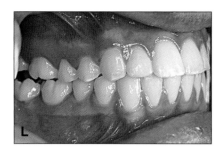
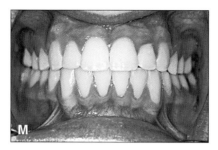
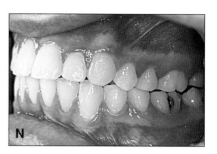

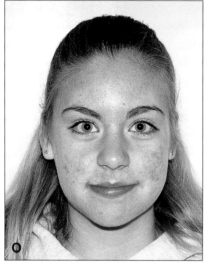
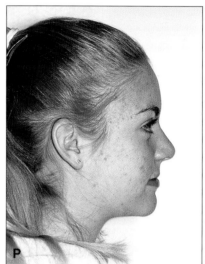

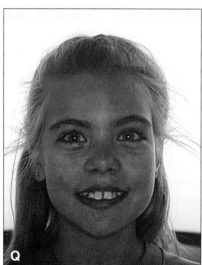
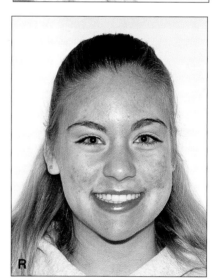

Fig. 7-22 *cont'd.* At this stage, CNA finishing arches show anterior and buccal views during the retention phase (**L-N**). **O** Frontal and **P** lateral views at the end of the treatment show lip contact. A significant improvement in the patient's smile is shown when comparing **Q** pretreatment and **R** post-treatment photos.

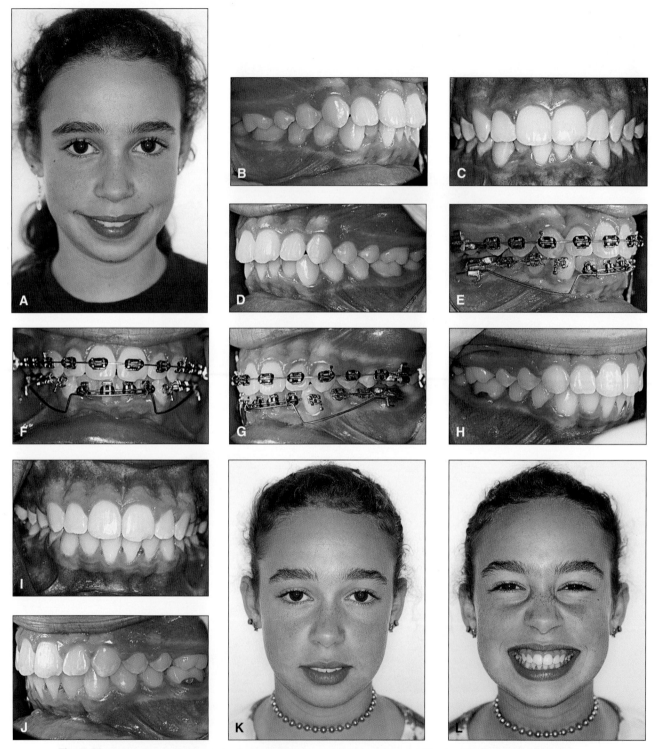

Fig. 7-23 Patient AD is a good example of when an intrusion arch in the maxillary dentition is not indicated at all. **A** Patient shows very minimal upper incisor even in smile. **B-D** Patient has moderate deep bite but an excellent interdigitation of the posterior teeth. The treatment plan is to maintain buccal occlusion and correct mandibular incisor crowding and occlusion. **E-G** CNA intrusion arch ligated to the mandibular anterior segment and a buccal segment on the posterior teeth to minimize any tipback of the molars. **H-J** Finished occlusion. Note the level of mandibular gingival margins compared to before treatment. **K** Incision–stomion distance after the treatment is maintained. **L** Patient in maximum smile. Although she shows gingival tissue in this view, the decision to intrude maxillary incisors is primarily based on the amount of incisor shown at the relaxed lip position.

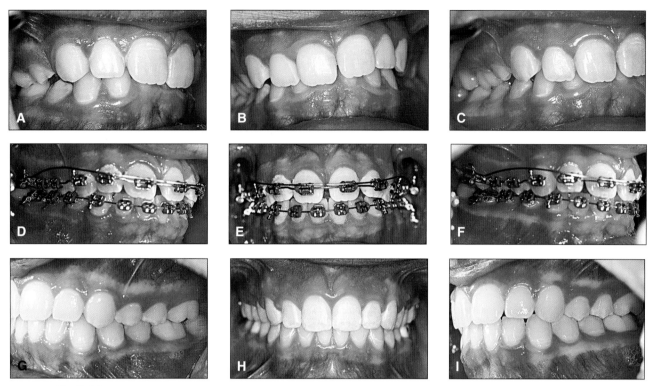

Fig. 7-24 Patient CC shows a canted upper occlusal plane and associated problem with gingival margin levels of the maxillary incisors (**A-C**). Patient received a CNA intrusion arch which was initially ligated asymmetrically to bring the incisor occlusal plane to one level. **D-F** Correction of deep bite and occlusal plane. The posterior occlusion is stabilized with a buccal segment. **G-I** Frontal and buccal occlusion during the retention phase.

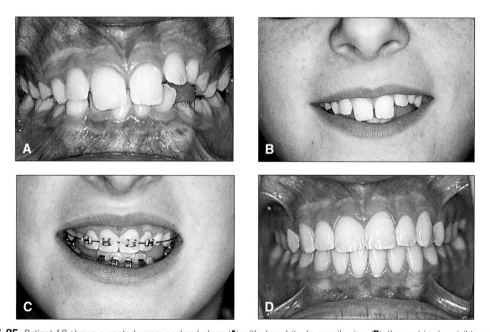

Fig. 7-25 Patient AC shows a canted upper occlusal plane (**A**) with deep bite. In a smile view (**B**), the cant is also visible and unattractive. The cant is corrected by the ligating intrusion arch on the right lateral for one visit and then the right lateral and between the central incisors at the next visit. Once the incisors are intruded, an ideal arch can be placed to bring the left lateral into the desired occlusal plane (**C**). **D** Finished treatment during the retention phase. *Continued*

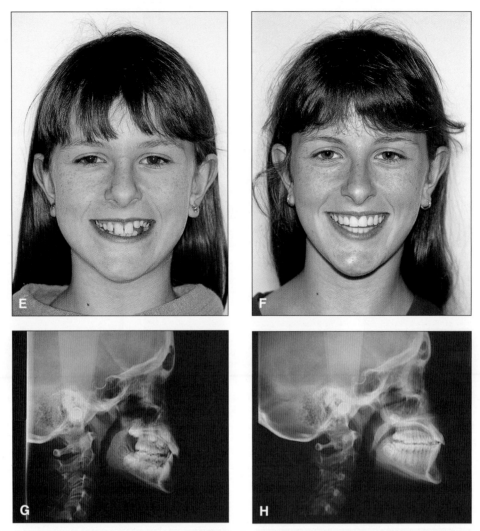

Fig. 7-25 *cont'd.* **E** and **F** Smile view before and after the treatment. Note the maxillary occlusal plane, upper lip, and gingival margins after the treatment (**F**). **G** and **H** Cephalometric radiographs of the patient before and after the treatment.

Clinical Concerns with Intrusion

Intrusion of Incisors and Apical Root Resorption

A major risk factor associated with orthodontic treatment is external apical root resorption.[36–40] While the prevalence of root resorption secondary to tooth movement appears to be high, reports average 1–2 mm for upper incisors with 2–3% of patients showing a loss of up to 4 mm. Of specific concern is the amount of root loss in response to the direction of movement, especially incisor intrusion. Many clinicians seem to have a subjective opinion that incisor intrusion increases the risk of apical root resorption. However, Baumrind et al found no significant associations between the directional variables of intrusion and root resorption.[41] In fact, this study showed an average of <0.06 mm of root shortening per millimeter of intrusion.

Deshields was unable to show a specific correlation between intrusion and root resorption.[36] Similarly, in a study of 200 consecutively treated patients, Kaley and Phillips did not show any cause and effect relationship related to intrusion and resorption of maxillary and mandibular root apices.[42]

Three studies have specifically looked at the effect of intrusion arches as described in this chapter. Goerigk and Wehrbein used intrusion arches on 31 patients for a mean treatment period of 4.3 months.[43] An average intrusion of 2–3 mm and apical root resorption of 1.0 mm was found. Dermaut and De Munck used a modified Burstone intrusion arch with Begg brackets in 20 patients for an average of 6–7 months.[44] The initial intrusion force on the maxillary incisors was 100 g. They showed an average intrusion of 3.6 mm with a mean apical resorption of 18% of root length. A prospective study by Costopoulos and Nanda showed a mean root resorption of 0.6 mm for the intrusion

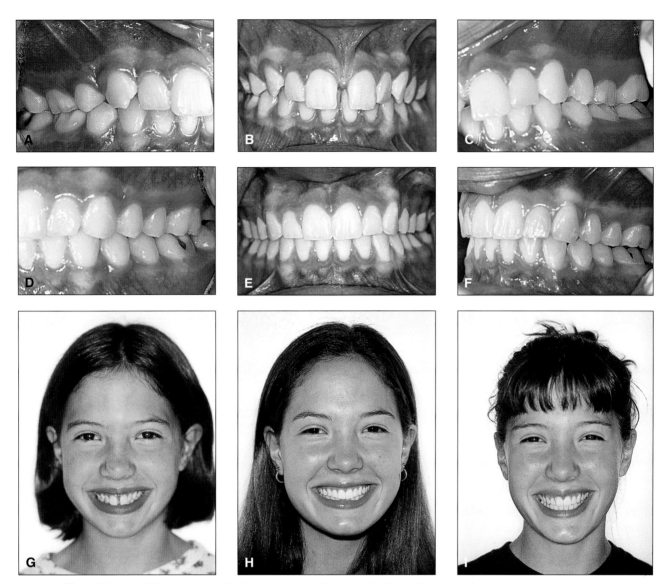

Fig. 7-26 Patient NK shows a deep bite (lower incisors touching the palatal tissue, flared upper incisors, and edge-to-edge molar relationship and Class II cuspids) (**A-C**). **D-F** show correction of malocclusion following 7-month use of a CIA maxillary intrusion arch to correct deep bite and posterior occlusion. A significant improvement in smile is shown before and after the treatment (**G, H**). **I** Two years following completion of the treatment.

group compared to 0.2 mm for controls.[45] This study used beta-titanium intrusion arches with an initial force of 60 g on four maxillary incisors. Faber, in a recent clinical study using CIA* intrusion arches with an average force of 38 g found negligible root resorption of incisors.[31] These studies confirm that lower force values provide a healthy biologic response. Based on the evidence, the risk of root resorption in response to a lower intrusion force does not appear to be any greater than with other types of orthodontic movement.[46,47]

Stability and Relapse of Deep Overbite Correction

The stability of deep overbite correction may be dependent on the specific nature of its correction (intrusion, extrusion, or flaring). Additionally, various factors, such as growth and neuromuscular adaptation, may play a role in relapse.

*Ortho Organizers Inc, San Marcos, CA

Simons and Joondeph, in a 10-year postretention study of deep overbite correction, reported that proclination of lower incisors and a clockwise rotation of the occlusal plane during treatment were significant relapse factors.[48] The stability of posterior extrusion is controversial, with conflicting reports of favorable longterm results versus high relapse potential.[49] Variables such as the amount of growth and the patient's age during treatment, muscle strength, adaptation, and the original malocclusion have all been postulated as factors contributing to the longterm stability of deep overbite correction.

Burzin and Nanda specifically investigated the stability of incisor intrusion.[34]

In this study, the average treatment time was 2.3 years and the average post-treatment observation period was 2 years. Overbite showed a mean reduction of 3.5 mm during treatment and a mean post-treatment relapse of 0.8 mm. The maxillary incisors were intruded an average of 2.3 mm and an insignificant relapse was noted (0.15 mm). This study showed that intrusion of maxillary incisors appears to be a stable procedure.

Summary

Deep overbite is a common form of malocclusion that may be addressed in many ways, including posterior extrusion, anterior intrusion, and incisor flaring. The specific approach to bite opening should be selected based on each patient's needs. Soft tissue, crown–gingival relations, occlusal plane, and skeletofacial concerns are among the special considerations for treatment planning for deep overbite correction. Selecting the method and mechanism of bite opening based on these considerations affords the opportunity to deliver goal-oriented treatment. Understanding the biomechanics of the appliances chosen improves the clinician's ability to achieve the desired results. With intrusion mechanics, the spring design allows attention to the magnitude of force, force constancy, the point of force application, and the molar tipback moment. Further control can be gained with careful wire selection and anchorage control techniques.

REFERENCES

1. Brunelle JA, Bhat M, Lipton JA. Prevalence and distribution of selected occlusal characteristics in the U.S. population, 1988–1991. J Dent Res 1996;**75**:706–713.
2. Dermaut LR, De Pauw G. Biomechanic aspects of Class II mechanics with special emphasis on deep bite correction as a part of the treatment goal. In: Nanda R, ed. Biomechanics in clinical orthodontics. Philadelphia: WB Saunders, 1996:86–98.
3. Fleming H. Investigation of the vertical overbite during the eruption of the permanent dentition. Angle Orthod 1961;31:53–62.
4. Moorrees C. The dentition of the growing child. A longitudinal study of dental development between 3 and 18 years of age. Cambridge, MA: Harvard University Press, 1959.
5. Nanda R. The differential diagnosis and treatment of excessive overbite. Dent Clin North Am 1981;25:69–84.
6. Otto RL, Anholm JM, Engel GA. A comparative analysis of intrusion of incisor teeth achieved in adults and children according to facial type. Am J Orthod 1980;77:437–446.
7. Weiland FJ, Droschl H. Evaluation of continuous arch and segmented arch leveling techniques in adult patients—a clinical study. Am J Orthod Dentofacial Orthop 1996;110: 647–652.
8. Burstone CJ. Deep overbite correction by intrusion. Am J Orthod 1977;72:1–22.
9. Case CS. A practical treatise on the techniques and principles of dental orthopedia and prosthetic correction of cleft palate, 2nd edn. Chicago: CS Case Company, 1921:480.
10. Ball JV, Hunt NP. The effect of Andresen, Harvold, and Begg treatment on overbite and molar eruption. Eur J Orthod 1991;13:53–58.
11. Callaway G. The use of bite plates. Am J Orthod Oral Surg 1940;26:120–124.
12. Dahl BL, Krogstad O. The effect of a partial bite-raising splint on the inclination of upper and lower front teeth. Acta Odont Scand 1983;41:311–314.
13. Hemley S. Bite plates: Their application and action. Am J Orthod 1938;24:721–736.
14. Sleichter C. Effects of maxillary bite plane therapy in orthodontics. Am J Orthod 1954;40:850–870.
15. Cooper RB. Indirect-bonded bite plate to prevent impingement on ceramic brackets. J Clin Orthod 1992;26:253–254.
16. Burstone CJ, Koenig HA. Creative wire bending—the force system from step and v bends. Am J Orthod Dentofacial Orthop 1988;**93**:59–67.
17. McNamara JA, Carlson DS, Yellich GM, Hendrickson RP, eds. Musculoskeletal adaptation following orthognathic surgery. Muscle adaptation in the craniofacial region, Monograph 8. Ann Arbor, 1978.
18. Nanda R, Marzban R, Kuhlberg A. The Connecticut Intrusion Arch. J Clin Orthod 1998;32:708–715.
19. Melsen B, Agerback N, Eriksen J, Terp S. New attachment through periodontal treatment and orthodontic intrusion. Am J Orthod Dentofacial Orthop 1988;94:104–116.
20. Melsen B. Tissue reaction following application of extrusive and intrusive forces to teeth in adult monkeys. Am J Orthod 1986;89:469–475.
21. Begg PR, Kesling PC. The differential force method of orthodontic treatment. Am J Orthod 1977;71:1–39.
22. Ricketts RM. Bioprogressive therapy as an answer to orthodontic needs. Part I. Am J Orthod 1976;70:241–268.
23. Greig DG. Bioprogressive therapy: overbite reduction with the lower utility arch. Br J Orthod 1983;10:214–216.
24. Kokich VG, Nappen DL, Shapiro PA. Gingival contour and clinical crown length: their effect on the esthetic appearance of maxillary anterior teeth. Am J Orthod 1984;86:89–94.

25. Tjan AM, The J. Some estetic factors in a smile. J Prosthet Dent 1984;51:24–28.

26. Janzen E. A balanced smile—A most important treatment objective. Am J Orthod 1977;72:359–372.

27. Levin RI. Deep bite treatment in relation to mandibular growth rotation. Eur J Orthod 1991;13:86–94.

28. Burstone CJ. Rationale of the segmented arch. Am J Orthod 1962;48:805–822.

29. Shroff B, Lindauer SJ, Burstone CJ, Leiss JB. Segmented approach to simultaneous intrusion and space closure: biomechanics of the three-piece base arch appliance. Am J Orthod Dentofacial Orthop 1995;107:136–143.

30. Shroff B, Yoon WM, Lindauer SJ, Burstone CJ. Simultaneous intrusion and retraction using a three-piece base arch. Angle Orthod 1997;67:455–461.

31. Faber ZT. The relationship of tooth movement to measured force systems: A prospective analysis of the treatment effects of orthodontic intrusion arches, Thesis. Department of Orthodontics, University of Connecticut, Farmington, 2001:1–77.

32. Vanden Bulcke MM, Dermaut LR, Sachdeva RCL, Burstone CJ. The center of resistance of anterior teeth during intrusion using the laser reflection technique and holographic interferometry. Am J Orthod Dentofacial Orthop 1986;90:211–220.

33. Gottlieb BS. The effects of an intrusive base arch on tooth position: A radiographic study, Thesis. Department of Orthodontics, University of Connecticut, Farmington, 1979.

34. Burzin J, Nanda R. The stability of deep overbite correction. In: Nanda R, ed. Retention and stability. Philadelphia: WB Saunders, 1993.

35. Dermaut LR, Kleutghen JP, De Clerck HJ. Experimental determination of the center of resistance of the upper first molar in a macerated, dry human skull submitted to horizontal headgear traction. Am J Orthod Dentofacial Orthop 1986;90:29–36.

36. DeShields RW. A study of root resorption in treated Class II, Div 1 malocclusions. Angle Orthod 1969;39:231–245.

37. Harris E. Root resorption during orthodontic therapy. Semin Orthod 2000;6:183–194.

38. Linge BO, Linge L. Apical root resorption in upper anterior teeth. Eur J Orthod 1983;5:173–183.

39. Harry MR, Sims MR. Root resorption in bicuspid intrusion. A scanning electron microscope study. Angle Orthod 1982;52:235–258.

40. Ketcham A. A progress report of an investigation of apical root resorption of vital permanent teeth. Int J Orthod Oral Surg Rad 1929;25:310–328.

41. Baumrind S, Korn EL, Boyd RL. Apical root resorption in orthodontically treated adults. Am J Orthod Dentofacial Orthop 1996;110:311–320.

42. Kaley JP, Phillips C. Factors related to root resorption in edgewise practice. Angle Orthod 1991;61:125–132.

43. Goerigk BD, Wehrbein H. Intrusion of anterior teeth with the segmented arch technique of Burstone—a clinical study. Fort der Kieferorthopadie 1992;53:16–25.

44. Dermaut LR, De Munck A. Apical root resorption of upper incisors caused by intrusive tooth movement: a radiographic study. Am J Orthod Dentofacial Orthop 1986;**90**:321–326.

45. Costopoulos G, Nanda R. An evaluation of root resorption incident to orthodontic intrusion. Am J Orthod Dentofacial Orthop 1996;109:543–548.

46. O'Hea C. A prospective investigation of maxillary incisor root resorption incident to orthodontic therapy, Thesis. Department of Orthodontics, University of Connecticut, Farmington, 1999.

47. McFadden WM, Engstrom C, Engstrom H, Anholm JM. A study of the relationship between incisor intrusion and root shortening. Am J Orthod Dentofacial Orthop 1989;96:390–396.

48. Simons ME, Joondeph DR. Change in overbite: a ten-year postretention study. Am J Orthod 1973;64:349–367.

49. Berg R. Stability of deep overbite correction. Eur J Orthod 1983;5:75–83.

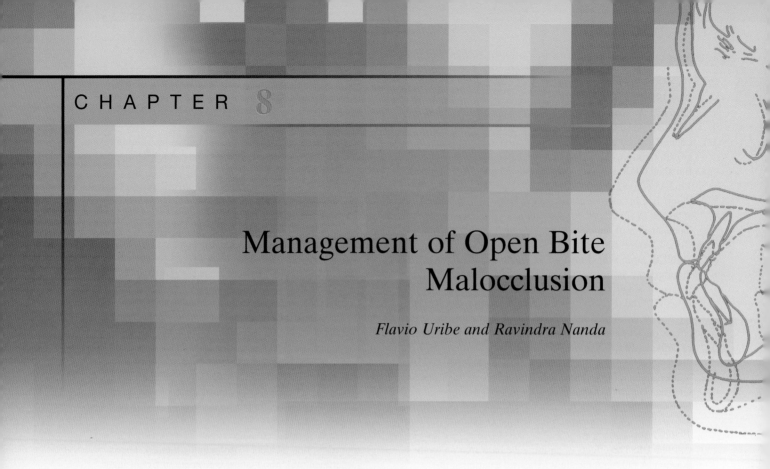

CHAPTER 8

Management of Open Bite Malocclusion

Flavio Uribe and Ravindra Nanda

The open bite malocclusion is one of the most difficult dentofacial deformities to treat. The complexity of this malocclusion is attributed to a combination of skeletal, dentoalveolar, functional, and habit related factors. Accurate diagnosis is essential for proper treatment planning, which, in combination with patient-specific mechanics, is needed to achieve stable results.

Open bite is an occlusal characteristic where the upper and lower teeth are not in contact and vertical overlap does not exist. Although this type of malocclusion can occur unilaterally or bilaterally in the buccal segments, it is mostly seen in the anterior segment. The anterior open bite malocclusion is most obvious when a clearance is observed between the upper and lower incisors from the frontal view. Of course, clinical diagnosis of an anterior open bite then becomes quite subjective, as it is based on the clinician's plane of evaluation (Fig. 8-1) and/or the patient's angulation of the occlusal plane. Taking the occlusal plane into consideration, a defined anterior open bite may or may not be evident from the frontal view; the steeper the occlusal plane, the less evident the anterior open bite becomes. Both issues are responsible for the numerous definitions of open bite in the literature.

The incidence of anterior open bite varies among races and with dental age. It is more common in African Americans (6.6%) than in Caucasians (2.9%) or Hispanics (2.1%).[1] Chronologically, as children develop dentally, the incidence of anterior open bite decreases, as it tends to self-correct during the mixed dentition phase.[2]

Although the term open bite typically refers to a dental malocclusion, it can be the result of a dental discrepancy, skeletal discrepancy, or a combination of the two. Terms such as skeletal open bite, vertical growth, hyperdivergent, and long-face pattern have been used to describe open bites that may be caused, at least partially, by a skeletal problem.

Most of the skeletal and dental characteristics commonly seen in open bite patients were initially described by Bjork.[3] This paper discussed the morphologic characteristics associated with downward and backward mandibular rotation during growth. These skeletal and dental characteristics include: distal condylar inclination, short ramus, antegonial notching, obtuse gonial angle, excessive maxillary height, straight mandibular canal, thin and long symphysis, long anterior facial height, short posterior facial height, steep mandibular plane, divergent occlusal planes, acute intermolar and interincisal angulation, anteriorly tipped-up palatal plane, and extruded molars. Of all these characteristics, the steepness of the mandibular plane has been considered the key skeletal finding associated with a skeletal anterior open bite.[4]

In terms of soft tissue characteristics, most parallel those of the hard tissues (long lower facial height, steep mandibular plane, and short posterior facial height). In addition, a large interlabial gap is most evident on clinical examination of a skeletal open bite patient (Fig. 8-2).[5]

Although all the above mentioned skeletal characteristics are associated with an anterior open bite, only 10% of patients with these features present with a clear anterior open bite evidenced as a negative overbite.[6] In many instances the skeletal open bite has been camouflaged by over eruption of the anterior teeth. This very issue makes classification of an open bite as either skeletal or dentoalveolar difficult. Often this malocclusion is the result of a combination of both factors.

It has been reported that skeletal open bites are often related to excessive vertical growth of the dentoalveolar complex, especially in the posterior molar region (Fig. 8-3A). Conversely, dental anterior open bites are primarily due to reduced incisor dentoalveolar vertical height (Fig. 8-3B).[7] The difference between these two types of open bites is

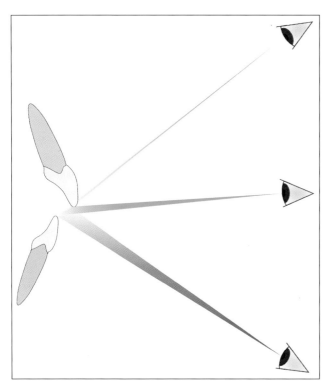

Fig. 8-1 Evaluation of an anterior open bite from different planes. No anterior open bite is evident from the upper most view. The lower most view angle reflects an extensive open bite not evident from the top view. The apparent magnitude of the open bite depends on the steepness of the occlusal plane and/or the plane of evaluation.

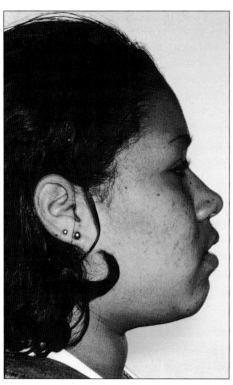

Fig. 8-2 A large interlabial gap (>3 mm) is the most significant soft tissue characteristic of a skeletal open bite.

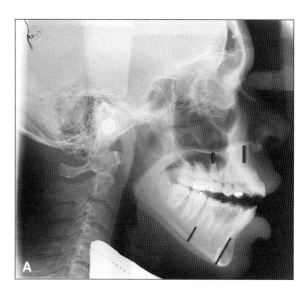

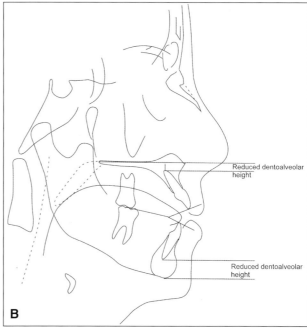

Fig. 8-3 A Excessive vertical height of the buccal segments is a common characteristic of skeletal anterior open bite patients. **B** Reduced anterior dentoalveolar height characterizes a dental anterior open bite.

also reflected in the occlusal planes. The skeletal type of malocclusion generally has occlusal contacts only at the molar level, with both occlusal planes diverging anteriorly (Fig. 8-4A), while the occlusal planes in the dentoalveolar open bite usually diverge from the first premolar forward (Fig. 8-4B).[8]

Even though the skeletal and dental characteristics of an anterior open bite are specifically related to the vertical dimension, these are also reflected in the anteroposterior

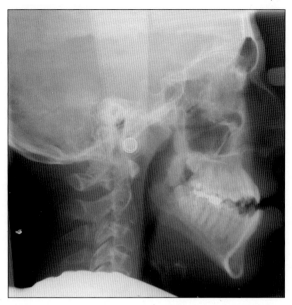

Fig. 8-5 Anterior open bite may also be found in patients with mandibular prognathism and Class III occlusion.

dimension. Open bite patients commonly have mandibles that are rotated down and back, with poor anterior chin projection and skeletal Class II patterns. However, although less common, some patients with skeletal anterior open bite may present with a Class III pattern (Fig. 8-5).[9–11]

Etiology

The etiology of any type of malocclusion is a combination of genetic and environmental factors. Although the genetic component of skeletal open bites is not well understood, the environmental factors that may contribute to this malocclusion have been reported extensively.

Environmental Factors

A major etiologic factor that reportedly contributes to open bites is an imbalance between the tongue and the perioral musculature.[12] Various habits such as tongue thrust, thumb and finger sucking, as well as anatomic conditions such as macroglossia have been reported as causative factors. These factors contribute to the development of an open bite malocclusion by adversely affecting the development of the anterior dentoalveolar complex and inhibiting the normal eruption of teeth.[13] Concurrent flaring of the upper anterior teeth is also observed as a result of the tongue or finger force against the lingual surface of the incisors.[14]

The clinician should carefully consider the role that the tongue plays in the etiology of open bite. Both the function and anatomy of the tongue must be evaluated. From an anatomic point of view, a large tongue (macroglossia) can be responsible for splaying the anterior teeth, and thus causing an open bite. Unfortunately, it is difficult to

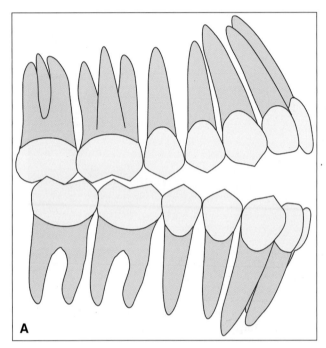

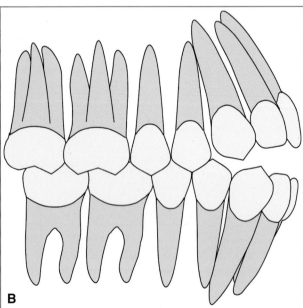

Fig. 8-4 Occlusal characteristics of skeletal and dental open bites. Occlusal planes **A** generally diverge from the first molar anteriorly in skeletal open bites and **B** generally diverge from the first premolars anteriorly in dental open bites.

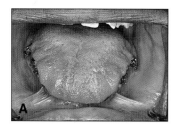

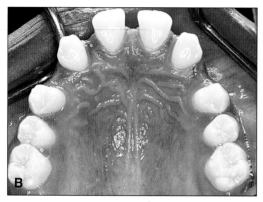

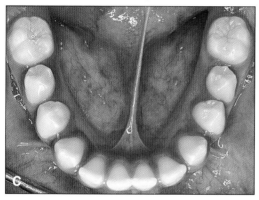

Fig. 8-6 Patient with a large tongue. **A** Intraoral clinical examination showing indentations on the lateral borders of the tongue and coverage of the occlusal surfaces of all the lower teeth. **B** and **C** Upper and lower arches depict generalized spacing.

that patients with long-face morphology tend to have weaker musculature.[18,19] Extreme examples of these skeletal characteristics are seen in patients with medical conditions such as muscular dystrophy.[20] Patients with this neuromuscular disorder cannot properly use their masticatory muscles to close the jaws. As a result the posterior buccal segments tend to supra-erupt, leading to an anterior open bite.

Another environmental factor that may contribute to open bites through a different mechanism of action is mouth breathing as a result of upper airway obstruction. Anatomic conditions such as enlarged adenoids and/or tonsils, deviated nasal septums, and swollen nasal turbinates may impair normal upper respiratory nasal function.[21] These patients maintain a low tongue and mandibular posture. Supra-eruption of the posterior teeth is considered to be the cause of the open bite. However a direct cause-and-effect relationship of mouth breathing and open bite has not been proven.[22]

Skeletofacial and dentoalveolar trauma have also been identified as etiologic factors of anterior open bite. Skeletal trauma involving the condyles has been shown to cause severe anterior open bites.[23] Arrested condylar growth or ankylosis of the condyle results in altered vertical growth of the mandible, clinically evidenced as an anterior open bite. Trauma to the dentition, particularly the incisors, can result in an anterior open bite if the damaged teeth become ankylosed before the patient finishes growing (Fig. 8-7).[24]

Finally, patients with degenerative diseases involving the condyles may develop anterior open bites. Idiopathic condylar resorption[25] and juvenile rheumatoid arthritis[26] are two pathologic conditions that involve condylar resorption. Clinically, an anterior open bite is evident as the disease progresses (Fig. 8-8).

diagnose macroglossia as there is no simple method available to quantify the volume of the tongue.[15] Certain features noted during the clinical examination that are indicative of macroglossia include: spacing and flaring of the anterior teeth, indentations on the lateral borders of the tongue, and lateral extension of the tongue onto the occlusal surface of the lower teeth (Fig. 8-6).[16]

From a functional point of view, the tongue may contribute to the development of an open bite by a continuous anterior posturing during swallowing.[17] Some controversy surrounds this point as the total amount of time during the day that swallowing occurs is very small to produce such a significant tooth movement. It has been proposed that the resting posture of the tongue is a more significant factor contributing to the open bite.

Neuromuscular deficiencies also contribute to the skeletal characteristics of an open bite. It has been reported

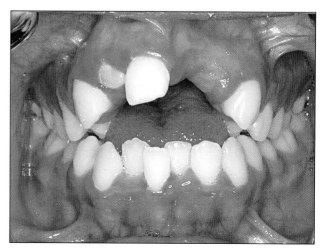

Fig. 8-7 Patient presented with ankylosed upper right lateral incisor due to previous trauma. Localized anterior open bite due to the arrested vertical dentoalveolar growth in this area.

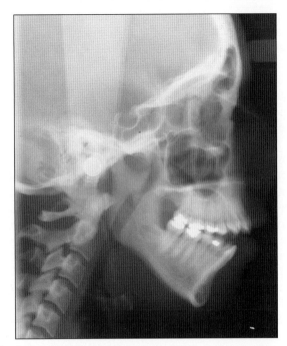

Fig. 8-8 A 21-year-old patient reporting progressive opening of her bite. The lateral cephalogram reveals a significant anterior open bite with shortened condylar morphology. Tomograms confirmed the resorptive condylar changes. The patient was diagnosed with idiopathic condylar resorption.

Genetics

The genetic component of an open bite is related primarily to the patient's inherent growth potential. Studies have shown that traits such as anterior facial heights are, to a high degree, inherited.[27] Obtaining a thorough family history will help the clinician predict a patient's growth potential.

Although the main goal in a child is to predict the vertical skeletal relationships at the end of growth, it has been shown that growth patterns are established early in life and maintained in the majority of individuals.[28,29] Therefore, a skeletal open bite pattern could be evident in the early mixed dentition. Numerous cephalometric planes have been used independently and combined to detect the early skeletal open bite pattern. Recently it has been suggested that the overbite depth indicator (ODI) index could be a good predictor in the primary dentition of a skeletal open bite tendency in the adolescent.[30] This index is a composite of cephalometric measurements involving the mandibular and palatal plane angles in relation to the A–B line and Frankfort horizontal, respectively.

Another useful method to help predict vertical growth patterns is the previously mentioned Bjork indicators. However, it is important to remember that these indicators are based on patients with extreme variations in vertical facial growth; they may be of limited value in patients with less severe open bite skeletal patterns.[31,32]

The genetic component is a very important contributing factor to the malocclusion. Control of the vertical growth pattern is difficult by orthodontic means alone. However, changes in the dentoalveolar complex may directly affect the most representative skeletal features of an anterior open bite. For example, controlling the vertical eruption of the molars allows the mandible to rotate in a counterclockwise direction, reducing the excessive vertical skeletofacial pattern.

Treatment Strategies

As described earlier in Chapter 3, treatment strategies should address the etiology of the malocclusion. Environmental factors contributing to a patient's malocclusion, such as digit sucking, should be identified during the clinical examination and eliminated. Other functional factors such as tongue thrust and airway obstruction need to be addressed in order to expect longterm stability of the anterior open bite correction.

Digit Sucking

It is common for children to have a finger or thumb habit. Many children stop this habit on their own, while others need assistance. Children should be encouraged by their parents to stop their habit before the age of 4 years. Prior to this age, most adverse dental and skeletal effects from the habit usually revert, creating a favorable environment for the eruption of permanent teeth.[13] Communication and positive reinforcement by the parents may help to modify any undesirable behaviors, but unless the child is willing to stop the habit, these attempts may not be successful.[33]

To aid the child in stopping a habit, it is important for the parents to note the time of the day the behavior is occurring, and then try to intervene. For example, if the habit occurs during sleep, mechanically obstructing the hand with a sleeping gown may be helpful.[34] If initial attempts are unsuccessful, an intraoral appliance that acts as a mechanical obstruction and reminder may be given. Different intraoral appliances are available for behavior modification. These consist of a stiff archwire with a series of loops that sit close to the anterior portion of the palate, and attach to two upper molar bands. The loops act as a mechanical obstruction/reminder of the pernicious habit. Spontaneous correction of any dentoalveolar or eruption problem is usually obtained after 3 months without using any other appliance (Fig. 8-9).

Tongue Thrust

Patients with tongue thrusts can be treated effectively in the same manner as digit suckers (Fig. 8-10), although different appliances such as the habit appliance with lingual spurs have been suggested for these cases (Fig. 8-11). It has been reported that spurs, rather than loops, result in better longterm stability.[35] Other devices aimed at retraining the tongue posture, known as myofunctional appliances, have also proven effective at treating tongue thrusts.

Myofunctional therapy aids in muscle retraining by using a series of tongue exercises to correct the deleterious resting and functional posture.[36] The results of this type of therapy have been mixed and no longterm studies are available. Additionally, it is difficult to assess the value of this therapy as orthodontic correction of the anterior open bite may produce the necessary seal during swallowing that the tongue was originally compensating for.[13]

Macroglossia

If macroglossia is diagnosed, surgical resection may be performed to reduce its volume. The open bite can then be corrected by retraction of the anterior teeth. Post-treatment, stability will most likely be enhanced, as the reduced tongue volume will better match the reduced arch length obtained after incisor retraction (A Kuhlberg, personal communication, 2003).

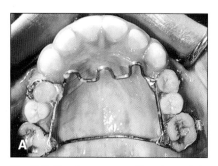 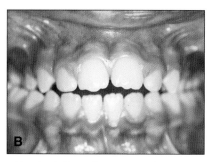 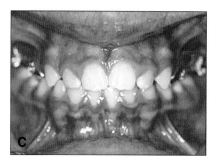

Fig. 8-9 Spontaneous correction of an anterior open bite after habit appliance delivery. **A** Habit appliance with loops acting as a mechanical obstruction in close approximation to the anterior portion of the palate. **B** Frontal view before appliance placement. **C** Three months after appliance placement.

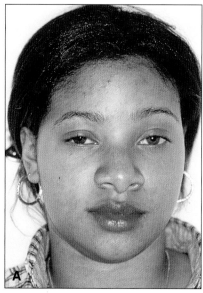 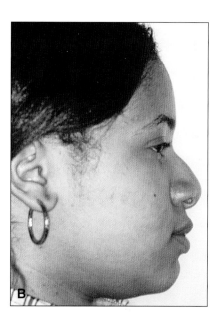 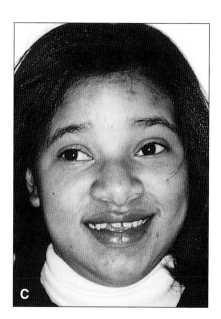
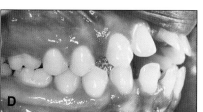 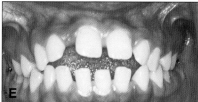 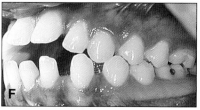

Fig. 8-10 An 18-year-old patient with a tongue thrust. **A-C** Extraoral views. On smile (**C**), only 50% of the incisors are displayed and an anterior tongue posture is evident. A reverse smile arc is consistent with the tongue thrusting habit. **D-F** Intraoral views showing a 3 mm anterior open bite with divergent occlusal planes from the first premolars. *Continued*

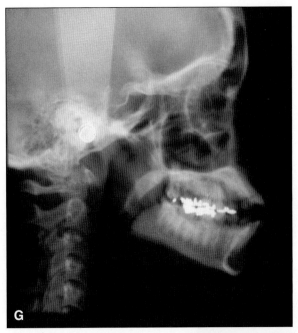

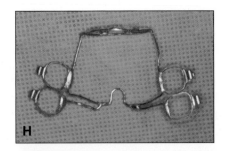

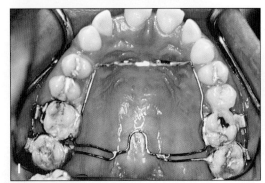

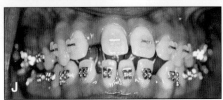

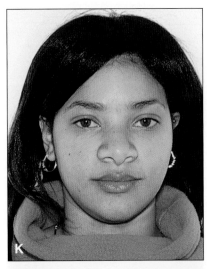

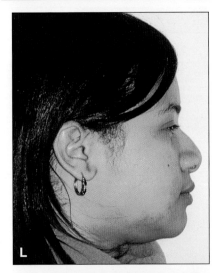

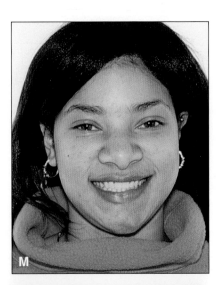

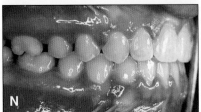

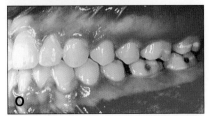

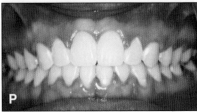

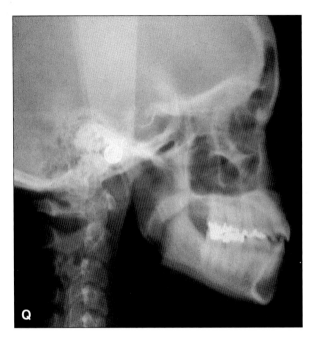

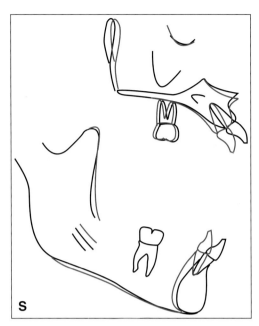

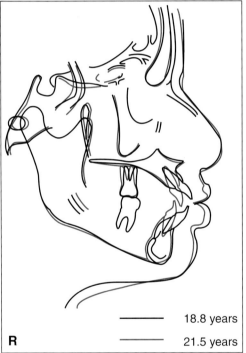

——	18.8 years
——	21.5 years

Fig. 8-10 *cont'd.* **G** Lateral cephalogram showing a dental anterior open bite with dentoalveolar protrusion. **H** Habit appliance with first and second molar bands, and anterior loop design close to the palate. **I** Intraoral view of the cemented habit appliance. **J** Brackets are placed after 6 months of exclusive treatment with the habit appliance. Fifty percent of the negative open bite self corrected. **K-M** Finished extraoral views. A positive smile arc (**M**) is obtained with approximately 90% incisor show on smile. **N-P** Adequate overbite is achieved with a good Class I relationship. **Q** Final lateral cephalogram showing the overbite correction. **R** General superimposition showing no maxillary or mandibular growth. Controlled lingual tipping of the upper and lower incisors reducing the dentoalveolar protrusion and anterior open bite. **S** Regional maxillary and mandibular superimpositions showing the same dental movements described above.

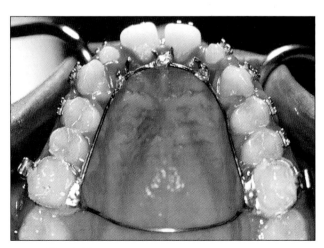

Fig. 8-11 Habit breaking appliance with lingual spurs.

Airway Obstruction

Procedures that allow for better nasal breathing (turbinate surgery, adenoid and tonsil removal, allergy treatment) may help to re-establish normal growth patterns.[37] However, research has shown great variability in the growth direction of the mandible after any of these procedures are performed.[38] This variability makes the decision to intervene with a resective surgical procedure difficult. Therefore, diagnosis of upper airway obstruction and the decision for surgical intervention should always be made by an appropriate team of specialists.

Correction of Open Bite by Incisor Extrusion

Extrusion of the upper and lower incisors is a common orthodontic treatment for anterior open bites. This treatment strategy is appropriate if the patient has an open bite with a normal skeletal pattern; although this treatment may also be applied to patients with vertical dysplasias that present with deficient incisor display at rest and smile. However, the vast majority of patients with long-face morphology and anterior open bite present with posterior as well as anterior vertical maxillary excess (Fig. 8-12).

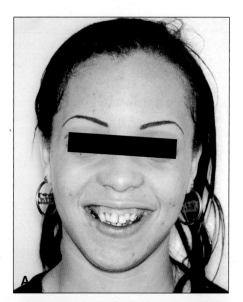
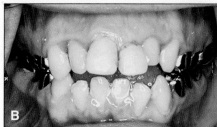

Fig. 8-12 A and **B** Patient with vertical maxillary excess and anterior open bite due to a digit sucking habit. Correction of the anterior open bite by extrusion of the anterior teeth will accentuate the anterior vertical maxillary excess to the biodetriment of facial esthetics.

Thus, correction of the malocclusion in these patients by extrusion of the upper incisors may result in an excessive display of the incisors and gingival tissues compromising not only the esthetic results but also the longterm stability. Nonetheless, the short-term occlusal results are usually satisfactory.

Different methods have been used to extrude the upper and lower incisors. These can be divided into compliant and noncompliant methods. Vertical elastics are the most common method for incisor extrusion in the compliant patient; extrusion arches are used in the noncompliant patient.

Extrusion Arches

Extrusion arches* are efficient tools used to correct upper and lower occlusal planes that diverge anterior to the first premolars. These archwires are indicated (1) when spontaneous correction of an anterior open bite does not occur following tongue crib therapy; (2) when a constant extrusive force is desired in the anterior teeth with minimal posterior side effects, and (3) in noncompliant patients who will not wear anterior vertical elastics.

The extrusion arch* is a one-couple force system (Fig. 8-13) that applies a single extrusive force to the anterior teeth, and a tip forward moment and intrusive force to the posterior segment. Often, the tip forward moment is undesirable.[39] First, to negate this side effect, a buccal segment from the upper first molar to the first premolar is added. Second, the magnitude of the extrusive force should be kept low (extrusion of the incisors requires very light forces) to maintain the posterior moment at a minimal level. Finally, adding vertical elastics off the posterior segment to negate this tip forward moment is also helpful (Fig. 8-14).[40]

The extrusive force of an extrusion arch applied to divergent occlusal planes anterior to the premolars is favorable, especially if the upper incisors are flared. As this force is

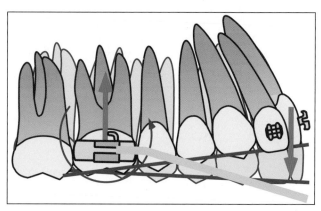

Fig. 8-13 Extrusion arch force system; a one couple system with an anterior extrusive and a posterior intrusive force. The couple on the molar produces a tip forward moment.

*Ortho Organizers Inc, San Marcos, CA

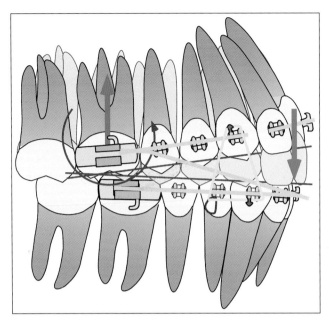

Fig. 8-14 Vertical elastic added to the upper buccal segment to negate the tip forward tendency produced by the couple system in the extrusion arch.

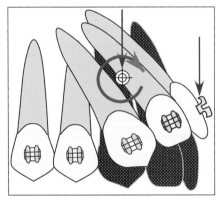

Fig. 8-15 Effects of the anterior force of the extrusion arch on the upper incisors. The applied force at the bracket will produce at the center of resistance of the incisors a clockwise moment plus an extrusive force of equal magnitude.

applied labially to the center of resistance of the incisors, the moment of the force will produce an uprighting movement (crown lingual) (Fig. 8-15).

Figure 8-16 shows a patient with anterior open bite that was corrected using upper and lower extrusion arches.

Vertical Elastics
Traditionally, vertical elastics have been used for open bite closure. Interarch mechanics with vertical elastics are indicated in anterior open bite cases with occlusal planes diverging anteriorly. Vertical elastics from the lower incisors to the upper incisors result in a consistent force system of equal and opposite forces (Fig. 8-17). Reduction of the overbite by extrusion of the incisors is the end result.

Although vertical elastics are a common method for incisor extrusion, certain problems are inherent in this type of treatment. First, response to this therapy varies greatly among patients due to poor control of the force magnitude and different degrees of compliance. Second, specific goals defined in the treatment plan (occlusal plane, incisor position objectives) can not be predictably achieved because good mechanical control is difficult with indiscriminate use of elastics.

Multiloop Edgewise Archwire Appliance
The multiloop edgewise archwire (MEAW) appliance is a combination of compliant and noncompliant mechanics where archwires with specific shapes in conjunction with vertical elastics correct the anterior open bite. It has been reported recently that most of the negative overbite reduction is achieved by extrusion of the anterior teeth with negligible molar intrusion.[41] Additionally, some correction of the intermolar angle is obtained which may aid in post-treatment stability.

Correction of Skeletal Open Bite
As mentioned above, although some patients may have the skeletal characteristics of an open bite, they may not exhibit a negative overbite in the occlusion (Fig. 8-18). If the anterior open bite is not evident, these patients must be treated with caution because the open bite can be expressed during treatment if not managed properly. In these patients the occlusion may have camouflaged the open bite skeletal pattern by excessive extrusion of the upper and lower incisors.[6]

Proper diagnosis of patients with skeletal open bite is essential. Key features to consider in the treatment of these patients are: the amount of incisor display at rest and smile, overbite, upper and lower occlusal planes, vertical molar height, interlabial gap, and mandibular plane angle. As mentioned in Chapter 3, all the dimensions (anteroposterior, vertical, and transverse) are closely related to each other. This is evident between the vertical and anteroposterior dimensions where a considerable number of patients with vertical maxillary excess not only exhibit a long facial height, but a mandible that swings back posteriorly. Additionally, it is common to find patients who present with a transverse discrepancy and an anterior open bite (this is most often seen in patients who have a finger habit or adenoid facies) (Fig. 8-19).[13]

Adult Versus Growing Patients
The treatment of skeletal open bites varies in growing versus adult patients. Treatment strategies in growing patients with skeletal open bites are geared towards vertical growth modification. In adult patients, the options are more limited, and a correction of the skeletal dysplasia usually involves surgery.

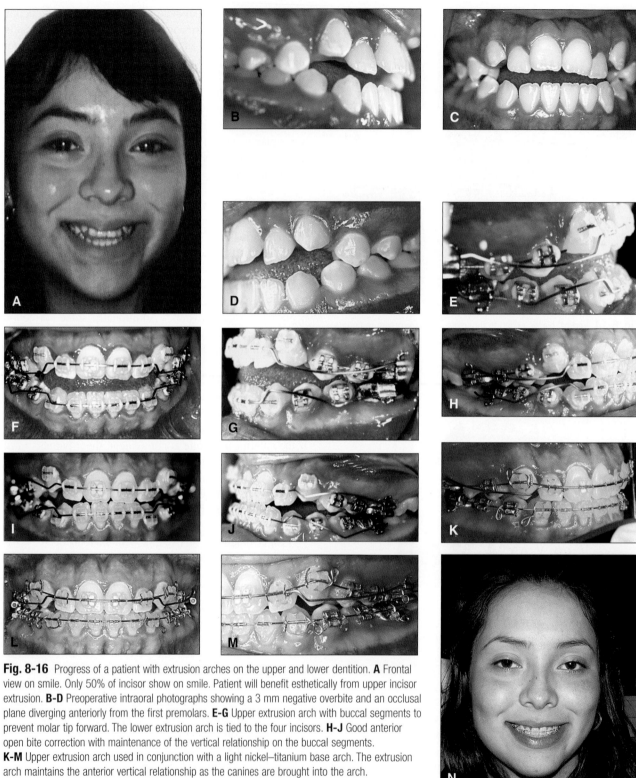

Fig. 8-16 Progress of a patient with extrusion arches on the upper and lower dentition. **A** Frontal view on smile. Only 50% of incisor show on smile. Patient will benefit esthetically from upper incisor extrusion. **B-D** Preoperative intraoral photographs showing a 3 mm negative overbite and an occlusal plane diverging anteriorly from the first premolars. **E-G** Upper extrusion arch with buccal segments to prevent molar tip forward. The lower extrusion arch is tied to the four incisors. **H-J** Good anterior open bite correction with maintenance of the vertical relationship on the buccal segments.
K-M Upper extrusion arch used in conjunction with a light nickel–titanium base arch. The extrusion arch maintains the anterior vertical relationship as the canines are brought into the arch.
N Esthetically a good smile arc and approximately 95% incisor display on smile are achieved.

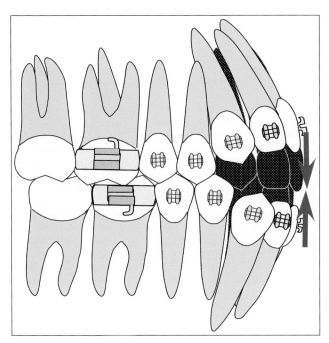

Fig. 8-17 Force system of anterior vertical elastics (equal and opposite forces).

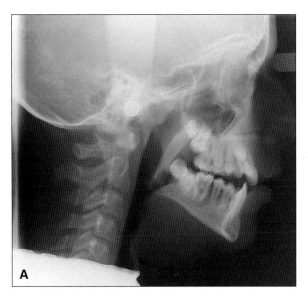

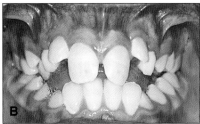

Fig. 8-18 A Cephalogram of a patient with skeletal anterior open bite characteristics but no negative overbite. **B** Anterior teeth have supraerupted, compensating for the vertical skeletal pattern.

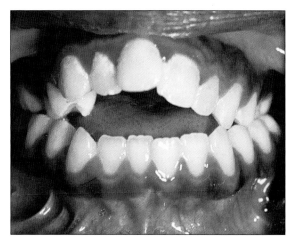

Fig. 8-19 Transverse dimension affected by a low tongue posture which is characteristic of patients with upper respiratory obstruction. This patient shows a maxillary constriction with bilateral cross bite.

The overall goal of treatment in growing patients should be vertical control of the molars to allow for correction of the open bite or open bite tendency.[42] Some of the direct methods that have been proposed are high-pull headgear or cervical-pull headgear to the mandible.[43] The rationale for this treatment is to prevent the eruption of the upper or lower molars and to allow the mandible to autorotate.

Other indirect methods, such as the vertical chin cap[43] and occlusal splint,[44] have been used to prevent molar alveolar vertical growth. The rationale for these treatment approaches is to prevent the eruption of the posterior teeth by delivering a vertical force via the occlusion. The occlusal splint is built with sufficient thickness (approximately 3–4 mm) to impinge on the freeway space. The chin cap and occlusal splint can also be used together for maximal effect.[45] Combining direct methods of force application, such as vertical-pull headgear, with indirect methods, such as occlusal splints, has also been reported.[46]

The active vertical corrector (AVC) appliance, which is considered to be a modified occlusal splint, may also be used for vertical control of the molars. This appliance uses repelling magnets embedded in acrylic to produce an additional posterior occlusal force.[47] Favorable effects have been observed in animal models.[48] Good vertical control was also seen in growing patients,[49] although there were limitations to the amount of vertical control such as the retromolar pad of the erupting second molar.[50] It is important to note that these appliances cause only a relative intrusion of the molar by preventing their eruption as the face grows vertically.

Other indirect methods used to control molar vertical growth include an acrylic button on the roof of the palate (see Ch. 9),[51] occlusally positioned palatal arches,[52] and lower lingual arches.[53] In all three methods the tongue acts indirectly to prevent vertical dentoalveolar growth of the molars.

Molar intrusion in nongrowing patients has always been a topic of interest. The rationale for this treatment method is based on the expectation of mandibular autorotation as the molars intrude, resulting in anterior open bite closure. For every millimeter of molar intrusion, approximately 3 mm of open bite reduction is seen in the anterior region.[54] Previous to absolute anchorage with implants, molar intrusion studies were limited to case reports. Most early attempts resulted in a reciprocal extrusion of the anchor teeth instead. The magnitude of the intrusion, if it occurred at all, was very small and generally difficult to verify in cephalograms.

Muscle exercises (clenching) as a means of closing anterior open bites have shown favorable results in growing and adult patients.[55] Although most of the published literature has been limited to case reports, it has been shown that the muscle force in hyperdivergent face patterns is reduced.[56] Although muscle exercises do not strengthen the masticatory muscles, intermittent forces applied to the opposing teeth appear to contribute to open bite closure.[19]

Recently, there has been increased interest in skeletal anchorage and the extended range of tooth movements previously unachievable with dental anchorage. Anterior open bites can be successfully corrected by intrusion of the posterior teeth with the help of skeletal anchorage.[57] Chapters 14 and 15 describe novel orthodontic movements achievable with skeletal anchorage.

Surgical Treatment

The decision between a surgical or nonsurgical approach to the treatment of a moderate-to-severe anterior open bite in an adult patient is not clear-cut. Longterm stability has been the deciding factor in the treatment decision, usually favoring the surgical approach. However, studies have shown that longterm stability results are very similar between the two treatment modalities.[58] Surgery is typically indicated if an esthetic objective is to be achieved (i.e. excessive incisor display pretreatment with vertical maxillary excess)[59] in patients in whom the open bite magnitude is so severe that orthodontic tooth movements would be outside the range of incisor extrusion (excessive occlusal plane divergence), and in patients where a pathologic problem (mostly at the temporomandibular joint level) needs to be addressed.

Surgery provides a consistent and esthetic result in patients who have anterior open bite with diverging occlusal planes, moderate-to-excessive incisal display, and a steep mandibular plane with a posteriorly positioned mandible. An optimal surgical outcome can be achieved only with maxillary impaction in these patients. Moreover, the stability of this type of surgery is very good because the pterygomasseteric sling and soft tissues are not stretched.[59]

Extractions for Open Bite Closure

Different types of extraction patterns have been suggested to correct anterior open bites. These extraction patterns include extracting: the second molars, first molars, second premolars, or first premolars.[60] The various extraction modalities for the correction of an open bite are tailored towards extruding the anterior segment, moving the posterior teeth anteriorly (wedge effect),[61,62] or a combination of the two.

Second Molar Extractions

The extraction of second molars has been suggested as a viable option in patients who have an anterior open bite with contact only on these teeth, and divergent occlusal planes (wedge effect).[62] Although this is a feasible option, the magnitude of the occlusal plane divergence is the limiting factor in full overbite correction (Fig. 8-20). A potential problem, depending on the age of the patient, is the necessary continuous monitoring of the third molars until full eruption and correct positioning in the arch is achieved.[63] However, this method provides an advantage over the other extraction patterns since no space closure is needed and vertical forces are not likely to be generated (see section on space closure in premolar extractions below). Interestingly, patients who present with this anterior open bite pattern (divergent occlusal planes with second molars only contacting) are generally viewed as surgical patients.

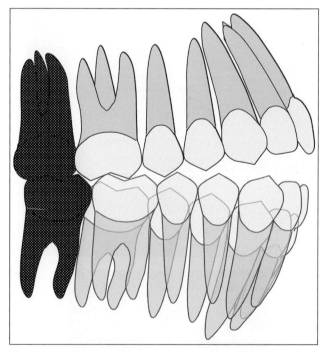

Fig. 8-20 Anterior open bite with occlusal planes diverging from the second molars anteriorly. All second molars are extracted for correction of the open bite. The magnitude of the open bite correction is dependent on the angle of divergence of the upper and lower occlusal planes. Full correction of the anterior open bite may not be obtained in extremely divergent occlusal planes.

First Molar Extractions

First molar extractions are typically performed only if these teeth are compromised by extensive decay. In theory, this treatment alternative should contribute to anterior open bite closure, and it has been reported that this extraction pattern maintains or slightly reduces the vertical skeletal relationships.[64] However, in the majority of patients, the second molar replaces the first molar and the anterior open bite is not resolved. As the molar is protracted into the extraction space, extrusion of the distal aspect usually results due to poor mechanics, thereby increasing or maintaining the anterior open bite. Overall, if this extraction option is considered, space closure mechanics is the deciding factor in the success of the overbite correction.[4,61]

This treatment alternative would be most effective if proper timing is considered. If the second molars have not erupted, and if the patient is only contacting on the first molars, extraction of the first molars would eliminate the increased vertical height and the second molars would only be able to erupt up to the new established vertical height (A Kuhlberg, 2003, personal communication).

Extractions of Premolars

Extractions of the first or second premolars are the most commonly considered procedures for the treatment of anterior open bites associated with crowding and/or overjet. The decision between extracting the first or second premolars depends on the amount of incisor retraction. In these patients the open bite is closed with the help of extrusion of the anterior segment instead of the "wedge effect." This treatment alternative works very well in patients with occlusal planes that diverge anteriorly from the first or second premolar. The mechanics are easier when the anterior teeth are flared (as is usually the case with this type of occlusal plane divergence).[65] A single distal force (ideally controlled tipping) will produce lingual tipping of the incisor crowns. Since the center of rotation is close to the apex, the net effect is extrusion and retraction of the incisors to close the bite (Fig. 8-21).

Biomechanics of Space Closure in Open Bites

Although the biomechanics of space closure is better discussed in Chapter 10, specific aspects as they pertain to anterior open bite will be reviewed here.

Group A Space Closure

Group A space closure is most difficult to perform in anterior open bite patients if intraoral anchorage is desired. The use of differential moments to maintain anchorage in this force system results in a large moment and an extrusive force posteriorly. Anteriorly a smaller moment and an intrusive force are generated. This force system is highly undesirable in an open bite patient.[66] Figure 8-22 shows that the vertical forces are antagonistic with this space closure strategy. An alternative would be to use a single couple system (intrusion arch*) where a couple is created at the level of the molar and an additional base arch

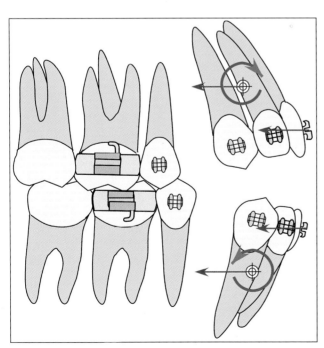

Fig. 8-21 Controlled tipping of the upper incisors produced by a distal force results in extrusion of the incisal edge and reduction of the amount of labial incisor inclination.

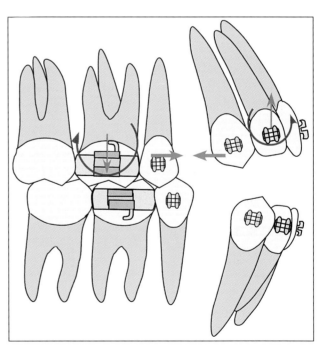

Fig. 8-22 Differential moment force system in group A space closure is unfavorable for anterior open bite correction. Vertical forces tend to accentuate the open bite.

*Ortho Organizers Inc, San Marcos, CA

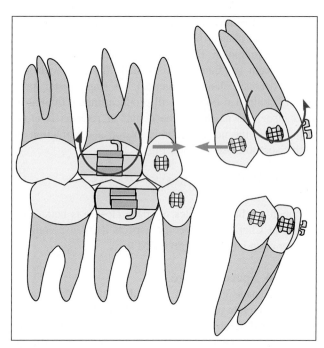

Fig. 8-23 Mechanics for group B anchorage with equal and opposite moments is favorable in anterior open bite patients since no vertical forces are generated. Adequate moment/force ratios of 10/1 are desired to prevent tipping of the posterior segments that may accentuate the open bite.

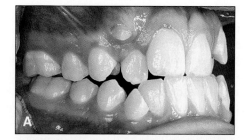

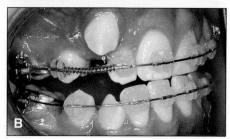

Fig. 8-24 Inadequate moment/force ratio in group space closure in an anterior open bite patient. **A** Preoperative right buccal view. **B** Patient showing tipping of the lower first molar and extrusion of the distal marginal ridge. Lateral open bite is developed.

(0.018 SS) is placed for canine sliding mechanics. The base arch would minimize the intrusive force in the anterior teeth while the intrusion arch would contribute to anchorage in the posterior end.

Group B Space Closure

Mechanically, group B space closure is the simplest.[67] No vertical forces are generated and only two equal and opposite moments are needed (Fig. 8-23). Careful monitoring is essential to ensure that equal moment/force ratios are delivered to the anterior and posterior segments. If a high force magnitude in relation to the moment is delivered in the posterior end, excessive crown tipping will result, extruding the distal cusps of the molar, and possibly increasing the open bite (Fig. 8-24).

Group C Space Closure

Group C space closure mechanics is the most favorable for anterior open bite correction. Intraoral anchorage by means of differential moments obtains a consistent force system. Figure 8-25 shows a larger moment in the anterior segment and an extrusive force that will maintain the anteroposterior incisor position. A smaller moment in the posterior and an intrusive force will allow this segment to tip as a mesial force is applied. The vertical forces will aid in the anterior open bite closure. The delivery of these mechanics is somewhat more complicated, as additional wires are needed if a sliding system is used. The progress using these mechanics is shown in the patient in Fig. 8-26.

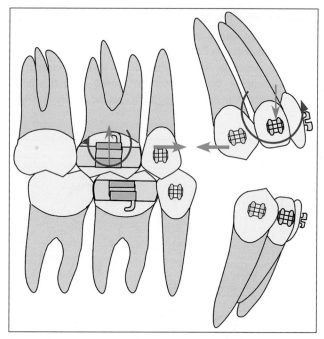

Fig. 8-25 Mechanics for group C space closure are the most favorable for open bite correction. Vertical forces are consistent with open bite correction in the anterior (extrusive) and posterior (intrusive) segments.

Bonding Second Molars

Traditionally it has been considered that bonding the second molars in a patient with an open bite tendency will result in an increased open bite.[68] The reason for this is that as the second molar is incorporated into the arch, it is usually more gingival than the first molar in the upper arch,

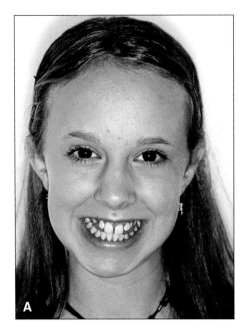
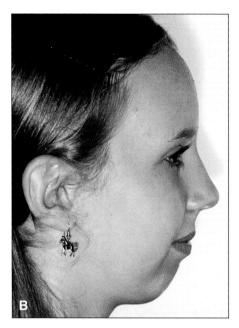
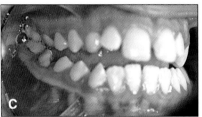
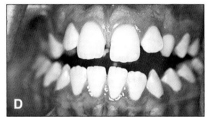
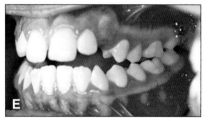
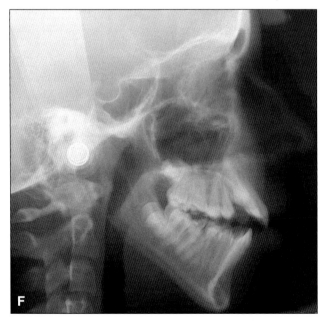

Fig. 8-26 Anterior open bite closure by molar extractions and group C mechanics. **A** Initial smile view showing an adequate amount of incisor show. **B** Profile view showing a retrognathic mandible and long facial height. **C-E** Preoperative photographs showing molar-to-molar open bite. All first molars have significant carious decay, except for the upper left. **F** Initial lateral cephalogram showing a retrognathic mandible with a skeletal anterior open bite and divergent occlusal planes from molar to molar. **G-I** Differential moment approach for group C space closure. A 19 x 25 stainless steel base archwire from 5 to 5 is used as the anchor unit to protract the lower 7s after extraction of the carious first molars. Sectional 17 x 25 CNA wires x with a V-bend offset anteriorly (Class V geometry) generate a larger anterior moment and extrusive force, and a smaller moment and intrusive force posteriorly. The sectional wire is connected to the base archwire by a vertical tube soldered to a horizontal tube. *Continued*

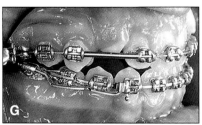
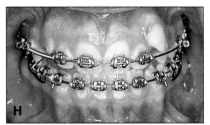
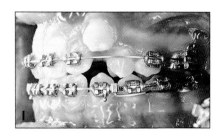

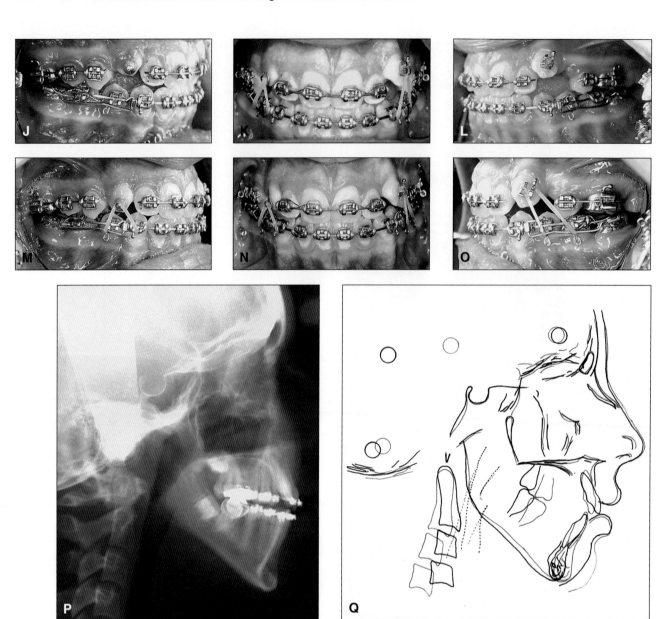

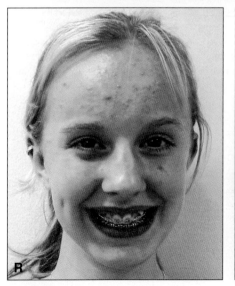

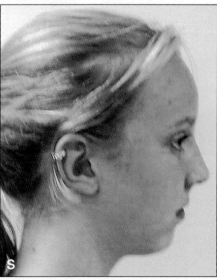

Fig. 8-26 *cont'd.* **J-O** Upper left first premolar extracted and upper canines brought into the arch using equal and opposite forces by means of an intermaxillary elastic. **P** Progress lateral cephalogram showing the anterior open bite closure. **Q** General superimposition showing the adequate vertical molar control with group C mechanics responsible for the anterior open bite closure. Mandibular autorotation evidenced with anterior positioning of the chin. **R** Smile view showing unaltered incisor display and open bite correction through molar vertical control as the second molars were protracted. **S** Profile view shows the positive skeletofacial change with the mandibular autorotation and reduction of the anterior facial height.

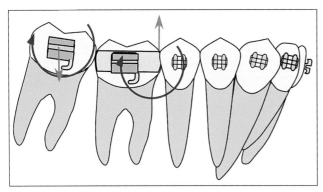

Fig. 8-27 Force system resulting from bonding the lower second molars. The vertical forces and moments are antagonistic to the open bite correction.

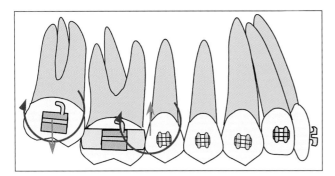

Fig. 8-28 Force system resulting from bonding the upper second molars. The extrusive force generated in the upper molars will accentuate the open bite. The anterior moment can cause over eruption of the incisors to the detriment of the esthetics.

and more occlusal in the lower arch (curve of Spee). When a straight wire is placed, a step geometry is generated. This causes the lower first molar to supra-erupt. Although the second molar experiences an intrusive force, this intrusion seldom occurs, probably due to the magnitude of the force, which is lower than the threshold needed for intrusion. Additionally, a tip forward moment is generated in the anterior segment that can open the bite (Fig. 8-27). In the upper arch the effect is extrusion of the second molar. If this extrusive force is not negated by the muscle forces, the mandible will rotate downward and backward (aggravating the open bite). The anterior moment generated is favorable for the open bite closure, but may be unfavorable to the esthetic objective as the incisor show will increase (Fig. 8-28). In summary, if alignment of the second molar is needed, care must be taken to engage the second molar passively in the second order.[68]

Esthetics and Open Bite

The three major esthetic factors to consider when planning the correction of an open bite are: incisor display, occlusal plane, and interlabial gap. In patients where anteriorly

divergent occlusal planes are present, it is important to decide which occlusal plane to treat.[69] Depending on this decision, the treatment will either be orthodontics or a combination of surgery and orthodontics.

The functional occlusal plane in an open bite patient with two divergent occlusal planes anterior to the premolars is the limiting factor in the amount of correction that can be obtained with orthodontics. This functional occlusal plane dictates the upper incisor position within a 1–2 mm range vertically. It is to this level that the incisors are to be erupted in order to achieve a positive overbite. If there is a reduced amount of incisor display at rest and smile, extrusion of the upper incisors is done until an acceptable level of display is achieved. The remaining amount of overbite correction can be achieved by extruding the lower incisors. In some instances this extrusion will accentuate the lower curve of Spee in an effort to obtain positive overbite but avoiding excessive upper incisor extrusion.

To achieve additional vertical correction of the anterior segments, the functional occlusal plane needs to be modified either by a clockwise (steepening) or a counterclockwise movement. Steepening the occlusal plane can be fairly easily achieved, although it is rarely desired. The reverse movement (counterclockwise rotation) is often indicated in skeletal open bites, but unfortunately it can rarely be achieved by orthodontic means alone (Fig. 8-29). The long-face patient with excessive gingival display and anterior open bite is a good example of a patient in whom a counterclockwise rotation of the occlusal plane is recommended

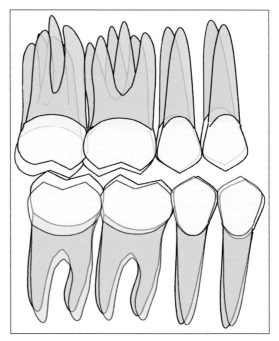

Fig. 8-29 Counterclockwise rotation of the lower occlusal plane by intruding the lower molars. Slight clockwise rotation of the upper occlusal plane is obtained by upper molar intrusion. The net result is anterior open bite reduction with mandibular autorotation.

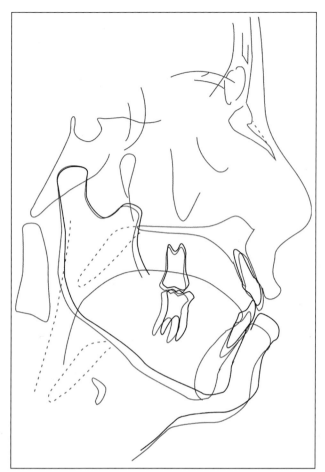

Fig. 8-30 Divergent occlusal planes on the buccal segment. Intrusion of the molar with counterclockwise rotation of the buccal segments results in upward and anterior mandibular autorotation. Esthetically, the incisor display can be maintained or reduced. Note that incisor intrusion can be attempted in anterior open bite patients by molar intrusion and counterclockwise rotation of the occlusal plane. This movement can be done by a Leforte I osteotomy or by using implants to intrude the molars.

movement, two-jaw surgery is usually done. The maxilla is impacted posteriorly with a center of rotation around the upper incisal edge. Some autorotation of the mandible follows and a minimal additional surgical counterclockwise rotation is done to correct the anterior open bite. These movements can also be achieved to a lesser degree with the use of implants and orthodontics for molar intrusion.

The final major aspect of esthetics in open bite patients is the interlabial gap. An excessive interlabial gap is one of the most notorious soft tissue characteristics of the skeletal open bite patient. This problem can be addressed in two ways. First, the interlabial gap can be reduced by retraction of the upper and lower incisors, although the magnitude of the vertical lip change in response to the incisor retraction can be unpredictable. The other alternative is to reduce the posterior facial height.

During growth, the posterior facial height can be decreased by the methods described above that control the dentoalveolar molar eruption. Once growth ceases, reduction of the interlabial gap can be obtained by molar intrusion (via maxillary impaction with mandibular autorotation or implants), or by a sliding genioplasty. The sliding genioplasty provides an additional advantage in vertical dysplasia patients. This procedure not only reduces the anterior vertical height but allows a more anterior positioning of the chin (limited invasive surgical procedure with good esthetic result).

Finally, it is important to note that the interlabial gap per se is not an indication of vertical skeletal dysplasia. It is important to evaluate the length and characteristics of the lips, as a lip lengthening procedure can be used to reduce the interlabial gap in the absence of vertical skeletal excess.[70]

Stability and Retention

The high relapse rate seen in patients with anterior open bites makes treating these cases frustrating. Relapse may result in negative esthetic characteristics such as a reverse smile line, and in some instances, interproximal anterior spacing.

A significant challenge to the longterm stability of anterior open bite treatment is the mechanical difficulty of retaining the vertical correction, especially if incisor extrusion is involved. Retention in the vertical dimension is complicated as it generally involves some sort of compliance with intermaxillary mechanics.

Open bites tend to relapse in approximately 20% of surgical and nonsurgical corrections.[58] The reasons for this instability are unclear due to the complex interaction of all possible etiologic factors. If the treatment plan does not address the etiologic factor(s), relapse is more prone to occur. Furthermore, even if the etiologic factor is identified, therapy may only change the environment temporarily. The result obtained may later revert due to a re-establishment of the etiologic factor(s). As a general rule, overcorrection is highly recommended for this type of malocclusion.

(see Fig. 8-11). In such patients the upper incisors should be maintained or intruded, and the upper occlusal plane either intruded or rotated in a counterclockwise direction to match the incisal plane (Fig. 8-30).

Treatment planning for a patient with divergent occlusal planes from molar to molar requires careful consideration of the esthetics and the occlusion. A treatment occlusal plane must be selected between the upper, lower, or an intermediate plane of occlusion. Generally, the upper plane, or a constructed one bisecting the upper and lower occlusal planes is considered. The lower occlusal plane is seldom used since it usually results in excessive incisal display and considerable extrusion of the upper buccal segments.

The upper occlusal plane is selected if a good vertical relationship is observed at the incisor (incisor display) and molar level. A surgical procedure is needed to rotate the mandible in a counterclockwise direction to match the upper plane. Due to the longterm instability of this surgical

Retention of this malocclusion should incorporate upper and lower fixed retainers that include the first premolars. In patients with divergent occlusal planes anterior to the premolars, this type of retention is ideal. The only problem is the high debonding rate of upper fixed retention, especially as the number of bonded teeth increases.[71]

Summary

The etiology of anterior open bite malocclusions is multifactorial. It is important to distinguish between a dentoalveolar and a skeletal open bite. Treatments to correct this malocclusion rely mainly on the molar vertical control and/or extrusion of the anterior segments in the growing patient. With the advent of implant anchorage, skeletofacial changes can also be obtained with molar intrusion in nongrowing patients. If esthetic results are desired in patients with severe long-face morphology, surgical options should be explored. Although all these treatments provide the possibility of attaining satisfactory outcomes, longterm stability remains the major challenge for the orthodontist, regardless of the therapy chosen.

REFERENCES

1. Proffit WR, Fields HW Jr, Moray LJ. Prevalence of malocclusion and orthodontic treatment need in the United States: estimates from the NHANES III survey. Int J Adult Orthod Orthognath Surg 1998;13:97–106.
2. Worms F, Meskin LH, Isaacson RJ. Open-bite. Am J Orthod 1971;59:589–595.
3. Bjork A. Prediction of mandibular growth rotation. Am J Orthod 1969;55:585–599.
4. Vaden JL. Nonsurgical treatment of the patient with vertical discrepancy. Am J Orthod Dentofacial Orthop 1998;113:567–582.
5. Mizrahi E. A review of anterior open bite. Br J Orthod 1978;5:21–27.
6. Dung DJ, Smith RJ. Cephalometric and clinical diagnoses of open bite tendency. Am J Orthod Dentofacial Orthop 1988;94:484–490.
7. Cangialosi TJ. Skeletal morphologic features of anterior open bite. Am J Orthod 1984;85:28–36.
8. Subtenly JD, Musgrave KS. The why of success or failure. In: Cook JT, ed. Transactions of the Third International Orthodontic Congress, London. St Louis: Mosby, 1973:432–445.
9. Magness MJ, Shanker SV, Vig KW. Interaction of the sagittal and vertical dimensions in orthodontic diagnosis and treatment planning. In: Bishara SE, ed. Textbook of orthodontics. Philadelphia: WB Saunders, 2001: 415–430.
10. Ellis E 3rd, McNamara JA Jr. Components of adult Class III open-bite malocclusion. Am J Orthod 1984;86:277–290.
11. Sassouni V, Nanda SK. Analysis of dentofacial vertical proportions. Am J Orthod 1964;50:801–823.
12. Winders RV. Forces exerted on the dentition by the perioral and lingual musculature during swallowing. Angle Orthod 1958;28:226–235.
13. Proffit WR. The etiology of orthodontic problems. In: Proffit WR, ed. Contemporary orthodontics. St Louis: Mosby, 2000:113–144.
14. Larsson E. Dummy- and finger-sucking habits with special attention to their significance for facial growth and occlusion. 4. Effect on facial growth and occlusion. Sven Tandlak Tidskr 1972;65:605–634.
15. Welch KC, Foster GD, Ritter CT, et al. A novel volumetric magnetic resonance imaging paradigm to study upper airway anatomy. Sleep 2002;25:532–542.
16. Wolford LM, Cottrell DA. Diagnosis of macroglossia and indications for reduction glossectomy. Am J Orthod Dentofacial Orthop 1996;110:170–177.
17. Kydd WL, Akamine JS, Mendel RA, Kraus BS. Tongue and lip forces exerted during deglutition in subjects with and without an anterior open bite. J Dent Res 1963;42:858–866.
18. Ingervall B, Thilander B. Relation between facial morphology and activity of the masticatory muscles. J Oral Rehab 1974;1:131–147.
19. English JD. Early treatment of skeletal open bite malocclusions. Am J Orthod Dentofacial Orthop 2002;121:563–565.
20. Kiliaridis S, Katsaros C. The effects of myotonic dystrophy and Duchenne muscular dystrophy on the orofacial muscles and dentofacial morphology. Acta Odontol Scand 1998;56:369–374.
21. Watson WG. Open–bite–a multifactorial event. Am J Orthod 1981;80:443–446.
22. Vaden JL, Pearson LE. Diagnosis of the vertical dimension. Semin Orthod 2002; 8:120–129.
23. McElroy S. Bjork predictors of mandibular rotation and their relationship to anterior open bite treatment. Farmington: Department of Orthodontics, University of Connecticut, 1998:187.
24. Proffit WR, Fields HW. Orthodontic treatment planning: From problem list to specific plan. In: Proffit WR, ed. Contemporary orthodontics. St Louis: Mosby, 2000:196–239.
25. Wolford LM, Cardenas L. Idiopathic condylar resorption: diagnosis, treatment protocol, and outcomes. Am J Orthod Dentofacial Orthop 1999;116:667–677.
26. Ronchezel MV, Hilario MO, Goldenberg J. Temporomandibular joint and mandibular growth alterations in patients with juvenile rheumatoid arthritis. J Rheumatol 1995;22:1956–1961.
27. Hartsfield JK. Development of the vertical dimension. Semin Orthod 2002;8:113–119.
28. Nanda SK. Patterns of vertical growth in the face. Am J Orthod Dentofacial Orthop 1988;93:103–116.
29. Bishara SE. Facial and dental changes in adolescents and their clinical implications. Angle Orthod 2000;70:471–483.
30. Klocke A, Nanda RS, Kahl-Nieke B. Anterior open bite in the deciduous dentition: longitudinal follow-up and craniofacial growth considerations. Am J Orthod Dentofacial Orthop 2002;122:353–358.

31. Ari-Viro A, Wisth PJ. An evaluation of the method of structural growth prediction. Eur J Orthod 1983;5:199–207.
32. Lee RS, Daniel FJ, Swartz M, Baumrind S, Kam EL. Assessment of a method for the prediction of mandibular rotation. Am J Orthod Dentofacial Orthop 1987;91:395–402.
33. Klein ET. The thumb-sucking habit: meaningful or empty? Am J Orthod 1971;59:283–289.
34. AlEmran SE. A new method in reminder therapy technique for ceasing digit sucking habit in children. J Clin Pediatr Dent 2000;24:261–263.
35. Justus R. Correction of anterior open bite with spurs: Long-term stability. In: American Association of Orthodontics Annual Meeting, 2004, Orlando, Florida.
36. Cayley AS, Tindall AP, Sampson WJ, Butcher AR. Electropalatographic and cephalometric assessment of myofunctional therapy in open-bite subjects. Aust Orthod J 2000;16:23–33.
37. Linder-Aronson S, Woodside DG, Lundstrom A. Mandibular growth direction following adenoidectomy. Am J Orthod 1986;89:273–284.
38. Linder-Aronson S, Woodside DG, Hellsing E, Emerson W. Normalization of incisor position after adenoidectomy. Am J Orthod Dentofacial Orthop 1993;103:412–427.
39. Nanda R, Marzban R, Kuhlberg A. The Connecticut intrusion arch. J Clin Orthod 1998;32:708–715.
40. Isaacson RJ, Lindauer SJ. Closing anterior open bites: The extrusion arch. Semin Orthod 2001;7:34–41.
41. Kim YH, Han UK, Lim DD, Serraon ML. Stability of anterior open bite correction with multiloop edgewise archwire therapy: A cephalometric follow-up study. Am J Orthod Dentofacial Orthop 2000;118:43–54.
42. Pearson LE. Vertical control in treatment of patients having backward-rotational growth tendencies. Angle Orthod 1978;48:132–140.
43. Pearson LE. Vertical control in fully-banded orthodontic treatment. Angle Orthod 1986;56:205–224.
44. Iscan HN, Sarisoy L. Comparison of the effects of passive posterior bite-blocks with different construction bites on the craniofacial and dentoalveolar structures. Am J Orthod Dentofacial Orthop 1997;112:171–178.
45. Basciftci FA, Karaman AI. Effects of a modified acrylic bonded rapid maxillary expansion appliance and vertical chin cap on dentofacial structures. Angle Orthod 2002; 72:61–71.
46. Fotis V, Melson B, Williams S, Droschl H. Vertical control as an important ingredient in the treatment of severe sagittal discrepancies. Am J Orthod 1984;86:224–232.
47. Dellinger EL. A clinical assessment of the Active Vertical Corrector—a nonsurgical alternative for skeletal open bite treatment. Am J Orthod 1986;89:428–436.
48. Woods MG, Nanda RS. Intrusion of posterior teeth with magnets. An experiment in growing baboons. Angle Orthod 1988;58:136–150.
49. Meral O, Yuksel S. Skeletal and dental effects during observation and treatment with a magnetic device. Angle Orthod 2003;73:716–722.
50. Kalra V, Burstone CJ, Nanda R. Effects of a fixed magnetic appliance on the dentofacial complex. Am J Orthod Dentofacial Orthop 1989;95:467–478.
51. Deberardinis M, Stretesby T, Sinha P, Nanda PJ. Evaluation of the vertical holding appliance in treatment of high-angle patients. Am J Orthod Dentofacial Orthop 2000;117:700–705.
52. Chiba Y, Motoyoshi M, Namura S. Tongue pressure on loop of transpalatal arch during deglutition. Am J Orthod Dentofacial Orthop 2003;123:29–34.
53. Villalobos FJ, Sinha PK, Nanda RS. Longitudinal assessment of vertical and sagittal control in the mandibular arch by the mandibular fixed lingual arch. Am J Orthod Dentofacial Orthop 2000;118:366–370.
54. Kuhn RJ. Control of anterior vertical dimension and proper selection of extraoral anchorage. Angle Orthod 1968;38:340–349.
55. Lindsey CA, English JB. Orthodontic treatment and masticatory muscle exercises to correct a Class I open bite in an adult patient. Am J Orthod Dentofacial Orthop 2003;124:91–98.
56. Garcia-Morales P, Buschang PH, Throckmorton GJ, English JD. Maximum bite force, muscle efficiency and mechanical advantage in children with vertical growth patterns. Eur J Orthod 2003;25:265–272.
57. Sugawara J, Baik UB, Umemori M. Treatment and posttreatment dentoalveolar changes following intrusion of mandibular molars with application of a skeletal anchorage system (SAS) for open bite correction. Int J Adult Orthod Orthognath Surg 2002;17:243–253.
58. Huang GJ. Long-term stability of anterior open-bite therapy: A review. Semin Orthod 2002;8:162–172.
59. Proffit WR, White RP, Sarver D. Long face problems. In: Proffit WR, ed. Contemporary treatment of dentofacial deformity. St Louis: Mosby, 2003:464–506.
60. Cusimano C, McLaughlin RP, Zernik JH. Effects of first bicuspid extractions on facial height in high-angle cases. J Clin Orthod 1993;27:594–598.
61. Kusnoto B, Schneider BJ. Control of vertical dimension. Semin Orthod 2000;6:33–42.
62. Kim YH. Anterior open bite and its treatment with multiloop edgewise archwire. Angle Orthod 1987;57:290–321.
63. Bishara SE, Ortho D, Burkey PS. Second molar extractions: a review. Am J Orthod 1986;89:415–424.
64. Aras A. Vertical changes following orthodontic extraction treatment in skeletal open bite subjects. Eur J Orthod 2002;24:407–416.
65. Sarver DM, Weissman SM. Nonsurgical treatment of open bite in nongrowing patients. Am J Orthod Dentofacial Orthop 1995;108:651–659.
66. Braun S. Biomechanic considerations in the management of the vertical dimension. Semin Orthod 2002;8:149–154.
67. Nanda R, Kuhlberg A. Biomechanic basis of extraction space closure. In: Nanda R, ed. Biomechanics in clinical orthodontics. Philadelphia: WB Saunders, 1996:156–187.
68. Beane RA Jr. Nonsurgical management of the anterior open bite: a review of the options. Semin Orthod 1999;5:275–283.
69. Burstone CJ, Marcotte MR. The treatment occlusal plane. In: Problem solving in orthodontics. Chicago: Quintessence, 2000:31–50.
70. Sarver D, Rousso D, White R. Adjunctive esthetic surgery. In: Proffit WR, ed. Contemporary treatment of dentofacial deformity. Mosby: Saint Louis, 2003: 394–415.
71. Segner D, Heinrici B. Bonded retainers–clinical reliability. J Orofac Orthop 2000;61: 352–358.

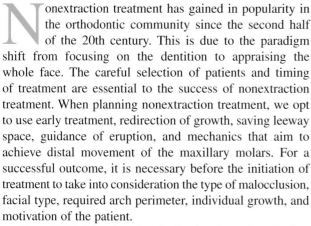

Biomechanic Strategies for Nonextraction Class II Malocclusions

Ram S Nanda, Tarisai C Dandajena, and Ravindra Nanda

Nonextraction treatment has gained in popularity in the orthodontic community since the second half of the 20th century. This is due to the paradigm shift from focusing on the dentition to appraising the whole face. The careful selection of patients and timing of treatment are essential to the success of nonextraction treatment. When planning nonextraction treatment, we opt to use early treatment, redirection of growth, saving leeway space, guidance of eruption, and mechanics that aim to achieve distal movement of the maxillary molars. For a successful outcome, it is necessary before the initiation of treatment to take into consideration the type of malocclusion, facial type, required arch perimeter, individual growth, and motivation of the patient.

Class II, Division 1 malocclusion has been described as the most frequent treatment problem in orthodontic practice. It is estimated that about 35% of American children have Class II malocclusions. Distal movement of the maxillary first molars is a common goal in the treatment of the Class II molar relationship and in the resolution of tooth size/arch length discrepancy in the maxillary arch.

Early treatment is the key to successful treatment of Class II malocclusions. During the 1940s and 1950s, Kloehn[1] suggested the use of headgear during the transitional dentition to correct molar relations. In the 1960s, Ricketts et al[2] promoted the bioprogressive philosophy, which utilized utility arches, quad helix, and cervical facebow headgear among several other innovative appliance systems. However, the real impetus behind nonextraction treatment was the realization that for far too long

orthodontists had focused on the placement of the denture on the basal bone without sufficient regard to the facial integument. Research findings on long term retention of treated dentitions revealed that relapse was common in both extraction and nonextraction treatment modalities. Cetlin and ten Hoeve[3] showed stable results for nonextraction treatment of patients with severe malocclusions. The thickness of facial soft tissue integument varies among individuals and its growth pattern is specific to individuals throughout their lifespan and not just during the period of active growth.[4] In view of these findings, the nonextraction treatment modality has become a treatment of choice for select groups of patients.

Patient Selection

Patients need to be carefully selected for nonextraction treatment. Prospective patients to be treated using maxillary molar distalization techniques should exhibit a Class II dental relation or a minor skeletal Class II relation. A Class II relationship with mesial migration of maxillary molars due to premature loss of the primary molar is preferred. The patient should have minimal or no mandibular arch length discrepancy, preferably with meso- or brachi-facial types, and potential remaining growth. A low mandibular plane angle is most suitable because in high angle the distal movement of molars will tend to open the bite due to the extrusive force component. Even a full Class II relationship can be corrected if treated earlier. Recently, Kim et al[5] have shown that an occlusion established at an early age is more likely to be maintained despite the differential growth of the jaws.

A variety of appliances have been used, including those that require patient cooperation and those that do not.

Biomechanic Principles

The adequate force for distal movement of the molars is in the range of 150–250 g. The type of movement can either be translation or controlled tipping followed by uprighting. Translation movement requires the force to pass through the center of resistance (see Ch. 1). Therefore, when using any type of appliance, it is necessary to evaluate the force system of that appliance and to be informed about the side effects. Anchorage considerations include extrusion of molars and mesial movement of the anterior segment. To obtain the maximum benefit the distal resistance (the presence of second or third molars), growth in the tuberosity region, and functional interferences should be checked.

Treatment Modalities for Maxillary Molar Distalization

Several treatment modalities exist for the distal movement of the maxillary molars. These can be either with fixed or removable appliances, and intra- or extra-oral. The extraoral approach can use cervical, occipital, or high-pull headgear. The intraoral mechanics can be inter- or intra-arch. Of the interarch appliances, the Herbst, twin force bite corrector, Jasper jumper, and "Saif" spring constitute fixed functional appliances that do not require patient compliance. Class II elastics with the jig and bimetric arch (Wilson appliance) require patient compliance. The transpalatal arch, coil springs, repelling magnets, K-loop,[7] pendulum, Jones jig, and distal jet are intra-arch appliances. These appliances can be used as single entities or combined with another appliance. Some of these appliances are discussed below.

Headgear

Kingsley[8] first introduced the extraoral method of applying traction to the maxillary arch to retract maxillary incisors. Later, Angle[9] described and illustrated the headgear he used in the treatment of patients with Class II, Division 1 malocclusion. Both Kingsley and Angle used astonishingly modern-looking appliances, apparently with reasonable success. At the beginning of the 20th century, the introduction of intermaxillary elastics resulted in the discontinuation of extraoral anchorage. This was not due to its ineffectiveness, but rather it was considered an unnecessary complication.

By 1920, Angle and his followers were convinced that Class II and III elastics not only moved teeth but also caused significant skeletal changes, stimulating the growth of one jaw while restraining the other. If intraoral elastics could produce a true stimulation of mandibular growth while simultaneously restraining the maxilla, there would be no reason either to ask a patient to wear an extraoral appliance or to initiate treatment while waiting for the permanent teeth to erupt.

When cephalometric evaluations became available, in the 1940s, they did not support the idea that significant skeletal changes occurred in response to intraoral forces. In 1936, Oppenheim[10] strongly advocated extraoral anchorage therapy. Later, Kloehn[1] demonstrated impressive results with headgear in the early treatment of Class II malocclusion. He stated that, during the transitional dentition, cervical traction can retard or even halt the forward growth of the maxilla and assist in moving maxillary teeth distally to correct developing Class II relationships.

While the distal movement of the molars by headgear may not be questionable, the changes that take place within the temporomandibular joint (TMJ) complex have not been well explained. Animal studies have shown remodeling of the condyle-glenoid fossa complex; apposition in the posterior compartment and resorption in the anterior.[11–13] Cephalometric studies have shown little or no change in the size of the mandible with the use of functional appliances such as headgear. It is possible that the lateral cephalogram is not sensitive enough to isolate these changes. The orthopedic forces applied by headgear cannot however be ignored.

Extraoral traction has some demonstrable important advantages. These include maximum anchorage, ability to adjust the force levels, and control of bodily or tipping movement. It can assist in correcting transverse deficiencies by expanding the inner bow. The extrusive component of the cervical headgear will allow for bite opening in deep bite patients. If vertical control is a concern in a high-angle patient, a high-pull facebow headgear will control the extrusive force component.

There are limitations in the use of extraoral traction, of which the need for patient compliance is perhaps the most important. Besides compliance, the type of force delivered by the appliance is intermittent, with tooth movement usually being slower. We have found that prolonged use of headgear can delay the eruption of maxillary second molars, or even lead to their impaction. This may not be a problem if treatment is initiated at the appropriate age of 9 years and for a limited time. In such cases, the second molars need to be monitored if treatment is completed prior to their eruption. Extraction of the second molars may be considered if the presence of the third molars is radiographically documented. Despite these limitations, extraoral traction is perhaps one of the most effective ways to obtain distal movement of maxillary molars and a successful nonextraction treatment plan.

A decision to extract the second molars may be made in severe Class II cases where maximum retraction of the first molars is required. As mentioned above, radiographic documentation for the presence of the third molars is important. Figure 9-1 documents a case where extraction of the maxillary second molars was performed prior to their eruption. A mandibular lip bumper engaged to the mandibular first molar bands was used to align and unravel the minor mandibular crowding. The maxillary premolars were allowed to passively drift back. Retraction of the anterior segment, however, required active mechanics and this was accomplished using a T-loop. Class II elastics were used for 1 month. During this process, the headgear was used as anchorage, and the patient wore it only at bedtime.

The headgear may effectively be used in cases of asymmetrical Class II correction. In such cases, there is asymmetrical adjustment of the outer bow, one side being longer than the other.[14,15] The longer arm of the outer bow will be placed on the side where correction of the Class II molar relationship is desired. Asymmetrically positioning the center of the outer bows while the arms are kept the same length may not achieve the same results as altering the lengths of the outer bows. This is because in the first instance, the force applied will pass through the center, while in the latter there is an asymmetrical distribution of the moments. The greater moment is applied to the

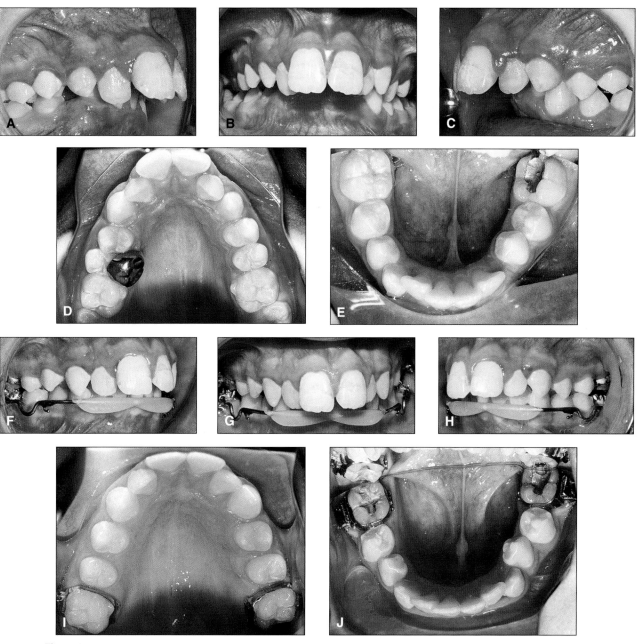

Fig. 9-1 Headgear treatment. **A-E** Pretreatment intraoral photographs. A stainless steel crown is present on the exfoliating maxillary left second primary molar. **F-J** Progress photographs showing the lip bumper in place. *Continued*

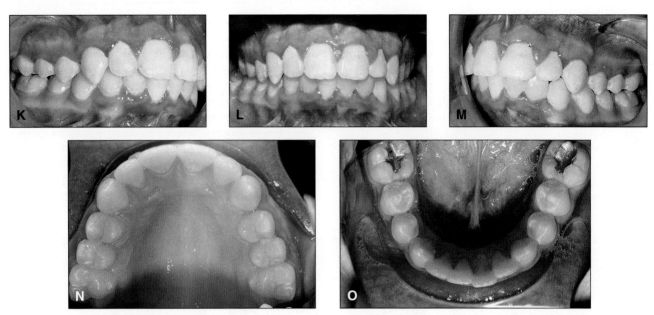

Fig. 9-1 *cont'd.* **K-O** Intraoral photographs 1 month post-treatment. Total treatment time was 23 months.

longer side.[14,15] Of importance, however, is the need for patient compliance.

Care should be taken to adjust the facebow so as to achieve the desired result. In open bite, for example, care should be taken to avoid extrusion of the molars while in cases of low mandibular plane angle, extrusion of the molars may be a desired consequence. In such patients then, application of the force above the center of resistance with the strap pulling down and backward will produce extrusion with distal movement.[16] Figure 9-2 shows the various movements that can be obtained using the facebow headgear depending on the point of force application.[16]

Vertical Holding Appliance

Some clinicians and investigators have sought ways to augment the extraoral traction. One method is the combined use of a vertical holding appliance (VHA)[17,18] and high-pull headgear. The VHA (Fig. 9-3) has been recommended for treatment of high-angle patients where there is an important need to control the vertical dimension. It is fabricated from a 0.040″ wire with a helix just distal to each maxillary first molar. Two more helices are placed at the center of the appliance, and these are separated by a V-bend to which is molded an acrylic button the size of a dime. The most mesial portion of this appliance, i.e. the acrylic button, should lie on a line that connects the mesial margins of the maxillary first molars. The button should also be 2–5 mm away from the palate. The VHA achieves the treatment objectives by way of an intrusive and distally directed force. The result is intrusion and distal movement of the molars. This is a fixed functional appliance since the forces are achieved from the functional activity of the tongue.

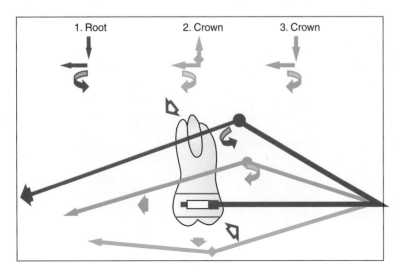

Fig. 9-2 Forces and moments generated by the facebow headgear. **1** Force is above the center of resistance—the result is extrusion, mesial moment, and distal movement of the root. **2** Force is below the center of resistance in an upward direction—the effect is distal crown movement, clockwise moment, and an intrusive effect. **3** Force is below the center of resistance in a downward direction—the effect is extrusion, distal crown movement, and clockwise moment.

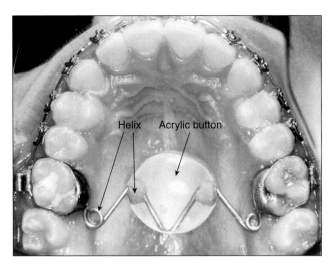

Fig. 9-3 Vertical holding appliance (VHA). The first set of helices is positioned distal to the maxillary first molar, and the second set is under the acrylic, but not inside it. Only the V-bend attaches the 0.040" wire onto the acrylic.

In a study conducted at the University of Oklahoma,[19] excellent results were achieved using the VHA compared to other methods.

Though initially recommended for use in combination with headgear, we have noted that the VHA on its own is useful for correction of Class II malocclusion. Figure 9-4

documents a patient whose initial treatment plan was for treatment with a straight-pull facebow headgear, but she declined to use it. The patient was put under observation for 6 months while the VHA was cemented to the maxillary first molars. A fixed lingual arch (FLA) was also cemented to the mandibular arch for maintenance of the leeway space. Even though the leeway space may not always be available,[19] the FLA can be used to control the vertical during the growth period.[20] After 6 months, correction of the Class II malocclusion was observed. No other appliance was used during this period.

Although the forces generated by the VHA have not been measured, measurement of the forces applied to the transpalatal arch (TPA) from the tongue[20] suggest that these forces may reach very high levels considering the size of the Nance button to which the 0.040" wire is attached. Chiba et al[21] noted that maximum pressure was applied to the TPA during deglutition when the appliance was engaged to the maxillary second molars. Also, this pressure was at its maximum when the TPA was positioned 6 mm away from the palate.

Cervical Facebow with Removable Maxillary Plate

Cetlin has proposed the treatment of Class II relationships using a combination of TPAs (Fig. 9-5), cervical headgear, and a removable maxillary plate with auxiliary springs. This treatment modality requires correction of maxillary

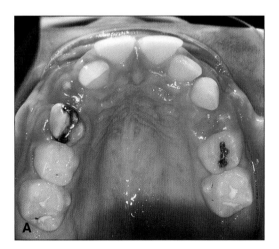

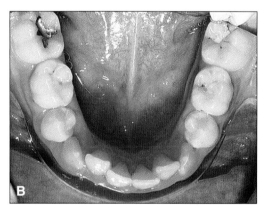

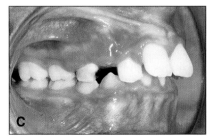

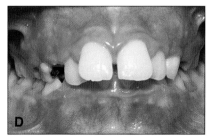

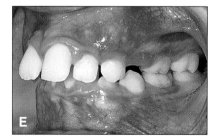

Fig. 9-4 Class II, Division 1 malocclusion treated with a vertical holding appliance (VHA). **A-E** Pretreatment intraoral photographs of a Class II, Division 1 subdivision left malocclusion.   *Continued*

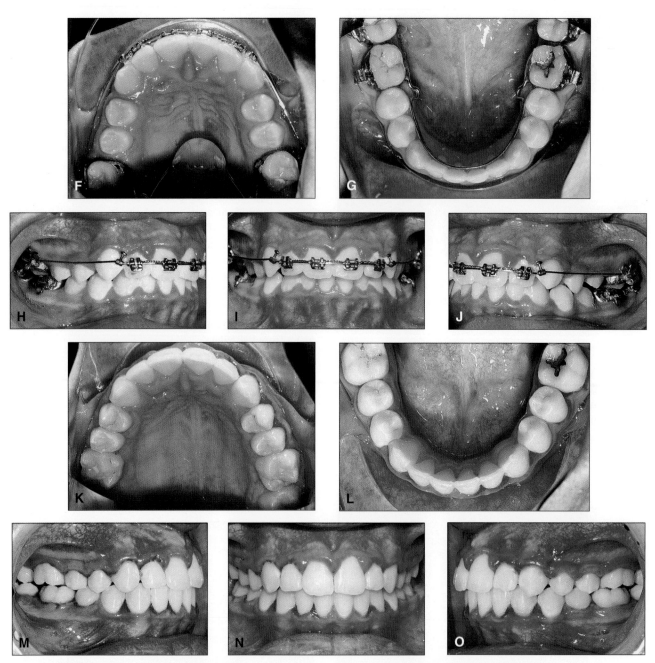

Fig. 9-4 *cont'd.* **F-J** Progress photographs showing a VHA cemented to the maxillary first molars, and a fixed lingual arch cemented to the mandibular first molars. These photographs were taken 6 months post delivery of the VHA and fixed lingual arch. **K-O** Final records at completion of treatment.

molar rotations (which in Class II are usually rotated mesiolingually) prior to distal movement, and then distalization. The derotation of the molars in a distobuccal direction may produce a space gain of as much as 2–3 mm on each side. Once the rotations are corrected, distal movement can be initiated. The distal movement of the maxillary molars is achieved by means of a removable maxillary plate to which is attached some auxiliary springs. The springs deliver a distally directed force of approximately 30 g that is augmented by a cervical-pull facebow headgear with approximately 150 g of force. Once again,

the outer bows of the facebow have to be positioned such that the side effects from the headgear are minimized. No extrusive forces should be applied when extrusion is not desired as these will result in opening of the bite from extrusion of the molars and clockwise rotation of the mandible.

Cervical Facebow Headgear

Some studies on molar distalization with cervical facebow headgear have reported negative effects, including extrusion of maxillary first molars, downward anterior tipping

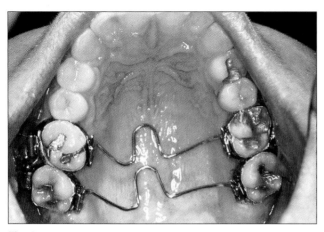

Fig. 9-5 Transpalatal arches for molar derotation prior to distalization. (Reproduced courtesy of Dr Cetlin.)

of palatal and occlusal planes, posterior rotation of the mandible with resultant steepening of the mandibular plane, and an increase in the anterior lower face height. Many of these clinical studies are of variable duration, some have small patient samples, and some lack information on compliance and usage of the appliance. The credibility of these studies is further compromised by poor documentation of force magnitude, direction of force, duration of force application, physiologic age of the patients, and biologic response.

Kloehn popularized and reported the successful usage of the cervical face bow headgear.[1] He demonstrated in many patients that this was an important and useful method of maxillary molar distalization and correction of Class II molar relation in developing dentitions. Along with the molars, the premolars also drifted distally through the pull of the trans-septal fibers. In a retrospective study conducted on the records of patients treated by Dr John S Kloehn,[22,23] 85 pre- and post-treatment records were selected from 125 patients based on the Class II first molar relationship prior to treatment on the transitional or permanent dentition, nonextraction treatment, and good cooperation. A common treatment protocol that was followed for successful treatment of these patients was alternate adjustment of the outer facebow below or above the line of occlusion every 6–12 weeks. The outer bow is bent down during the first 6–12 weeks, and then it is bent up for another period of equal duration. The rationale for this treatment protocol can be appreciated from looking at Figure 9-2 which analyzes the forces and moments applied to the maxillary first molars with each adjustment. With this treatment regimen, there was no change in the anterior face height. An average tipping of the palatal plane of 1.5° was however observed, an indication of the orthopedic effect of the headgear. It was concluded that the cervical pull headgear can effectively be used for maxillary molar distalization without detrimental effects. However, patient compliance with the treatment regimen is a serious issue as social and peer

pressures on children make it almost impossible for them to accept the facebow headgear regimen.

Jig

Another appliance that can be used either with patient compliance or noncompliance is the jig. The jig can be easily fabricated at chairside and used to correct either bilateral or unilateral Class II, Division 1 malocclusions (Fig. 9-6). In patients where there is poor compliance, the appliance can be tied in using long nickel-titanium coil springs with an external tubing to minimize patient discomfort. These springs are very small in diameter and do not cause more discomfort than the Saif springs. The Saif spring, compared to the nickel–titanium springs (Fig. 9-7), is bulky, and it can be tied either from the mandibular first or second molar to the maxillary canine hook. Figure 9-6 is an example of a patient treated with a unilateral jig.

Bimetric (Wilson) Arch

Wilson[24] introduced the bimetric arch into the orthodontic literature in 1955 at a time when there was considerable argument between proponents of extraction and of non-extraction with expansion. The appliance consists of a labial arch made of a 0.040" posterior section and a 0.020" anterior section. Hooks for Class II elastics are soldered on to the anterior end of the 0.040" section, and an adjustable omega loop is placed in the premolar region of the 0.040" section. The appliance is activated by placement of an open coil-spring between the omega loop and the maxillary first molar. Continued activation of the appliance can be achieved by opening the omega loop, thereby compressing the open coil against the molar. The bimetric arch, as it would look in the mouth, is shown in Fig. 9-8.

With patient compliance, a limitation to the use of the appliance, a Class I molar relationship can be achieved in as little as 6–12 weeks.[25–27] In a noncompliant patient, side effects can lead to flaring of the incisors.[27] Both distal movement and distal tipping of the maxillary molars are observed with the Wilson appliance.[25,27] Upon achievement of a Class I relationship, the second premolar can be allowed to drift back and the appliance may not be removed until this relationship is achieved.[27] Of importance during the use of Class II elastics is stability of the mandibular molars, which can be achieved in one of three ways: FLA, removable lingual arch (RLA), or lip bumper. The lip bumper has the added advantage of uprighting the mandibular molars and unraveling mandibular anterior crowding, if present.

Fixed Noncompliance Appliances

To overcome the problems of patient compliance, several fixed noncompliance appliances have been introduced, especially during the past two decades. These include

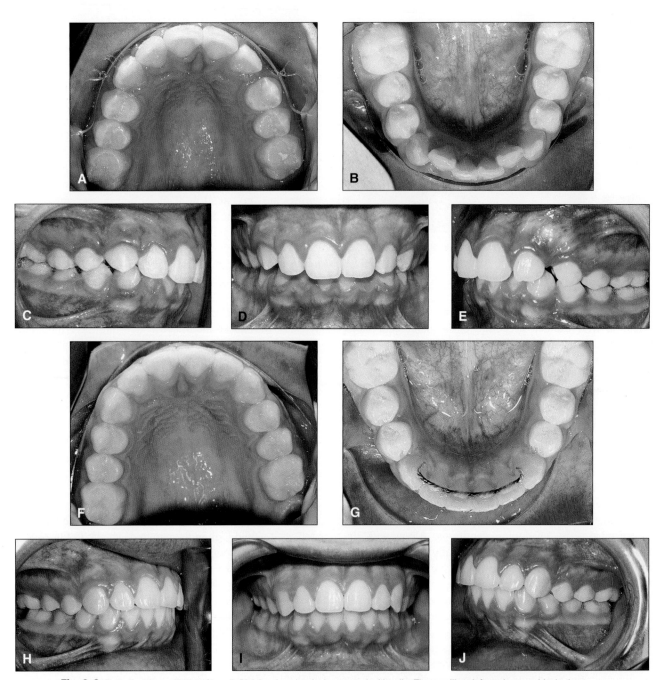

Fig. 9-6 Patient with a unilateral Class II, Division 1 malocclusion treated with a jig. The maxillary left canine was blocked out and could not erupt. **A-E** Pretreatment records showing Class II, Division 1 subdivision left. **F-J** Final records after 12 months of treatment. No exposure of the unerupted canine was performed, and the canine erupted as soon as space was created.

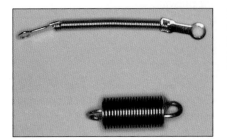

Fig. 9-7 Size difference between the "Saif" (bottom) and nickel–titanium springs (top). These springs can be tied in in the case of the noncompliant patient to correct a Class II malocclusion. The "Saif" spring is more bulky compared to the nickel–titanium spring.

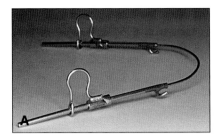 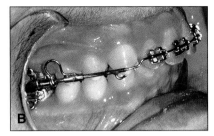 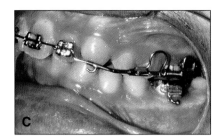

Fig. 9-8 A Bimetric arch (Wilson appliance). **B** and **C** Bimetric arch engaged and activated.

the Herbst, twin force bite corrector, repelling magnets, the pendulum appliance, compressed stainless steel or nickel–titanium springs, Jones jig, and distal jet. The majority of these appliances have been reported to achieve the same amount of molar distalization as the headgear. They also have side effects that need to be considered.

Pendulum Appliance

Hilgers[28] introduced an appliance for Class II correction in the noncompliant patient to expand the maxilla and simultaneously rotate and distalize the maxillary first molars. The pendulum appliance provides the clinician with the ability to distalize molars unilaterally and bilaterally. The type of force delivered is continuous and it requires minimal patient cooperation.

The appliance consists of a palatal acrylic button of about 25 mm in diameter with distalization springs made out of 0.032" beta-titanium wire, and that originate from the palatal acrylic and are engaged in lingual sheaths on maxillary first molar bands (Fig. 9-9). It is bonded to the first and second premolars with wires embedded in the acrylic. It only needs a one-time activation of 60–70°, producing a force of 230 g per side. It produces a swinging arch, or pendulum of force, from the palate to the molars. A loop within each spring can be adjusted to allow for expansion and prevent any tendency for the maxillary molar to move lingually into a crossbite. Once the molars are distalized, they may be stabilized with either a Nance button attached to the maxillary first molars, a headgear, or a fixed appliance, along with a maxillary utility archwire or a stopped continuous archwire. Usually after molar distalization, the second premolar is released from the anchor unit and allowed to drift distally. According to

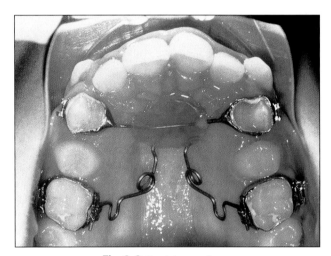

Fig. 9-9 Pendulum appliance.

Hilgers,[28] it is not unusual to see as much as 5 mm of distal molar movement in 3–4 months of treatment with this appliance.

Evaluation of the treatment effects has shown that there is a difference in response between patients with erupting second molars and those with second molars in occlusion. Patients with erupted second molars will experience an extrusion of these teeth with subsequent opening of the bite, which is observed by an increase in the mandibular plane angle, increased lower anterior face height, and a reduced overbite.[29,30] Table 9-1 shows some of the results observed from a cephalometric analysis of patients treated with the pendulum appliance. The response differs between individuals with a low and a high mandibular plane angle. In another study, patients in the angle >25° group showed

Table 9-1	Effects of the pendulum appliance (adapted from Ghosh and Nanda[10])		
		Sagittal change	Vertical change
Tooth		Mesial mvt (mm) Tipping (degrees)	Extrusion (mm)
First premolar	2.55 ± 1.9	1.29 ± 7.52	1.7 ± 1.36
	Distal mvt (mm)		
First molar	3.37	8.36 ± 8.37	0.1 ± 1.29
Second molar	2.27 ± 1.44	11.99 ± 1.9	0.47 ± 1.36

mvt = movement.

an increase in the lower anterior vertical height (4.13 mm) that was greater than in the patients in the low and average groups (1.97 and 2.84 mm, respectively).[29]

A common finding in studies that have evaluated the pendulum is distal tipping of the maxillary first molars and anterior tipping of the premolars.[29,30] An important side effect of this appliance is undesirable anterior displacement of anterior teeth. This appliance, however, presents an effective method for molar distalization with minimal dependence on patient compliance.[31] Other advantages include ease of fabrication, one-time activation, adjustment of the springs if necessary to correct minor transverse and vertical molar positions, and patient acceptance. Modifications of the pendulum appliance with removable arms have been introduced.[32–34] Such a modified appliance makes it easier to adjust and stabilize the appliance upon completion of molar distal movement.

Distal Jet

Carano and Testa[35] first described the distal jet as a fixed lingual appliance that required no compliance from the patient. They claimed that it could produce translatory movement of the maxillary molars in 4–6 months.

The original appliance[35] has had some modification[36,37] and now consists of a bilateral piston and tube arrangement (Fig. 9-10). The tube is embedded in an acrylic palatal button supported by attachments to the first or second premolars. This tube extends distally, adjacent to the palatal tissues and parallel to the occlusal plane, to the first molars. A bayonet wire inserted into the lingual sheath on the first molar bands extends into the tube, much like a piston. A superelastic nickel–titanium open coil-spring is placed around this piston and tube arrangement, along with an activation collar used to compress the spring distally. This collar is pushed distally to compress the coil-spring once every 4–6 weeks during distalization. The mesial set-screw in the collar is locked onto the tube with a small Allen wrench in an aluminum handle.

Upon completion of distalization of the molars, the appliance is converted to a palatal holding arch by removal of the coil-spring (peeling it off the tube with utility pliers) and locking the activation collar over the junction of the tube and piston; the mesial set-screw is locked onto the tube, and the distal set-screw is locked onto the piston, thereby creating a solid support from the first molars to the Nance button. The supporting wire is then sectioned from the premolars and the Nance button with a dental handpiece and a burr.

Other than clinical reports from users of the appliance,[36–38] no research has clearly documented the effects of the appliance. Studies conducted at the University of Oklahoma[39,40] revealed that the distal jet was indeed a good tool for distalizing maxillary molars but there could also be anchorage loss during its use, although less than reported for other appliances such as the pendulum. Minimal tipping

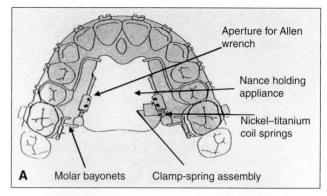

Aperture for Allen wrench

Nance holding appliance

Nickel–titanium coil springs

A Molar bayonets   Clamp-spring assembly

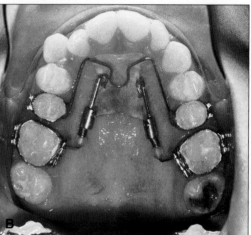

Fig. 9-10 A Schematic and **B** photograph of the distal jet appliance in a patient's mouth.

of the maxillary molars was observed during the treatment period due to the force application near the center of resistance of the maxillary molars. The patients evaluated were in their growth period, and some of the distalization achieved was lost during retraction of the anterior teeth. This was, however, compensated for by anterior movement of the mandibular molars. Upon completion of distalization of the molars and during the rest of the treatment phase, it is necessary to use some other appliance to hold the molars back.[37,38] A Jasper jumper[41,42] or a short twin force bite corrector[6] may serve this purpose well since they do not require compliance from the patient.

Jones Jig Appliance

The Jones jig appliance[43] is an intraoral noncompliance distalization appliance (Fig. 9-11). It has a modified Nance appliance banded to the second bicuspids, with the Jones jig assemblies tied in place. It consists of a palatal acrylic button of 0.5″ diameter anchored to the second premolar with a bonded 0.036″ wire. One arm of the jig fits into a 0.045″ headgear tube and the second arm fits into a 0.018″ tube on the first molar. The activation is delivered from the nickel–titanium coil-spring tied to the second premolar bracket. The force applied is between 70 and 75 g, and average treatment time is 6.35 ± 2.75 months.

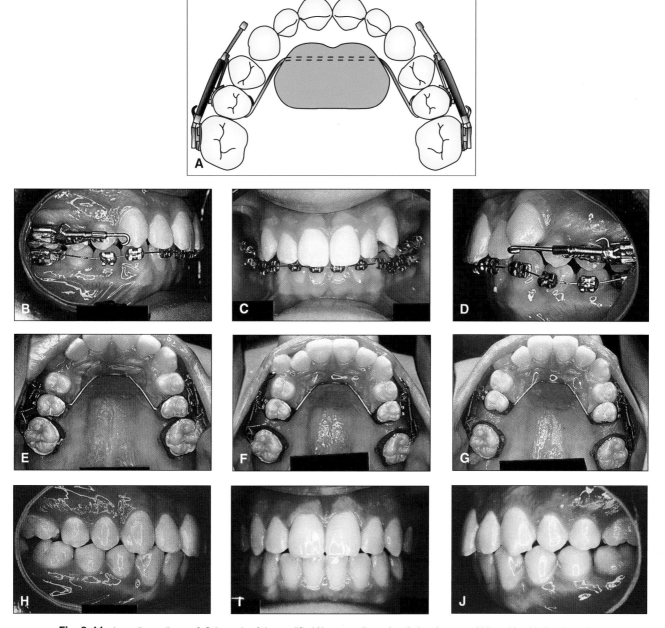

Fig. 9-11 Jones jig appliance. **A** Schematic of the modified Nance appliance banded to the second bicuspids with the Jones jig assemblies tied into place. **B-D** Pretreatment photographs of a patient with a Class II, Division 1 malocclusion, showing the activated appliance. **E-G** Intraoral palatal photographs at, from left to right: initial delivery (0 months), 2 months, and 4 months of appliance activation. **H-J** Treatment completion. Total treatment time was 24 months. The majority of the time was spent distalizing the premolars, canines, and incisors.

Despite reports of successful correction of Class II malocclusions with the Jones jig, there has been no comprehensive study of molar movement and loss of anchorage during the use of this appliance. To validate its effectiveness, a study was conducted on the patients treated in Dr Richard Jones' office, the clinician credited with the design and use of this appliance.[44] The sample of 72 patients (26 male and 46 female) was unique. The average age before treatment was 13.8 ± 4.38 years. The results showed

molar correction for Class II to Class I malocclusions due primarily to distal movement of the molars. The mean maxillary first molar distal movement was 2.51 mm, with distal tipping of 7.53°. The mean reciprocal mesial movement of the maxillary premolar was 2.0 mm, with mesial tipping of 4.76°. The maxillary first molar extruded 0.14 mm while the maxillary premolar extruded 1.88 mm. The maxillary second molars also moved and tipped distally 2.02 mm and 7.89°, respectively. Table 9-2 shows

Table 9-2	Sagittal and vertical changes with Jones jig treatment		
	Sagittal change		Vertical change
Tooth	Distal mvt (mm)	Tipping (degrees)	Extrusion (mm)
First molar	2.16 ± 1.35	7.53 ± 4.57	0.1 ± 1.3
Second molar	1.79 ± 1.55	8.03 ± 6.65	0.71 ± 1.96
	Mesial mvt (mm)		
Second premolar	2.36 ± 1.99	5.89 ± 5.19	1.82 ± 1.44
			1.46 ± 1.61 Increase anterior lower face height

mvt = movement.

the sagittal and vertical movements that accompany the molar distalization procedure with the Jones jig. The changes are highly variable, a factor that should be noted when considering treatment options.

Although the Jones jig appliance can effectively distalize maxillary first molars, it has negative effects on the anchor unit.[44,45] Compared to the headgear, however, it has the advantage of accelerated distal molar movement within a short timespan.[45] Upon completion of distalization, proper anchorage has to be used to maintain the molar relationship. Suitable anterior retraction mechanics have to be used to achieve this goal. The use of full palatal coverage combined with short Class II elastics to reinforce posterior anchorage could possibly minimize the reciprocal anchorage loss of the molar anchor units during anterior segment retraction. An option that should be considered is night-time headgear wear, which can be tolerated, especially by the young patient.

Intermaxillary Class II Malocclusion Correction Appliances

Several intermaxillary fixed noncompliant appliances have been proposed and used over the past two decades.[6,12,13,41,42,46–48] The advantage of these appliances is that they allow forward displacement of the mandible and a distal force on the maxillary teeth as well as an anterior force on the mandibular dentition. The net result of these three force vectors is correction of a Class II malocclusion. The common disadvantages of intermaxillary appliances is undesirable steepening of the occlusal plane with concomitant flaring of the lower incisors, and distal tipping along with extrusion of the maxillary incisors.

Herbst Appliance

The Herbst appliance was developed in the early 1900s and it was reintroduced by Pancherz[46,47] in the mid 1970s. Pancherz showed that a 6-month Herbst treatment in

prepeak pubertal patients with a Class II, Division 1 malocclusion resulted in a Class I occlusion relationship. He reported, however, that improvement in occlusion was equally due to skeletal and dentoalveolar changes: a Class II molar correction averaging 6.7 mm resulted from a 2.2 mm increase in mandibular length, a 1.8 mm mesial movement of mandibular incisors, and a 2.8 mm distal movement of maxillary molars.

Pancherz and Hagg[48] found that sagittal growth at the condyle in patients treated with the Herbst appliance at the peak in pubertal growth was twice that observed in patients treated 3 years before or 3 years after the peak. Other studies[49,50] have shown that greater percentages of molar and overjet correction were dentoalveolar in nature in postpubertal patients with greater lower incisor flaring.

Jasper Jumper

Fixed intermaxillary appliances such as the Jasper jumper incorporate active pushing force on the maxillary molars and mandibular dentition. Rankin[51] in a clinical study reported greater dentoalveolar effects as compared to skeletal. The Class II correction was obtained from mesial movement of lower molars and a significant flaring of the lower incisors. Jasper and McNamara[42] concluded that the skeletal and dental components of Class II correction were approximately equal, whereas Weiland and Bantleon[41] attributed only 38% of molar correction to skeletal changes. The majority of the studies on this appliance have shown that Class II correction is attributed to a slight increase in mandibular length, a significant posterior movement of the maxillary posterior segments, and proclination of the lower incisors.[52,53]

Twin Force Bite Corrector*

The twin force bite corrector (TFBC) is a fixed push type intermaxillary appliance which delivers a force from nickel–titanium coil-springs through the point of attachment to both the maxillary and mandibular archwires along

*Ortho Organizers Inc, San Marcos, CA

the long axis of the appliance.[6,54] Like other fixed inter-maxillary appliances its use is full time and not subject to patient compliance. The TFBC incorporates two plunger/tube telescopic assemblies per side, each of which contains a nickel–titanium coil-spring delivering a full compression force of approximately 200 g. Campbell[6] used the TFBC in a prospective clinical trial at the University of Connecticut on 20 adolescent patients between the ages of 10 and 16 years. He showed that the TFBC is a valuable tool in correcting a Class II dental relationship between half and full cusp during a 3-month period followed by Class II vector seating elastics. The molar correction was achieved by dental (64%) and skeletal (36%) changes. He also noted that the TFBC displayed a propensity for advantageous vertical changes, i.e. intrusion of maxillary posterior and mandibular anterior teeth and extrusion of mandibular posterior teeth favoring a Class II correction (Fig. 9.12).

Summary

Headgear is perhaps the most useful appliance for maxillary molar distalization if used in the early treatment of Class II malocclusions. Kim et al[5] have shown that the occlusion established early during the growth phase is most likely to be maintained throughout life. Based on this and the premise that children are more compliant before adolescence, the headgear becomes a versatile appliance for treatment of Class II malocclusions. Its effect is twofold: (1) distal movement of the maxillary molars; and (2) an orthopedic effect on the maxilla that restrains growth.

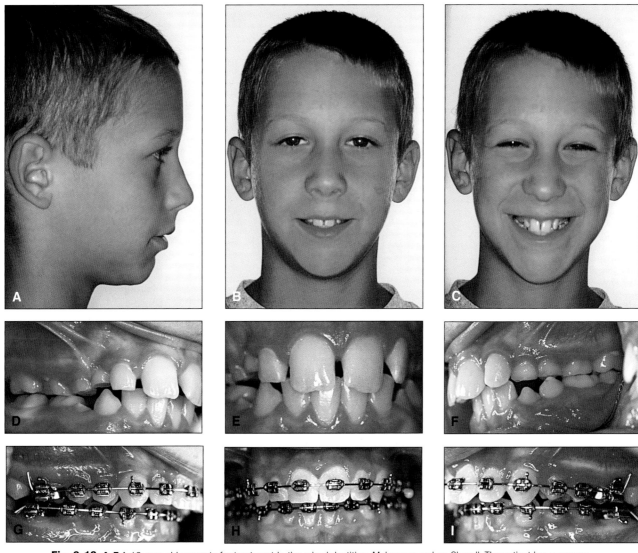

Fig. 9-12 A-F A 13-year old presents for treatment in the mixed dentition. Molars are end on Class II. The patient has a convex soft tissue profile. **G-I** After 18 months of treatment, the patient is in permanent dentition and shows a full-cusp Class II molar and canine relationship. Maxillary 0.019" × 0.025" and mandibular 0.021" × 0.025" stainless steel archwires are cinched distal to the first molars.

Continued

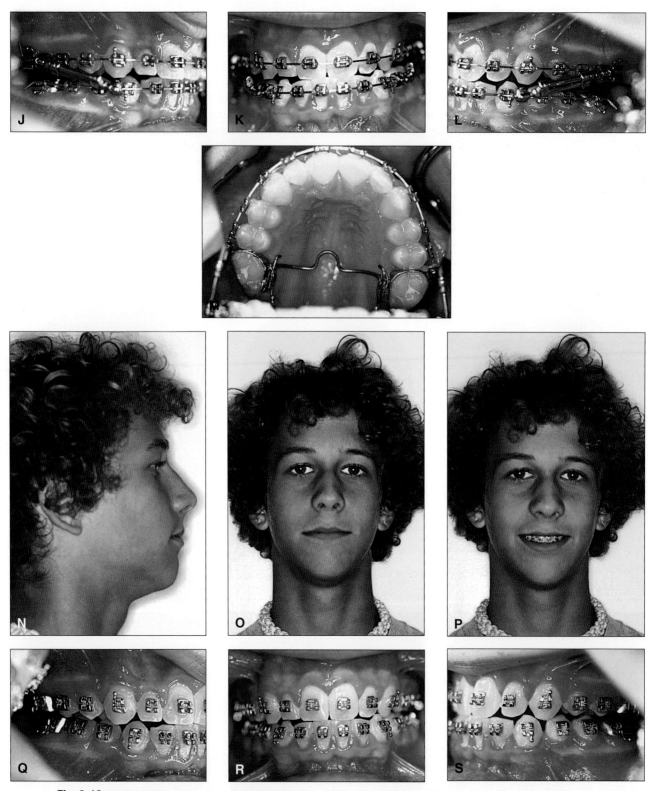

Fig. 9-12 *cont'd.* **J-M** Insertion of a twin force bite corrector (TFBC) postures the mandible forward into edge-to-edge occlusion; a passive 0.032" CNA beta-titanium transpalatal arch counteracts the distobuccal forces of the TFBC. **N-S** After 3 months of TFBC therapy, the patient is Class I molar and canine on the right and left, edge-to-edge, and has an improved soft tissue profile.

Continued

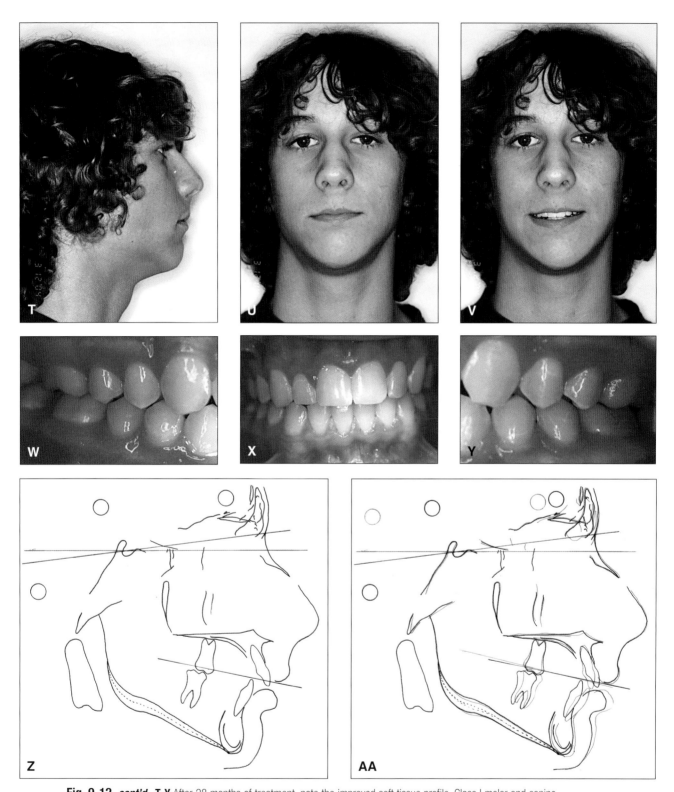

Fig. 9-12 *cont'd.* **T-Y** After 28 months of treatment, note the improved soft tissue profile, Class I molar and canine relationships, coincident midlines, and ideal overbite. **Z-AB** Cephalometric tracings and superimpositions. **Z** T1 (black) prior to TBC insertion. **AA** Superimposition T2 (blue) after TFBC removal.   *Continued*

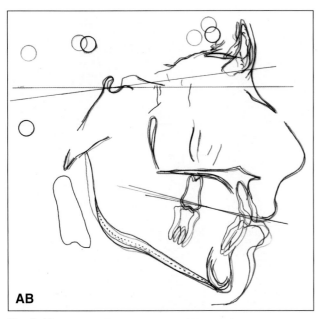

Fig. 9-12 *cont'd.* **AB** Superimposition of T3 (red), 6 months later. Note the relapse of the flared lower incisor (blue) during post TFBC (red).

Both extra- and intra-oral interarch appliances require patient compliance, which may sometimes pose difficulty. Intermaxillary appliances that use the mandibular arch as anchorage may have protrusive effects on the mandibular teeth. All investigations that have evaluated intraoral arch noncompliance appliances for molar distalization have come to surprisingly similar conclusions on the behavior of both the distal segment and the anterior anchor unit. The intramaxillary arch appliances that have gained in popularity because they do not require patient compliance to distalize molars, show loss of anchorage whereby the premolars move mesially with concomitant protrusion of the maxillary incisors. This suggests that no matter which intraoral appliance is used, it behooves the clinician to avoid round tripping in retraction of maxillary anterior teeth.

It is necessary that the molars are held back with some other form of appliance upon completion of distalization. The use of a Nance palatal arch or transpalatal arches has proven not to resist the anchorage loss during the subsequent retraction of the anterior segment.

REFERENCES

1. Kloehn SJ. Orthodontics – Force or persuasion. Angle Orthod 1953;23:56–66.
2. Ricketts RM, Bench RW, Gugino CF, Hilgers JJ, Schulhof RJ. Bioprogressive therapy. Rocky Mountain Orthodontics, 1979.
3. Cetlin NM, Ten Hoeve A. Nonextraction treatment. J Clin Orthod 1983;17:396–413.
4. Macho GA. Cephalometric and craniometric age changes in adult humans. Ann Hum Biol 1986;14:49–61.
5. Kim YE, Nanda RS, Sinha PK. Transition of molar relationships in different skeletal growth patterns. Am J Orthod Dentofacial Orthop 2002;121:280–290.
6. Campbell E. A prospective clinical trial and mechanical analysis of a push type fixed intermaxillary Class II correction appliance. Master of Dental Science Thesis, University of Connecticut, 2003.
7. Kalra V. The K-loop distalizing appliance. J Clin Orthod 1995;29:298–301.
8. Kingsley NW. Treatise on oral deformities. New York: Appleton & Co, 1880.
9. Angle EH. Treatment of malocclusion of the teeth. Philadelphia: SS White Dental Manufacturing Co, 1907.
10. Oppenheim A. Biologic orthodontic therapy and reality. Angle Orthod 1936;6:69–79.
11. Rabbie ABM, Leung FYC, Chayanupatkul A, Hägg U. The correlation between neovascularization and bone formation in the condyle during forward mandibular positioning. Angle Orthod 2002;72:431–438.
12. Voudouris JC, Donald G. Woodside DG, et al. Condyle–fossa modifications and muscle interactions during Herbst treatment, Part 1. New technological methods. Am J Orthod Dentofacial Orthop 2003;123;604–613.
13. Voudouris JC, Donald G. Woodside DG, et al. Condyle–fossa modifications and muscle interactions during Herbst treatment, Part 2. Results and conclusions. Am J Orthod Dentofacial Orthop 2003;124:13–29.
14. Haack DC, Weinstein S. The mechanics of centric and eccentric cervical traction. Am J Orthod 1958;44:346–357.
15. Hershey GH, Houghton CW, Burstone CJ. Unilateral face-bows: A theoretical analysis. Am J Orthod 1981;79:229–249.
16. Contasti GI, Legan HL. Biomechanic guidelines for headgear application. J Clin Orthod 1982;16:308–312.
17. Wilson MD. Vertical control of maxillary molar position with a palatal appliance, Thesis. Oklahoma City: Health Sciences Center, University of Oklahoma, 1996.
18. DeBerardinis M, Stretesky T, Sinha PK, Nanda RS. Evaluation of the vertical holding appliance in treatment of high-angle patients. Am J Orthod Dentofacial Orthop 2000;117:700–705.
19. Nanda RS, Chawla JM. Variability of leeway space in Lucknow children. Ind Dental J 1973;45:99–108.
20. Villalobos FJ, Sinha PK, Nanda RS. Longitudinal assessment of vertical and sagittal control in the mandibular arch by the mandibular fixed lingual arch. Am J Orthod Dentofacial Orthop 2000;118:366–370.
21. Chiba Y, Motoyoshi M, Namura S. Tongue pressure on loop of transpalatal arch during deglutition. Am J Orthod Dentofacial Orthop 2003;123:29–34.
22. Hubbard GW. A cephalometric evaluation of non-extraction cervical headgear treatment in Class II malocclusion, Thesis. Oklahoma City: Health Sciences Center, University of Oklahoma, 1992.
23. Hubbard GW, Nanda RS, Currier GF. A cephalometric evaluation of non-extraction cervical headgear treatment in Class II malocclusion. Angle Orthod 1994;60:359–370.

24. Wilson WL. Variations of labiolingual therapy in Class II cases. Am J Orthod 1955;41:852–871.

25. Muse DS, Fillman MJ, Emmerson WJ, Mitchell RD. Molar and incisor changes with Wilson rapid molar distalization. Am J Orthod Dentofacial Orthop 1993;104:556–565.

26. Harnick DJ. Case report: Class II correction using a modified Wilson bimetric distalizing arch and maxillary second molar extraction. Angle Orthod 1998;68:275–280.

27. Ücem TT, Yüksel S, Okay C, Gülsen A. Effects of a three-dimensional bimetric maxillary distalizing arch. Eur J Orthod 2000;22:293–298.

28. Hilgers JJ. The pendulum appliance for Class II non-compliance. J Clin Orthod 1992;26:706–714.

29. Ghosh J, Nanda RS. Evaluation of an intraoral maxillary molar distalization technique. Am J Orthod Dentofacial Orthop 1996;110:639–646.

30. Bussick TJ, McNamara JA Jr. Dentoalveolar and skeletal changes associated with the pendulum appliance. Am J Orthod Dentofacial Orthop 2000;117:333–343.

31. Wong AMK, Rabie ABM, Hägg U. The use of pendulum appliance in the treatment of Class II malocclusion. Br Dent J 1999;187:367–370.

32. Scuzzo G, Pisani F, Takemoto K. Modified molar distalization with a modified pendulum appliance. J Clin Orthod 1999;33:645–650.

33. Scuzzo G, Takemoto K, Pisani F, Della VS. The modified pendulum appliance with removable arms. J Clin Orthod 2000;34:244–246.

34. Byloff FK, Kärcher H, Clar E, Stoff F. An implant to eliminate anchorage loss during molar distalization: a case report involving the Graz implant-supported pendulum. AOOS 2000;15:129–137.

35. Carano A, Testa M. The distal jet for upper molar distalization. J Clin Orthod 1996;30:374–380.

36. Bowman SJ. Modifications of the distal jet. J Clin Orthod 1998;32:549–556.

37. Quick AN, Harris AMP. Molar distalization with a modified distal jet appliance. J Clin Orthod 2000;34:419–423.

38. Bowman SJ. Class II combination therapy (distal jet and jusper jumpers): a case report. J Orthod 2000;27:213–218.

39. Patel A.Analysis of the distal jet appliance for maxillary molar distalization, Thesis. Oklahoma City: Health Sciences Center, University of Oklahoma, 1999.

40. Ngantung V, Nanda RS. Posttreatment evaluation of the distal jet appliance. Am J Orthod Dentofacial Orthop 2001;120:178–185.

41. Weiland FJ, Bantleon H. Treatment of Class II malocclusions with the Jasper Jumper appliance—a preliminary report. Am J Orthod Dentofacial Orthop 1995;108:341–350.

42. Jasper JJ, McNamara JA. The correction of interarch malocclusions using a fixed force module. Am J Orthod Dentofacial Orthop 1995;108:641–650.

43. Jones RD, White MJ. Rapid Class II molar correction with an open-coil jig. J Clin Orthod 1992;26:661–664.

44. Brickman CD, Sinha PK, Nanda RS. Evaluation of the Jones jig appliance for distal molar movement. Am J Orthod Dentofacial Orthop 2000;118:526–534.

45. Haydar S, Üner O. Comparison of Jones jig molar distalization with extraoral traction. Am J Orthod Dentofacial Orthop 2000;117:49–53.

46. Pancherz H. Treatment of Class II malocclusions by jumping the bite with the Herbst appliance: Acta Odotol. Scand 1980;38:187–200.

47. Pancherz H. The mechanism of Class II correction in Herbst appliance treatment: a cephalometric investigation. Am J Orthod 1982;82:104–113.

48. Pancherz H, Hagg U. Dentofacial orthopedics in relation to chronologic age, growth period and skeletal development: an analysis of 72 male patients with Class II division 1 malocclusion treated with Herbst appliance. Eur J Orthod 1988;10:169–176.

49. Croft RS, Buschang PH, English JD, Meyer R. A cephalometric and tomographic evaluation of Herbst treatment in the mixed dentition. Am J Orthod Dentofacial Orthop 1999;116:435–443.

50. Konik M, Pancherz H, Hansen K. The mechanism of Class II correction in late Herbst treatment. Am J Orthod Dentofacial Orthop 1997;112:87–91.

51. Rankin T. Correction of Class II malocclusions with a fixed functional appliance, Thesis. University of Connecticut, 1990.

52. Cash RG. Adult non-extraction treatment with Jasper Jumper. J Clin Orthod 1991;25:443.

53. Cope JB. Quantitative evaluation of craniofacial changes with Jasper Jumper therapy. Angle Orthod 1994;64:113.

54. Rothenberg J, Campbell ES, Nanda R. Class II correction with the Twin Force Bite Corrector. J Clin Orthod 2004;38:232–240.

CHAPTER 10

Biomechanic Basis of Extraction Space Closure

Ravindra Nanda, Andrew Kuhlberg, and Flavio Uribe

Extraction space closure is a particularly interesting aspect of orthodontic treatment with respect to the principles of biomechanics due to the large movement distances involved. The technical features of the appliances, including loop or spring shape, bracket–wire interactions, and the types of forces, are important treatment considerations. However, understanding the biomechanic basis of space closure leads to a better ability to determine the anchorage and treatment options and the prognosis of various alternatives, and to decide on the specific adjustments that can improve the outcome of care.

Orthodontic space closure should be individually tailored based on the diagnosis and treatment plan. The selection of any treatment, involving any technique, stage, spring, or appliance design, should be based on the desired tooth movement. Consideration of the force system produced by an orthodontic device aids in determining the utility of the device for correcting any specific problem.

There has been a decline in the frequency of premolar extraction in orthodontic treatment with the development of various nonextraction modalities, including maxillary molar distalization, interarch fixed devices to attain dentoalveolar changes, expansion of dental arches, and stripping of mesiodistal dimensions of teeth. However, the need for premolar extraction treatment plans remains when good occlusion, esthetics, and stability are the major objectives.

This chapter will discuss various theoretic aspects of space closure and two methods to close extraction sites based on biomechanic concepts. One approach employs a two-step space closure, namely single canine retraction followed by en-masse retraction of four incisors; the second method uses en-masse retraction of the anterior six teeth.

Anchorage Classification

To anchor is to hold or resist the movement of an object; anchorage is the gaining of that hold. In orthodontics, terms such as "critical anchorage", "noncritical anchorage", or "burning anchorage" are often used to describe the degree of difficulty of space closure. Anchorage may be defined as the amount of movement of the posterior teeth (molars, premolars) to close the extraction space (Fig. 10-1A) in order to achieve selected treatment goals. Therefore, the anchorage needs of an individual treatment plan could vary from absolutely no permitted mesial movement of the molars/premolars (or even distal movement of the molars required) to complete space closure by protraction of the posterior teeth.

Anchorage can be classified as:
- *Group A anchorage.* This category describes the critical maintenance of the posterior tooth position. Seventy-five percent or more of the extraction space is needed for anterior retraction (Fig. 10-1B).
- *Group B anchorage.* This category describes relatively symmetric space closure with equal movement of the posterior and anterior teeth to close the space. This is often the least difficult space closure problem (Fig. 10-1C).
- *Group C anchorage.* This category describes "noncritical" anchorage. Seventy-five percent or more of the space

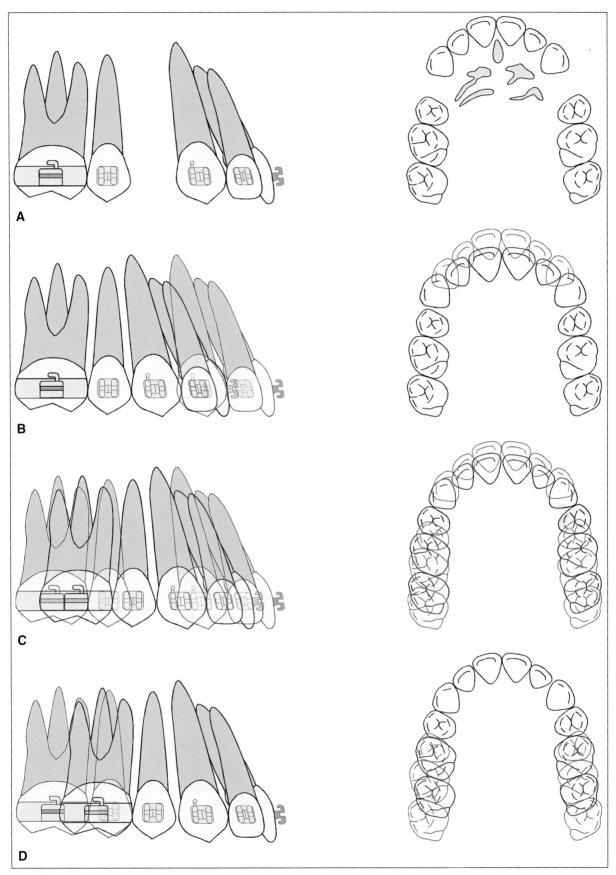

Fig. 10-1 Anchorage classification. **A** Teeth before space closure. **B** Group A anchorage. Group A space closure is characterized by anterior retraction. **C** Group B anchorage. Group B space closure involves equivalent amounts of anterior retraction and posterior protraction. **D** Group C anchorage. Group C space closure requires posterior protraction (maintenance of anterior anchorage).

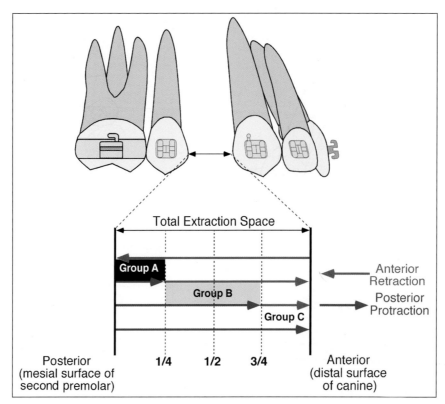

Fig. 10-2 Anchorage classification. Dividing the total extraction space into quarters aids in visualizing the anchorage classification. The shaded areas represent the final position of the interproximal contact between the canine and premolar. Group A space closure includes 100% (no posterior anchorage loss) to 75% anterior retraction (25% of space closure from posterior anchorage movement). Group B space closure includes more equal amounts of anterior and posterior tooth movement. Group C space closure includes 75–100% posterior protraction.

closure is achieved through mesial movement of the posterior teeth. This could also be considered to be "critical" anterior anchorage (Fig. 10-1D).

This classification helps in the design of mechanics plans that are individualized for specific patient needs. Figure 10-2 shows the extraction space divided into these classifications.[1,2]

Space Closure: A Biomechanic Perspective

The end result of space closure procedures should be upright, well-aligned teeth with ideal root angulations and positions in accordance with the treatment objectives. This implies that the tooth movement will almost always require some degree of bodily tooth movement or even root movement. Figure 10-3 demonstrates a typical sagittal view of space closure treatment. In this case, the space closure is shown as group B anchorage, or symmetric space closure. The space is closed while maintaining coincident occlusal planes and molar–premolar–canine root parallelism. The tooth movement from Figure 10-3A to 10-3B requires translation of the anterior and posterior teeth. The force

system necessary to achieve such movement requires the application of equal and opposite forces and moments. Figure 10-4 represents the general force system needed for this movement. Since the moments and forces are of equal magnitude and only opposite in direction, vertical force couples would not be present; therefore, the biomechanic side effects (from this view) would be negligible. The moment/force ratios acting on the anterior and posterior teeth should approximate 10/1, which is the ratio needed for bodily tooth movement.

Space closure requiring precise anchorage control is more difficult. For group A anchorage, or critical posterior anchorage, the mesial forces acting on the posterior teeth must be minimized or neutralized. Figure 10-5 shows this type of space closure along with the most desirable force system, with no forces or moments acting on the posterior teeth. Unfortunately, the force system shown can be achieved only with nondental anchorage. According to Newton's third law, any forces acting on the anterior teeth must be opposed by equal and opposite forces acting somewhere else, typically the posterior teeth, head, or neck (via fulltime headgear use). If intraoral anchorage is used, the forces and moments *must* be present on the posterior teeth. To obtain differential tooth movement (i.e. anchorage

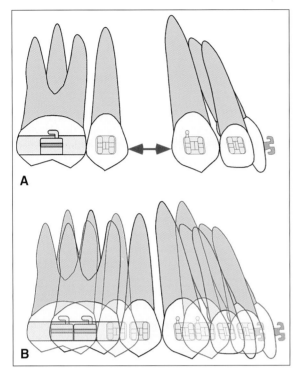

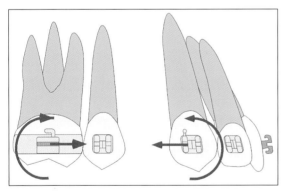

Fig. 10-3 Ideal space closure. **A** Before closure of extraction space. **B** Following space closure, the canine contacts the second premolar, the roots are parallel, and the occlusal plane is level.

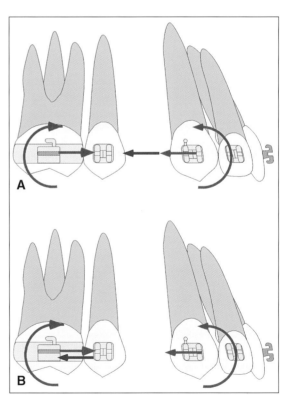

Fig. 10-4 Force system for group B space closure. Translation of the anterior and posterior teeth is required to achieve ideal space closure. A moment/force ratio approximating 10/1 is needed for translation.

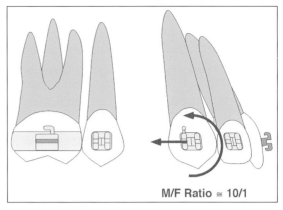

M/F Ratio ≅ 10/1

Fig. 10-5 Ideal force system for group A space closure. For perfect maintenance of the posterior anchorage, no forces should act on the posterior teeth; only a force system resulting in anterior translation is desired. *This force system cannot exist unless all the anchorage units are extraoral or in the opposite arch.*

Fig. 10-6 A and **B** Alternative approaches to obtaining group A anchorage through varying the magnitude of force acting on either the anterior or posterior teeth. The solid arrow represents the forces and moments generated by the archwire/retraction device (i.e. archwire and elastic chain). In **A** the blue arrow represents an additional force acting on the anterior teeth (i.e. Class II elastics or J-hook headgear). In B the blue arrow represents the force from a headgear acting on the posterior teeth. In both cases the change in the force magnitude results in a lower moment/force ratio on the anterior teeth and an increased moment/force ratio on the posterior teeth.

control), biomechanic strategies must be incorporated into the appliance design. Figure 10-6 shows two possible approaches for this strategy.

As Figure 10-6 demonstrates, the distal force on the anterior teeth must allow maximum potential for tooth movement while the mesial force on the posterior teeth must be minimized or counteracted. Regarding the force system required for such movement, group A anchorage requires a relative increase in the posterior moment/force ratio (reducing the force results in a higher ratio) and/or a decrease in the anterior moment/force ratio (increasing force results in a lower ratio). Unfortunately, within a single intra-arch appliance, the mesiodistal forces must be equal (rules of static equilibrium); thus, the forces can be increased or decreased only by utilizing extraoral appliances or the opposite dental arch. This is the differential force strategy achieved by headgears or intermaxillary elastics (Class II elastics). The use of headgear or intermaxillary elastics is dependent on good patient compliance and is not without other side effects. Class II elastics also result in forces acting on the mandibular teeth and exert a vertical (extrusive) force on the upper anterior teeth. Either of these side effects may be detrimental to the outcome of the treatment.

The strategy for group A space closure suggests another approach, as shown in Figure 10-7. The key feature is the differential moment/force ratio. The scheme described above (Fig. 10-6) obtains a difference in the anterior and posterior moment/force ratios by varying the force through the use of headgear and/or intermaxillary elastics. The moments can also be varied. Figure 10-7 depicts the application of a higher moment on the posterior compared to the applied moment on the anterior teeth. Increasing the posterior moment while decreasing the anterior moment results in an equivalent change in the moment/force ratios. Increasing the moment on the posterior teeth increases the moment/force ratio and decreasing the moment on the anterior teeth decreases the ratio; the force on the anterior and posterior teeth is equal. Additionally, increasing the posterior moment/force ratio encourages root movement (ratio ~ 12/1) while decreasing the anterior moment/force ratio causes a tipping type of tooth movement (ratio ~ 7/1). If the posterior moment were large enough, the moment/force ratio would approach infinity as the force is negligible in relation to the moment, consistent with the application of a pure couple on the posterior teeth. That couple would

result in rotational tooth movement around the center of the resistance of the anchor unit, moving the crowns distally (potentially increasing the size of the extraction space). Furthermore, the clinical expression of tipping tooth movements regularly occurs more quickly than root movement, so that the anterior teeth retract distally into the space before any mesial molar movement is seen.

Differential moments are not without side effects. The unequal moments must be "balanced" by a third moment or couple. This couple is a pair of vertical forces, intrusive to the anterior teeth and extrusive to the posterior (Fig. 10-7). The magnitude of these vertical forces is dependent on the difference between the anterior and posterior moments. No matter what the strategy, some biomechanic side effects will result. The proper selection of appliance design depends on the comparative risks or benefits of those side effects.

The difficulty of group C anchorage mirrors that of group A anchorage. The difference is that the anterior teeth become the effective "anchor unit". Therefore, the anterior moment is of greater magnitude and the vertical force side effect is an extrusive force on the anterior teeth. Due to the difficulty of this type of space closure in the lower arch, extraction treatment should be re-evaluated carefully and great awareness of the possible side effects is needed.

From the perspective of the biomechanic force system, analyzing any space closure technique increases awareness of potential side effects or unwanted tooth movements. Selecting the mechanics best suited to obtaining the planned goals improves both the efficiency of treatment and the probability of successful results.[1-11]

Determinants of Space Closure

Treatment planning in orthodontics involves far more than deciding on extraction versus nonextraction. Simplistic approaches to treatment planning, such as extraction versus nonextraction, fail to consider the individual patient's problems, interests, and welfare. Numerous factors must be considered when determining the need for extraction of teeth for orthodontic treatment. Along with the following factors, the minimum considerations must include esthetics, the general health of the teeth, and the patient's chief complaint.

Many details of the diagnosis and treatment objectives determine the tooth movement required during space closure, including:

- Amount of crowding
- Anchorage
- Axial inclination of canines and incisors
- Midline discrepancies and left/right symmetry
- Vertical dimension.

Amount of Crowding

Extractions are usually done to relieve dental crowding. In cases of severe crowding, anchorage control becomes

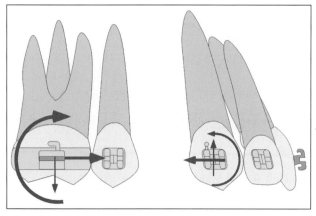

Fig. 10-7 Biomechanic strategy for group A space closure using differential moments. The posterior (beta) moment is increased relative to the anterior (alpha) moment. The moment differential reduces the moment/force ratio on the anterior teeth while increasing the moment/force ratio on the posterior teeth. Vertical forces occur due to the difference in the alpha and beta moments, intrusive to the anterior teeth, extrusive to the posterior teeth.

very important. Maintenance of anchorage while creating space for incisor alignment is necessary in order to meet the treatment objectives.

Anchorage

Anchorage classification and the concept of differential anchorage are very important (see above). Using the same mechanics for different anchorage needs limits the ability to achieve goal-oriented results. Traditional anchorage reinforcement methods (headgear, increasing the number of teeth in the anchor unit, lip bumpers, or palatal arches) may be suitable. However, if the concepts of biomechanics are applied to anchorage control, more predictable results with minimal patient cooperation may be achieved.

Control of the molar position is an obvious necessity in space closure. Inadvertent anchorage loss can prevent correction of anteroposterior malocclusions (Class II/III). This can be especially important in extraction space closure associated with Class II correction. Mesial movement of the maxillary posterior teeth may make it very difficult to obtain correction of the malocclusion. Utilizing a determined force system appliance design can improve the chances of success.

Axial Inclination of Canines and Incisors

The same force and/or moment applied to a tooth or a group of teeth with different axial inclinations will result in different types of tooth movements. The axial inclination of the teeth is an important consideration in the type of tooth movement needed during space closure. Figure 10-8 shows the effect of a single force acting on teeth at different axial inclinations. In these examples, the root would move mesially, opposite to the desired direction of movement. Figure 10-9 shows the relative force system required to retract and upright these teeth.[10]

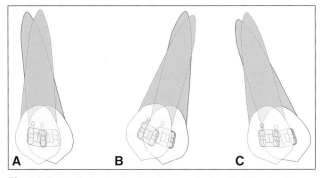

Fig. 10-8 Effect of a single, distal force on teeth with different axial inclinations. **A** Tooth is tipped distally; a simple distal force would result in further tipping, with the root moving more mesially. **B** A single force on an upright tooth also results in tipping and the root moving mesially. **C** A single force acting on a mesially tipped tooth will result in an uprighting tooth movement; however, this simple force system does not control the root position.

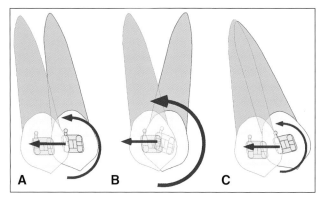

Fig. 10-9 Force systems needed for retraction of teeth shown in Figure 10-7. **A** Translation requires a moment/force ratio of 10/1. **B** Root movement is needed to upright this tooth. A moment/force ratio of approximately 12/1 is needed. **C** Controlled or apical tipping occurs with a moment/force ratio of about 7/1

Midline Discrepancies and Left/Right Symmetry

Midline discrepancies with or without an asymmetric left and right occlusal relationship should be corrected as early as possible in treatment. Eliminating asymmetries early in treatment allows the remainder of the therapy to be completed symmetrically (i.e. the left and right sides receive the same mechanics). Asymmetric forces on the left and right sides could result in unilateral vertical forces, skewing of the dental arch(es), or asymmetric anchorage loss. Completing as much of the treatment as possible using symmetric mechanics minimizes the potential impact of any of these side effects.

Vertical Dimension

Attention to vertical forces is essential for the control of the vertical dimension in space closure. Undesired vertical extrusive forces on the posterior teeth may result in backward mandibular rotation with increased lower facial height and increased interlabial gap. The vertical forces associated with Class II elastics may not only result in these problems, but in excessive gingival display ("gummy" smiles). Understanding the vertical forces associated with differential space closure prepares the orthodontist to deal with these difficulties.

Space Closure: Considerations for Anchorage Control and Differential Tooth Movement

Biologic Variables

Ultimately, it is the biologic response to the orthodontic force system that results in tooth movement. The mechanical stimulus that the appliances exert on the teeth induces physiologic activity that promotes bone resorption and/or deposition and the resulting tooth movement. The force system acting on the teeth produces a stress in the periodontium (the structures of the periodontal ligament [PDL] "feel" a level of force per unit area). The stresses within the PDL strain or distort the cells, fibers, and other structures. The biologic response is due to the stress/strain characteristics in the periodontium.

The term *optimal force* is the idea that there is a force level which will promote the most efficient treatment response without untoward side effects (i.e. root resorption). Unfortunately, little is known about what constitutes an optimal force level. Quinn and Yoshikawa[12] discussed hypothetical models characterizing optimal force. One model views the relationship between tooth movement and force magnitude as linear: the greater the force, the greater the tooth movement. An alternative model represents the relationship as a threshold. The tooth movement response varies with force magnitude to a threshold, and once the threshold is reached, tooth movement occurs at a constant rate regardless of any increases in force levels.

Ideally, the force magnitudes produced by orthodontic devices could be accurately measured and prescribed based on individual, specific treatment objectives. The levels of force magnitude generated have been reported only for a few appliance designs. Since ideal force levels needed for different types of tooth movements are unknown, descriptions of specific force magnitudes are of limited value. However, knowledge of the force levels applied to teeth via the appliance is at least a step in the direction of understanding optimal forces.[13–16]

Size of Anchorage Units

A popular approach to improving anchorage is to increase the number of teeth in the anchorage unit. Increasing the number of teeth disperses the load over a greater root surface area. This decreases the strain or distortion of the periodontal structures within the anchorage unit.

A fundamental presumption is that the rate of tooth movement varies with the force or load such that increasing the force magnitude results in an increased rate of tooth movement. The rate of tooth movement may vary with force only up to a threshold level (see above). Once the threshold force magnitude is reached, tooth movement occurs. Since the true relationship between force levels and the rate of tooth movement is unknown, this approach to anchorage control should be used with caution.

Differential Force Systems: Variable Moments and Forces

The force system of an orthodontic appliance determines the type of tooth movement expressed. The forces act in all three planes of space (first, second, or third order). Most space closure concerns are second order, or the sagittal

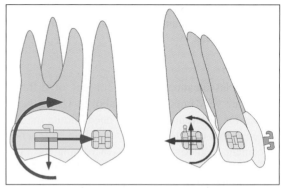

Fig. 10-10 Components of the space closure force system. Forces and moments acting on the anterior tooth are shown by blue arrows, and those acting on the posterior tooth shown by red arrows. The alpha moment is shown smaller in magnitude than the beta moment; thus the vertical forces are intrusive on the anterior and extrusive on the posterior tooth. If the alpha moment were greater than the beta, the vertical forces would be in the opposite direction.

view. The components of any force system (Fig. 10-10) in this view are[1–8]:

- *Alpha moment.* This is the moment acting on the anterior teeth (often termed anterior torque).
- *Beta moment.* This is the moment acting on the posterior teeth. An example is tipback bends placed mesial to the molars that produce an increased beta moment.
- *Horizontal forces.* These are the mesiodistal forces acting on the teeth. The distal forces acting on the anterior teeth always equal the mesial forces acting on the posterior teeth.
- *Vertical forces.* These are intrusive–extrusive forces acting on the anterior or posterior teeth. These forces generally result from unequal alpha and beta moments. When the beta moment is greater than the alpha moment, an intrusive force acts on the anterior teeth while extrusive forces act on the posterior teeth. When the alpha moment is greater than the beta moment, extrusive forces act on the anterior teeth while intrusive forces act on the posterior teeth. The magnitude of the vertical forces is dependent on the difference between the moments and the interbracket distance. Futhermore, higher forces are associated with decreased interbracket distances (for equivalent alpha-beta moment differences).

Space Closing Appliance Designs

Despite the variety of appliance designs available to the orthodontist, space closure is usually accomplished with either sliding mechanics or closing loops. Each technique has its advantages and disadvantages.

Sliding Mechanics

The attractiveness of sliding mechanics is its clinical simplicity. In addition, many clinicians feel that sliding mechanics offer predictable results since the preformed archwire helps maintain the occlusal plane and chosen arch form. Regardless of its simplicity, however, the efficiency of sliding mechanics may be compromised due to the effects of friction.

The importance of friction is not fully understood, but suffice to say that many practitioners would agree that it impedes tooth movement. With sliding mechanics, space closure is slowed as the bracket undergoes a "stick–slip" action along the archwire. This erratic movement occurs as the tooth tips and the bracket then binds against the archwire.[17–22] On binding, movement ceases until the deflected archwire forces the tooth upright wherein the tipping/binding action begins anew. In addition, the frictional forces occurring during sliding mechanics compromise the delivery of the desired force levels.

The "stick–slip" action of tooth displacement during sliding mechanics may promote rapid changes in the magnitude, location, and direction of periodontal strains. Periodontal strain magnitudes may vary significantly and lead to ambiguous stimuli to the cellular tissues responsible for orthodontic remodeling. Furthermore, the patient may not tolerate the fluctuating inflammatory-like pain responses.

Finally, poorly managed sliding mechanics are associated with several unwanted side effects such as uncontrolled tipping, deepening of the overbite, and loss of anchorage (Fig. 10-11). The frequency and severity of these effects depends on the archwire composition and dimensions, magnitude of the traction force, and interbracket distance.[18,23] These limitations of sliding mechanisms suggest an alternative approach needs to be considered.

Closing Loops

Well-designed closing loops promote a more continuous type of tooth movement by eliminating the intermittent ("stick–slip") force delivery seen in sliding mechanics. Additionally, since closing loops deliver frictionless forces, the tissues of the periodontium experience more continuous stresses. While historic reports suggest otherwise,[24] contemporary studies on force constancy suggest that continuous forces promote greater rates of tooth displacement.[25–27] Nevertheless, there are several advantages to the use of closing loops as well as numerous design options.

While loop designs are numerous,[28–30] there are many reasons for choosing one configuration over another. Preference for a particular closing loop is often based on its simplicity of fabrication and delivery. While simplicity is a goal of practice management, it may be at odds with the desired biomechanic properties of the appliance. Three important criteria in the use of closing loops are: (1) loop position; (2) loop preactivation or gabling; and (3) loop design.

Loop Position

An often overlooked but important aspect of closing loops is the *position* of the loop within the interbracket space.[31,32] Traditionally, when retracting anterior teeth, continuous closing loops are typically placed immediately distal to the lateral incisors or canines (Fig. 10-12). The rationale for placing the loops adjacent to the teeth anterior to the extraction space is that it allows for repeated activation of the loop as the space closes. Recent research, however, has shown that a change in the location of the loop can augment or reduce the posterior anchorage needed for a given patient.[32] To understand the effects of loop positioning, the forces that occur when a closing loop is activated must first be considered.

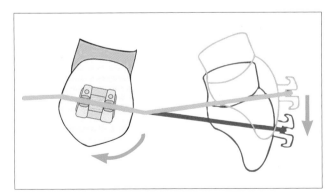

Fig. 10-11 Wire deflection with canine retraction on light wire. Canine root anterior tipping, deepening overbite, and molar anchorage loss are the most remarkable undesirable effects.

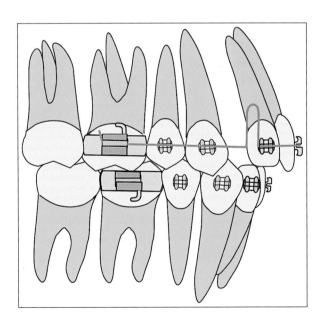

Fig. 10-12 Vertical loop placed distal to the upper lateral incisors. The loop shape provides a very low moment/force ratio with inadequate root control. The main advantage of this loop position is the possibility of numerous activations on the same wire as the space closes.

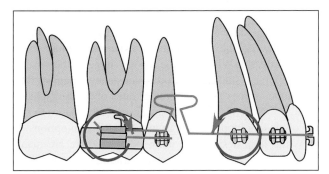

Fig. 10-13 T-loop positioned midway between the first molar and the canine. The preactivation bends provide equal and opposite moments in this position.

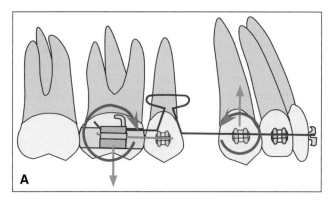

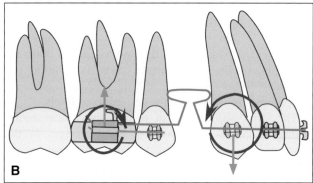

Fig. 10-14 **A** and **B** Off-centered T-loop between the molar and the canine. There are differential moments, with the higher moment on the shorter leg and an opposite moment of lower magnitude on the other end. An extrusive force is found on the side with the larger moment and an intrusive force on the opposite end.

Force System of Loop Activation. When an activated closing loop is situated between the brackets spanning a space in the arch, equal and opposite activation moments are delivered to the adjacent teeth (Fig. 10-13).[16] Equal moments encourage *reciprocal* space closure, since the anterior and posterior moments are equal in magnitude but opposite in direction. In contrast, *asymmetric* or off-center placement of the loop results in *unequal* moments (Fig. 10-14). The moment magnitudes are greatest at the teeth closest to the loop and smallest at the more distant teeth. Since the type of tooth movement (e.g. tipping or translation) is determined by the moment/force ratio at the bracket, differential tooth movement is encouraged with asymmetrically placed closing loops.[10,31]

It is important to be aware, however, of the vertical effects produced by differential moment force systems.[10,33–36] Extrusive forces act at the attachments nearest the loop (greater moment) and intrusive effects act at the more distant attachment (see Fig. 10-14). The magnitudes of the forces are proportional to the moment differential and are nearly constant.[32] These vertical force may be beneficially used, moreover, to meet treatment objectives (e.g. correction of excessive overbite during space closure).

The effects of asymmetric loop placement can be explained by the fact that the addition of a loop in an archwire essentially creates two sections of wire, an anterior and a posterior section. If the loop is placed asymmetrically between the anterior and posterior teeth, the anterior and posterior sections of the wire become unequal in length (which is inversely proportional to the third power of the length). The greater stiffness of the shorter section of an off-centered loop acts to create greater moments relative to the longer section. Since the magnitude of the moment (relative to the force) determines the type of tooth movement,[10,14,31,37–38] one tooth or segment of teeth is initially encouraged to translate and the other is initially encouraged to tip. In this way, *differential* tooth movement and anteroposterior anchorage may be established by producing *differential moments* through careful placement

of the closing loop.[36] To apply these concepts clinically, space can be closed while meeting anchorage objectives by simply *offsetting* the loop to the posterior for *posterior anchorage* (Fig. 10-15), or conversely, to the anterior for *anterior anchorage*. (Reflecting back to the traditional technique of placing the closing loop as far anterior as possible, it may be appreciated that the anterior teeth may actually act as the anchorage teeth!). Figure 10-16 shows an adult patient in whom a group A anchorage strategy was employed for space closure with a posteriorly placed continuous arch T loop.

Loop Preactivation

When a closing loop is activated, the anterior and posterior portions of the archwire deflect away from a parallel orientation. When the closing loop archwire is engaged into the brackets, a second- and/or third-order couple (moment) is felt by the anterior and posterior sections of the wire (Fig. 10-17). The moments acting on the archwire, in turn, are delivered to the teeth as the wire deactivates.[31] Depending on the loop design, these moments (termed *activation moments*) encourage varying degrees of root control during space closure and are directly affected by the position of the loop within the interbracket space.

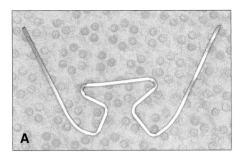

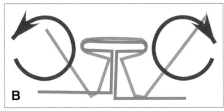

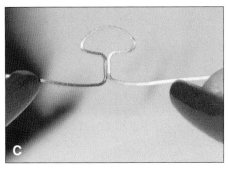

Fig. 10-15 A and **B** Preactivation bends on a T-loop. **C** Loop in the neutral position. Equal and opposite moments are present without horizontal forces.

Although loop position is critical in delivering the proper force system, research at the University of Connecticut[2,31,32] suggests that the moments occurring through activation alone are insufficient to produce an adequate force system necessary for root control. Indeed, generations of orthodontists have empirically recognized this and have placed gable bends in the archform adjacent to the loops to increase root control and, thus, avoid "dumping" of the teeth as the space closes. From a biomechanic standpoint, the gable bends act to increase the moments delivered to the teeth and augment the moments that occur during activation of the closing loop.[31] The two act in concert to promote root control and anchorage.

Loop Design

Proper positioning and gabling are essential features of controlled space closure using closing loop mechanics. The final key, however, to efficiency and space closure control is loop design. Ideal loop designs should meet a number of criteria, most notably closing loops should accommodate a large activation, deliver relatively low and nearly constant forces (i.e. exhibit low load/deflection characteristics), be comfortable to the patient, and be easily fabricated.[2,31]

Although many loop designs are available, few meet all these criteria. For example, consider a standard vertical loop, 6 mm in height, fabricated from 0.018" by 0.025" stainless steel.[2] While this is easy to fabricate, this design delivers very high forces (in the order of 1000 g or more) when activated by only 2 or 3 mm. These force values may cause a good deal of discomfort to the patient and will tend to "overpower" the moments, resulting in loss of anchorage and root control. "Dumping" of the teeth toward the extraction site may be a common side effect. Moreover, simple vertical loops are associated with small activations, rapid force decay, and intermittent force delivery. These characteristics may have a negative impact on the efficiency of treatment.[25,27]

To meet the above criteria of an ideal closing loop, several design components could be altered.[31] Notably, incorporating additional wire in the design will reduce the amount of force produced when the loop is activated. As a consequence, lower, more optimal forces are delivered and the moments required for root control increase in a relative fashion. Several options are available to the orthodontist to increase the amount of wire in the loop: the horizontal dimension of the loop itself may be increased, the diameter of the bend may be increased, helices may be added, or the height of the loop may be increased. Benchtop tests have shown that the latter, increasing the height of the loop, has the greatest effect on reducing the force while simultaneously increasing the moment.[15]

Anatomic constraints such as the depth of the vestibule, however, limit how high the loop can be made. One way to overcome this problem is by adding wire *horizontally*. As such, the T-loop[31] was developed to deliver optimal space closure. A recent adaptation is the mushroom shape (M-loop),* which is more patient friendly as it reduces the horizontal part near the vestibule.

Beta-Titanium CNA Mushroom Loop. * The M-loop (Fig. 10-18) is desirable because the apical addition of the wire in the archial configuration decreases the load-deflection rate, and therefore produces lower and more continuous forces compared to simpler designs. Additionally, the archival shape has the added advantage of increasing the applied moment when the spring is activated.[6] The decreased force and increased moment, when activated, increases the moment/force ratio and, therefore, allows for greater root control and anchorage. Moreover, the CNA* beta-titanium recommended for use in the M-loop has a much lower stiffness than steel and promotes a more constant force delivery.

The beta-titanium M-loop may be "set up" for a number of space-closing strategies while meeting planned anchorage objectives.[36] Space closure with this appliance takes advantage of the effects of loop placement. If posterior anchorage is the objective, the loop is offset to

*Ortho Organizers Inc, San Marcos, CA

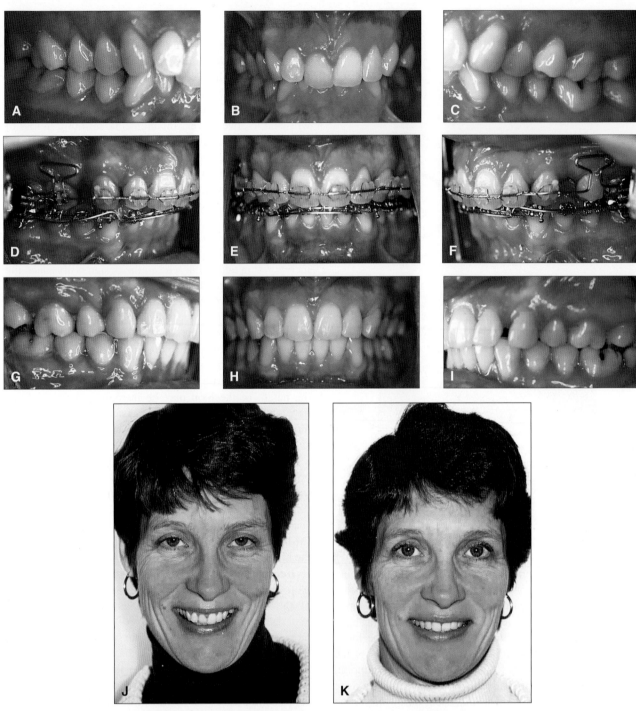

Fig. 10-16 Adult patient with Class II malocclusion treated with upper first bicuspid extractions. The upper continuous T-loop arch is positioned off center (loop closer to the molar) for a group A space closure strategy. **A-C** Class II, Division 2 malocclusion with 100% overbite. **D-F** Continuous off-center T-loop in the upper arch and lower intrusion arch for deep overbite correction. **G** and **H** Finished Class I canine occlusion and coincident midlines. Slight anterior tooth size discrepancy is present with space distal to the upper left lateral incisor. **I** Initial and **J** final frontal photographs showing maintenance of the vertical position of the upper incisors achieving an esthetic smile. Overbite was corrected through lower incisor intrusion.

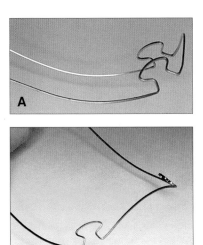

Fig. 10-17 A and **B** M-loop 17 × 25 CNA archwire with preactivation bends giving anterior and posterior moments.

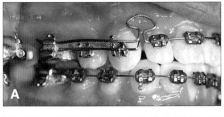

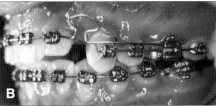

Fig. 10-18 A and **B** Intraoral buccal views showing the M-loop distal to the laterals bypassing the canine and premolar brackets and engaging the first molars.

the posterior. If simple reciprocal tooth movements are required, the loop is placed equidistantly between the bracket anterior to the extraction site and the molar tube.

To take advantage of the positional effects of the loop, bypassing the premolar(s) and directly engaging the molar auxiliary tube is recommended (see Fig. 10-18). This practice allows for force/moment delivery to the active (anterior) and reactive (molar) teeth directly rather being "lost" to the canines and premolars. Additionally, the increased interbracket distance has the effect of reducing errors in loop placement and helps maintain force constancy.[2] It is often advisable, however, to stabilize the posterior teeth with a transpalatal arch and buccal segments.

Wire dimensions of T- and M-loop archwires are 0.017" × 0.025" CNA;* although, for adults requiring lower force values, a 0.016" × 0.022" may be preferred.[7] Care should be taken to make a trial activation and correct any distortions that may occur under initial loading. Once engaged, the loop may be activated up to 5 mm. This activation will deliver enough force to simultaneously retract all the anterior teeth *en masse*[4] with little impact on posterior anchorage. Reactivation is necessary approximately every 6–8 weeks.

Single Cuspid Retraction with En-Masse Anterior Retraction

At the University of Connecticut we have designed multifunctional orthodontic wires capable of simultaneously performing different orthodontic tooth movements. Since the force system, along with the side effects, of these wires is well understood it becomes easier to use noncompliant mechanics. These "smart" wires minimize the need for headgear and Class II elastics.

The two-step space closure described here allows the introduction of biomechanic principles to the sliding mechanics commonly used to retract a cuspid on an archwire. Cuspid retraction on an archwire often poses a catch-22 situation. If a light wire is used to retract the cuspids, the apparent tooth movement is faster as primarily uncontrolled tipping occurs. Various notable side effects may occur with this practice. At the posterior end, this movement will produce anchorage loss and extrusion with possible bite opening, and in the anterior segment, a loss of control of the axial inclination of the incisors with possible bite deepening. Additionally, loss of control of the canine root is usually observed. On the other hand, a heavier wire increases friction and results in a slower tooth movement

To eliminate the side effects of bite deepening and loss of anchorage, an intrusion arch (see Ch. 7) can be used as a piggyback archwire. This wire also allows simultaneous intrusion of the incisors during cuspid retraction. Once the cuspids are retracted the anterior retraction can be accomplished with CNA* M-loop archwires.

Sliding Canine Retraction with Simultaneous Use of Intrusion Wires

To retract canines, a stainless steel round base archwire is used to slide the canines distally. To prevent the side effects of deepening of the incisor bite due to change in the inclination of the canines (see Fig. 10-11) an intrusion arch* is tied as a piggyback wire on top of the stainless steel wire (Fig. 10-19). The intrusion arch* is ligated at

*Ultimate Wireforms, Bristol, CT

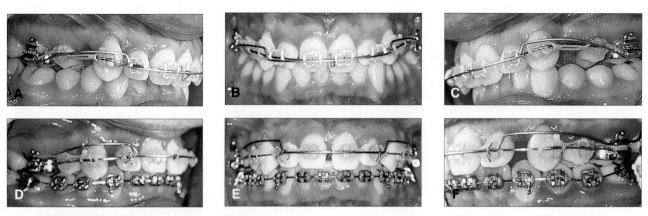

Fig. 10-19 Canine retraction using an intrusion arch to control for the undesirable side effects seen in Figure 10-11. **A-C** Class II, Division 2 patient treated with upper first premolar extractions. A 16 × 25 stainless steel base archwire with a nickel–titanium intrusion arch. An elastic chain was used to retract the canines separately. **D-F** Canines retracted to a Class I relationship. Good overjet and overbite are achieved with proper third-order inclination of the upper incisors, and excellent anchorage control is observed.

the level of the lateral incisors and between the central incisors. The intrusion arch delivers a distal crown tipback moment on the molars to effectively control the loss of distal anchorage often associated with sliding mechanics (Fig. 10-20). These mechanics are especially ideal for patients where anchorage is critical. In adults it also eliminates the need for headgear or Class II elastics. With an intrusive force on the incisors and a moment on the molars, the base archwire does not deflect as much as it is often seen with the retraction of canines using light wires. The intrusive force and the moment counteracts the archwire deflection generated by friction during canine retraction.

M-Loop Space Closing Archwires

Once the canine retraction has been completed, the anterior segment is retracted. In the majority of patients at this stage, the four incisors either need translation or controlled movement of crowns and root apices. For translatory movement a high constant moment/force ratio of approximately 10/1 is recommended.[10] If this ratio is too low (very commonly observed with straight wire mechanics) the incisors crowns move lingually, reducing the overjet and giving

the erroneous impression of a tooth size discrepancy as the space distal to the laterals appears to be enormous. To correct this side effect, the bite needs reopening or the incisor crowns need to be torqued bucally, thereby creating an unnecessary stress at the root apices as well as increasing the treatment time.

To achieve this moment/force ratio, the preformed M-loop space closing archwires are ideal. The mushroom shape of the loop allows no interference with gingival tissue and an activated loop does not distort in shape, thereby giving a better force delivery. The archwire size of choice for a 0.022 bracket prescription is a preformed M-loop 0.017 × 0.025 CNA* available with standardized interloop distances from 26 to 46 mm (in 2 mm increments) (Fig. 10-21). This measurement represents the distance from the distal surface of one lateral incisor to the other across the midline. Once the proper archwire has been selected it is preactivated outside the mouth.

Preactivation of the archwire achieves the necessary moment/force ratio. This preactivation starts by carefully separating the legs of both M-loops by approximately 3 mm. Additional gable bends may be placed, as needed, mesially to increase the anterior moment (torque) and distal to the M-loop to increase anchorage moment. Next,

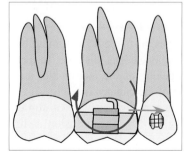

Fig. 10-20 Tipback on the upper molar obtained with the intrusion arch. This tipback moment aides in anchorage control.

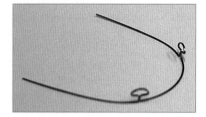

Fig. 10-21 Mushroom loop arches made of CNA without preactivations.

*Ortho Organizers Inc, San Marcos, CA

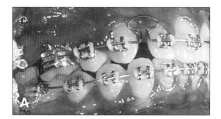 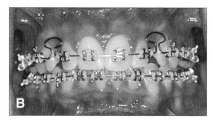 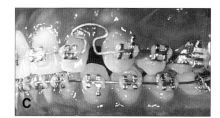

Fig. 10-22 A-C Mushroom loop for anterior incisor retraction. Preactivation of the loop helps to maintain the incisor inclination during space closure. The archwire is engaged on every bracket from first molar to first molar.

the torque on the distal legs is eliminated to make the wire passive in the third order in the buccal segments. The archwire is now placed in the mouth and engaged across the arch from first molar to first molar (Fig. 10-22). The archwire is ready to be activated approximately 4 mm (3 mm of preactivation plus 1 mm of additional activation).

The loop should not be reactivated until there is at least 3 mm of space closure. In this manner a more constant moment/force ratio is maintained. Once the space is closed the wire should be left in the mouth for one or two additional visits so that the residual moments can be utilized for correction of the root axial inclination of anterior and posterior teeth. This completely eliminates the need for root uprighting and torquing springs and significantly reduces the treatment time.

Figure 10-23 shows the progress of a patient from the initial phase to the placement of the M-loop archwire. Single canine retraction with sliding mechanics was used as the first stage, and an M-loop archwire with gable bends was used to close the spaces distal to the upper laterals.

Finishing

The finishing phase of treatment only involves use of coordinated 0.017 × 0.025 or 0.018 × 0.025 CNA wires.

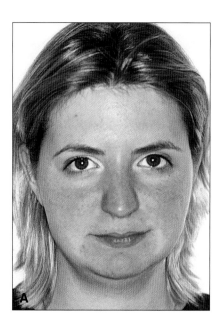 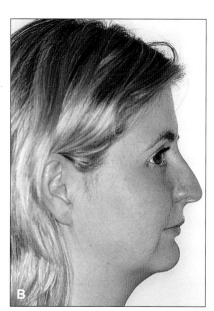

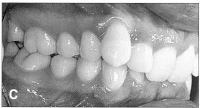 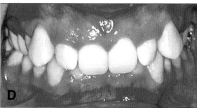 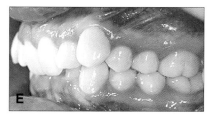

Fig. 10-23 Adult patient treated with upper first premolar extractions and separate canine retraction using intrusion arch and elastic chain. M-loop archwires are used to retract the upper anterior teeth. **A** and **B** Extraoral preoperative views. **C-E** Preoperative intraoral views. Bilateral full cusp Class II molar relationship with a deep overbite and lingual inclination of the upper incisors.

Continued

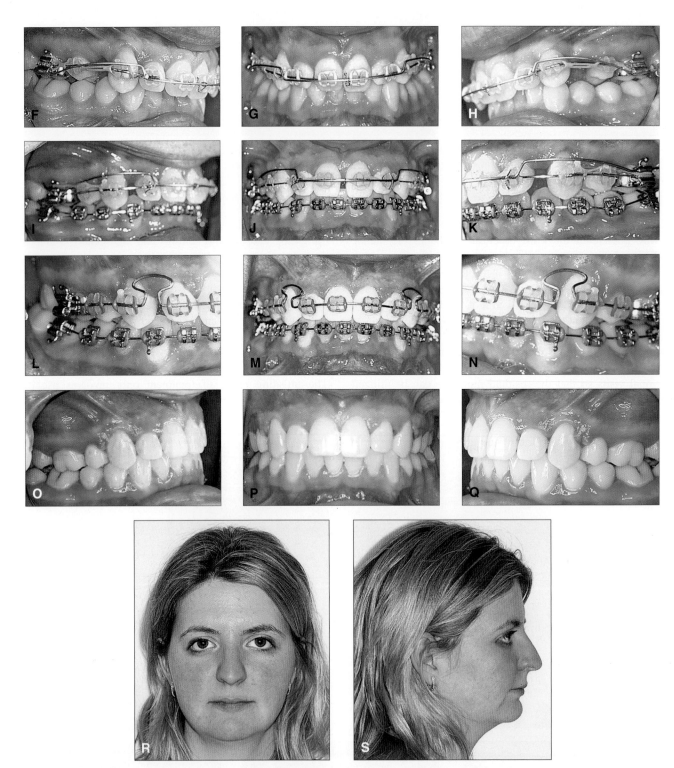

Fig. 10-23 Adult patient treated with upper first premolar extractions and separate canine retraction using intrusion arch and elastic chain. M-loop archwires are used to retract the upper anterior teeth. **A** and **B** Extraoral preoperative views. **C-E** Preoperative intraoral views. Bilateral full cusp Class II molar relationship with a deep overbite and lingual inclination of the upper incisors. **F-K** Separate canine retraction on a light base archwire with a nickel–titanium overlay intrusion arch tied anteriorly. **L-N** M-loop tied to all the teeth to retract the four upper anterior teeth. **O-Q** Final intraoral views showing the good occlusal result, with a minimum of anchorage loss and proper incisor buccolingual inclination. **R** and **S** No significant changes in the frontal or profile views are observed after upper premolar extractions. (Reproduced with permission from Uribe F, Nanda R. Treatment of Class II Division 2 Malocclusion in Adults. JCO 2003; 37:599-606).

Minor bends can be placed in these beta-titanium wires for finishing details in the alignment and occlusion. It should be noted that the finishing stage is usually of short duration due to the correct positioning of the incisors following retraction.

Retention

For adult patients a maxillary modified Hawley retainer (wrap-around) is usually ideal as there is no interference in the occlusion. For a lower arch a bonded retainer from canine to canine is ideal. It is important to stress that intrusion is a very stable movement[10] and minimal overbite relapse should be expected as the deep bite correction with this method involves minimal posterior buccal extrusion.

Summary

Extraction is a common treatment option in orthodontics. Proper space closure mechanics are necessary to achieve the desired treatment objectives and outcomes. Anchorage control is one of the most difficult tasks in extraction patients. Differential moment strategies for maximum anchorage space closure are necessary if non compliance intra arch anchorage is desired. A method for critical anchorage (group A) space closure in two stages (canine retraction followed by incisor retraction) is presented. Intrusion arches and Mushroom loop archwires are very useful aides in space closure to maintain maximum anchorage with minimum side effects.

REFERENCES

1. Burstone CJ. Rationale of the segmented arch. Am J Orthod 1962;48:805–822.
2. Burstone CJ. The segmented arch approach to space closure. Am J Orthod 1982;82:361–378.
3. Burstone CJ, Hanley KJ. Modern edgewise mechanics segmented arch technique. Farmington: University of Connecticut Health Center, 1985.
4. Burstone CJ. The mechanics of the segmented arch techniques. Angle Orthod 1966;36:99–120.
5. Burstone CJ, Koenig HA. Optimizing anterior and canine retraction. Am J Orthod 1976;70:1–19.
6. Faulker MG, Fuchshuber P, Haberstock D, Mioduchowski A. A parametric study of the force/moment systems produced by T-loop retraction springs. J Biomechanics 1989;22:637–647.
7. Manhartsberger C, Morton JY, Burstone CJ. Space closure in adult patients using the segmented arch technique. Angle Orthod 1989;59:205–210.
8. Kusy RP, Tulloch JF. Analysis of moment/force ratios in the mechanics of tooth movement. Am J Orthod Dentofac Orthop 1986;90:127–131.
9. Sachdeva RC. A study of force systems produced by TMA T-loop retraction springs. Master's thesis, University of Connecticut School of Dental Medicine, 1985.
10. Smith RJ, Burstone CJ. Mechanics of tooth movement. Am J Orthod 1984;85:294–307.
11. Kuhlberg AJ. Force systems from T-loop orthodontic space closure springs. Master's thesis, University of Connecticut School of Dental Medicine, 1992.
12. Quinn RS, Yoshikawa DK. A reassessment of force magnitude in orthodontics. Am J Orthod 1985;8:252–260.
13. Nikolai RJ. On optimum orthodontic force theory as applied to canine retraction. Am J Orthod 1975;68:290–302.
14. Tanne K, Koenig HA, Burstone CJ. Moment to force ratios and the center of rotation. Am J Orthod 1988;94:426–431.
15. Hixon EH, Aasen TO, Arango J, et al. On force and tooth movement. Am J Orthod 1970;57:476–488.
16. Nanda R, Goldin B. Biomechanic approaches to the study of alterations of facial morphology. Am J Orthod 1980;78:213–226.
17. Tselepis M, Brockhurst P, West VC. The dynamic frictional resistance between orthodontic brackets and arch wires. Am J Orthod Dentofacial Orthop 1994;106:131–138.
18. Schlegel V. Relative friction minimization in fixed orthodontic bracket appliances. J Biomech 1996;29:483–491.
19. Nanda RS, Ghosh J. Biomechanic considerations in sliding mechanics. In: Nanda R, ed. Biomechanics in clinical orthodontics. Philadelphia: WB Saunders, 1997:188–217.
20. Kusy RP, Whitley JQ. Influence of archwire and bracket dimensions on sliding mechanics: derivations and determinations of the critical contact angles for binding. Eur J Orthod 1999;21:199–208.
21. Kusy RP, Whitley JQ. Assessment of second-order clearances between orthodontic archwires and bracket slots via the critical contact angles for binding. Angle Orthod 1999;69:71–80.
22. Loftus BP, Artun J, Nicholls JI, Alonzo TA, Stoner JA. Evaluation of friction during sliding tooth movement in various bracket-archwire combinations. Am J Orthod Dentofacial Orthop 1999;116:336–345.
23. Ogata RH, Nanda RS, Duncanson MG Jr, Sinha PK, Currier GF. Frictional resistances in stainless steel bracket-wire combinations with effects of vertical deflections. Am J Orthod Dentofacial Orthop 1996;109:535–542.
24. Reitan K. Some factors determining the evaluation of forces in orthodontics. Am J Orthod 1957;43:32–45.
25. Owman-Moll P, Kurol J, Lundgren D. Continuous versus interrupted continuous orthodontic force related to early tooth movement and root resorption. Angle Orthod 1995;65:395–401.
26. Daskalogiannakis J, McLachlan KR. Canine retraction with rare earth magnets: an investigation into the validity of the constant force hypothesis. Am J Orthod Dentofacial Orthop 1996;109:489–495.
27. Iwasaki LR, Haack JE, Nickel JC, Morton J. Human tooth movement in response to continuous stress of low magnitude. Am J Orthod Dentofacial Orthop 2000;117:175–183.
28. Storey E, Smith R. Force in orthodontics and its relation to tooth movement. Aust J Dent 1952;56:11–18.
29. Siatkowski RE. Continuous arch wire closing loop design, optimization, and verification. Part I. Am J Orthod Dentofacial Orthop 1997;112:393–402.

30. Siatkowski RE. Continuous arch wire closing loop design, optimization, and verification. Part II. Am J Orthod Dentofacial Orthop 1997;112:487–495.

31. Burstone CJ, Koenig HA. Optimizing anterior and canine retraction. Am J Orthod 1976;70:1–19.

32. Kuhlberg AJ, Burstone CJ. T-loop position and anchorage control. Am J Orthod Dentofacial Orthop 1997;112:12–18.

33. Burstone C. Application of bioengineering to clinical orthodontics. In: Graber T, Vanarsdall R, eds. Orthodontics: current principles and techniques. St Louis: Mosby, 2000.

34. Burstone CJ, Koenig HA. Force systems from an ideal arch. Am J Orthod 1974;65:270–289.

35. Burstone CJ, Koenig HA. Creative wire bending—The force system from step and V-bends. Am J Orthod Dentofac Orthop 1988;93:59–67.

36. Nanda R, Kuhlberg AJ. Biomechanics of extraction space closure. In: Nanda R, ed. Biomechanics in clinical orthodontics. Philadelphia: WB Saunders, 1997.

37. Burstone C. The rationale of the segmented arch technique. Am J Orthod 1962;48:805–822.

38. Burstone CJ, Pryputniewicz RJ. Holographic determination of centers of rotation produced by orthodontic forces. Am J Orthod 1980;77:396–409.

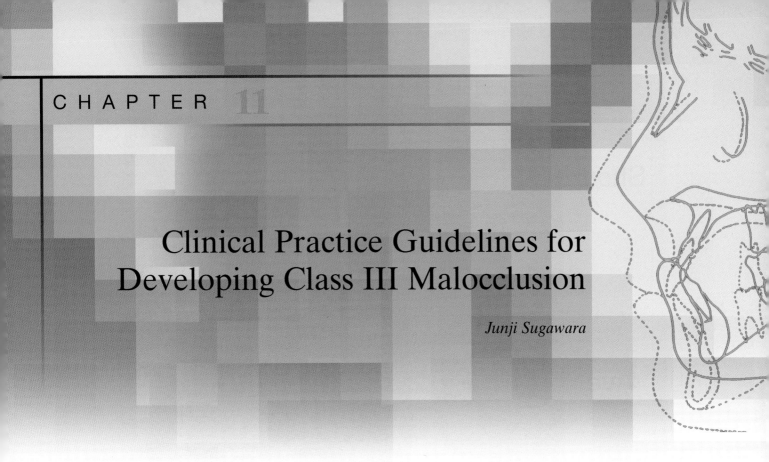

CHAPTER 11

Clinical Practice Guidelines for Developing Class III Malocclusion

Junji Sugawara

Class III malocclusion can be defined as a skeletal facial deformity characterized by a forward mandibular position with respect to the cranial base and/or maxilla (Fig. 11-1). This facial dysplasia can be classified into mandibular prognathism, maxillary retrognathism, or a combination of both, depending on the variation of the anteroposterior jaw relationships. Vertically, they can also be divided into three basic types depending on the vertical disproportions: long, average, and short face (Fig. 11-1). In this chapter, Class III malocclusions will refer only to anteroposterior dysplasia. Class III malocclusion represents patients with anterior crossbite and a skeletal Class III jaw disharmony (Fig. 11-2). Pseudo Class III malocclusion, which is characterized by an anterior crossbite and a skeletal Class I relationship, is excluded from this category.

It has been believed that Class III malocclusion may be caused by excessive growth of the mandible with respect to the maxilla and/or cranial base. However, the results of our longitudinal studies show similar maxillary and mandibular incremental changes during the prepubertal, pubertal, and postpubertal period when compared to Class I subjects. Therefore, it would be rational to assume that the skeletal framework of Class III malocclusion must have been established early before the prepubertal growth period. In addition, the manner of mandibular growth during the postpubertal period seems to be quite critical in Class III treatment, because the maxillary growth changes are almost negligible and only the mandible is displaced in a downward–forward direction according to its growth potential.

Concerning mandibular growth control that can possibly alter the skeletal framework of Class III patients, our aftermentioned studies on the short- and long-term effects of chin cap force indicate that the skeletal framework is greatly improved during the initial stages of chin cap therapy. However, such changes are rarely maintained during the pubertal growth period and, when growth is complete, results suggest that treatment with chin cap force seldom alters the inherited prognathic characteristics of Class III profiles.

Considering the scientific evidence, we have produced a clinical practice guideline for managing Class III patients and practiced in accordance with this guideline for >10 years. The principal role of the guideline is to make provisions so that almost all patients achieve functional occlusion and esthetic dentition until adulthood, and lifelong stability thereafter. In addition, it aims to assure the quality of orthodontic treatment and to provide risk management strategies for unexpected situations occurring during treatment and management.

The clinical practice guideline for the correction of developing Class III malocclusion is outlined below, with particular consideration given to Class III facial growth and the long-term effects of chin cap orthopedic force for controlling Class III mandibular growth. In addition, treatment progress and the results of representative Class III patients who were managed in accordance with the clinical practice guideline are reported. Figure 11-3 shows the clinical practice guideline for growing and developing Class III patients and represents our present concept of their treatment and management.[1]

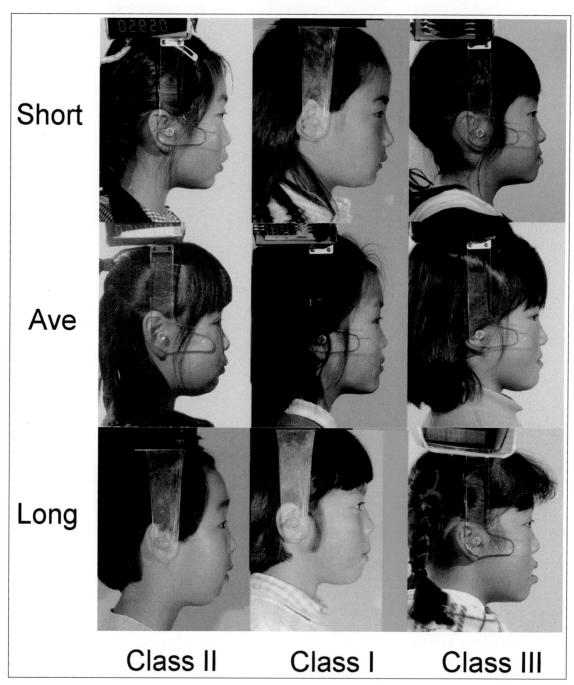

Fig. 11-1 Classification of facial types.

At the initial diagnosis in the deciduous dentition and/or early mixed dentition, patients receive a differential diagnosis and are divided into two groups according to the extent of their three-dimensional jaw disharmonies. Long-term management is usually recommended for patients diagnosed with mild or moderate skeletal Class III, and this management is clearly separated into two treatment phases (Fig. 11-3). The early mixed dentition is the most desirable time for the first phase of orthodontic treatment (although not all patients seek consultation early enough for this), and the second phase of treatment is generally applied during or after the postpubertal period. The growth observation period runs from the end of the first phase of treatment to the beginning of the second phase.

The treatment objectives of the first phase are:
1. To maintain good oral hygiene with the help of dental caries risk tests
2. To correct functional deviation of the mandible and to stabilize the jaw position
3. To improve the three-dimensional jaw deformity as far as possible
4. To correct and control the deviation of the dental midline

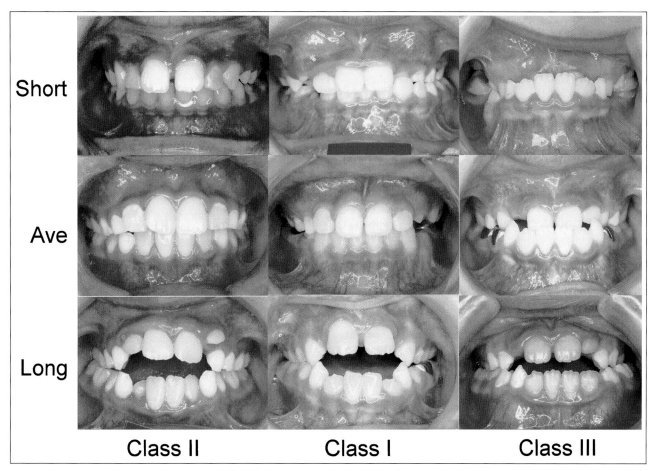

Fig. 11-2 Occlusion of each skeletal facial type.

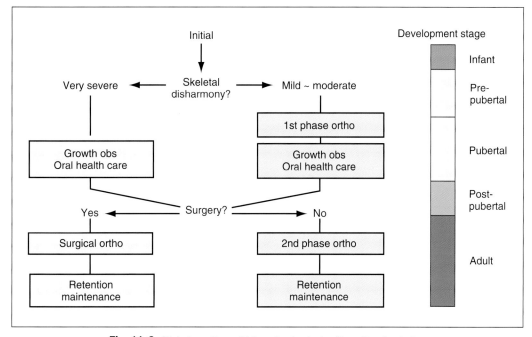

Fig. 11-3 Clinical practice guidelines for developing Class III malocclusion.

5. To accomplish desirable anterior occlusion for establishing anterior guidance in the future
6. To establish bilateral posterior support
7. To gain enough space for the buccal teeth
8. To normalize and enhance orofacial functions.

On the other hand, the treatment objectives of the second phase of treatment are:

• To achieve a balanced soft tissue profile
• To establish final functional occlusion
• To regulate temporomandibular joint (TMJ) and oral functions
• To prevent periodontal disease and promote oral health.

During the observation period, growth data is collected from the patient and his/her oral hygiene is professionally controlled. A very important point is that the quick completion of each phase will motivate the patient to comply throughout the longterm management period.

Patients with extremely severe skeletal Class III malocclusion, in whom orthognathic surgery is indicated, usually skip the first phase of treatment and their orthodontic problems cannot be addressed until the postpubertal period. It is important to collect growth data from these patients to establish an individual growth database for determining the timing of orthognathic surgery, and to professionally control oral hygiene during the observation period.

Most Class III patients are managed according to one of the two pathways described above, but occasionally a patient is managed in a modified manner. For instance, it is possible that patients diagnosed as requiring jaw surgery at the initial examination can be camouflaged with usual second-phase orthodontic treatment. Conversely, some patients may need to change from the right to the left side of the clinical practice guideline (Fig. 11-3) if they experience abnormal jaw growth.

The reasons for proposing this clinical practice guideline for the correction of growing Class III malocclusion can be narrowed down to two points: Class III facial growth, and chin cap orthopedic effects.

Class III Facial Growth

Most malocclusions and dentofacial deformities do not result from some pathologic process, but rather a moderate distortion of normal development. Class III malocclusion appears to develop from an interaction between environmental and innate factors. An understanding of craniofacial growth behavior in Class III patients will help in determining the treatment timing and biomechanics. However, little is known about the craniofacial growth pattern of Class III malocclusion in comparison to normal patients. Early studies were largely based on either cross-sectional[2] and semi-longitudinal samples,[3] or longitudinal data[4,5] that encompassed too few subjects to be statistically valid.

In 1981, Mitani[6] published a longitudinal study on Class III growth during the prepubertal period. Since then, our research group has conducted several longitudinal

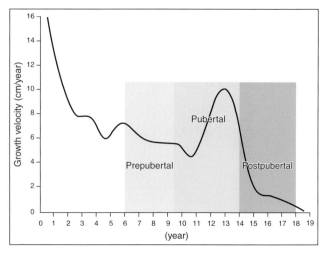

Fig. 11-4 Growth curve showing the development stages.

studies[7–12] utilizing growth records of patients who were waiting for orthognathic surgery. The craniofacial growth of skeletal Class III subjects in Japanese girls during the prepubertal, pubertal, and postpubertal periods, and which was one of the sources informing the development of the clinical practice guideline, is shown in Figure 11-4.

Prepubertal Growth Period

Mitani[6] compared growth changes between Class III and Class I patients during the prepubertal growth period. The investigation was based on two groups of Japanese girls: an experimental group of 18 girls (Class III group) and a control group of 22 (Class I group). Each set of serial lateral cephalometric head films consisted of a 4-year series from age 7 to 10 years. All Class III subjects exhibited Class III malocclusion and all Class I subjects showed excellent or mild Class I malocclusion. None of the Class III subjects underwent any growth-related orthopedic treatment before or during the study period.

Table 11-1 shows mean and standard deviations of linear and angular measurements at the age of 7 and 10 years and their overall changes during this period. No significant difference was found between the two groups with regard to the size of the maxilla (Ptm–A). However, the maxilla, as measured from basion to Ptm (Ba–Ptm), was more retruded for the Class III group (P<0.01). The incremental changes in both groups for these two measurements were relatively similar.

Comparison of the annual size increase in the mandible showed that the total mandibular length (Ar–Pog) of the Class III group maintained greater values than the Class I group until the age of 10 years. There was no significant difference between the means of the two groups for the total incremental changes in any measurements.

The ANPog angle showed a significant difference in facial convexity between the two groups. The amount of reduction in convexity was slightly greater in the Class I

Table 11-1	Results of measurements for Class III (n = 18) and Class I (n = 22) groups during prepubertal growth period in Japanese females														

| | 7 years old | | | | | 10 years old | | | | | Total change | | | | |
| | Class III | | Class I | | | Class III | | Class I | | | Class III | | Class I | | |
	x	SD	x	SD	Sig.	x	SD	x	SD	Sig.	x	SD	x	SD	Sig.
Maxilla															
Ptm–A (mm)	42.6	1.5	43.1	1.7	NS	44.0	1.9	44.7	1.8	NS	1.7	0.8	1.6	1.0	NS
Ba–A (mm)	83.3	2.7	85.7	2.3	**	86.1	2.9	89.4	2.3	**	3.0	1.4	3.7	1.7	NS
Ba–Ptm (mm)	40.5	2.0	42.5	2.4	**	42.1	2.4	44.6	2.5	**	1.5	1.0	2.1	1.4	NS
Mandible															
Ar–Pog (mm)	96.6	2.8	92.5	3.6	**	101.6	4.3	99.4	3.9	NS	7.0	1.5	7.1	1.5	NS
Go–Pog (mm)	68.8	2.5	66.6	3.0	*	73.1	3.4	71.7	3.5	NS	5.2	1.5	5.3	1.5	NS
Ar–Go (mm)	38.9	2.2	38.0	2.5	NS	41.7	2.7	41.5	2.9	NS	3.4	1.3	3.4	1.4	NS
Ba–Pog (mm)	79.0	3.3	76.5	3.0	*	83.2	3.7	81.9	3.8	NS	3.7	2.3	5.5	2.7	NS
Gonial angle (deg.)	126.5	3.8	128.4	5.3	NS	124.8	4.1	127.8	6.5	NS	−1.6	1.4	−0.6	2.5	NS
Mand. pl. (deg)	28.2	3.6	32.5	3.2	**	28.1	3.3	31.0	3.6	*	0.1	0.9	−1.5	2.3	NS
Intermaxillary															
ANPog (deg.)	1.0	1.2	6.3	1.8	**	0.6	0.9	4.9	1.8	**	−0.5	0.9	−1.4	0.9	NS

NS = Not significant; * = P < 0.05; ** = P < 0.01
Reprinted with permission from Mitani H. Prepubertal growth of mandibular prognathism. Am J Orthod 1981;80:546–553.

than in the Class III group with age, but there was no significant difference between the two groups.

In conclusion, skeletal Class III malocclusion showed an incremental growth change similar to the Class I group during the prepubertal period. These results suggest that the morphologic pattern of the prognathic face associated with mandibular excess is probably established in early life. Once established, the annual growth increment is quite similar to that in an individual with a normal or Class I face before puberty.

Pubertal Growth Period

Bandai et al[12] reported on the craniofacial growth pattern of skeletal Class III malocclusion during the pubertal growth period (9–14 years) in Japanese girls. The Class III group comprised 16 Class III girls selected from patients waiting for surgical orthodontic treatment. All patients exhibited a large reverse overjet and none underwent orthodontic or growth-related orthopedic therapy before or during the study period. The Class I group comprised 18 Class I girls who served as control subjects. A few of these patients underwent first-phase orthodontic treatment for the alignment of incisors only. The pubertal growth peak of all subjects, which was individually evaluated by ossification events of hand–wrist roentgenograms[12,13] and the incremental curve of body height,[14] was observed around the middle of the period studied. Serial lateral cephalometric head films were used over a period of 5 years from 9 to 14 years of age.

Table 11-2 shows the mean and standard deviations of linear and angular measurements at the age of 9 and 14 years and their overall changes during this period. Figure

11-5 depicts the longitudinal changes of the skeletal profile in each group. These skeletal profiles were constructed with 13 cephalometric landmarks measured in terms of the X–Y coordinates.

No significant difference between the two groups was found in the total increase of any cephalometric measurements or in any measurements regarding the maxilla at ages 9 and 14. Although the midfacial length (Cd–A) and upper facial height (N–ANS) of the Class III patients were significantly smaller (P<0.05) than those of the Class I, the average incremental changes in the maxillary length (A'–Ptm') showed no significant difference between the two groups.

The mean values of the total mandibular length (Gn–Cd) and the body length (Pog'–Go) of the Class III group were significantly greater (P<0.001) than the Class I group, whereas the ramus height (Cd–Go) was not. The average mandibular growth changes measured at Gn–Cd were 14.9 mm in the Class III group and 13.1 mm in the Class I group, showing no significant difference between the two groups.

The principal skeletal frameworks of the two groups were maintained during the pubertal period. The occlusal plane angle (SNOP) of Class III subjects remained unchanged. However, in Class I subjects it showed counterclockwise rotation during this growth period. There was a significant difference (P<0.001) in the total change of Wits appraisal between the two groups.

In conclusion, Class III malocclusion showed neither excessive mandibular growth nor deficient maxillary growth when compared to Class I subjects during the pubertal growth period. The skeletal malocclusion seems to have

Table 11-2 Measurements for Class III (n = 16) and Class I (n = 18) groups during pubertal growth period in Japanese females

| | 9 years old | | | | | 14 years old | | | | | Total change | | | | |
| | Class III | | Class I | | | Class III | | Class I | | | Class III | | Class I | | |
	x	SD	x	SD	Sig.	x	SD	x	SD	Sig.	x	SD	x	SD	Sig.
Cranial base															
S–N (mm)	61.6	1.8	62.3	2.2	NS	64.3	2.2	65.3	2.3	NS	2.7	0.9	3.0	0.9	NS
S–Ba (mm)	42.9	2.6	43.0	2.2	NS	45.9	2.2	47.0	2.6	NS	3.0	1.5	3.9	1.5	NS
Ba–S/FH angle (deg.)	123.8	4.0	124.2	3.3	NS	123.2	4.0	123.7	3.0	NS	−0.6	1.4	−0.4	1.3	NS
Maxilla															
A'–Ptm' (mm)	43.1	2.1	43.6	1.5	NS	46.0	2.3	47.3	2.1	NS	2.9	1.3	3.8	1.3	NS
Cd–A (mm)	77.4	3.3	77.4	2.5	NS	83.2	3.4	84.7	2.6	NS	5.8	1.9	7.2	1.8	*
N–ANS (mm)	49.4	2.3	49.5	2.1	NS	54.5	2.3	55.7	2.4	NS	5.1	0.8	6.2	1.0	*
SNA (deg.)	80.2	1.5	80.1	3.2	NS	81.1	1.5	81.0	2.7	NS	0.9	1.3	0.9	0.9	NS
Mandible															
Gn–Cd (mm)	106.8	3.9	101.0	4.1	***	121.7	4.8	114.1	5.1	***	14.9	2.5	13.1	2.6	NS
Pog'–Go (mm)	70.7	2.4	67.5	3.2	**	79.3	3.0	75.6	3.5	**	8.6	1.8	8.1	1.3	NS
Cd–Go (mm)	49.2	2.3	48.2	3.2	NS	57.7	2.4	56.2	4.3	NS	8.6	2.1	8.0	2.1	NS
SNB (deg.)	81.3	1.7	77.4	2.6	***	83.8	1.8	78.6	2.5	***	2.0	1.8	1.4	1.4	NS
SNPog (deg.)	80.1	2.0	77.0	2.7	***	82.4	2.2	77.8	3.3	***	2.2	1.5	0.8	2.9	NS
Gonial angle (deg.)	128.6	7.0	124.6	5.3	NS	127.9	6.8	122.5	5.8	*	−0.7	2.3	−2.1	3.0	NS
Mand. pl. (deg.)	38.0	5.5	37.0	3.3	NS	37.8	5.9	36.1	4.1	NS	−0.1	2.0	−0.9	2.4	NS
Intermaxillary															
Wits appraisal (mm)	−8.6	2.0	−3.0	1.4	***	−12.4	2.7	−3.0	1.3	***	−3.8	2.4	0.0	1.5	***
ANS–Me (mm)	61.1	3.9	61.2	4.3	NS	69.2	5.5	67.4	5.2	NS	8.1	2.5	6.2	1.6	*
ANB (deg.)	−1.1	1.7	2.7	1.6	***	−2.2	1.9	2.4	1.7	***	−1.1	1.6	−0.2	1.4	NS
SN to Occlusal (deg.)	20.2	3.3	22.2	2.5	NS	20.3	2.6	18.9	3.0	NS	0.2	2.7	−3.3	2.5	*

* = P < 0.05; ** = P < 0.01; *** = P < 0.001; Abbreviation: NS, Not significant

Reprinted with permission from Bandai (Sakamoto) E, Sugawara J, Umemori M, et al. Craniofacial growth of mandibular prognathism in Japanese girls during pubertal growth period – Longitudinal study from 9 to 14 years of age. Orthod Waves 2000;59:77–89.

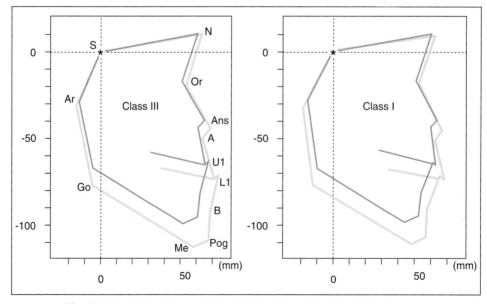

Fig. 11-5 Longitudinal changes in the skeletal profiles of Class III and Class I groups.

been established before the pubertal growth period and maintained thereafter. Meanwhile, the dentoalveolar disharmony is aggravated and becomes more severe during this period as shown by the difference in occlusal plane angle and the Wits appraisal.

Postpubertal Growth Period

Several studies[7-10] have reported on the craniofacial growth pattern of Class III malocclusion during the postpubertal period using longitudinal data. Mitani et al[10] studied the serial lateral cephalometric head films of skeletal Class III and Class I malocclusion in Japanese females over a period of 3 years during the postpubertal period. Cephalograms were taken at the age of 14 and 17 years. The Class III group comprised 20 female subjects selected from a file of patients waiting for surgical orthodontic treatment and 20 female subjects were used as control. The criteria for case selection were the same as in the studies described above, with the exception of maturational stage. Maturational stages and physiologic ages of all subjects were evaluated individually by the ossification events taken from hand–wrist radiographs.[13-17]

Table 11-3 shows mean and standard deviations of linear and angular measurements for female subjects. During the observation period, a comparison of the maxillary measurements showed that neither the size (Ptm–A) nor position (SNA, Ba–Ptm) of the maxilla showed any significant difference between the two groups. The total change in maxillary measurements also showed no significant difference between the two groups.

Comparison of the mandibular measurements showed that the total length (Gn–Cd) of the Class III group were significantly greater than those of the Class I, whereas the ramus height (Cd–Go) and the body length (Go–Pog) exhibited no significant difference between the two groups. There was no significant difference between the two groups in any of the changes in mandibular measurements during the time periods studied.

No significant difference was observed between the two groups in the total changes in ANB angle and Wits appraisal. Differential growth between the maxilla and the mandible was observed in each group, but the changes were minimal. The skeletal frameworks of the two groups were maintained during the postpubertal period.

Table 11-3 Results of measurements for Class III (n = 20) and Class I (n = 20) groups during postpubertal growth period in Japanese females

| | 14 years old | | | | | 17 years old | | | | | Total change | | | | |
| | Class III | | Class I | | | Class III | | Class I | | | Class III | | Class I | | |
	x	SD	x	SD	Sig.	x	SD	x	SD	Sig.	x	SD	x	SD	Sig.
Cranial base															
S–N (mm)	63.7	3.2	65.0	2.8	NS	64.4	3.0	65.3	2.9	NS	0.7	0.5	0.3	0.4	*
S–Ba (mm)	45.6	2.2	45.4	1.9	NS	46.0	2.3	45.9	1.9	NS	0.4	0.5	0.5	0.5	NS
Ba–S/FH angle (deg.)	120.7	4.0	129.9	3.4	**	120.0	3.8	123.8	3.6	**	−0.3	1.5	−0.1	1.0	NS
Maxilla															
Ptm–A (mm)	44.8	3.1	46.7	3.1	NS	45.2	2.9	47.2	3.3	NS	0.4	0.8	0.5	1.2	NS
Ba–A (mm)	86.5	4.3	90.7	5.4	**	86.9	4.2	91.3	5.5	**	0.4	0.8	0.6	1.3	NS
Ba–Ptm (mm)	41.7	3.4	44.0	3.2	*	41.7	3.5	44.1	3.2	*	0.1	0.8	0.1	0.7	NS
N'–ANS (mm)	54.9	3.3	53.8	2.4	NS	55.5	3.6	54.6	2.6	NS	0.6	1.0	0.9	1.2	NS
SNA (deg.)	81.5	4.3	81.9	4.0	NS	81.3	4.3	82.0	4.2	NS	−0.1	0.9	0.1	1.0	NS
Mandible															
Gn–Cd (mm)	120.1	7.8	113.4	4.9	**	123.0	8.6	116.2	5.0	**	2.9	1.9	2.8	1.8	NS
Go–Pog (mm)	76.3	6.0	73.4	3.5	NS	77.9	6.0	74.9	3.7	NS	1.6	0.9	1.5	1.4	NS
Cd–Go (mm)	56.0	3.6	55.3	5.3	NS	57.9	4.0	57.4	5.1	NS	1.9	1.8	2.1	1.0	NS
SNPog (deg.)	83.6	5.4	77.9	4.3	**	84.5	5.9	78.7	4.1	**	0.9	1.4	0.8	0.8	NS
Gonial angle (deg.)	132.3	6.2	125.0	6.5	**	132.2	5.8	124.7	6.4	**	0	1.6	−0.3	0.8	NS
Mand. pl. (deg.)	31.2	5.7	30.0	4.9	NS	30.7	6.1	29.8	4.8	NS	−0.5	1.8	−0.3	1.5	NS
Intermaxillary															
Wits appraisal (mm)	−11.4	4.3	−0.6	2.6	**	−12.7	4.9	−1.3	2.1	**	−1.6	1.9	−1.3	1.7	NS
ANS–Me (mm)	75.0	5.8	70.4	4.6	*	77.3	6.2	72.2	4.3	**	2.3	1.5	1.8	1.5	NS
ANB (deg.)	−2.9	2.7	3.0	1.8	**	−3.8	3.3	2.5	2.1	**	−1.3	2.0	−0.7	1.3	NS

* = P < 0.05; ** = P < 0.01; Abbreviation: NS, Not significant

Reprinted with permission from Mitani H, Sato K, Sugawara J. Growth of mandibular prognathism after pubertal growth peak. Am J Orthod Dentofac Orthop 1993;104:330–336.

In conclusion, the Class III group showed an incremental growth change similar to the Class I group. The morphologic characteristics of the skeletal Class III malocclusion are maintained during the postpubertal period.

Clinical Implications

The results of our longitudinal studies[6-12] on Class III facial growth suggest that Class III malocclusion is established early and before the prepubertal growth period. The authors[11,12] speculated the reason why Class I subjects with growth changes similar to those of Class III subjects could maintain a normal occlusion. This phenomenon may be attributed to the rotational change of the occlusal plane (Fig. 11-6). Namely, in the Class I group, the occlusal plane is displaced in a downward–forward direction with counterclockwise rotation. Therefore, the anteroposterior relationship between the bimaxillary apical bases evaluated on the occlusal plane (Wits appraisal) is harmoniously maintained in spite of differential jaw growth. However, in Class III subjects the amount of maxillomandibular differential growth is not compensated for by the counter-clockwise rotational change of the occlusal plane. The dentoalveolar disharmony evaluated by Wits appraisal is significantly aggravated due to lack of homeostasis of the neuromuscular system which functions to maintain a stable intercuspal position in normal occlusion. These results may point to the benefit of early orthodontic intervention that may minimize the amount of apical base discrepancy that seems to be aggravated with growth.

Orthopedic Effects of Chin Cap Therapy

The orthopedic effects of chin cap appliances, which were thought to improve facial growth in Class III patients with mandibular excess, became the object of orthodontists' attention in the 1960s. Since then, chin cap therapy has been widely recognized as a method for treating developing Class III malocclusion in young patients. A number of clinical and experimental studies[2,17-26] have reported that chin cap force has several short-term orthopedic effects: (1) redirection of mandibular growth; (2) backward repositioning of the mandible; (3) retardation of mandibular growth; and (4) remodeling of the mandible and the TMJ.

Sugawara et al[27] reported longterm growth changes in patients treated with chin cap therapy at different ages and with various treatment schedules. The possibility that these effects may induce permanent skeletal changes and alter the prognathic skeletal profile, particularly when applied at an early age,[20,28] has kept attention on chin cap therapy. However, little is known about whether the improved skeletal profile can be maintained until craniofacial growth is complete. Most studies have been based either

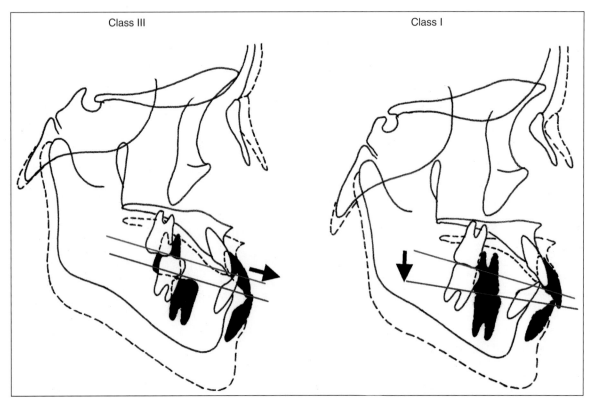

Fig. 11-6 Differences in facial growth changes between Class III and Class I groups.

on relatively short-term results, which are of too short a duration to determine the final result, or longterm results that encompass too few subjects to be statistically valid. The short- and long-term results of chin cap therapy on the developing Class III malocclusion are reviewed below.

In this study it was hypothesized that (1) early application of chin cap force is more effective for correction of skeletal discrepancies; and (2) the short-term effects of chin cap therapy are maintained after complete growth. This study involved 63 Japanese girls who showed anterior crossbite and Class III skeletal pattern before treatment and who were divided into three groups according to their age at the start of chin cap therapy: age 7 (before the pubertal growth spurt); age 9 (at the beginning of the growth spurt), and age 11 (around the peak of the growth spurt). The data were derived from lateral cephalometric head films taken serially at the ages of 7, 9, 11, 14, and 17 years for analysis of intercuspal position. All patients underwent chin cap therapy at the beginning of the treatment, but the length of time the chin cap was worn varied. Half the patients in the total sample were also treated with a multibracket system at a later stage. Basically the same type of chin cap was worn by all patients. The force applied on the chin was oriented along a line from the gnathion to the sella turcica and ranged from 250 to 300 g per side of the chin. Patients were instructed to wear the chin cap for at least 14 hours daily. All subjects attained a normal anterior bite with the initial chin cap treatment, but two cases showed anterior crossbite. Seven had edge-to-edge bites at the final observation.

The average skeletal profile diagram for each group was constructed from X–Y coordinates of 14 representative cephalometric landmarks using the same method as in the study by Bandai et al.[12] The results are summarized by the superimposition of the skeletal profile diagrams. Figures 11-7–11-9 show the longitudinal changes of the skeletal profiles in the groups that began chin cap therapy at ages 7, 9 and 11 years, respectively. Figures 11-10 and 11-11 represent the short- and long-term effects of chin cap therapy on the skeletal profiles, respectively.

Short-Term Effects

The skeletal profiles of patients were significantly improved and there was retrusion of the mandible during the initial stage of chin cap therapy for every group (Figs 11-7–11-9). In response to the orthopedic force, the skeletal profiles of patients who began treatment at age 7 changed more than those who began treatment at a later age. In addition, patients who began treatment at age 7 showed a more posterior positioning of the mandible than those who entered treatment at age 11. These results indicate that chin cap treatment is more effective before the pubertal growth spurt. In other words, it appears that the effects of chin cap force may be offset by rapid mandibular growth during puberty, if all patients receive treatment under the same conditions. This data supports

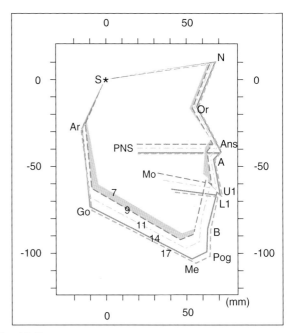

Fig. 11-7 Longitudinal changes in the skeletal profiles of the group that began chin cap treatment at age 7 and was observed at ages 9, 11, 14, and 17. (Reproduced with permission from Sugawara J, Asano T, Endo N, et al. Long-term effects of chincap therapy on skeletal profile in mandibular prognathism. Am J Orthod Dentofacial Orthop 1990;98:127–133.)

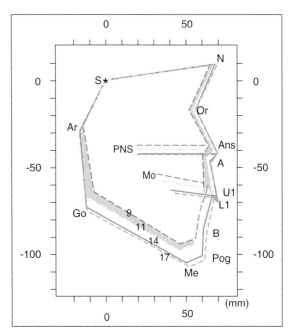

Fig. 11-8 Longitudinal changes in the skeletal profiles of the group that began chin cap treatment at age 9 and was observed at ages 11, 14, and 17. (Reproduced with permission from Sugawara J, Asano T, Endo N, et al. Long-term effects of chincap therapy on skeletal profile in mandibular prognathism. Am J Orthod Dentofacial Orthop 1990;98:127–133.)

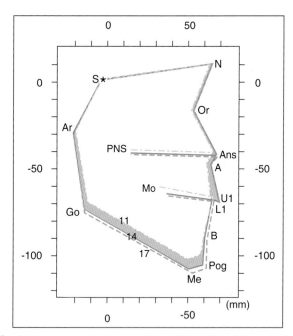

Fig. 11-9 Longitudinal changes in the skeletal profiles of the group that began chin cap treatment at age 11 and was observed at ages 14 and 17. (Reproduced with permission from Sugawara J, Asano T, Endo N, et al. Long-term effects of chincap therapy on skeletal profile in mandibular prognathism. Am J Orthod Dentofacial Orthop 1990;98:127–133.)

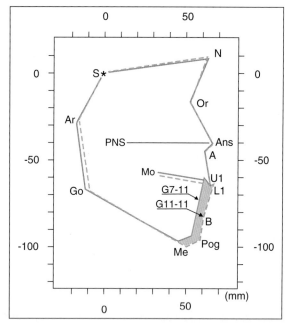

Fig. 11-10 Comparison of skeletal profiles at age 11 between a group of patients who began chin cap treatment at age 7 and a control group of patients who had no prior treatment. (Reproduced with permission from Sugawara J, Asano T, Endo N, et al. Long-term effects of chincap therapy on skeletal profile in mandibular prognathism. Am J Orthod Dentofacial Orthop 1990;98:127–133.)

the hypothesis that "the early application of chin cap force is more effective for correction of skeletal discrepancies."

Longterm Effects

Figure 11-10 shows the differences in skeletal profiles at age 11 for patients who had begun treatment at age 7 and those who were just entering treatment at age 11. The latter group had received no treatment up to this age. When comparing these two groups, significant differences were observed in the anteroposterior position of the mandible, but no significant difference in the maxillary region was apparent. The mandible of the first group had apparently been displaced in a backward direction during the 3 years of treatment. Moreover, a significant reduction in the gonial angle was observed during this period. Figure 11-10 shows that chin cap treatment had significant orthopedic effects (short term) on the mandible in patients who began treatment at age 7.

Figure 11-11 shows the differences in skeletal profiles at age 17 between patients who began treatment at age 7 and at age 11, compared with the control group of 19 year olds. For the group that began treatment at age 11, the position of the mandible was relatively more forward than the group who began treatment at age 7. Statistically, there was no significant difference between these two groups with respect to any of the landmarks. Although a great difference was observed in the position of the mandible

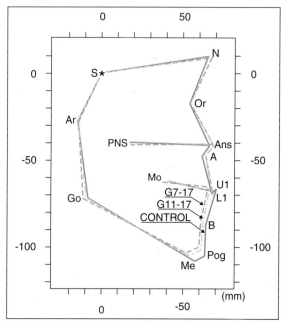

Fig. 11-11 Comparison of skeletal profiles at age 17 between a group of patients who began chin cap treatment at age 7, a group of patients who began chin cap treatment at age 11, and a control group of patients who had no prior treatment. (Reproduced with permission from Sugawara J, Asano T, Endo N, et al. Long-term effects of chincap therapy on skeletal profile in mandibular prognathism. Am J Orthod Dentofacial Orthop 1990;98:127–133.)

at age 11, these differences decreased gradually up to age 17 years. The control Class III group who received no treatment showed the mandible in a relatively more forward position than the other two groups, but anteroposteriorly there was no significant difference in any specific landmark. The changes in skeletal profile, although they represent significant improvement in the younger children, are not maintained in most cases. This finding suggests that skeletal profiles have a tendency to return to their original shapes, which may have been predetermined morphogenetically.[29,30] It has been speculated that some skeletal rebound may occur during or after the pubertal growth period. The significant rebound observed in this study indicates that the hypothesis that "the short-term effects of chin cap therapy are maintained after complete growth" should be rejected.

Two cases manifest the effects and the limitations of chin cap orthopedic force. Figure 11-12 shows the changes with treatment of a patient from the group that began chin cap therapy at age 7. She received chin cap treatment for 3 years and at age 10, her prognathic profiles were drastically altered into a rather retrognathic profile by the short-term effects of the chin cap orthopedic force. At age 17, after the second phase of treatment with a multibracket system, her profile changed from retrognathic to a straight type, mainly due to skeletal rebound during the pubertal and postpubertal growth period. Despite orthopedic relapse, recurrence of anterior crossbite was avoided by dentoalveolar compensation in the second phase of orthodontic treatment.

The patient shown in Figure 11-13 also belonged to the group that began chin cap therapy at age 7. By age 10, her skeletal profile had changed into a straight type. However, at age 19, recurrence of anterior crossbite was observed, probably due to skeletal rebound and postpubertal differential growth.

Clinical Implications

Short- and long-term studies on the effects of chin cap force indicate that the skeletal profile is greatly improved during the initial stages of chin cap therapy, but such changes are often not maintained thereafter. In other words, chin cap force seldom alters the inherited prognathic characteristics of Class III profiles after growth.

Based on these findings, the following recommendations can be made on the use of chin cap therapy. First, the chin cap appliance should be considered only as an option to correct anterior crossbite in the first phase of treatment for Class III patients who are still growing. Second, indications for chin cap therapy should be limited to mild-to-moderate skeletal Class III malocclusions that can be camouflaged by dentoalveolar compensation in the second phase of orthodontic treatment, even if anterior crossbite recurs after the first phase of treatment. Third,

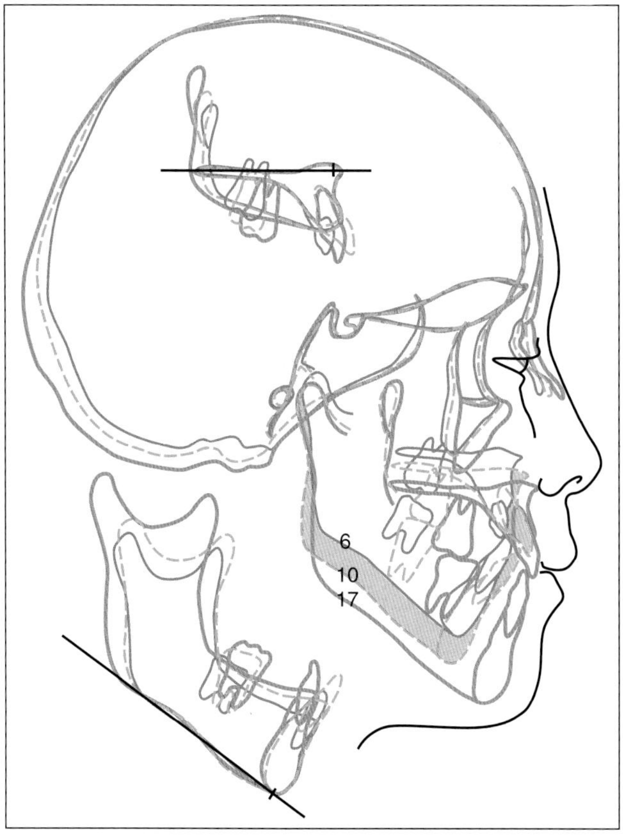

Fig. 11-12 Cephalometric superimpositions for patient MS from the group that began chin cap therapy at age 7; observed at age 10 and 17.

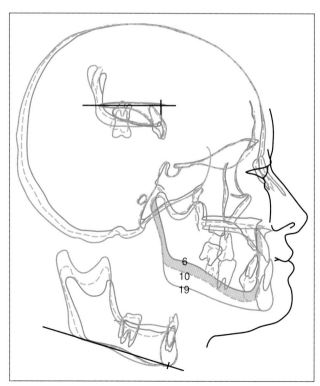

Fig. 11-13 Cephalometric superimpositions for patient TS from the group that began chin cap therapy at age 7; observed at age 10 and 19.

chin cap therapy is contraindicated in Class III patients with apparent mandibular excess. For such cases, surgical orthodontic treatment is recommended to construct stable and functional occlusion after growth.

Class III Correction in Accordance with Clinical Practice Guidelines

The clinical practice guidelines help practitioners to decide the best treatment options in consultation with their patients. The guidelines for growing Class III patients were derived from studying numerous reported clinical studies. However, there is a significant gap between the guidelines and evidence-based medicine (EBM), because almost all the clinical studies did not undergo critical examination by EBM specialists. The deficit of evidence in the guidelines is supplemented with empirical knowledge that had been accumulated over a long time in clinical orthodontic practice.

The only way to verify the effectiveness of the proposed clinical guidelines is to statistically evaluate the outcome in longterm follow-up cases, because orthodontic treatment mostly targets symptoms rather than cause.

We have been managing Class III patients in accordance with the clinical practice guidelines and practicing post-treatment evaluation for >10 years. No fundamental problems with the guidelines have been identified.

The treatment progress and results of three cases who have undergone orthodontic management in accordance with the guidelines are reported below.

CASE REPORT 1

This patient was a 7-year-old girl. Although she did not complain about her profile and occlusion, her mother seriously worried about her anterior crossbite and prognathic profile. Figure 11-14 shows her facial and oral photographs at the initial examination.

Problem List

Her principal problems identified from various analyses were:

- Forward position of the mandible
- Mild Class III jaw relationship
- Short face tendency
- Occlusal interference at incisors
- Gingival recession at lower left central incisor
- Anterior crossbite
- Deep bite
- Class III denture
- Excessive interaction between the upper and lower lips at the intercuspal position.

She was diagnosed as having a good prognosis because her mild anteroposterior jaw disharmony would allow downward–backward rotation of the mandible to correct the anterior crossbite and deep bite. Her treatment plan was established by following the right-hand pathway in the clinical practice guidelines (see Fig. 11-3).

First phase of treatment

Figure 11-15 shows the progress of her first phase of orthodontic treatment. A jumping plate was applied to the lower dentition and a partial bracket system to the upper dentition. The roles of the jumping plate were: (1) to stabilize her mandibular position; (2) to raise her bite to allow the placement of brackets at the upper incisors; (3) to promote the eruption of the first molars by cutting the jumping plate off at the distal end of the lower second deciduous molars; (4) to inhibit lingual tipping of the lower incisors during jumping of the anterior bite; and (5) to smoothly correct the anterior crossbite without occlusal interference at the incisors. A partial bracket system in the upper dentition was applied to expand and intrude the upper incisors.

Figure 11-16 shows the girl at age 8 years, immediately after the first phase of treatment. The cephalometric superimpositions during the first phase of treatment show that her anterior crossbite was corrected by labial movement of the upper incisors and a clockwise rotation of the mandible (Fig. 11-17). In addition, the short face tendency and excessive interaction of the lips were simultaneously improved.

Growth Observation Period

After the first phase of treatment, growth observation and control of oral hygiene were performed every 6 months until the postpubertal period.

Figure 11-19 shows the patient at the age of 16 immediately before the second phase of treatment. Figure 11-18 shows the cephalometric superimposition during the growth observation period from 8 to 16 years old.

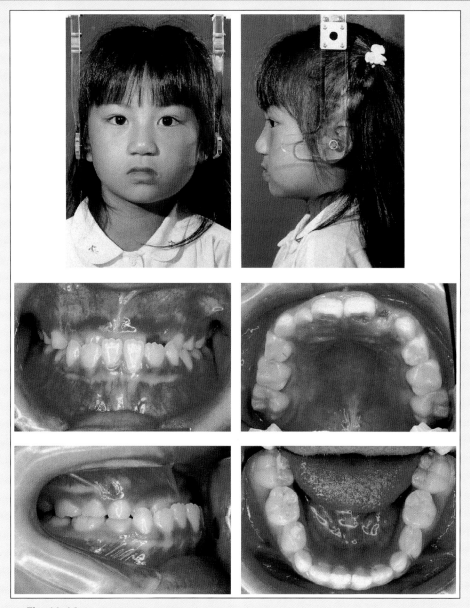

Fig. 11-14 Case 1. Facial and intraoral photographs at initial examination (age 7 years, 3 months).

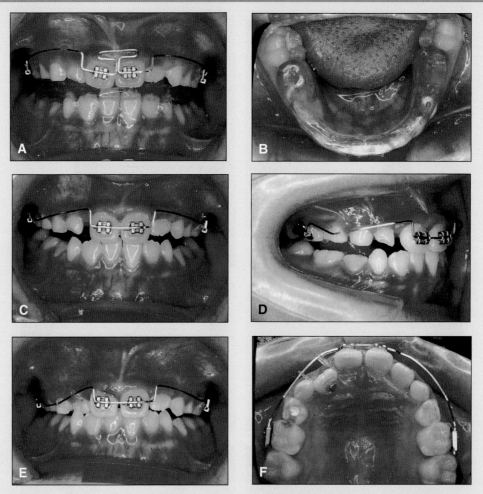

Fig. 11-15 Case 1. Biomechanics for the first phase of treatment. **A** and **B** Partial brackets and jumping plate. **C** and **D** Jumped with upper utility arch and vertical stop at first molars. **E** and **F** Utility arch and labial movement of the upper right lateral incisor.

The current clinical practice guidelines do not recommend applying a chin cap to inhibit mandibular growth and alter skeletal profile. Although a chin cap orthopedic force was not applied in this case, her mandible mostly showed downward growth and eventually her anteroposterior jaw relationship was not aggravated (Fig. 11-18).

Second Phase of Treatment

Figure 11-20 shows her progress during the second phase of treatment, which lasted just a year. A multibracket system was first applied only to the upper dentition to intrude the upper incisors and to enable the placement of brackets at the lower incisors. The upper incisors were significantly intruded with the application of a basal arch

(Fig. 11-20A and B). Then brackets were bonded to the lower dentition and leveling was performed (Fig. 11-20C and D). After detailing and finishing, all the brackets were debonded and a wraparound type of retainer and lingual bonded retainer were applied to the upper and lower dentition, respectively (Fig. 11-20E and F).

Figure 11-22 shows the patient 1 year after debonding. She has maintained a balanced profile, function, occlusion, and a caries-free status.

The cephalometric superimpositions indicate dentofacial changes during the second phase of treatment (Fig. 11-21). Regarding skeletal changes, her mandible showed slight downward growth, but the maxilla did not change at all. It is obvious that her orthodontic problems were improved by

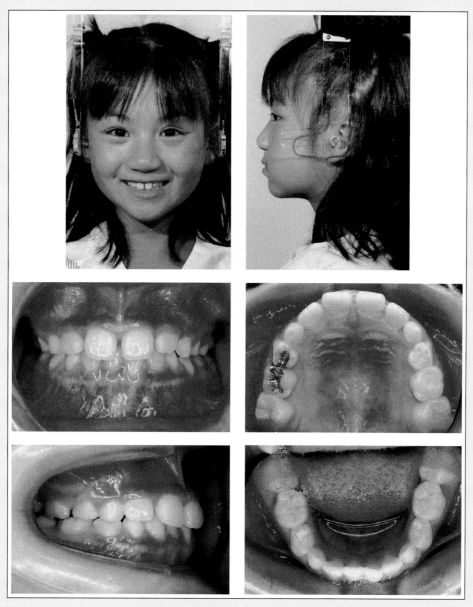

Fig. 11-16 Case 1. Facial and intraoral photographs after the first phase of treatment (age 8 years, 3 months).

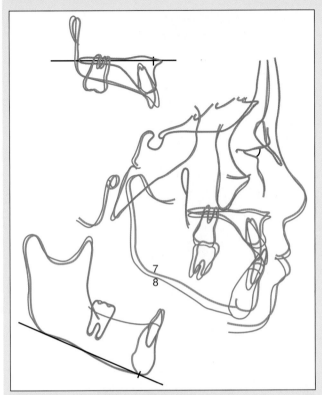

Fig. 11-17 Case 1. Cephalometric superimpositions show the dentofacial changes during the first phase of treatment. Thick solid line: age 7 years, 3 months (initial); thin solid line: age 8 years, 3 months (immediately after the first phase of treatment).

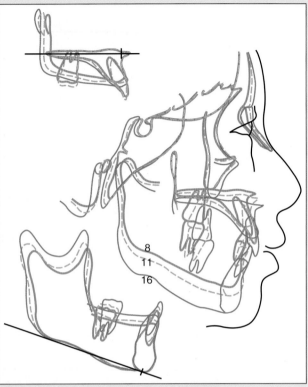

Fig. 11-18 Case 1. Cephalometric superimpositions show the dentofacial changes during the growth observation period. Thick solid line: age 8 years, 3 months (immediately after the first phase of treatment); dotted line: age 11 years, 3 months (during growth observation); thin solid line: age 16 years, 3 months (immediately prior to the second phase of treatment).

intrusion of the upper incisors and labial inclination of the bimaxillary incisors.

Summary

This patient exhibited anterior crossbite with short face, and overclosured bite. However, as her antero-posterior jaw disharmony was quite mild, she could be diagnosed as skeletal Class I. In cases with good prognosis, such as this one, therapeutic intervention should be as minimal as possible. In this case the total treatment period (first and second phases) was only 1 year 5 months. "The minimum intervention and the maximum profit for each patient" is one of the important mottos in the clinical practice guidelines. In keeping with this, the length of time orthodontic appliances, which can injury teeth and periodontal tissue, are worn should be shortened.

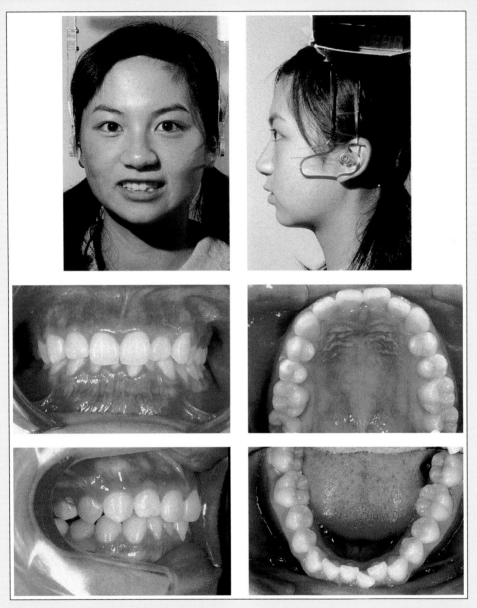

Fig. 11-19 Case 1. Facial and intraoral photographs before the second phase of treatment (age 16 years, 3 months).

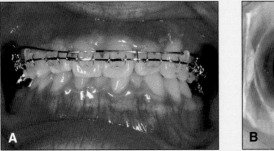
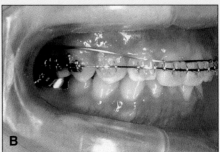

Fig. 11-20 Case 1. Biomechanics for the second phase of treatment. **A** and **B** Upper multibracket system and a basal arch for incisor intrusion.

Continued

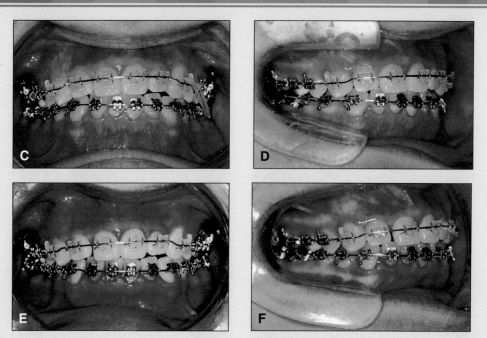

Fig. 11-20 *cont'd.* **C** and **D** Lower multibracket system. **E** and **F** Overcorrection for deep bite.

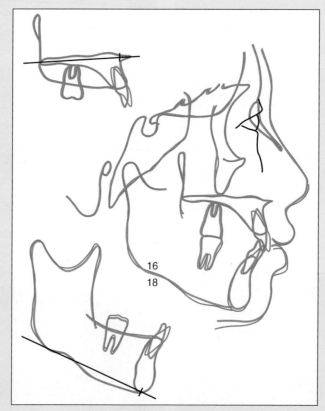

Fig. 11-21 Case 1. Cephalometric superimpositions show the dentofacial changes during the second phase of treatment. Thick solid line: age 16 years, 3 months (immediately prior to the second phase of treatment); thin solid line: 18 years, 4 months (at debonding).

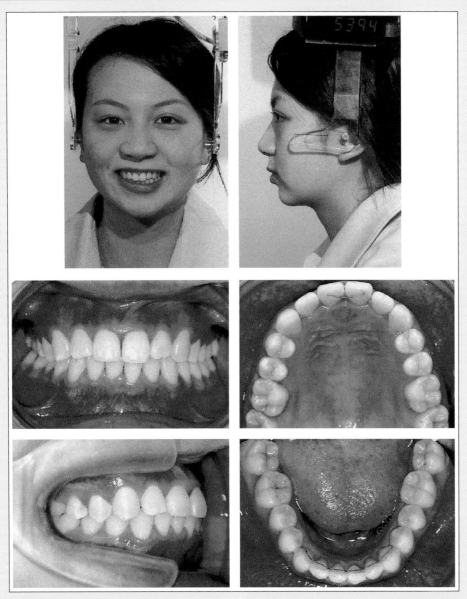

Fig. 11-22 Case 1. Facial and intraoral photographs 2 years after completion of the second phase of treatment (age 19 years, 4 months).

CASE REPORT 2

This patient was a 7-year-old girl who complained about anterior crossbite and winging of the upper central incisors (Fig. 11-23). Regarding family history, her mother underwent orthognathic surgery for correction of severe mandibular prognathism approximately 30 years ago.

Problem List

Her orthodontic problems at the initial examination were:

- Large mandible and forward position of the mandible
- Moderate Class III jaw relationship (Wits appraisal: –8.5 mm)
- Long face tendency
- Occlusal interference at the incisors
- Anterior crossbite
- Class III denture
- Diastema and winging of upper central incisors.

Considering her skeletal disharmony and genetic background, she could have been managed surgically, skipping the first phase of treatment. However, it was decided, tentatively, to apply first-phase

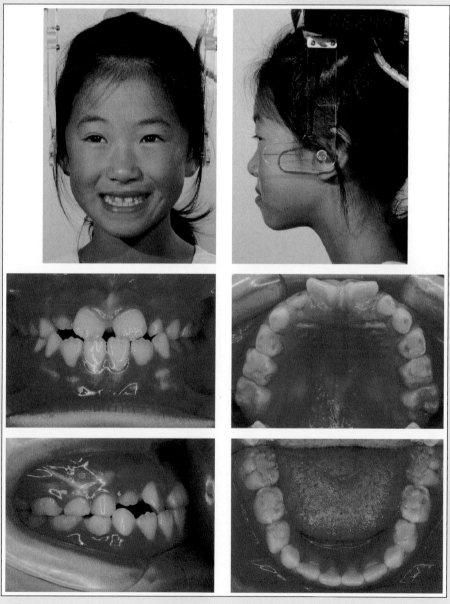

Fig. 11-23 Case 2. Facial and intraoral photographs at initial examination (age 7 years, 10 months).

CASE REPORT 2—cont'd

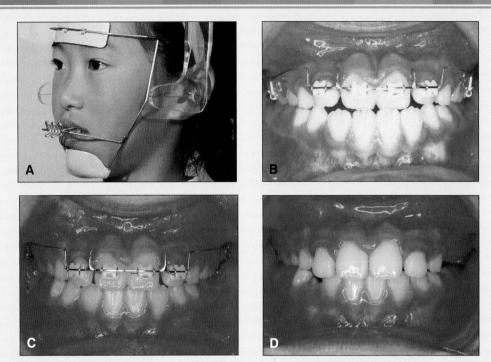

Fig. 11-24 Case 2. Biomechanics for the first phase of treatment. **A** Face mask (maxillary incisors protraction [MIP]). **B** Oral appliance (upper utility arch). **C** Correction of anterior crossbite. **D** Immediately after the first phase of treatment (age 9 years, 4 months).

mechanics, because she was not a clear case for surgery at that time.

First Phase of Treatment

After eruption of the upper lateral incisors, the first phase of treatment began at the age of 8 and the progress is shown in Figure 11-24. Because the long-term effects of chin cap orthopedic force for alteration of skeletal profile were already being questioned at that time, protraction of the upper incisors using a face mask (referred to as maxillary incisors protraction [MIP])[31] was applied (Fig. 11-24A). A 2 × 4 partial bracket system was used as an oral appliance (Fig. 11-24B and C). Her anterior crossbite was corrected within 1 month with the application of those first-phase mechanics (Fig. 11-24C). After stabilizing the occlusion, all appliances were removed (Fig. 11-24D). The first phase of treatment lasted just 5 months.

The cephalometric superimpositions show the dentofacial changes during the first phase of treatment (Fig. 11-25). Her anterior crossbite was corrected by labial movement of the upper incisors and lingual inclination of the lower incisors; following these dental changes the mandible showed downward growth and displacement.

Growth Observation Period

Between the age of 9 and 16 years, growth observation and oral hygiene management were performed every 6 months and no orthodontic appliances needed to be worn. Figure 11-27 shows the patient's facial and oral photographs immediately before the start of the second phase of treatment at 16 years old, and Figure 11-26 shows the cephalometric superimpositions during the growth observation period. As a chin cap orthopedic force for controlling mandibular growth was not applied, her mandible appeared to grow excessively in a downward and forward direction. However, the amount of mandibular growth measured at Cd–Gn was 13.0 mm during the growth observation period, which is the same average mandibular growth change as in the Class I girls (13.1 mm) and less than in the Class III girls (14.9 mm) described in Table 11-2.

The patient's problem list immediately before the second phase of treatment was:

- Mandibular asymmetry
- Large mandible and forward displacement
- Skeletal Class III jaw relation (Wits appraisal: −9.0 mm)
- Deviation of lower dental midline

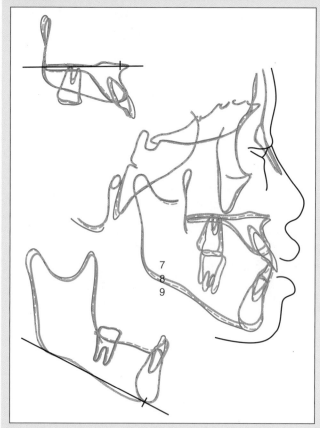

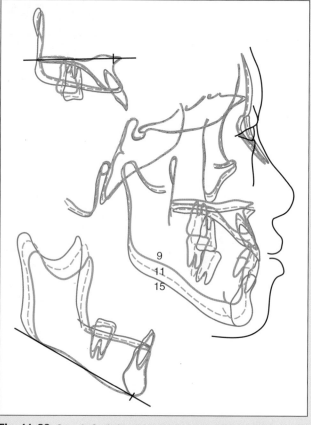

Fig. 11-25 Case 2. Cephalometric superimpositions show the dentofacial changes during the first phase of treatment. Thick solid line: age 7 years, 10 months (initial); dotted line: age 8 years, 10 months (during the first phase of treatment); thin solid line: age 9 years, 4 months (immediately after the first phase of treatment).

Fig. 11-26 Case 2. Cephalometric superimpositions show the dentofacial changes during the growth observation period. Thick solid line: age 9 years, 4 months (immediately after the first phase of treatment); dotted line: age 11 years, 10 months (during the growth observation period); thin solid line: age 15 years, 10 months (immediately prior to the second phase of treatment).

- Anterior crossbite
- Open bite tendency
- Class III denture.

In comparison to the problem list at initial examination, mandibular asymmetry became obvious. However, her skeletal disharmony was still not severe enough to indicate orthognathic surgery, and camouflage treatment using the skeletal anchorage system (SAS) (see Ch. 15)[31,32] was chosen for the second phase of orthodontic mechanics without extraction of the bicuspids (Fig. 11.28).

Second Phase of Treatment

Figure 11-29 shows the treatment progress during the second phase. Subsequent to extraction of the bilateral mandibular third molars, leveling and aligning of the upper and lower dentition began (Fig. 11-29A). Four months later, orthodontic anchor plates were bilaterally implanted beneath the apices of the molars at the mandibular body. Then the lower molars were distalized utilizing SAS[32-34] in which the anchor plates are implanted as absolute anchorages (Fig. 11-29B). Deviation of the mandibular dental midline was improved within 1 month, and the major problems with occlusion were mostly corrected within 2 months (Fig. 11-29C and D).

Figure 11-30 shows the facial and oral photographs 1 year after debonding. Her skeletal problems were successfully camouflaged with the application of SAS mechanics. As shown in the cephalometric superimpositions (Fig. 11-31), the entire mandibular dentition was distalized asymmetrically. Therefore, the post-treatment evaluation of this case suggested

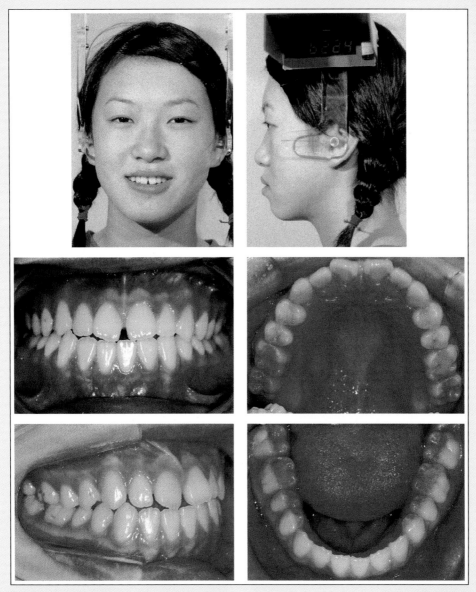

Fig. 11-27 Case 2. Facial and intraoral photographs before the second phase of treatment (age 15 years, 11 months).

that SAS is very effective as second-phase mechanics and will be widely used for Class III correction and revision.

Summary

Throughout the treatment it was difficult to determine this orthognathic surgery was indicated. It appears that the first phase of treatment made almost no significant difference to the final result. However, it is easy to be wise after the event; therefore, in borderline cases such as this, the decision as to which management pathway to follow should be left to the patient's choice and doctor's discretion. It is very important to recognize that the second phase of orthodontic treatment after the postpubertal growth period places a great deal of weight on such a borderline Class III case. The first phase of treatment must be completed quickly, and not allowed to continue aimlessly, so that the effective and reliable camouflage biomechanics of SAS can be applied.

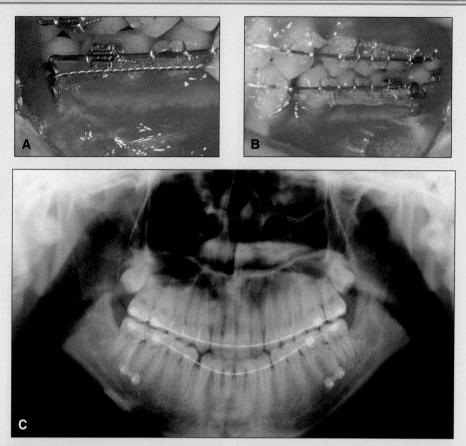

Fig. 11-28 Case 2. Skeletal anchorage system (SAS). **A-C** Anterior crossbite and asymmetric mandibular dentition were corrected by asymmetric distalization of the lower molars with titanium anchor plates.

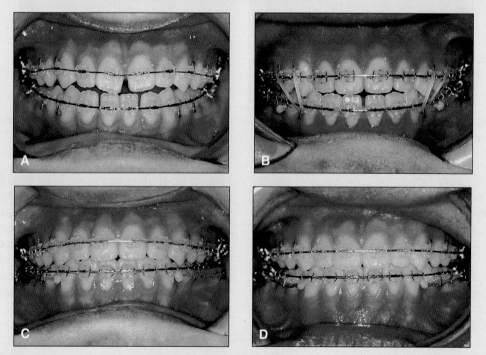

Fig. 11-29 Case 2. Treatment progress of the second phase of treatment. **A** Leveling and aligning of the upper and lower arches. **B** Distalization of the lower molars. **C** Anterior crossbite and asymmetric dentition were corrected. **D** Immediately prior to debonding.

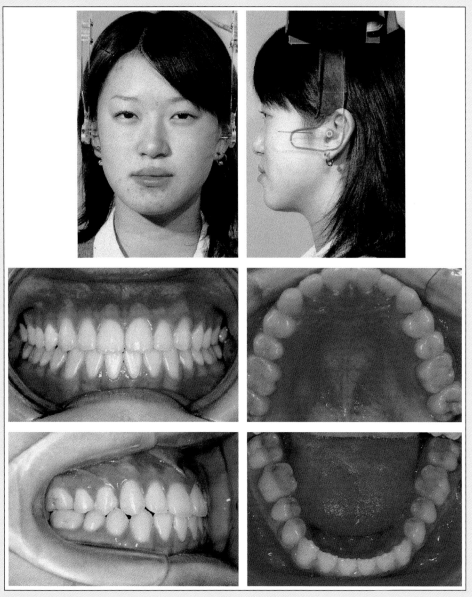

Fig. 11-30 Case 2. Facial and intraoral photographs 1 year after completion of the second phase of treatment (age 18 years, 1 month).

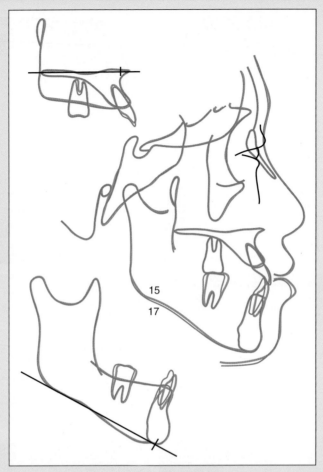

Fig. 11-31 Case 2. Cephalometric superimpositions show dentofacial changes during the second phase of treatment. Thick solid line: age 15 years, 10 months (immediately prior to the second phase of treatment); thin solid line: age 17 years, 1 month (at debonding).

CASE REPORT 3

The final patient was a 6-year-old girl who complained of anterior crossbite at the initial consultation (Fig. 11.32). Regarding her family history, her father had anterior crossbite.

Problem List

Her problem list at the initial examination was:

- Extremely large mandible and forward position of the mandible
- Severe Class III jaw relationship (Wits appraisal: –13.5 mm)

- Hypodontia
- Total crossbite
- Deviation of maxillary dental midline
- Class III denture
- High risk of dental caries.

Considering her severe skeletal disharmony, genetic background, hypodontia, and high risk of caries, following the left-hand pathway of the clinical practice guidelines (see Fig. 11-3) was proposed to her parents, because it was thought to be very difficult to control her mandibular

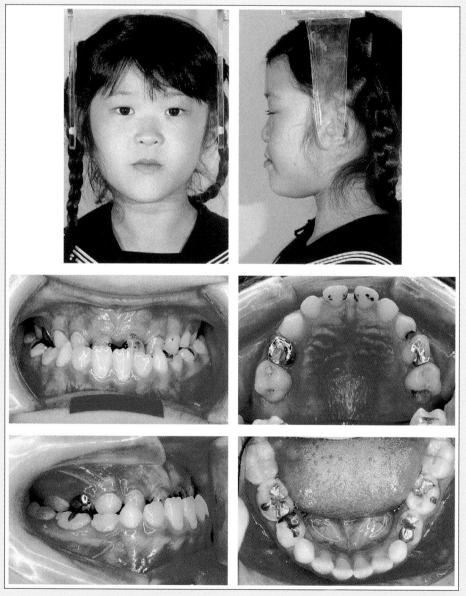

Fig. 11-32 Case 3. Facial and intraoral photographs at initial examination (age 6 years, 5 months).

excess even by means of chin cap orthopedic force. After a growth observation period without having received any first-phase treatment, surgical orthodontic treatment was to be undertaken depending on the final differential diagnosis. It was, however, important to inform her parents of the possibility of a nonsurgical approach. Her parents understood the meaning of the clinical guidelines and accepted the comprehensive treatment plan.

Growth Observation Period

Figure 11-33 shows the facial and oral photographs at the age of 15 and immediately before presurgical orthodontic treatment. It was cephalometrically confirmed that her facial growth almost ceased after 15 years of age. The observation period lasted 9 years. During this period, the maxilla showed a downward growth tendency, but the mandible showed downward–forward growth. Consequently, anteroposterior jaw disharmony seemed to become more severe (Fig. 11-34). Her problem list at that time was:

- Mild facial asymmetry
- Severe Class III jaw relationship (Wits appraisal: –14.5 mm)
- Deviation of the mandibular dental midline (2 mm to the right)

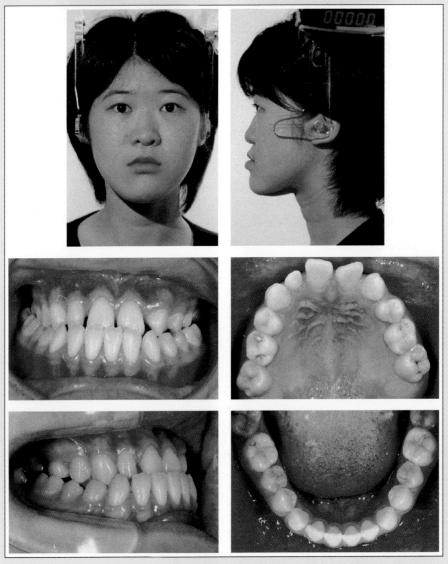

Fig. 11-33 Case 3. Facial and intraoral photographs before presurgical orthodontic treatment (age 15 years, 4 months).

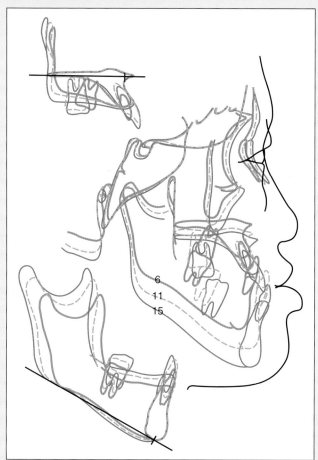

Fig. 11-34 Case 3. Cephalometric superimpositions show the dentofacial changes during the growth observation period. Thick solid line: 6 years, 5 months (initial examination); dotted line: age 11 years, 7 months (during the growth observation period); thin solid line: age 15 years, 4 months (immediately prior to the presurgical orthodontics).

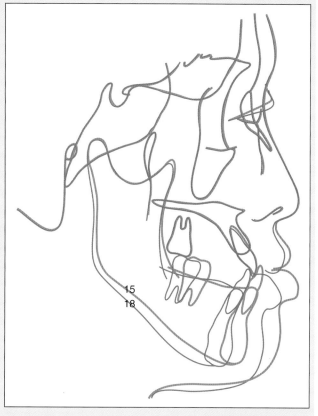

Fig. 11-35 Case 3. Cephalometric superimpositions show dentofacial changes during the surgical orthodontic treatment. Thick solid line: age 15 years, 4 months (immediately prior to presurgical orthodontics); thin solid line: age 18 years, 5 months (at debonding).

- Total crossbite
- Dental compensation of the upper and lower incisors
- Class III denture
- Hypodontia (UL2, UL5, UL7).

Given this problem list, especially considering her severe skeletal disharmony, she was finally diagnosed as having an indication for surgical orthodontics.

Surgical Orthodontics

Figure 11-36 shows the treatment progress with surgical orthodontics. First, leveling and aligning began using a multibracket system (Fig. 11-36A). Then space regaining for the upper left lateral incisor that was congenitally missing, decompensation of the lower incisors, and coordination of upper and lower arches were performed as presurgical orthodontic treatment (Fig. 11-36B). Figure 11-36C shows the occlusion immediately after orthognathic surgery. Sagittal splitting ramus osteotomy (SSRO) was bilaterally applied and proximal and distal segments were semi-rigidly fixed with titanium bone plates and screws. Following orthognathic surgery, rehabilitation and post-surgical orthodontics were carried out (Fig. 11-36D). Brackets were debonded 5 months after surgery. A wraparound retainer in the upper dentition and lingual bonded retainer in the lower dentition were placed for retention. The total length of the active treatment was 1 year and 9 months.

Figure 11-37 shows her facial and oral photographs at the age of 19, 1 year after debonding. Figure 11-35 shows the dentofacial changes with

CASE REPORT 3-cc

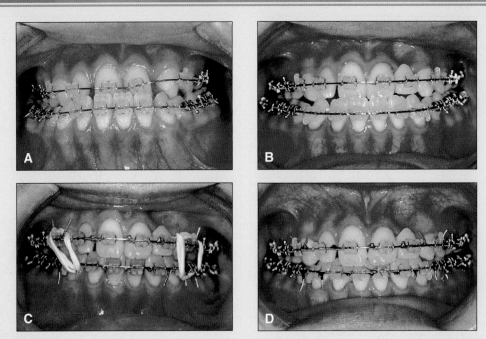

Fig. 11-36 Case 3. Treatment progress of surgical orthodontic treatment. **A** Leveling and aligning of the upper and lower arches. **B** Immediately prior to jaw surgery. **C** Immediately following sagittal splitting ramus osteotomy (SSRO). **D** Immediately prior to debonding.

cephalometric superimpositions before presurgical orthodontics (15 years, 4 months) and debonding (18 years, 5 months). It can be seen that her orthodontic problems were mostly improved with the application of surgical orthodontics. In addition, her awareness of oral health was significantly promoted during a longterm management period, and good oral health conditions have been maintained.

Summary

Generally, the prognathic profile and anterior crossbite in patients with very severe skeletal disharmony are not corrected until the postpubertal period. Some orthodontists criticize the clinical practice guidelines on the basis that it does not allow all orthodontic problems to be addressed during the growth period and psychosocial disorders may occur as a result. However, from our clinical survey,[35] on interview after surgical orthodontic treatment, most patients said they had not worried about their profiles and occlusions during the observation period, because they believed that surgical orthodontics would solve their orthodontic problems in the future. As mentioned above, the longterm effects of orthopedic force are quite limited and surgical orthodontics must be the first treatment option for patients with very severe Class III malocclusion.

Orthodontists should be cautioned against continued unpredictable therapy with a multibracket system because of the risk of dental cavities and iatrogenic side effects. The left-hand pathway of Figure 11-3 for severe Class III patients seems to be a relatively passive strategy, but it is the most realistic considering the cost, and the need to eliminate iatrogenic factors and maintain the masticatory system lifelong. Of course, this pathway should not be forced on patients by practitioners, but chosen by informed patients.

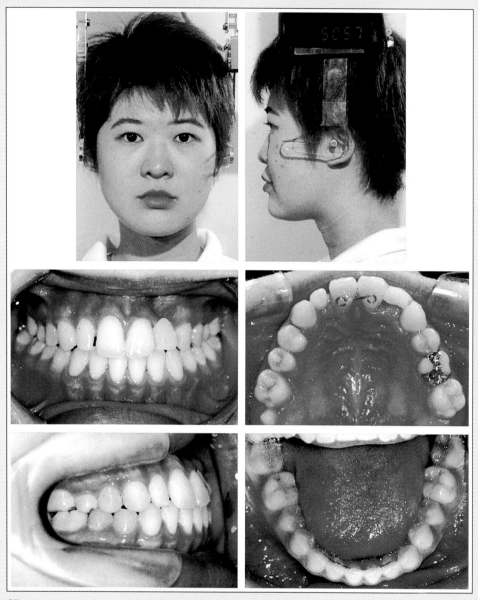

Fig. 11-37 Case 3. Facial and intraoral photographs 1 year after debonding (age 19 years, 1 month).

REFERENCES

1. Sugawara J, Asano T. The clinical practice guideline for treatment of developing Class III malocclusion, In: Sugawara J and Asano T, ed. Seeking a consensus for Class III treatment. Osaka: Tokyo Rinsho Shuppan, 2002:21–30.

2. Susami R. A cephalometric study of dentofacial growth in mandibular prognathism. Jpn J Orthod Soc 1967;26:1–34.

3. Sawa S. Roentgeno-cephalometric study on the dentocraniofacial growth of the individuals with reversed occlusion. J Jpn Orthod Soc 1978;37:237–268.

4. Yamazaki O, Sawa S, Hayashi M, et al. Studies on the longitudinal and individual growth of children with anterior reversed occlusion. J Jpn Orthod Soc 1979;38:8–13.

5. Takeuchi U, Genba Y, Suzuki S, et al. Longitudinal growth study of untreated cases with reversed occlusion. J Jpn Orthod Soc 1979;38:14–29.

6. Mitani H. Prepubertal growth of mandibular prognathism. Am J Orthod 1981;80:546–553.

7. Sugawara J, Tsuchikawa T, Soya T, et al. Late adolescent growth of skeletal Class III craniofaces in Japanese girls—Average growth from 14 to 17 years of age based on longitudinal data. J Jpn Orthod Soc 1983;42:399–408.

8. Sato K, Sugawara J, Mitani H. Longitudinal study on average craniofacial growth of skeletal Class III girls in the late adolescent period—Possibility of early orthognathic surgery. J Jpn Orthod Soc 1989;48:21–28.

9. Sato K, Sugawara J, Mitani H. Longitudinal study on average craniofacial growth of skeletal Class III males in late adolescent period—Possibility of early orthognathic surgery. J Jpn Orthod Soc 1992;51:25–30.

10. Mitani H, Sato K, Sugawara J. Growth of mandibular prognathism after pubertal growth peak. Am J Orthod Dentofacial Orthop 1993;104:330–336.

11. Sakamoto M, Sugawara J, Umemori M, et al. Craniofacial growth of mandibular prognathism during pubertal growth period in Japanese boys—Longitudinal study from 10 to 15 years of age. J Jpn Orthod Soc 1996;55:372–386.

12. Bandai (Sakamoto) M, Sugawara J, Umemori M, et al. Craniofacial growth of mandibular prognathism in Japanese girls during pubertal growth period—Longitudinal study from 9 to 14 years of age. Orthod Waves 2000;59:77–89.

13. Houston WJB, Miller JC, Tanner JM. Prediction of the timing of the adolescent growth spurt from ossification events in hand–wrist films. Br J Orthod 1979;6:142–152.

14. Houston WJB. Relationship between skeletal maturity estimated from hand–wrist radiographs and the timing of the adolescent growth spurt. Eur J Orthod 1980;2:81–93.

15. Sato K. A study on growth timing of mandibular length, body height, hand bones and cervical vertebrae during puberty. J Jpn Orthod Soc 1987;46:517–533.

16. Grave KC. Timing of facial growth: a study of relations with stature and ossification in the hand around puberty. Aust J Orthod 1973;3:117–122.

17. Hagg U, Taranger J. Skeletal stages of the hand and wrist as indicators of the pubertal growth spurt. Acta Odontol Scand 1980;38:187–200.

18. Suzuki N. A cephalometric observation on the effect of the chin cap. J Jpn Orthod Soc 1972;31:64–74.

19. Irie M, Nakamura S. Orthopedic approach to severe skeletal Class III malocclusion. Am J Orthod 1975;67:377–392.

20. Graber LW. Chin cup therapy for mandibular prognathism. Am J Orthod 1977;72:23–41.

21. Nukatsuka S. The longitudinal study of orthopedic effect caused by chin cap treatment. Tohoku Univ Dent J 1982;1:1–17.

22. Janzen EK, Bluher JA. The cephalometric, anatomic, and histologic changes in *Macaca nulatta* after application of a continuous-acting retraction force on the mandible. Am J Orthod 1965;51:823–855.

23. Matsui Y. Effect of chin cap on the growing mandible. J Jpn Orthod Soc 1965;24:165–181.

24. Joho JP. The effects of extraoral low-pull traction to the mandibular dentition of *Macaca nulatta*. Am J Orthod 1973;64:555–577.

25. Petrovic AG, Stutzman JJ, Oudet CL. Contro processes in the postnatal growth of the condylar cartilage of the mandible: effect of orthopedic therapy on condylar growth. In: McNamara JA Jr (ed). Determinants of mandibular form and growth. Ann Arbor: University of Michigan, 1975.

26. Asano T. The effects of mandibular retractive force on the growing rat. Am J Orthod Dentofacial Orthop 1986;90:464–474.

27. Sugawara J, Asano T, Endo N, Mitani H. Long-term effects of chincap therapy on skeletal profile in mandibular prognathism. Am J Orthod Dentofacial Orthop 1990;98:127–133.

28. Wendell PD, Nanda R. The effects of chin cap therapy on the mandible: a longitudinal study. Am J Orthod 1985;87:265–274.

29. Tsuchikawa T, Sugawara J, Nakamura H, et al. Long-term results of skeletal profile changes occurred in the chin cap therapy of Japanese male skeletal Class III cases. J Jpn Orthod Soc 1985;44:644–659.

30. Endo N. A study on the variation and formation of vertical skeletal facial patterns in skeletal Class III cases. J Jpn Orthod Soc 1987;46:50–70.

31. Oyama A, Sugawara J. Maxillary incisors protraction (MIP). In: Sugawara J, Asano T, eds. Seeking a consensus for Class III treatment. Osaka: Tokyo Rinsho Shuppan; 2002:148–155.

32. Umemori M, Sugawara J, Mitani H, Nagasaka H, Kawamura H. Skeletal anchorage system for open-bite. Am J Orthod Dentofacial Orthop 1999;115:166–174.

33. Sugawara J. JCO interviews, Dr Junji Sugawara on the skeletal anchorage system, J Clin Orthod 2000;33:689–696.

34. Sugawara J, Baik UB, Umemori M, et al. Treatment and posttreatment dentoalveolar changes following intrusion of mandibular molars with application of a skeletal anchorage (SAS) for open bite correction. Int J Adult Orthod Orthognath Surg 2002;17:1–11.

35. Kawauchi M. Evaluation for psycho-social problems in patients who have possibility to undergo orthognathic surgery after completion of jaw growth. In: Sugawara J, Asano T, eds. Seeking a consensus for Class III treatment. Osaka: Tokyo Rinsho Shuppan; 2002:368–375.

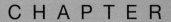

CHAPTER 12

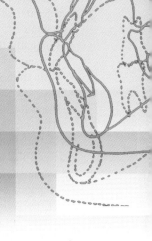

Treatment Strategies for Developing Class III Patients

Frank Hsin-Fu Chang and Jenny Zwei-Chieng Chang

There are many definitions of Class III malocclusions.[1–5] The most common is "an occlusion in which the buccal groove of the mandibular permanent first molar occludes mesial to the mesiobuccal cusp of the maxillary permanent first molar." A Class III malocclusion may also be classified simply as an anterior crossbite. Clinically, a skeletal class III malocclusion denotes a straight or concave profile.

To obtain an accurate diagnosis of Class III malocclusions, a thorough evaluation of the clinical data is necessary. The following information should be assessed:

1. Age, sex, and family history of the patient.
2. Molar relationship: careful assessment of caries, missing teeth, tooth size discrepancies, or any mesial drift of the posterior teeth.
3. Craniofacial morphogenic characteristics: in addition to determining a patient's maxillary and mandibular relationship relative to the cranial base, evaluation of the intermaxillary relationship, mandibular plane angle, gonial angle, and vertical facial dimension is also helpful.
4. Position of the maxillary and mandibular incisors: dental aberrations in patients with skeletal Class III relationships manifest as protrusion of the maxillary incisors and linguoversion of the mandibular incisors. From the inclination of the upper and lower incisors, any dental compensation can be identified.
5. Soft tissue appearance: evaluating a patient's frontal view and lateral profile helps to identify the components of the skeletal Class III problem. Is the problem maxillary retrusion, mandibular prognathism, or a combination of the two? Correct diagnosis is essential in determining the proper treatment plan and estimating the future prognosis of the case.
6. Functional shift: some anterior crossbite patients and skeletal Class III patients suffer from a functional shift. This may be the result of a premature contact between the maxillary and mandibular incisors, resulting in a forward displacement of the mandible. Correction of patients with Class III malocclusions and a functional shift of the mandible is considered to be easier to achieve than correction of patients with Class III malocclusion but no functional shift. However, longterm follow-up of Class III patients with or without a functional shift shows that some initially successfully treated cases develop into skeletal Class III malocclusions at a later stage. Many Class III patients with a functional shift are, in fact, true skeletal Class III cases; only a few fall into the pseudo Class III group.

Sometimes patients are not initially diagnosed with a Class III malocclusion, yet over time (during treatment, or even in the retention phase), their malocclusion becomes more obvious. The failure to properly diagnose these patients may be due to inadequate analysis of pretreatment data or to unpredictable jaw growth. Details concerning these situations will be discussed in the following section.

Since most Class III subjects have an anterior crossbite, several treatment methods for this will be described. Treatment modalities include:

• Incline plane
• Modified incline plane

- Chin cap
- Face mask
- Fixed appliances.

Clinical cases will be presented to illustrate the indication, mechanism, and prognosis of these appliances.

Incline Plane

For patients who have an anterior dental crossbite, with or without a mandibular functional shift, an incline plane is a good treatment choice. These patients are characterized as having:
- Lingually inclined upper anterior teeth with an anterior crossbite
- Well-aligned lower anterior teeth without labioversion
- Deep-to-normal overbite
- Normal-to-low mandibular plane angle.

The incline plane is fixed onto the lower anterior teeth with temporary cement. The appropriate angulation between the incline plane and the upper anterior teeth in crossbite should be determined by considering the vertical discrepancy between the teeth in crossbite and the adjacent teeth, as well as the degree of overbite of the teeth in crossbite. By adjusting the different contact angulations, it is possible to control the labial inclination of the maxillary anterior teeth in crossbite. Most anterior dental crossbites can be corrected within 3–4 weeks using an incline plane.

Comparing pre- and post-treatment cephalometric radiographs, the following treatment effects of the incline plane can be seen:
1. The pretreatment lingually inclined upper anterior teeth now tip labially with biting force.
2. The lower anterior teeth tip slightly lingually, even though they are used for anchorage as a whole.
3. The mandible rotates downward and backward and the mandibular plane angle increases during correction of the anterior crossbite. After correction, the mandible will recover to its original downward and forward position and the mandibular plane angle will return to its original angulation or even less.
4. In terms of the incisor positions, most patients show lingually inclined lower incisors; upper incisor positions exhibit greater variation.

An example of a patient treated with an incline plane is shown in Figure 12-1.

Modified Incline Plane

For patients with an anterior dental crossbite, where the upper and lower incisors are lingually and labially inclined, respectively, an incline plane is contraindicated. In these circumstances, a modified incline plane is a better choice.[6] A modified incline plane is a removable appliance which structurally resembles a Hawley appliance with an incline plane placed at the anterior portion. The incline plane portion covers the lower anterior teeth up to their incisal third. When the patient bites, the incline plane portion raises the bite and proclines the upper anterior teeth labially. The metal wire parts consist of a labial bow and occlusal rests or Adam's clasps. Occlusal rests and Adam's clasps are made from 0.7 mm diameter round wire. They are placed on the first molars for appliance retention and stability. The labial bow is placed on the labial side of the lower incisors, near the cervical third, to make the force application closer to the center of resistance of the lower anterior teeth. The acrylic resin lingual to the lower incisors may be trimmed to allow lingual movement of the lower anterior teeth when the labial bow is activated.

Anterior crossbite problems can be corrected within 3–4 weeks using a modified incline plane. The anterior incline plane portion can be trimmed away by the time the anterior crossbite has been corrected, allowing the appliance to serve as a retainer. Superimposition of the pre- and post-treatment cephalometric radiographs will show:
1. Improvement of the soft tissue profile
2. Labial inclination of the upper incisors
3. Lingual inclination of the lower incisors
4. Downward and backward rotation of the mandible with an increase in the mandibular plane angle.

Longterm follow-up of these patients shows that mandibular growth returns to its original forward and downward direction, and the mandibular plane angle decreases to its original angulation or even less. Since many anterior crossbite patients with mandibular functional shift appear to have a skeletal Class III craniofacial pattern, it is suggested that combined treatment with both a modified incline plane and a chin cap to redirect mandibular growth is used. Even after the anterior crossbite has been corrected, continual wear of the chin cap is suggested to control the direction of mandibular growth.

An example of a patient treated with a modified incline plane is shown in Figure 12-2.

Chin Cap

Chin cap therapy is indicated for young patients with mandibular prognathism. Clinical studies by several researchers found that the chin cap does not restrain mandibular growth, but rather redirects the mandible to grow in a more vertical direction.[7-10] This change in the direction of mandibular growth helps to improve the skeletal Class III malocclusion. If chin cap treatment is discontinued before growth is completed, the mandible will resume its original forward and downward growth direction. Since mandibular growth persists for a longer period of time than maxillary growth, it is understandable why many Class III patients resume their Class III growth pattern following chin cap treatment. It is recommended that the patient wear the chin cap until growth is completed in order to maintain any effects that were achieved during treatment. The forces applied on the chin are oriented along the lines from the chin point to the condylar heads,

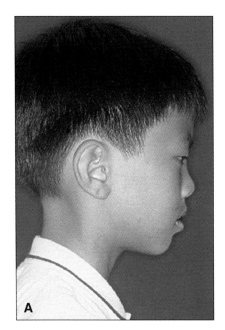

Fig. 12-1 A-D A 9-year-4-month-old patient with anterior crossbite. The lower anterior teeth are well aligned. **E** An incline plane was temporarily cemented on to the lower anterior teeth. **F** Positive overjet was achieved within a few weeks, and the incline plane was discontinued. A transient posterior open bite problem was noted at the time of appliance removal. Four months later, as shown, positive overbite was maintained and the posterior bite settled down. **G-I** One year and 10 months follow-up after treatment with the incline plane. The overjet, overbite, and occlusion of this patient appear to be stable. The patient did not undergo treatment with a fixed orthodontic appliance.

Continued

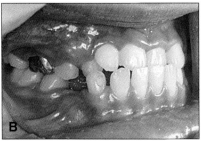
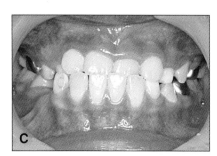
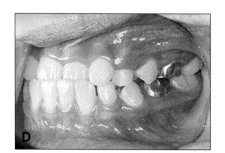
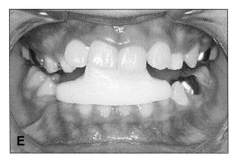
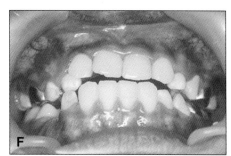
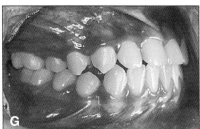
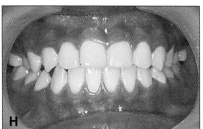
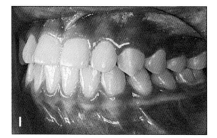

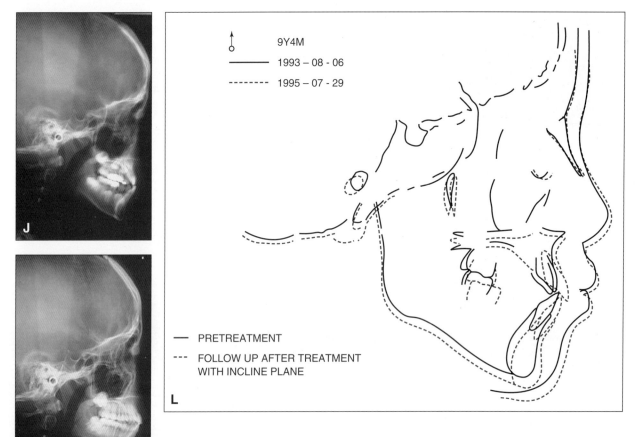

Fig. 12-1 *cont'd.* **J-L** One year and 10 months follow-up cephalometric radiographs and a superimposition of the pretreatment cephalometric radiograph show that the upper incisors have flared out labially, the lower incisors have tipped lingually, and the mandibular plane angle has remained unchanged.

bilaterally. The force magnitude used for this therapy ranges from 400 to 500 g. Patients are instructed to wear the chin cap for at least 10–14 h daily. Care should be taken to avoid the chin cap impinging on the lower lip as this will cause the lower incisors to tilt lingually and sometimes cause recession of the labial gingiva. Although the chin cap may be used to treat children with mandibular prognathism, its longterm prognosis is unpredictable because there are always variations in mandibular growth. The patient's parents should be fully informed of this before treatment is started.

Examples of patients treated with a chin cap are shown in Figures 12-3 and 12-4.

Face Mask

Face mask therapy can correct an anterior dental crossbite problem in 1–3 months. Factors influencing treatment time include patient compliance and the pretreatment

craniofacial characteristics of the patient. Treatment effects can be summarized as:[11–13]

1. Maxillary forward displacement: increase in SNA angle
2. Mandibular downward and backward rotation: decrease in SNB angle, increase in MP–SN angle, and increase in ANS–Me length
3. Improvement of intermaxillary relationship: increase in ANB angle
4. Labial inclination of upper incisors: increase in U1–SN angle
5. Lingual inclination of lower incisors: decrease in L1–MP angle.

Clinical observations show significant enhancement of the facial profile and achievement of positive overjet.

If satisfactory improvement is achieved during the first phase of orthopedic treatment, many clinicians continue with a second phase of treatment with fixed orthodontic appliances and without supplementary use of extraoral orthopedic forces. Mandibular growth will resume its

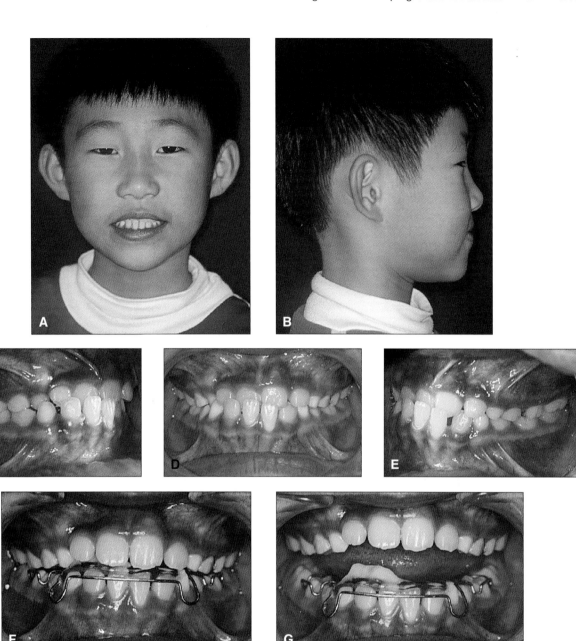

Fig. 12-2 **A-E** An 8-year-2-month-old boy whose chief complaint was anterior dental crossbite. The lower incisors were slightly inclined labially. **F** and **G** Modified incline plane with acrylic incisal capping, labial bow, and Adam's clasp. The incline plane portion tended to tilt the right upper central and lateral incisors labially. *Continued*

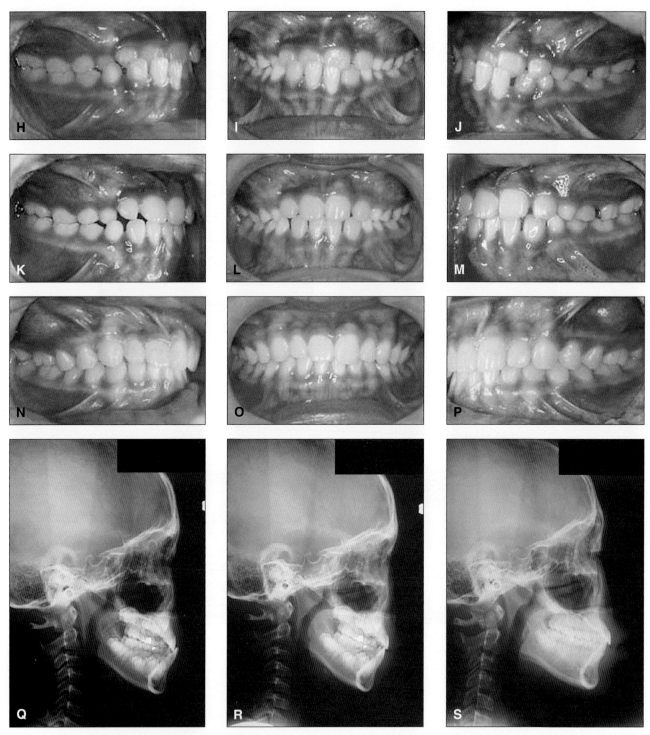

Fig. 12-2 *cont'd.* **H-J** Pretreatment intraoral photographs. **K-M** Six weeks after the start of treatment with the modified incline plane. **N-P** Follow-up photographs at 3 years and 10 months post-treatment. **Q-S** Pretreatment, post-treatment, and follow-up cephalograms.   *Continued*

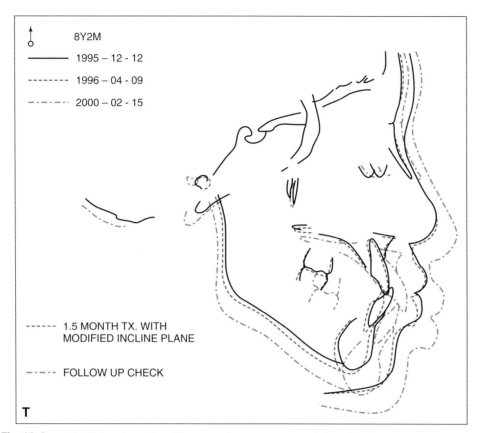

Fig. 12-2 *cont'd.* **T** Superimposition of the pre- and post-treatment cephalometric radiographs shows labial inclination of the upper anterior teeth, lingual inclination of the lower incisors, and downward and backward rotation of the mandible. Longterm follow-up showed that the mandibular growth returned to its original forward and downward direction.

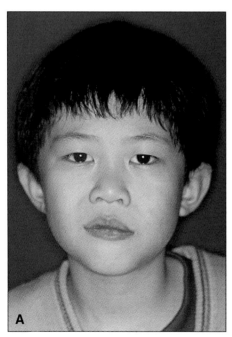
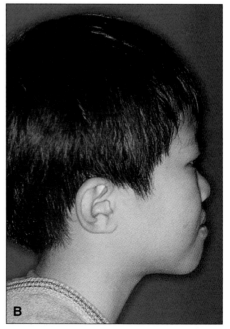

Fig. 12-3 **A** and **B** A 7-year-7-month-old boy with a straight lateral profile.

Continued

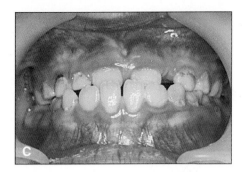

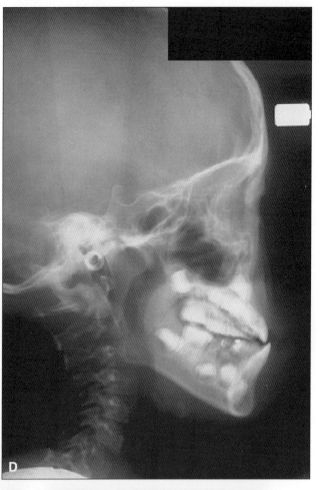

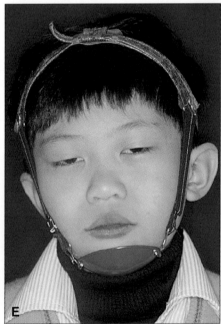

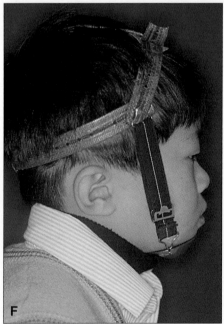

Fig. 12-3 *cont'd.* **C** Intraoral frontal view shows anterior crossbite. The patient was in his early mixed dentition stage. **D** Pretreatment lateral cephalometric radiograph shows a skeletal Class III pattern with a slightly high mandibular plane angle and upper incisor proclination. **E** and **F** Forces applied on the chin were oriented anterior to the lines from the chin point to the condyle heads bilaterally to provide a more vertical vector in order to control the vertical dimension and the forward growth of the mandible.

Continued

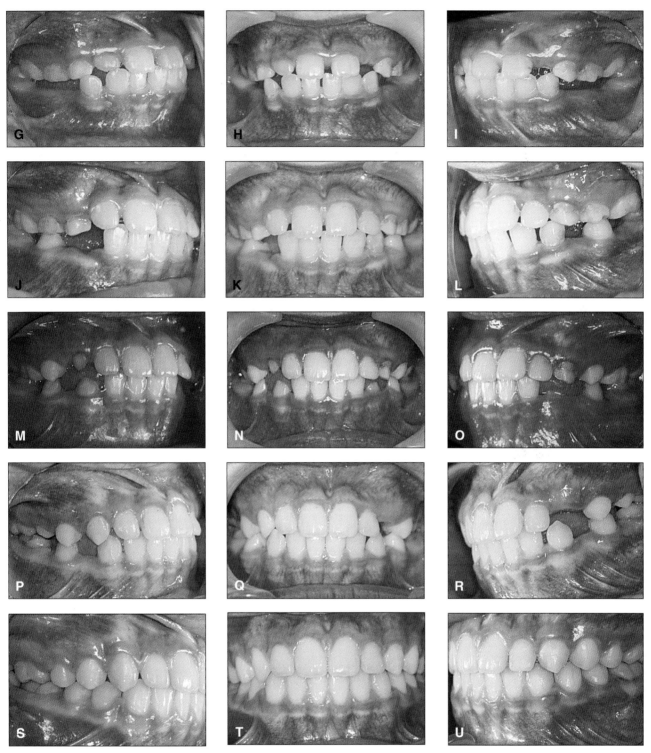

Fig. 12-3 *cont'd.* **G-I** Six months post-treatment with an incline plane and chin cap. The incline plane was discontinued soon after correction of the crossbite; chin cap treatment continued. **J-L** After 1 year and 10 months of chin cap treatment, the overbite and overjet were kept positive. **M-O** Positive overbite and overjet were maintained throughout the 2 years and 11 months of chin cap treatment. **P-R** Three years and 5 months of chin cap treatment. **S-U** Patient underwent the fixed orthodontic appliance combined with chin cap treatment. Six years and 3 months after the start of chin cap therapy (which included 3 weeks of incline plane treatment in the beginning and 2 years of fixed appliance treatment in the final stage), an ideal occlusion was achieved.

Continued

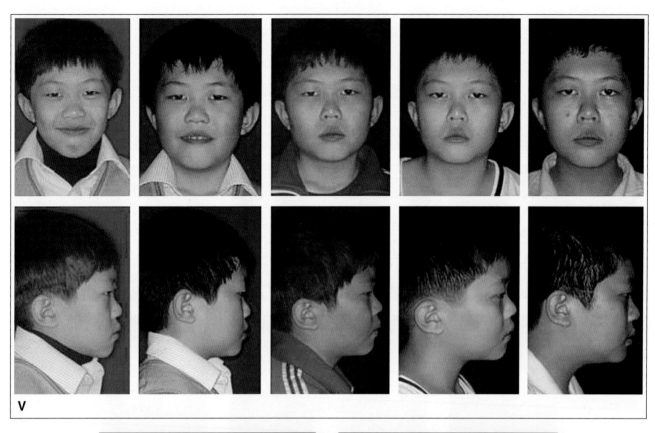

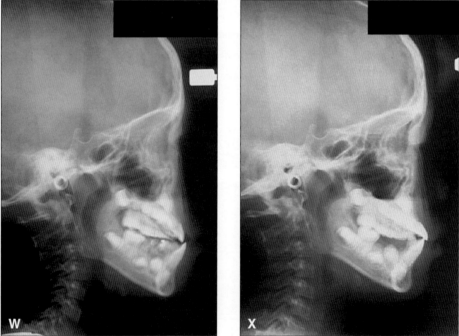

Fig. 12-3 *cont'd.* **V** Profile change during the 6 years from the start of chin cap treatment. From left to right: after 6 months, 1 year and 10 months, 2 years and 11 months, 3 years and 5 months, 6 years and 3 months. **W-Z** Successive cephalometric radiographs following chin cap treatment.

Continued

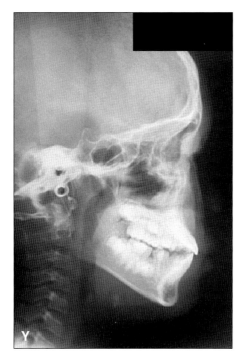
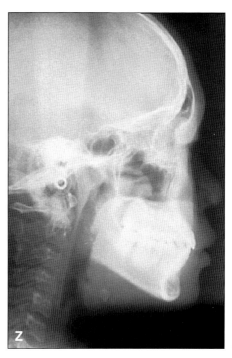
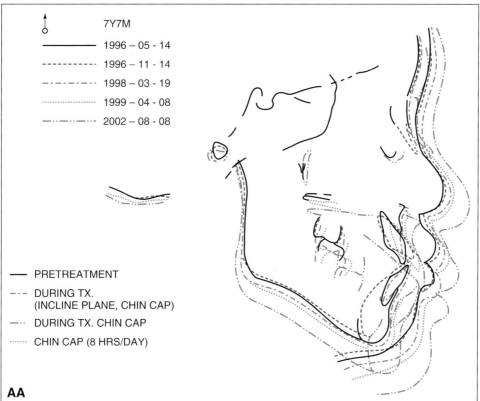

7Y7M
——————— 1996 – 05 - 14
- - - - - - - 1996 – 11 - 14
-·-·-·-· 1998 – 03 - 19
············· 1999 – 04 - 08
—·—·—·· 2002 – 08 - 08

—— PRETREATMENT
- - - DURING TX.
(INCLINE PLANE, CHIN CAP)
—·· DURING TX. CHIN CAP
······ CHIN CAP (8 HRS/DAY)

AA

Fig. 12-3 *cont'd.* **W-Z** Successive cephalometric radiographs following chin cap treatment. **AA** Superimposition of successive lateral radiographs shows improvement of the skeletal discrepancy and maintenance of the vertical facial proportion. The upper incisors flared labially after the incline plane therapy but were corrected to a more upright position during the fixed appliance phase.

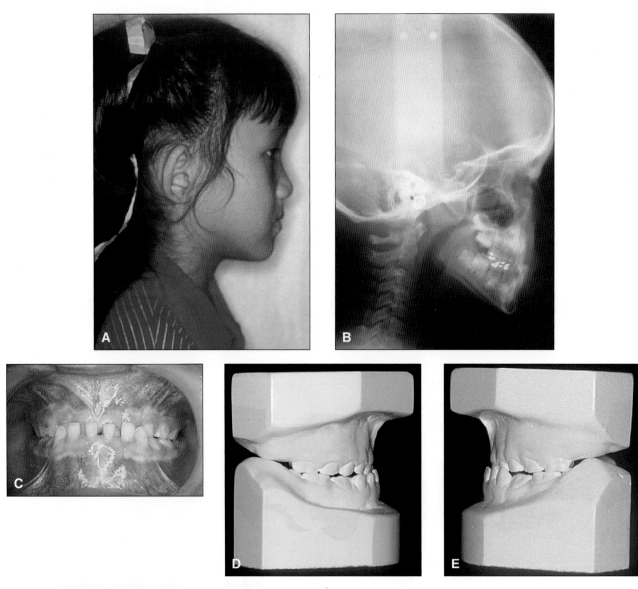

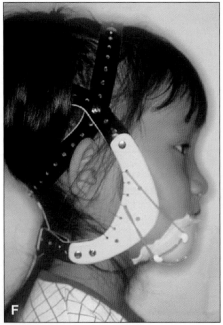

Fig. 12-4 **A** and **B** A 5-year-10-month-old girl. Her pretreatment lateral cephalometric radiograph shows skeletal Class III discrepancy with a high mandibular plane angle. **C-E** Intraorally she had anterior dental crossbite and Class III buccal occlusion. **F** Chin cap therapy was indicated. The forces applied on the chin are oriented along the lines from the chin point to the condyle heads bilaterally. *Continued*

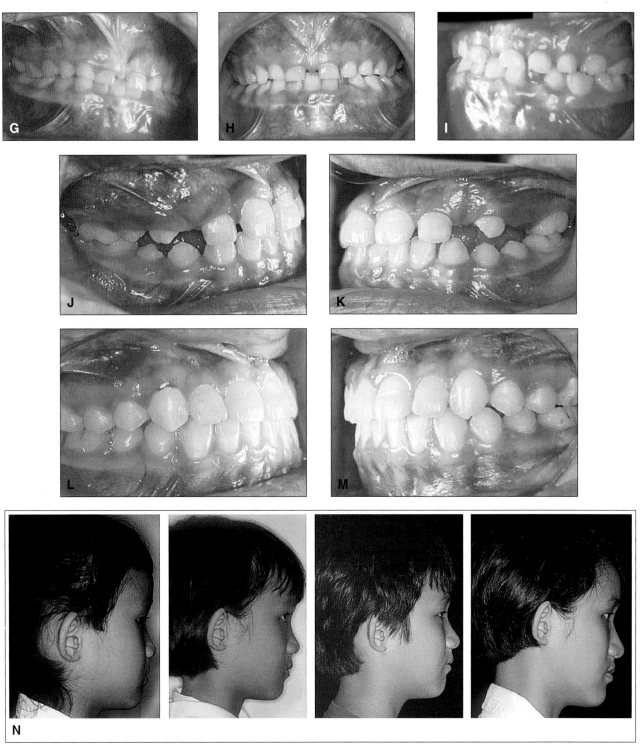

Fig. 12-4 *cont'd.* G-I One year and 3 months since the start of chin cap treatment. Positive overjet and overbite were achieved. Buccal occlusion was in Class I relationship. **J** and **K** Four years and 6 months from the start of treatment, in late mixed dentition stage. Positive overjet and overbite were maintained. **L** and **M** Eight years and 3 months later, with continual wear of the chin cap and second-phase fixed orthodontic appliance therapy, satisfactory occlusion was achieved. **N** Lateral profile change. From left to right: 3 months of chin cap therapy, 1 year and 3 months, 5 years and 1 month, 8 years and 3 months. *Continued*

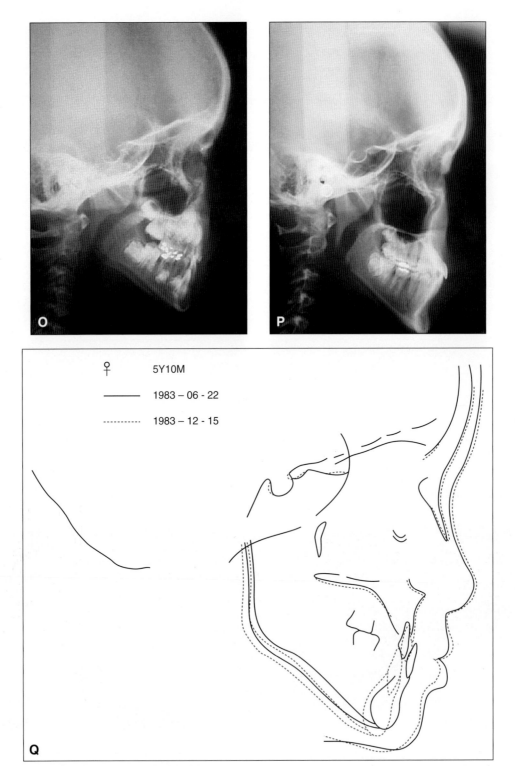

Fig. 12-4 *cont'd.* Cephalometric radiographs with chin cap treatment of 6 months, negative overjet corrected (**O**), and 8 years and 3 months following chin cap and fixed appliance treatment (**P**). **Q** Positive overjet achieved during the initial 6 months from the start of chin cap treatment. Superimposition of the lateral cephalometric radiographs illustrates backward and downward rotation of the mandible with the lower deciduous incisors lingually tilted and the upper deciduous incisors labially inclined. **R** For the next 6 months, the mandibular plane angle decreased, which indicated that the mandible tended to grow into its original direction. **S** Skeletal relationship worsened during the pubertal growth spurt period, as the ANB angle decreased significantly. A second-phase fixed orthodontic appliance treatment helped to camouflage the jaw discrepancy by flaring out the upper incisors and rotating the mandible backward and downward, as shown in the superimpositions of the lateral tracings.   *Continued*

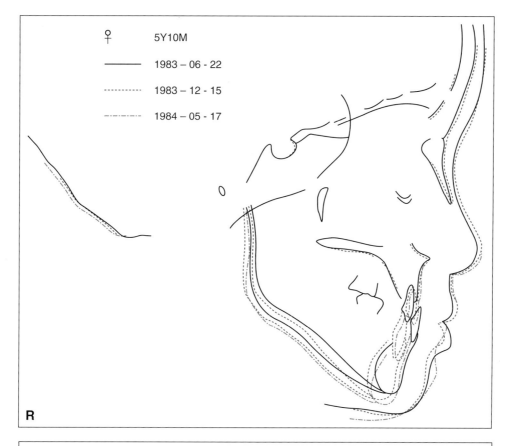

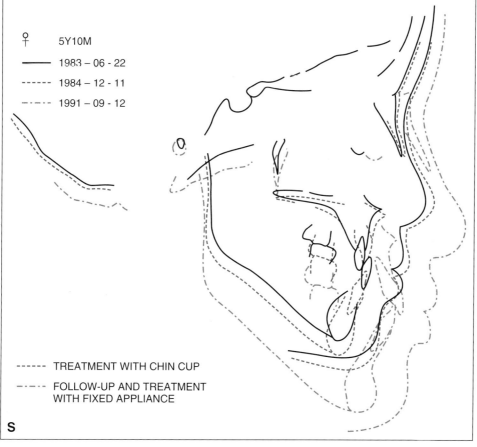

Fig. 12-4 *cont'd.*

original downward and forward direction; hence, many patients tend to have a more Class III molar relationship and smaller anterior overjet during the second phase of treatment. Combined use of extraoral orthopedic appliances, such as a chin cap, with fixed orthodontic appliances may effectively control the mandibular growth direction, keeping it mainly vertical, while the maxilla maintains its forward and downward growth, thus retaining the effects of the first phase of treatment with the face mask.

Longterm follow-up data shows that some treated patients maintain positive overjet and Angle's Class I occlusal relationship while others relapse. Cephalometric analysis discloses maxillary protraction and mandibular downward and backward rotation during the initial treatment stage. As treatment continues, the mandible tends to grow vertically. Even longer observation shows that the mandible reverts toward its original downward and forward growth direction.

Post-treatment cephalometric radiographs reveal skeletal Class III craniofacial patterns in all patients after longterm follow-up. For those who maintain a positive overjet, the amount of dental change is capable of compensating for the intermaxillary jaw discrepancy. For those who relapse to an anterior crossbite, the amount of dental compensation is not enough to overcome the discrepancy caused by the mandibular growth. If the relapse is too great, it is better to wait until growth is completed. Further evaluation of the severity of the Class III malocclusion, the amount of anterior crossbite, the soft tissue profile, and the patient's chief complaint helps with the decision to proceed with an orthodontic camouflage or a surgical intervention.

An example of a patient treated with a face mask is shown in Figures 12-5.

Fixed Orthodontic Appliance

Fixed orthodontic appliance treatment without additional orthopedic forces or combined surgical intervention is indicated for mild Class III patients with acceptable facial appearance and completed growth. If the diagnosis is accurate, the treatment result may be quite favorable.

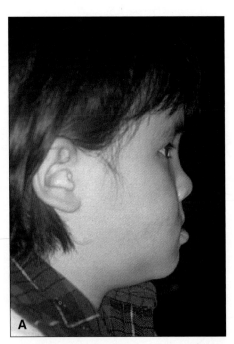
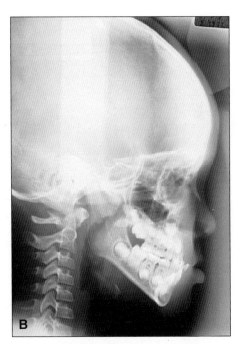

Fig. 12-5 **A** and **B** A 5-year-7-month-old girl with maxillary deficiency and slightly high mandibular plane angle.   *Continued*

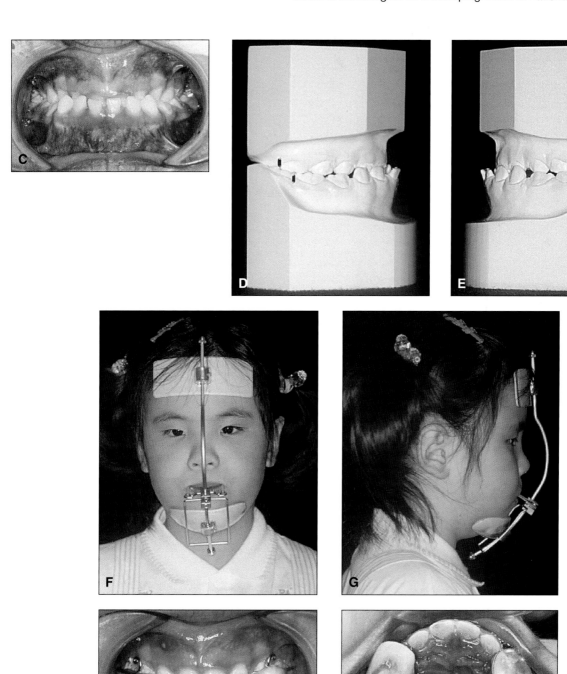

Fig. 12-5 *cont'd.* **C** Intraorally she had anterior crossbite with deep overbite and maxillary transverse deficiency. **D** and **E** Buccal segment shows a mesial step of primary molars that corresponds to a Class III molar relationship. **F** and **G** Patient wearing face mask according to the design of Petit. The face mask comprised a single midline rod connected to a chin pad and a forehead pad. Elastics are connected bilaterally to an adjustable midline crossbow. **H** and **I** Bonded appliance with acrylic resin covering the occlusal surfaces of the maxillary posterior teeth. The midline expansion screw of the bonded maxillary expander was activated once per day until the desired change in the transverse dimension was achieved (the lingual cusps of the upper posterior teeth approximating the buccal cusps of the lower posterior teeth).

Continued

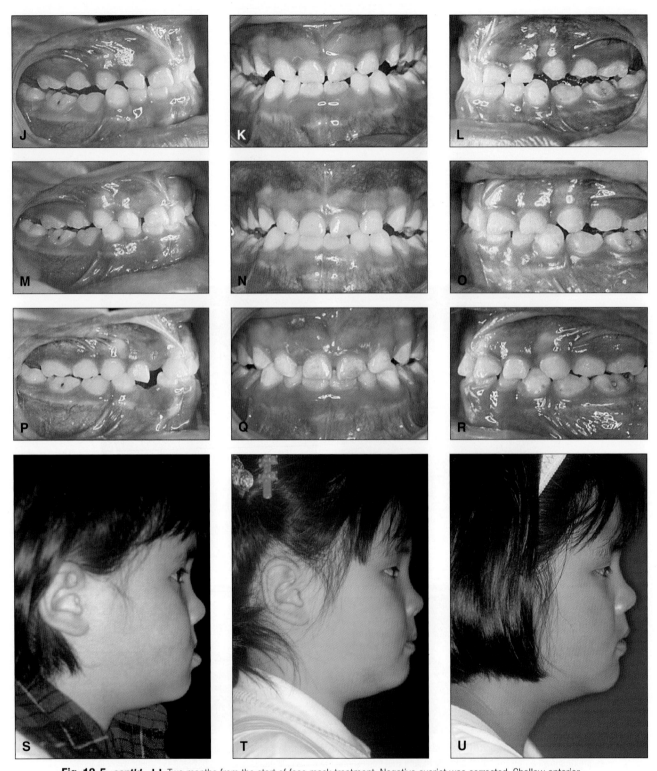

Fig. 12-5 *cont'd.* **J-L** Two months from the start of face mask treatment. Negative overjet was corrected. Shallow anterior overbite and posterior open bite were noted. Bonded type expander and the face mask were discontinued at this time. **M-O** Bite settled down by itself within the next 3 weeks without additional treatment. **P-R** Six weeks follow-up after discontinuation of the face mask and expander. Lateral profile before treatment (**S**), after 2 months of treatment with a bonded type rapid palatal expansion (RPE) device and protraction face mask (**T**), and 4 years post-treatment follow-up (**U**). *Continued*

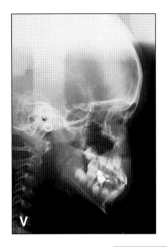
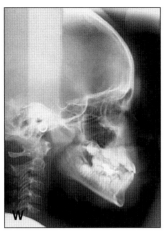
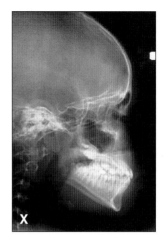
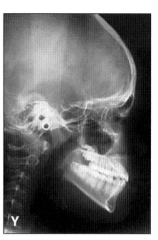

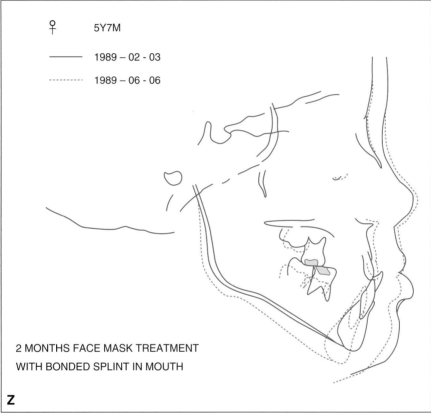

♀　5Y7M

——— 1989 – 02 - 03

---------- 1989 – 06 - 06

2 MONTHS FACE MASK TREATMENT
WITH BONDED SPLINT IN MOUTH

Fig. 12-5 *cont'd.*

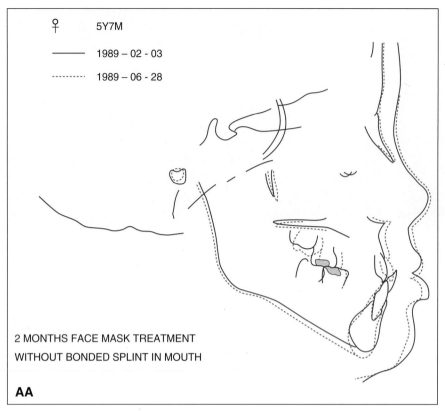

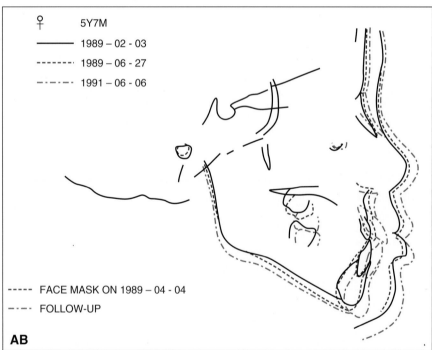

Fig. 12-5 *cont'd.* **V-Y** Successive cephalograms following face mask therapy with bonded expander. **Z** and **AA** Superimpositions of cephalometric tracings. 2 weeks of face mask and bonded type RPE treatment shows downward and backward rotation of the mandible and retroclination of the mandibular incisors (**Z**). Two months of treatment shows maxillary forward displacement, mandibular downward and backward rotation, and retroclination of the mandibular incisors (**AA**). **AB** At 2-year follow-up after treatment, positive overjet was retained but the mandible reverted toward its original downward and forward growth direction.

REFERENCES

1. Hellman M. Morphology of the face, jaws, and dentition in Class III malocclusion of the teeth. J Am Dent Assoc 1931;18:2150–2173.
2. Stapf WC. A cephalometric roentgenographic appraisal of the facial pattern in Class III malocclusions. Angle Orthod 1948;18:20–23.
3. Sanborn RT. Differences between the facial skeletal patterns of Class III malocclusion and normal occlusion. Angle Orthod 1955;25:208–222.
4. Dietrich UC. Morphological variability of skeletal Class III relationships as revealed by cephalometric analysis. Trans Eur Orthod Soc 1970;46:131–143.
5. Guyer EC, Ellis EE, McNamara JA, Behrents RG. Components of Class III malocclusion in juveniles and adolescents. Angle Orthod 1986;56:7–29.
6. Ash MM, Ramfjord S. Occlusion, 4th edn. Philadelphia: WB Saunders, 1995:377–378.
7. Sakamoto T, Iwase I, Uka A, Nakamura S. A roentgenocephalometric study of skeletal changes during and after chin cup treatment. Am J Orthod 1984;85:341–350.
8. Sugawara J, Asano T, Endo N, Mitani H. Long-term effects of chincap therapy on skeletal profile in mandibular prognathism. Am J Orthod Dentofacial Orthop 1990;98:127–133.
9. Uner O, Yuksel S, Ucuncu N. Long-term evaluation after chincap treatment. Eur J Orthod 1995;17:135–141.
10. Deguchi T, Kuroda T, Hunt NP, Graber TM. Long-term application of chincup force alters the morphology of the dolichofacial Class III mandible. Am J Orthod Dentofacial Orthop 1999;116:610–615.
11. Ngan P, Wei SH, Hagg U, Yiu CK, Merwin D, Stickel B. Effect of protraction headgear on Class III malocclusion. Quintessence Int 1992;23:197–207.
12. Macdonald KE, Kapust AJ, Turley PK. Cephalometric changes after the correction of class III malocclusion with maxillary expansion/facemask therapy. Am J Orthod Dentofacial Orthop 1999;116:13–24.
13. Baccetti T, Franchi L, McNamara JA Jr. Treatment and posttreatment craniofacial changes after rapid maxillary expansion and facemask therapy. Am J Orthod Dentofacial Orthop 2000;118:404–413.

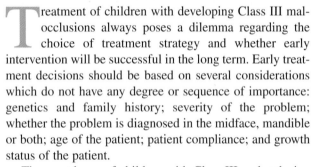

CHAPTER 13

Biomechanical Aspects of a Modified Protraction Headgear

Ravindra Nanda

Treatment of children with developing Class III mal-occlusions always poses a dilemma regarding the choice of treatment strategy and whether early intervention will be successful in the long term. Early treatment decisions should be based on several considerations which do not have any degree or sequence of importance: genetics and family history; severity of the problem; whether the problem is diagnosed in the midface, mandible or both; age of the patient; patient compliance; and growth status of the patient.

The prevalence of children with Class III malocclusion in the US is relatively small compared to Japan, Korea, and Taiwan. Two studies evaluating the incisor relationship in children have reported an anterior crossbite incidence of 0.8–1.0%.[1,2] One study reported a Class III molar relationship incidence of 3.8% in high school children.[3] However, a Class III malocclusion in a child deserves special attention due to the esthetic, occlusion, function, and psychosocial concerns it raises.

Treatment of developing Class III patients is often based on the orthodontist's expectations of treatment. The parents should be fully informed about the variability of results that can be expected. The wishful thinking is always to convert a Class III pattern to a Class I growth pattern. The reality is that treatment results range from 100% success to no change at all in the long term. The degree of success is based on the etiology of the Class III pattern, severity of malocclusion, age and growth status, choice of appliance used, and degree of patient cooperation. Other short-term goals should not be overlooked; i.e. to provide young Class III patients with a functioning occlusion, reduction in severity, and some esthetic improvement during their formative years.

Rationale of Protraction Headgear

Delaire et al[4–8] are credited with introducing the concept of protraction headgear to treat Class III malocclusions. We introduced a modified protraction headgear in 1980,[9] based on biomechanical concepts.

The rationale for protraction headgear is to apply heavy forces on the midface in order to advance the maxilla anteriorly. In patients with a normally sized mandible and retrusive maxilla, forward displacement of the maxilla is conceptually good. Several studies in the past three decades have shown that 25–41% of Class III problems in children are primarily the result of a retrognathic maxilla.[10–12]

The efficacy of protraction headgear is also supported by several studies in primates in the 1970s and 1980s.[13–17] These studies, using cephalometrics and histologic techniques, showed that treatment with an anterior force on the maxilla is capable of causing disassociation of sutural articulations by a resorption and apposition process at the sutural interfaces. Our own experience has also shown that the direction of midface protraction can be altered by changing the direction and point of delivery of the force.

In recent years noteworthy clinical studies have been reported regarding the use of protraction headgear.[18–25] The majority of these studies show an anterior movement of the maxillary dentition, a significant extrusion of the upper molars, anterior displacement of the maxillary dentition, 1–3 mm anterior displacement of the maxilla, and a significant rotation of the mandible downward and backward.

A conventional protraction headgear as described by Delaire et al[4–8] and its variations utilizes elastics from the molars (or other points at the occlusal plane level) to the facial mask. The interlabial gap and lips limit the ability to change the point of force application to attain predictable movement of the maxilla in the anterior direction.

Nanda[9] introduced a modified protraction headgear in 1980, which allowed changes in the direction of force and point of force application on the maxilla as well as the chin. The study showed that use of a modified protraction headgear for 4–8 months can displace the maxilla 1–3 mm and maxillary dentition 1–4 mm. These changes were accompanied by remodeling at the B point, lingual tipping of the mandibular incisors, and downward rotation of the mandible. The cumulative effect of these changes was the correction of the Class III malocclusion. This chapter describes the biomechanical aspects of this headgear, which allows modification of forces in Class III patients to achieve the desired changes, such as in long- and short-face Class III patients.

Components of Modified Protraction Headgear

There are two main components of a protraction headgear: intra- and extra-oral set-up.

Intraoral Components

The protraction headgear force is applied via elastics to teeth or other devices supported by teeth and/or the palate. The primary aim is to transmit the force to the midface sutural interfaces. To achieve this, it is important to stabilize the maxilla as one unit (Fig. 13-1). In the primary dentition, it is advisable to use a cemented acrylic occlusal bite block or a removable acrylic plate with occlusal coverage (see Ch. 12). In mixed dentition and early permanent dentition patients, a removable acrylic plate (Fig. 13-2) should be used supported by bands with headgear tubes on the molars or a rigid archwire with a palatal arch. Probably the best stabilization in patients with maxillary first molars is provided by a fixed rapid palatal expansion (RPE) device (Fig. 13-3). We prefer a Hyrax type of nonbonded device, as bonded RPEs (Fig. 13-4) interfere with the primary exfoliating teeth or teeth in the eruptive phase. Studies have also indicated that a simultaneous sutural expansion with an RPE at the start of protraction headgear treatment facilitates the anterior movement of the maxilla.[19,20,26,27]

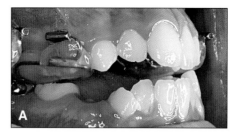

Fig. 13-1 **A** Left and **B** right lateral views of an intraoral stabilization appliance. An acrylic bite block includes a heavy archwire to which a headgear tube is soldered. The bite block provides disocclusion to facilitate forward displacement of the maxilla and is cemented on to posterior maxillary teeth.

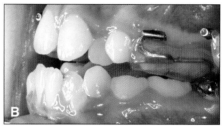

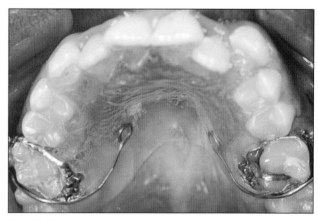

Fig. 13-2 Occlusal view of a removable intraoral stabilization appliance. The acrylic plate has a clasp which fits on a molar tube of a cemented band. This plate must be worn when the protraction appliance is in use.

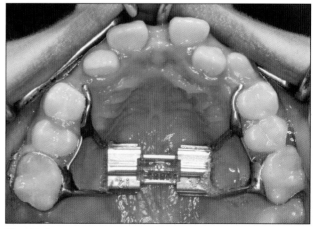

Fig. 13-3 Occlusal view of a rapid palatal expansion device used as a stabilization appliance. This is an ideal stabilization device if the first molars are fully erupted.

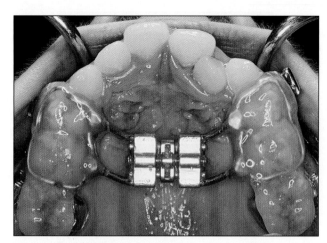

Fig. 13-4 Occlusal view of a bonded rapid palatal expansion device. In mixed dentition patients its use may interfere with the exfoliation of primary teeth and eruption of permanent teeth.

Extraoral Components

The extraoral components (Fig. 13-5) of a modified protraction headgear have two parts. The first is a face mask and the second is an intraoral-to-extraoral connecting force device which utilizes a modified headgear bow instead of intraoral elastics.

Commonly used face masks have chin and forehead support connected by a heavy metal arch which has a horizontal bar for attachment of a force module. The forehead and chin supports are adjustable. The horizontal bar also must be adjustable vertically to vary the point of force attachment (Figs 13-6 and 13-7).

A conventional headgear bow with a standard outer and inner bow without loops can be easily converted into a modified bow for use with the face mask. It is important

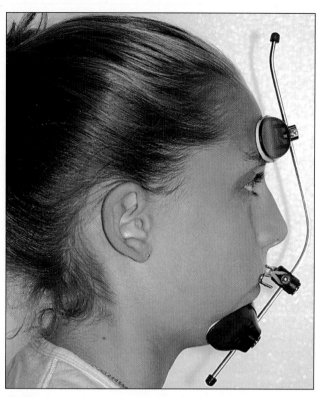

Fig. 13-6 Lateral view of a patient with the appliance shown in Figure 13-5 in place. The outer bow of the headgear is attached to the center bar of the face mask. The point of attachment on the mask can be moved up or down and the outer bow can be similarly positioned to achieve the desirable line of force.

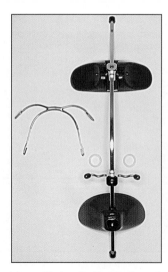

Fig. 13-5 Complete modified protraction headgear device. It includes a face mask, a modified inner bow of a headgear, and elastics.

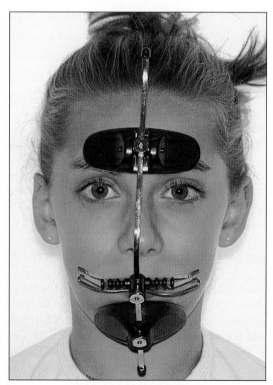

Fig. 13-7 Frontal view of the protraction headgear device.

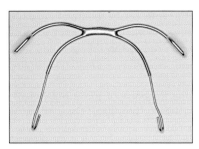

Fig. 13-8 Close up view of a modified headgear bow. The distal ends of the inner bow can be bent to achieve distal insertion of the appliance.

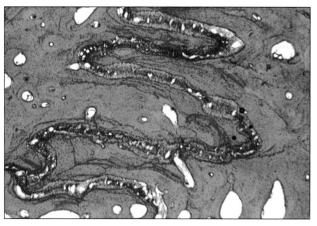

Fig. 13-9 Histologic photograph of an area of zygomaticomaxillary suture of a *Macaca nemestrina* monkey subjected to an anterior protraction force. Note the tortuous nature of the suture with areas of stress and strain and resting lines.

that the molar band has a headgear tube. In cemented acrylic stabilization devices, a headgear tube can be embedded in acrylic.

To construct a reverse headgear bow (Fig. 13-8), a U-shaped horizontal bend is made in such a way that it can be inserted into the molar tubes from the distal side. Anteriorly, the bow should clear the incisors and should be between the upper and lower lips. The outer bow is modified to make a hook in the premolar area in such a way that elastics can be attached to the horizontal bar of the face mask. The vertical position of the outer bow is adjusted to deliver the necessary force for a predictable maxillary displacement.

Protraction Headgear Force System

The following four components of force systems are important for proper adjustments of the protraction headgear.
1. Magnitude of force
2. Direction and point of force application
3. Duration of force
4. Force constancy.

Magnitude of Force
Hickory and Nanda[28] showed in an in vitro study of 2-day-old rat cranial sutures that very small forces (0.2–0.6 g) applied with wire springs are capable of generating cellular activity along with an increase in the suture width. For human studies, the force values used for protraction of the maxilla have ranged from 200 to 800 g. Most of the studies give no rationale for the magnitude of the force selected and in clinical practice the force used is often based on anecdotal experience.

Indeed there have been no prospective studies to determine the optimal force to protract the maxilla. However, based on clinical experience, studies in the literature, and sutural morphology changes related to age progression, certain observations regarding the desirable magnitude of force can be made.

The sutural articulations in children are simple; interdigitations interlock more with age. A clear example is the midpalatal suture. The suture remains patent long after growth is complete, but it becomes difficult to open with an RPE after the age of 15–16 years due to the complex interlocking of sutures. Conversely, in adolescents, midpalatal suture opening is very simple and can be accomplished with minimal tipping of the posterior teeth. A protraction force on the maxilla needs "disarticulation" at numerous sutures (Fig. 13-9), most notably zygomaticomaxillary, pterygopalatine, and nasomaxillary sutures of the midface. With age, these sutures not only become more mechanically intertwined, but also more tortuous in their orientation. Also, for the maxilla to advance forward in each affected suture, numerous areas of resorption and apposition have to take place due to their tortuous nature, quite unlike the midpalatal suture.

Thus, the sutural anatomy and age of the patient play a major role in determining the amount of force needed to bring the maxilla forward with protraction forces. For preadolescent patients (5–8 years), a force of 200–250 g on each side is adequate, and for early adolescent patients (8–11 years), a force of 300–450 g on each side may be desirable. In late adolescent patients (12 years and up), higher forces (450–600 g) can be used, but in our experience, protraction of the midface in the latter group is minimal. It is advisable to start with lower force values which can be increased if needed, especially in late adolescent patients.

Direction and Point of Force Application
Direction of the applied force is one of the most important force components for anterior displacement of the maxilla. Nanda[17] varied the point of force application in primates and showed that by changing the line of force on the midface, the center of rotation of the maxilla could be

altered. Later, Nanda and Hickory[16] speculated, based on different centers of rotation created by varying the line of protraction force, that the center of resistance of the midface is probably 5–10 mm below the orbitale on the zygomatic bone. Later, Tanne et al[29,30] reported that the center of resistance of the maxilla was located between the root tip of the maxilla first and second premolars. Miki[31] agreed with the previous two authors but added that in the vertical direction, the center of resistance of the midface was between the orbitale and the distal root apex of the first maxillary molars. Hata et al[32] and Lee et al[33] studied the effects of changing the level of force application on dried skulls and confirmed the findings of Nanda[17] in primates. They reported that a line of force 5 mm above the palatal plane and 15 mm above the occlusal plane did not result in counterclockwise movement of the maxilla and dentition.

Keles et al[34] studied the effects of varying the force direction on maxillary orthopedic protraction in two groups of patients. The first group received protraction headgear with a force applied by intraoral elastics and the second group received a force applied with a modified protraction headgear as described above.[9] They reported that in the first group, the maxilla rotated (Fig. 13-10) counterclockwise, resulting in downward and backward rotation of the mandible, while in the second group, an anterior translation

of the maxilla with no to minimal mandibular rotation occurred. This important study showed that predictable changes can be achieved in the direction of maxillary advancement with desired or without undesirable mandibular changes.

By changing the point of force attachment on the mask or outer bow of the headgear, the vertical dimension of the face can be very nicely controlled. This is especially important in Class III patients with a long vertical dimension and a steep mandibular plane. Similarly, in Class III patients with a flat mandibular plane and a deep bite, a force below the level of the occlusal plane may be more desirable to rotate the mandible downward and backward (see Fig. 13-10). A line of force closer to the center of resistance of the midface will deliver a translatory force (Fig. 13-11) and a line of force closer to the occlusal plane has a rotational force (Fig. 13-12).

The force delivered by the protraction mask on the chin is almost a "forgotten" force and is very rarely mentioned in the literature. An anterior force on the midface applies equal and opposite force on the forehead and chin (Figs 13-10). The direction of the force on the chin is distal and almost in a straight line, which can also cause a rotation of the mandible downward and backward. In Class

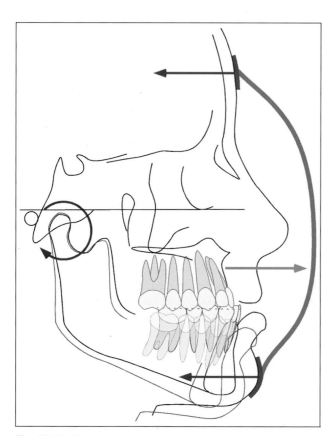

Fig. 13-10 Force diagram of a protraction device using intraoral elastics to deliver force. Note the clockwise moment on the midface and dentition resulting in a downward and backward rotation of the mandible.

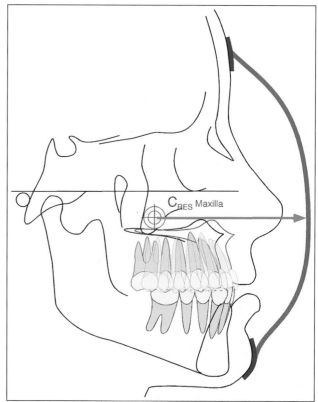

Fig. 13-11 Schematic representation of a line of force through the center of resistance of the maxilla, which will result in a translatory movement of the maxilla. The precise location of the center of resistance (C_RES) of the midfacial bones is difficult to locate but most studies point to the area 5–10 mm below the orbitale.

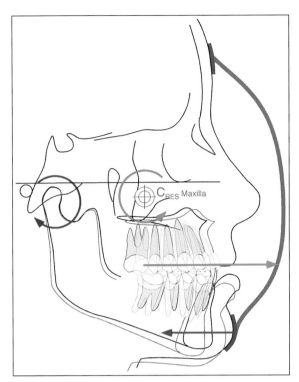

Fig. 13-12 Force diagram showing the nature of the maxillary and mandibular change when the point of force application is at the level of the root apices of the maxillary teeth. C$_{RES}$ = center of resistance.

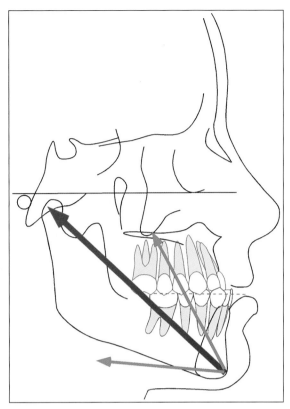

Fig. 13-14 Addition of a cervical strap or a vertical pull chin cap will change the resultant force vector of a chin cap.

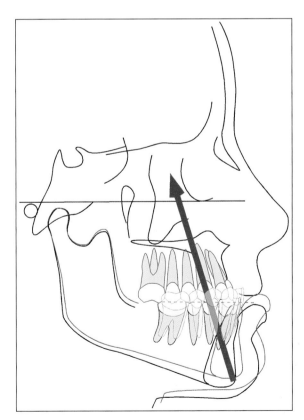

Fig. 13-13 Force diagram showing the line of force of an added chin cap. In the long vertical dimension of Class III patients, it is advisable to use a vertical pull chin cap to prevent downward rotation of the mandible.

III, long-faced patients, a vertical pull chin cap (Fig. 13-13) can be added to minimize the undesirable forces on the chin. A chin cap is especially desirable in Class III patients with a long vertical dimension and open bite tendency (Fig. 13-14).

Duration of Force

The majority of clinical studies recommend use of a protraction headgear anywhere from 3 to 12 months. Patient compliance beyond 6 months is difficult. Also, the older the patient, the less cooperative he/she will be. In our clinic, use of a protraction headgear is stopped after 6 months. In some patients, if necessary after an observation period, patients are asked to use the headgear again for 3–4 months.

The daily wear time depends also on the age of the patient. In preadolescent patients, 10–12 h of use per day is sufficient. In adolescent patients, it may be necessary to increase the wear time from 12 to 16 h per day. The latter group may also have problems with compliance.

Force Constancy

The force is applied with elastics from the outer bow of the headgear to the face mask. The elastic force should be measured at the beginning to determine the desired force level. Patients should be instructed to use fresh elastics as much as possible.

Two patient examples are presented. The first patient is unique because a decision was made to extract four premolars after protraction headgear use (Fig. 13-15). Clinical photographs are shown for the second patient 6 years after protraction (Fig. 13-16). In both patients a modified protraction headgear was used and the point of attachment and line of force was changed at various times during the protraction period.

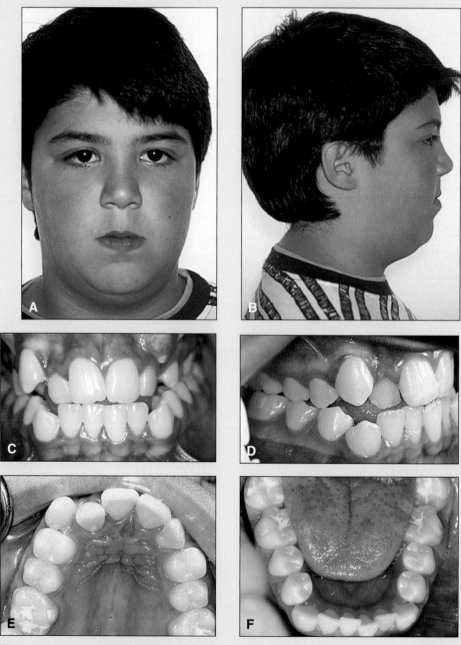

Fig. 13-15 A-F Frontal and lateral facial and intraoral views of an adolescent patient determined to have a developing Class III malocclusion after a careful examination of dental, facial, and family history findings, and a cephalometric analysis. **C** and **D** Edge-to-edge anterior bite and skeletal maxillary constriction. **E** and **F** Intraoral view of upper and lower arch. *Continued*

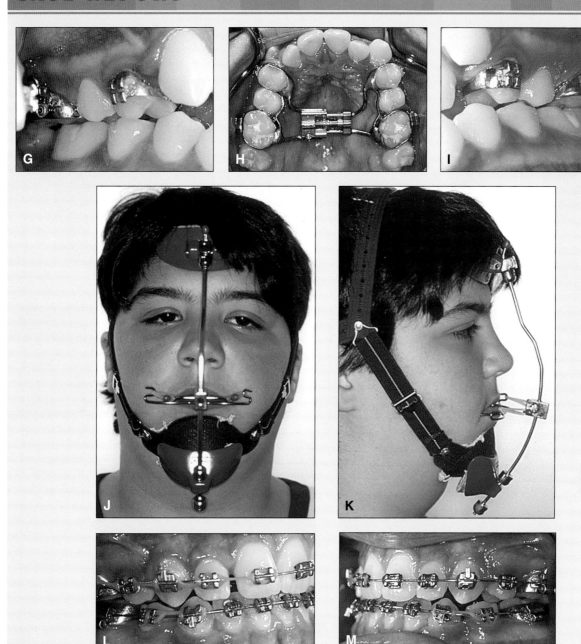

Fig. 13-15 *cont'd.* **G-I** Intraoral view showing a rapid palatal expansion (RPE) appliance at the end of the maxillary expansion. **J** Frontal and **K** lateral extraoral views with the protraction headgear in place. The chin cap component is added during the active RPE phase to prevent any extrusion of the maxillary posterior teeth. **L** and **M** Lateral intraoral views and **N** frontal view with smile after extraction of the four first premolars and completion of the space closure. Protraction headgear was used for 6 months prior to the extractions.

Continued

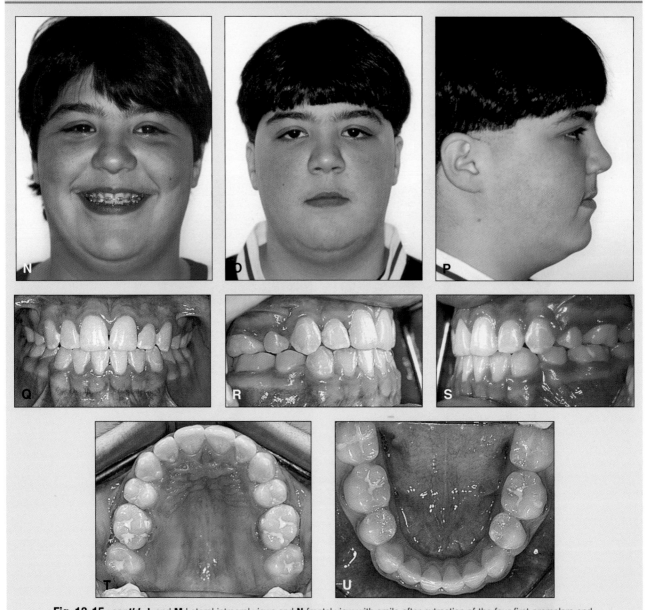

Fig. 13-15 *cont'd.* **L** and **M** Lateral intraoral views and **N** frontal view with smile after extraction of the four first premolars and completion of the space closure. Protraction headgear was used for 6 months prior to the extractions. **O-U** Facial and intraoral views at the end of the treatment.

Continued

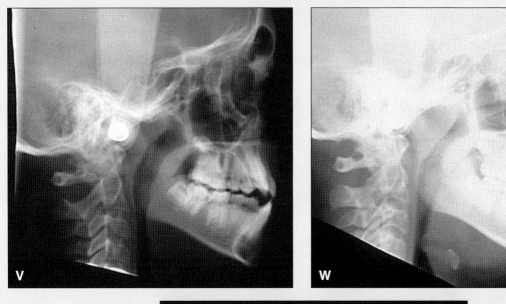

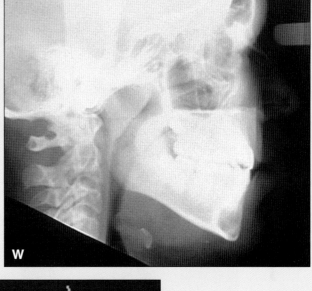

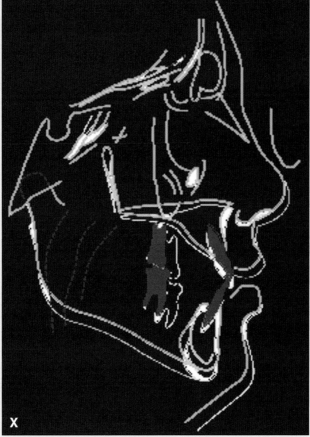

Fig. 13-15 *cont'd.* **V** Before and **W** after cephalograms, and **X** superimposition tracings showing cumulative changes over a 3-year treatment period.

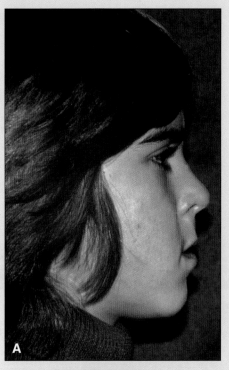

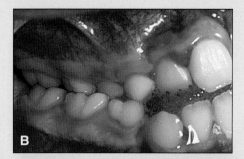

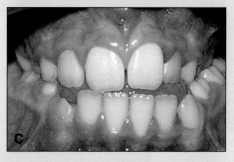

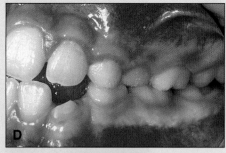

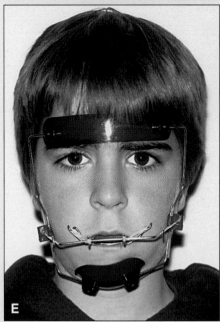

Fig. 13-16 **A-D** Extaoral and intraoral views of a developing Class III malocclusion in an early adolescent patient. **E** and **F** Extraoral frontal and lateral views of the protraction headgear appliance in place. Note the line of force in this patient is at the level of the root apices of the maxillary teeth. The line of force was adjusted at various times during the 6-month protraction headgear application to achieve the desired results. *Continued*

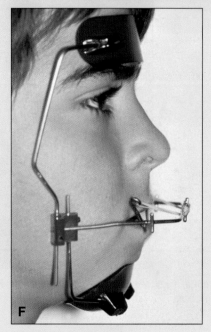

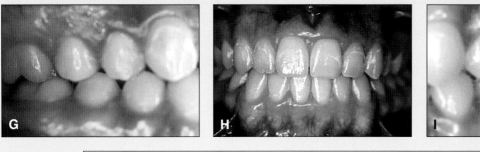

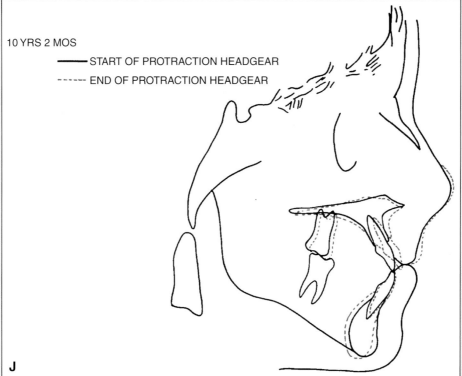

10 YRS 2 MOS

——— START OF PROTRACTION HEADGEAR

------ END OF PROTRACTION HEADGEAR

Fig. 13-16 *cont'd.* **G-I** Intraoral views of the dentition 6 years following the application of the protraction headgear and 3 years into the retention period. **J** Cephalometric superimposition tracings of the patient at the end of the protraction headgear period. **K** 6 years after the end of protraction. Note the amount of maxillary and mandibular growth.

Continued

CASE REPORT 1 and 2—cont'd

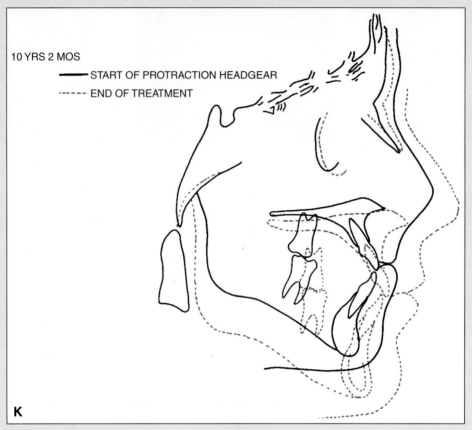

10 YRS 2 MOS

—————— START OF PROTRACTION HEADGEAR

- - - - - - END OF TREATMENT

K

Fig. 13-16 *cont'd.*

REFERENCES

1. Kelly JE, Sanchez M, Van Kirk LE. An assessment of the occlusion of the teeth of children. DHEW Publication No (HRA) 74-1612. Washington, DC: National Center for Health Statistics, 1973.
2. Proffit WR, Fields HW, Moray LJ. Prevalence of malocclusion and orthodontic treatment need in the United States: Estimates from the N-HANES III survey. Int J Adult Orthod Orthogn Surg 1998;13:97–106.
3. Mills LF. Epidemiologic studies of occlusion IV: the prevalence of malocclusion in a population of 1,455 school children. J Dent Res 1966;45:332–336.
4. Delaire J. Confection du masque orthopedique. Rev Stomat Paris 1971;72:579–584.
5. Delaire J. La croissance maxillaire. Trans Eur Orthod Soc 1971:81–102.
6. Delaire J. L'articulation fronto-maxillaire: Bases theoretiques et principles generaux d'application de forces extra-orales postero-anterieures sur masque orthopedique. Rev Stomat Paris 1976;77:921–930.
7. Delaire J, Verdon P, Lumineau JP, Cherga-Negrea A, Talmant J, Boisson M. Note de Tecnique. Rev Stomatol 1972;73:633–642.
8. Delaire VJ, Verdon P, Floor J. Moglichkeiten und Grenzen Extraoraler Kratie in Postereo-anterior Richtung unter Verwandung der Orthopadischen Maske. Forsch Keiferorthop 1978;39:27–45.
9. Nanda R. Biomechanical and clinical considerations of a protraction headgear. Am J Orthod 1980;78:125–139.
10. Dietrich UC. Morphological variability of skeletal Class III relationships as revealed by cephalometric analysis. Trans Eur Orthod Soc 1970;46:131–140.
11. Guyer EC, Ellis E, McNamara JA Jr, Behrents RG. Components of Class III malocclusion in juveniles and adolescents. Angle Orthod 1986;56:7–30.
12. Williams S, Andersen CE. The morphology of the potential Class III skeletal pattern in the growing child. Am J Orthod 1986;89:302–311.
13. Dellinger EL. A preliminary study of anterior maxillary displacement. Am J Orthod 1973;63:509–516.
14. Jackson GW, Kokich VG, Shapiro PA. Experimental and

postexperimental response to anteriorly directed extraoral force in young *Macaca nemestrina*. Am J Orthod 1979;75:318–333.

15. Kambara T. Dentofacial changes produced by extraoral forward force in the *Macaca irus*. Am J Orthod 1977;71:249–277.

16. Nanda R, Hickory W. Zygomaticomaxillary suture adaptations incident to anteriorly-directed forces in rhesus monkeys. Angle Orthod 1984;54:199–210.

17. Nanda R. Protraction of maxilla in rhesus monkeys by controlled extraoral forces. Am J Orthod 1978;74:121–141.

18. Baccetti T, Franchi L, McNamara JA Jr. Treatment and post-treatment craniofacial changes following rapid maxillary expansion and facial mask therapy. Am J Orthod Dentofac Orthop 2000;118:404–411.

19. Baccetti T, McGill JS, Franchi L, McNamara JA Jr, Tollaro I. Skeletal effects of early treatment of Class III malocclusion with maxillary expansion and face-mask therapy. Am J Orthod Dentofac Orthop 1998;113:333–343.

20. MacDonald KE, Kapust AJ, Turley PK. Cephalometric changes after correction of Class III malocclusion with maxillary expansion/facemask therapy. Am J Orthod Dentofac Orthop 1999;116:13–24.

21. McGill JS, McNamara JA Jr. Treatment and post-treatment effects of rapid maxillary expansion and facial mask therapy. In: McNamara JA Jr, ed. Growth modification: What works, what doesn't and why. Monograph 36, Craniofacial Growth Series. Ann Arbor: Center for Human Growth and development, University of Michigan, 1999.

22. Ngan P, Hagg U, Yiu C, Merwin D, Wei SH. Treatment response to maxillary expansion and protraction. Eur J Orthod 1996;18:151–168.

23. Ngan P, Yiu C, Hu A, Hagg U, Wei SH, Gunel E. Cephalometric and occlusal changes following maxillary expansion and protraction. Eur J Orthod 1998;20:237–254.

24. Pangrazio-Kulbersh V, Berger J, Kersten G. Effects of protraction mechanics on the midface. Am J Orthod Dentofac Orthop 1998;114:484–491.

25. Turley PK. Orthopedic correction of Class III malocclusion with palatal expansion and custom protraction headgear. J Clin Orthod 1988;22:314–325.

26. Ngan P, Hagg U, Yiu C, Wei H. Treatment response and long-term dentofacial adaptations to maxillary expansion and protraction. Semin Orthod 1997;3:255–264.

27. Shanker S, Ngan P, Wade D, et al. Cephalometric A point changes during and after maxillary protraction and expansion. Am J Orthod Dentofac Orthop 1996;110:423–430.

28. Hickory WB, Nanda R. Effect of tensile force magnitude on release of cranial suture cells into S phase. Am J Orthod Dentofac Orthop 1987;91:328–334.

29. Tanne K, Hiraga J, Kakiuchi K, Yamagata Y, Sakuda M. Biomechanical effect of anteriorly directed extraoral forces on the craniofacial complex: a study using the finite element method. Am J Orthod Dentofac Orthop 1989;95:200–207.

30. Tanne K, Sakuda M. Biomechanical and clinical changes of the craniofacial complex from orthopedic maxillary protraction. Angle Orthod 1991;61:145–152.

31. Miki M. An experimental research on the directional of the complex by means of the external force—two dimensional analysis on the sagittal plane of the craniofacial skeleton. J Tokyo Dent Coll 1979;79:1563–1597.

32. Hata S, Itoh T, Nakagawa M, et al. Biomechanical effects of maxillary protraction on the craniofacial complex. Am J Orthod 1987;91:305–311.

33. Lee K, Ryu Y, Park Y, Rudolph D. A study of holographic interferometry on the initial reaction of maxillofacial complex during protraction. Am J Orthod 1997;111:623–632.

34. Keles A, Erverdi N, Sezen S. Bodily distalization of molars with absolute anchorage. Angle Orthod 2003;73:471–482.

Orthodontic Anchorage
and Skeletal Implants

Nejat Erverdi, Ahmet Keles, and Ravindra Nanda

The importance of anchorage in orthodontics can best be described by the famous quote from the Greek philosopher Archimedes: "Give me a place to stand and I will move the earth." Orthodontic anchorage can also be explained by the third law of Newton, which states that every action creates a reaction, which is equal in size and opposite in direction. The anatomic unit, which antagonizes the active force, is called anchorage in orthodontics.

Anchorage preparation is a very important part of orthodontic treatment. The success of orthodontic treatment generally relies on the anchorage protocol planned for that particular case. When preparing anchorage, the clinician must be realistic enough to foresee the possibility of losing some anchorage. Anchorage loss can result from unrealistic anchorage construction as well as lack of patient cooperation. The type of anchorage is based on the desired type of tooth movement. Maximum anchorage is frequently required in the treatment of orthodontic cases and is usually obtained by extraoral appliances. Adults and teenagers are prone to reject extraoral appliances because of esthetic problems and the discomfort they cause.[1-3] Thus, different intraoral mechanics to gain maximum anchorage have been designed by various investigators.

The term maximum anchorage refers to the type of anchorage, in which up to one-quarter of the extraction space is taken up by the anchor teeth in the course of treatment. In some instances it is necessary to use 100% of the extraction space for the movement of the anterior teeth in order to reach the treatment goal. Such anchorage is termed stationary anchorage, which cannot be obtained by conventional mechanics in every case. It usually requires the use of extraoral appliances. In some cases even stationary anchorage may not be enough and to reach the treatment goal an extra space in the dental arch may be necessary. This can also be achieved with extraoral appliances or an intraoral appliance. It was shown by various investigators that intraoral molar distalization appliances create some anchorage loss, which manifests as an increase in incisor proclination.[4-7]

Recent developments in osseointegration have made it possible to use implants for orthodontic anchorage.[8-13] Since the implant is known to behave like an ankylosed tooth, it can be used as a reliable anchorage unit for orthodontic tooth movement. The use of implants in orthodontics involves tooth replacement or intraoral rigid anchorage assistance in the movement of teeth. Experimental biomechanic studies,[14,15] studies on animal models,[15-20] and clinical investigations[21-23] have shown that dental implants placed in the alveolar bone are resistant to orthodontic force application. However, orthodontic patients usually have an intact dentition with no available sites for implant placement. The retromolar area[11,24] and palatal region[25-30] have been suggested as alternative anatomic sites by different investigators.

This chapter discusses the use of some nonroot form implants and presents some biomechanic procedures and example cases.

Anatomic Sites for Orthodontic Implant Placement

In cases with multiple lost teeth in the dental arch, placement of implants at the beginning of treatment is a useful procedure.[31] These implants will serve first as anchor units during orthodontic treatment and then as abutments for the restorations after orthodontic treatment. In such cases, the implants must be positioned accurately prior to orthodontics so they can be used as restorative abutments following tooth movement. The overall treatment in these cases has to be planned by a team made up of a prosthodontist, an orthodontist, and an oral surgeon.

In cases without previous tooth loss in the dental arch, orthodontic implants are used only as anchorage units. These are nonroot form onplants and implants that can be placed in nonalveolar bone and explanted after treatment.[11,24–30]

Several criteria must be evaluated prior to the selection of the implant site for nonalveolar implants:

1. A location has to be selected that can be used as an indirect or direct anchorage for the planned biomechanics.
2. Care must be taken not to create any root, nerve, or artery injury.
3. The implant site must contain enough depth and thickness of bone material.
4. Areas rich in cortical bone are preferred as they improve the primary stability of the implant.

The hard palate, mandibular retromolar area, inferior border of zygomatic buttress, symphysis region, and labial or buccal interradicular bone are usually the sites of choice for orthodontic implant placement.

Palatal Implants

The hard palate is used as an anchorage site in most maxillary biomechanic procedures. The Nance appliance is a moderate anchorage appliance, which can be used in both extraction and nonextraction cases. The hard palate may serve also as an anchorage site for intraoral molar distalization. Anchorage loss can manifest as an increase in incisor overjet during intraoral molar distalization.[4–7] Palatal implants can be used as direct or indirect anchorage units for regular maxillary mechanics.

Anatomic Restrictions in Palatal Implant Placement

Bone Thickness for Implant Placement
The minimum bone thickness necessary for palatal implant placement is 4 mm. The hard palate is composed of a thin bone structure in the vertical direction. Generally, the bone thickness does not exceed 3 mm in the hard palate. The midpalatal suture, the area adjacent to the midpalatal suture, and the incisor region are the exceptions.

Incisive Nerve Injury
Implants placed in an anterior location along the midpalatal suture area can create incisive nerve injury. Bernhard et al[32] carried out a study in 22 patients using CT scans and reported that in order not to perforate the incisive canal, the implant must be placed 6–9 mm distal to it.[32]

Root Injuries
Palatal implants placed in the anterior slope of the hard palate can cause incisor root injuries. In some cases, the implant and incisor root may not be in contact but they can be in close proximity; if incisor retraction is carried out as a part of the treatment, root injuries can easily result.

Placing the Palatal Implant Paramedially
As the bone thickness is maximum in the midpalatal suture area, some clinicians recommend placing the palatal implants directly in the midpalatal suture.[29,30] In cases with complete suture ossification, this will not cause any problem. On the other hand, implant loss can result in cases with an unossified suture. As the implant will be in contact with the fibrous tissue in the suture, the chances of total osseointegration will be lower compared to implants with paramedial implantation. Melsen et al[33] concluded that ossification in the midpalatal suture is variable and is completed after the age of 27 years in males and even later in females. Schlegel et al[34] carried out a study on cadavers and reported that the thickness of the connective tissue in the midpalatal suture was 0.03 mm and the thickness of the implant was 0.4 cm. They concluded that this narrow band of connective tissue would not create a serious problem for osseointegration. Anyhow, we suggest a paramedial placement of palatal implants in order to avoid this minimal negative effect.

Palatal Artery Injury
There is always the possibility of causing an arterial injury in punch burr application. To prevent bleeding during the operation, infusion of an anesthetic with a vasoconstricting agent is recommended around the area where the implant is intended to be placed. In instances where there is aggressive bleeding, suturing of the artery is recommended.

To avoid the complications described above, an implant must be placed with special care. An acrylic resin template, including a cylindrical metal housing (similar to the stents that are used in implantology for prosthetic purposes), must be used. A method, which was developed for precise placement of palatal implants, is explained below.

Method for Palatal Implant Placement
Preparation of Acrylic Resin Template
A spherical metal marker is embedded in an acrylic resin template, which covers the occlusal surfaces of the maxillary teeth (Fig. 14-1). The metal marker is placed at

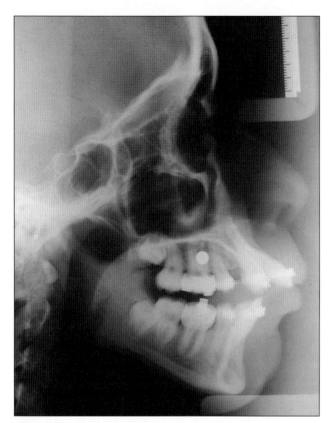

Fig. 14-1 Lateral cephalogram with the acrylic template including a metal marker.

the highest point of the palate in the midline. The purpose of placing a metal marker is to calculate the magnification of the radiograph when assessing the exact bony dimensions of the area where the implant is to be placed. At least 4 mm of bone thickness is required in this area. Moreover, the metal marker creates a reference point in the sagittal direction for identifying the location of the drilling site for implant placement.

Radiographic Evaluation
A lateral cephalogram with the patient wearing the maxillary acrylic template is obtained (see Fig. 14-1). Bone depth in the area where the implant is to be placed is measured in relation to the metal marker which has a diameter of 5 mm. Cases having at least 4 mm of bone height are accepted as suitable for palatal implant placement, and cases without enough bone thickness are candidates for onplant placement.

Preparation of the Surgical Template for Positioning the Implant
The plaster cast used for template preparation is cut along the paramedian line, passing through the mesial aspect of the central incisor. On the lateral cephalogram, radiographic views of the maxilla and central incisor are traced on tracing paper and then a cut is made along the pencil line and carried to the paramedian section of the plaster

cast. A drill insertion hole is prepared in the acrylic resin template, using a 2.5 mm diameter stainless steel burr. A cylindrical metal housing, 7 mm in length and 2.1 mm in diameter, which contains a pilot drill, is placed in the implant access hole. The extension of the implant drill is adjusted to 8 mm from the metal housing. In the sagittal plane, the desired implant inclination in relation to the incisor roots and the nasal cavity is defined. The implant axis is adjusted between 45 and 60° to the occlusal plane, pointing to the anterior nasal spine (ANS). Care is taken to place the implant at least 3–4 mm above the apices of the incisor roots. The metal housing is fixed to the acrylic plate by some cold curing acrylic. In the transverse plane, the metal housing should have a lateral orientation with 2 mm of distance from the palatine suture. Thus, a three-dimensional surgical template for accurate implant angulation is obtained (Fig. 14-2).

Surgical Method
After mouth rinsing for 1 min with 0.2% chlorhexidine gluconate, the palatal region is locally anesthetized using an agent that also has a vasoconstrictive effect. The three-dimensional surgical template is placed in the mouth to mark the implant position. A pilot drill is applied through the metal housing in the template. After this, mucosa is removed using a punch drill, and the standard surgical protocol for placing the chosen implant system is followed. Drilling is carried out at 1000 rpm under internal and external sterile saline cooling. Drills with 8 mm long stoppers are used in the following order: a pilot drill of 2 mm diameter, a twist drill of 3 mm diameter, and a spade drill of 4.5 mm diameter (Fig.14-3A-E).

In the standard surgical protocols for almost all implant systems, the implant carrier is removed after the initial placement of the implant in the cavity before screwing. The implant is placed transmucosally so that 4 mm of the implant will stay in the bone and 4 mm will stay in the palatal mucosa and serve as an extension to reach the oral cavity (Fig. 14-3F-K). Transmucosal placement of the implant has the advantage of avoiding the need for secondary surgery. To avoid postoperative pain, an analgesic agent is recommended and the patient is instructed to use an antiseptic mouth wash twice a day for 2 weeks. The recommended osseointegration period for palatal implants is 3 months and during this period the implant must not be loaded.

Testing Accuracy
The accuracy of the implant placement method was tested by superimposing the presurgical lateral cephalogram with the template and the postsurgical lateral cephalogram with the implant (Fig. 14-3L-N).

Evaluation
The method seems to be successful and practical, with only a few complications, like slight bleeding which can

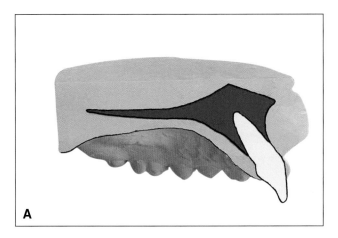

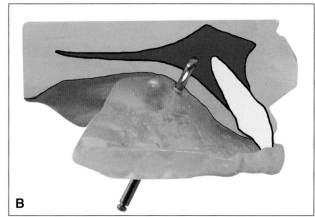

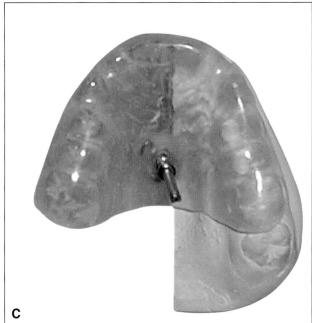

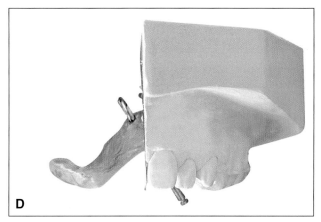

Fig. 14-2 **A** Lateral cephalometric tracing of the maxilla superimposed on the model. **B** Orientation of the pilot burr in relation to the incisor root. **C** Acrylic template and pilot burr. **D** Orientation of the pilot burr in frontal section.

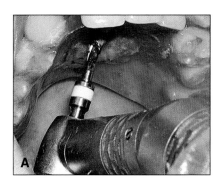

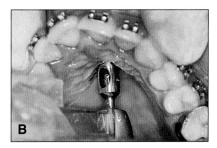

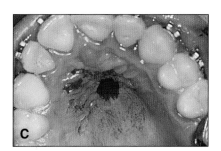

Fig. 14-3 **A** Pilot drill and **B** punch drill application. **C** Mucosa removed by punch drill.

Continued

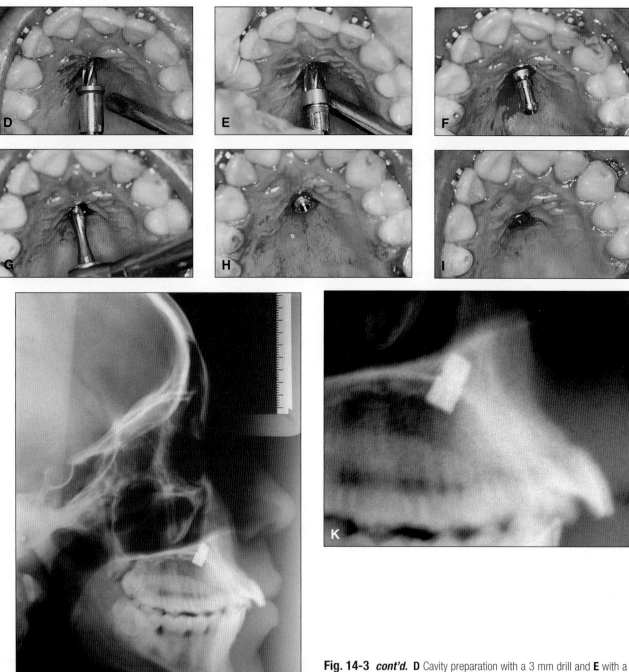

Fig. 14-3 *cont'd.* **D** Cavity preparation with a 3 mm drill and **E** with a 4.5 mm drill. **F** Implant placed in the cavity. **G** Screwing. **H** Implant carrier removed. **I** Transmucosal placement. **J** Radiologic evaluation. **K** Implant and incisor root relationship. *Continued*

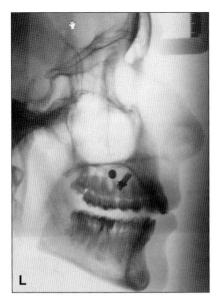 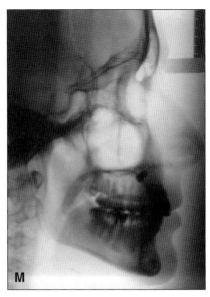 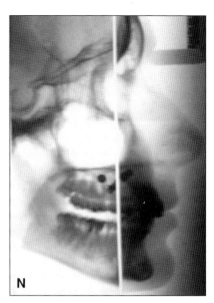

Fig. 14-3 *cont'd.* **L** Lateral cephalogram with template, including metal spherical marker and metal housing. **M** View of the palatal implant placed with the guidance of the metal housing in the template. **N** Cephalograms with metal housing and palatal implant were superimposed to test the accuracy of the method. On the superimposed radiographs, the implant looked like an extension of the metal housing, indicating the accurate positioning of the implant.

be easily controlled. Patient comfort during and after the operation is excellent and the procedure does not last >10 min. The only risk related to this procedure is the possibility of the implant carrier being swallowed by the patient while it is being removed in the conventional way. The location of the implant and possible vomiting reflex during the removal of the implant carrier are the two factors creating this risk. To avoid this risk, a safe method was developed especially for the removal of the implant carrier.

Safe Method for Removal of the Implant Carrier

To avoid the risk of the implant carrier being swallowed, it is recommended that it is removed when it is outside the mouth, and to carry the implant to the cavity while it is seated on the screwing instrument. Care must be taken to hold the implant by Weingart pliers from the polished band, which is designed normally for gingival attachment. The implant holder is removed while the implant is being held by Weingart pliers and the implant is seated on the screwing instrument. Then, the implant is carried to the cavity by the screwing instrument and screwed directly (Fig. 14-4).

Healing Cap Application

After waiting 3 months for osseointegration, a healing cap of proper length is screwed onto the implant. One week is usually enough for shaping of the palatal mucosa (Fig. 14-5).

Laboratory Procedures

After completion of the healing period, a transfer kit is screwed onto the implant and a plastic cap is mounted. Molar bands and an impression post are transferred to the plaster cast by a conventional impression technique. If needed, premolar bands are transferred too. An orthodontic abutment (Friadent, Mannheim, Germany) is fixed to the implant analog on the plaster (Fig.14.6).

Stationary Anchorage

On the plaster cast, a segment of stainless steel wire of 1.5 mm in diameter is bent to connect the anchor teeth to the orthodontic abutment and is then soldered to the bands (Fig. 14-7). Care is taken not to overheat the wire and not to create dead wire which can be a cause of anchorage loss.

Orthodontic Mechanics with Palatal Implants

Using this stationary anchorage supported by a palatal implant, various procedures like en masse retraction of six anterior teeth, canine distalization, and correction of excessive crowding, can be carried out without any anchorage loss.

For molar distalization with buccal mechanics, orthodontic abutment of the palatal implant can be connected to the first premolars. Molars can also be distalized using the Keles slider type of palatal mechanics supported by palatal anchorage.[35–39]

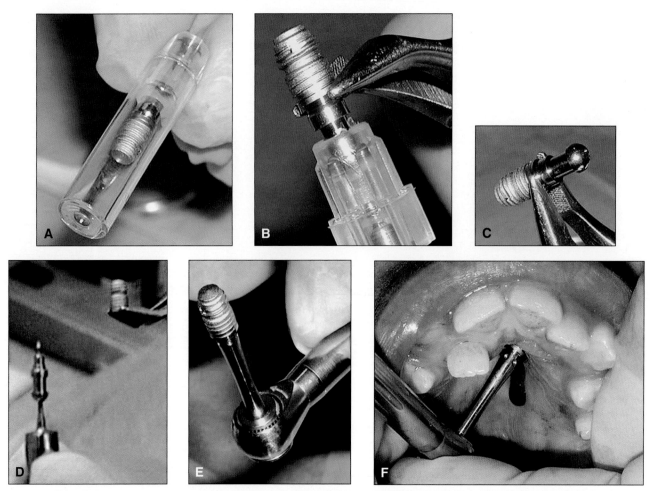

Fig. 14-4 A Frialit 2 implant. **B** Implant held from the polished surface by Weingart pliers. **C** Implant with its carrier. **D** Implant carrier removed. **E** Implant seated on the screwing device. **F** Implant carried to the cavity.

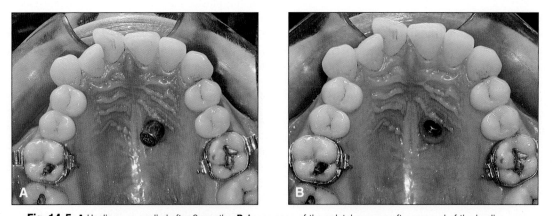

Fig. 14-5 A Healing cap applied after 3 months. **B** Appearance of the palatal mucosa after removal of the healing cap.

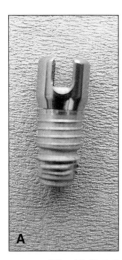
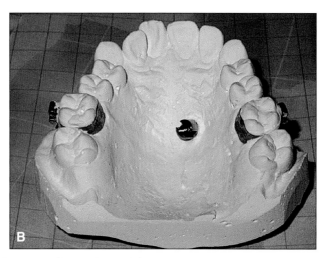

Fig. 14-6 A Special abutment for orthodontics. **B** Orthodontic abutment and bands.

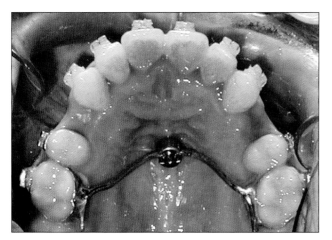

Fig. 14-7 Appliance for stationary anchorage.

Molar Distalization with Palatal Mechanics

Molar bands and implant abutment are transferred to the plaster cast as explained above. Teuscher tubes (Leone, Florence, Italy) are soldered to the palatal aspects of the molar bands in parallel orientation to the central sulcus of the molar crown. The Keles slider appliance is modified and the steel rods are prepared from 1 mm thick stainless steel round wire. Ten mm long nickel–titanium open coil-springs with a diameter of 2 mm and Gurin locks (3M Unitek, Monrovia, California) to fix these coil-springs are mounted on the molar slider bilaterally (Fig. 14-8). Figure 14-9 shows a patient treated with the modified Keles slider using palatal anchorage.

Explantation

The palatal implant is removed easily by first loosening the implant with the help of a hollow drill and then unscrewing it with a screwing instrument in the counterclockwise direction. The implant site heals rapidly within approximately 5 days (Fig. 14-10).

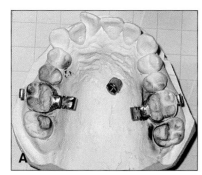
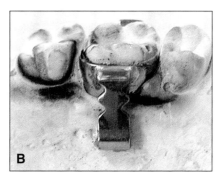
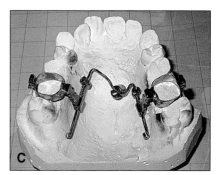

Fig. 14-8 A Bands with Teuscher tubes and orthodontic abutment. **B** Position of the tubes. **C** Keles slider appliance is modified for implant anchorage.

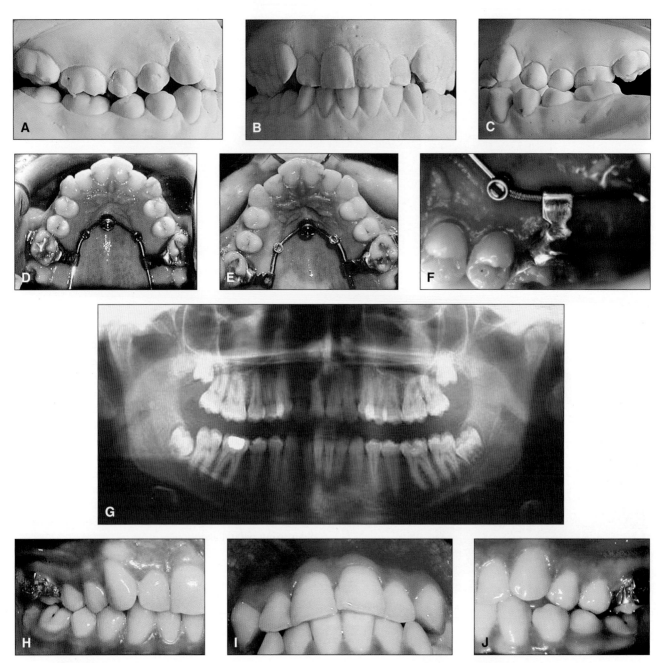

Fig. 14-9 A 16-year-old female patient with anterior crowding and Class II molar and canine relationship on both sides. **A** Right side posterior, **B** frontal, and **C** left side posterior views. **D** Before and **E** after molar distalization. **F** Point of force application is at the level of the first molar trifurcation. **G** Point of force application–center of resistance relationship. **H** Right side molars in super Class I relationship. **I** The overjet did not increase, indicating that there was no anchorage loss. **J** Left side molars in super Class I.   *Continued*

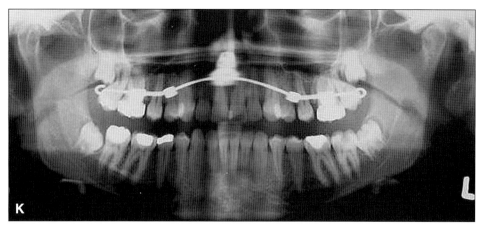

Fig. 14-9 *cont'd.* **K** Panoramic radiograph after distalization, showing that the molars were distalized without tipping.

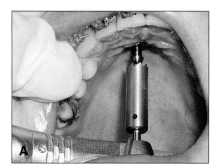
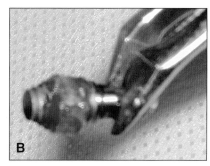
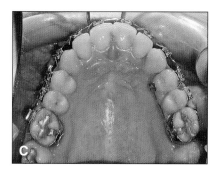

Fig. 14-10 **A** Application of the hollow drill. **B** Explanted implant. **C** Healed palatal mucosa after 1 week.

Zygomatic Anchorage

The maxilla is made up of thin cortical bone in its buccal and labial aspects. Bone thickness is not >2 mm except in the three buttress areas—the posterior buttress close to the tuber area; the zygomatic buttress; and the nasal buttress close to the nasal area. All these areas contain a thick and solid bony structure, which makes implant placement possible. The anatomic location of the posterior buttress prevents easy access to this area. The nasal buttress area is not suitable because of its close location to the infraorbital foramen and nasal cavity. The inferior border of the zygomaticomaxillary buttress is therefore the most suitable area for implant placement because of its anatomic location, which gives an opportunity for easy and direct access (Fig. 14-11). A second advantage of the zygomatic area is that it is distant from critical anatomic structures like nerves and blood vessels. Owing to its close location to the first molar, the zygomatic buttress can be used directly as anchorage or as an indirect anchorage to support the maxillary molar anchorage. Zygomatic buttress anchorage can also be used for the intrusion of maxillary dentoalveolar segments, which can otherwise only be achieved by orthognathic surgery.[40]

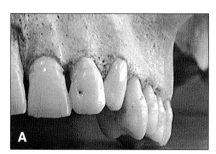
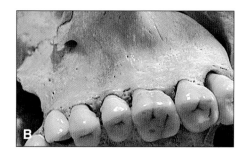
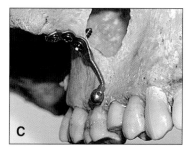

Fig. 14-11 **A-C** Location of the zygomaticomaxillary buttress on a dry skull.

As the zygomatic anchorage is located approximately in the middle of the maxillary half, it is possible to carry the anchor to any area where it is needed simply by bending the extension of the implant in the distal or mesial direction. A multipurpose implant (MPI) has been developed for use as an orthodontic anchorage unit.

Multipurpose Implant

An implant in the form of a surgical miniplate with a round bar extension has been developed from pure titanium for general use as an orthodontic anchorage unit (patented to Erverdi by Tasarim Med, Istanbul, Turkey) (Fig. 14-12). The MPI has two parts: a retentive part in the form of a surgical miniplate with three holes for miniscrews; and a round bar extension which is 20 mm long and bendable. Formability of the extension bar makes it possible to carry the anchor to the area where it is required. The extension bar has thick and thin types; the thick one has a diameter of 0.9 mm and is recommended for use during molar distalization, while the thin one has a diameter of 0.7 mm and is suitable for use during open bite treatment and consolidation.

Surgical Procedure

After mouth rinsing for 1 min with 0.2% chlorhexidine gluconate, the zygomatic buttress region is anesthetized using a local anesthestic with a vasoconstrictor agent. An L-shaped incision is made, beginning with a vertical incision passing 5 mm mesial to the inferior crest of the zygomaticomaxillary buttress. This incision is continued with a small horizontal incision in the mesial direction, along the intersection of the mobile and attached gingiva. The mucoperiosteum is elevated and the upper part of the MPI is adapted to the bony curvature using orthodontic

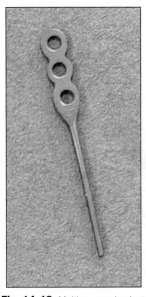

Fig. 14-12 Multipurpose implant.

pliers. The bar of the implant which extends into the oral cavity is bent to make a step at the level of the horizontal incision. Care is taken to adjust the length of the step so that it will not apply pressure on the attached gingiva. The round bar is bent differently according to the aim of the treatment.

Molar Distalization Using Multipurpose Implant Anchorage

For molar distalization, an MPI with a 0.9 mm bar thickness is used. The upper part of the MPI is adapted to the bony curvature, 5 mm mesial to the line passing from the mesial edge of the first molar tube. The round bar is extended in the downward direction to the level of the first molar tube and then bent in the mesial direction along the sulcus depth 3 mm apart from the vestibular mucosa. A 1 mm thick stainless steel round wire is soldered onto the lower surface of the custom fabricated metal sliding lock (Dentaurum), extending towards the archwire. A horizontal U bend is made in the wire to be used in adjusting the force vector. A segmental round tube is soldered to the lower edge of the round wire at the same level as the main archwire, to be used for compressing the open coil-spring (Fig. 14-13A). The metal sliding lock is engaged on the mesial extension of the zygomatic implant. A 0.016" stainless steel archwire is engaged passing through the segmental tube, a segmental nickel–titanium open coil-spring is placed on the archwire after the segmental tube, and the archwire is engaged in the main tube of the molar band. A metal sliding lock is slid in the distal direction so that sufficient activation of the open coil-spring is obtained and is fixed in that position (Fig. 14-13B).

Open Bite Treatment

Open bite is one of the most difficult malocclusions to treat and to maintain the treatment results. Several approaches for the treatment of open bite have been reported. Some investigators used fixed appliances with multilooped archwires and intermaxillary elastics,[41,42] while others used preformed reverse curved nickel–titanium arches and intermaxillary elastics.[43] Other investigators used posterior bite blocks with and without magnets[44–47] and others applied functional appliances[48] for the treatment of anterior open bite. In all these procedures anterior open bite was treated by the extrusion of anterior teeth rather than the intrusion of posterior dentition. Ohmae et al[49] in an animal model and Umemori et al[50] in humans applied titanium miniplates to the mandibular corpus area and used them as anchorage for the intrusion of mandibular posterior segments. They were able to intrude the mandibular posterior dentoalveolar segments and correct the anterior open bite. This can be an effective way of anterior open bite treatment in cases with overerupted mandibular molars.

In most anterior open bite cases, the malocclusion is morphologically characterized by overeruption of the maxillary posterior teeth and the resultant posterior rotation

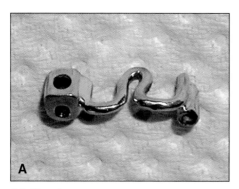
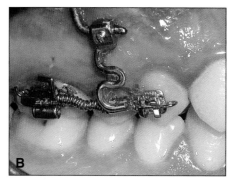

Fig. 14-13 A Sliding bar extension and segmental tube. **B** Sliding lock is fixed in the position activating the coil-spring.

of the mandible. True treatment of anterior open bite requires intrusion of the maxillary posterior segments and anterior rotation of the mandible. The only treatment modality in which this goal can be achieved effectively is orthognathic surgery.[40]

As the zygomatic anchor is located in a superior position in relation to the maxillary posterior dentition, it is possible by using its support to achieve maxillary posterior dentoalveolar intrusion and mandibular anterior rotation for the correction of anterior open bite.[51,52]

Before the development of MPIs, surgical miniplates were used as zygomatic anchors. A patient treated with this approach is shown in Figure 14-14. Miniplates were adapted and fixed with three miniscrews to the inferior border of the zygomatic buttress. The free end of the plate was extended to the oral cavity and exposed through the line of horizontal incision. Closed nickel–titanium coil-springs were applied between the free end of the miniplate and the maxillary posterior dentition (Fig. 14-14F-H). To prevent buccal tipping of the molars during intrusion, a transpalatal arch constructed from 1.5 mm stainless steel round wire was used (Fig. 14-14I). The transpalatal arch passed at least 3 mm from the palatal mucosa in order not to hinder molar intrusion.

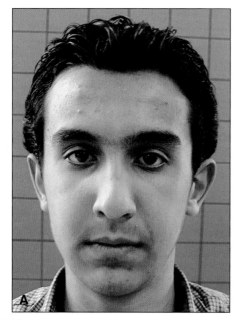
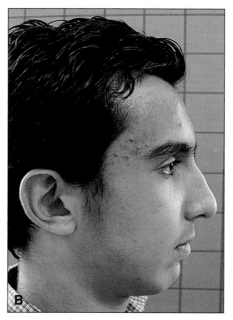

Fig. 14-14 A 21-year-old patient with a high angle growth pattern, Class II molar and canine relationship, anterior crowding, and open bite. The treatment plan involved extraction of the upper first premolars to resolve crowding and intrusion of the upper posterior segments to close the open bite. **A** and **B** Extraoral views. *Continued*

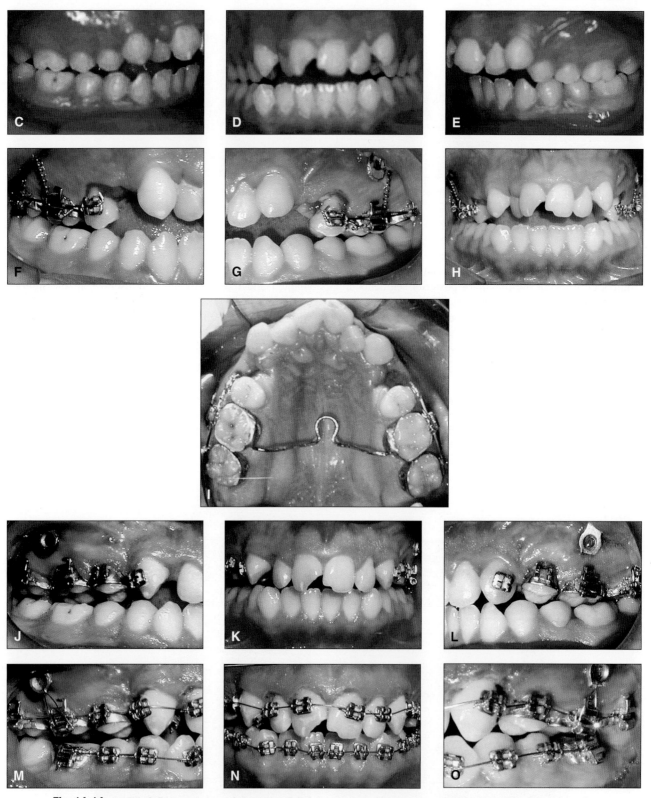

Fig. 14-14 *cont'd.* **C-E** Intraoral views of the patient. **F-H** Following upper first premolar extractions, intrusion of the right and left posterior segments was initiated using nickel–titanium closed coil-springs which were placed between the free ends of the miniplates and the first molar tubes. **I** Transpalatal arch to prevent buccal tipping of the molars. **J-L** Intraoral views of the patient after 5 months of posterior intrusion. **M-O** Intraoral views of the patient after 8 months of treatment. *Continued*

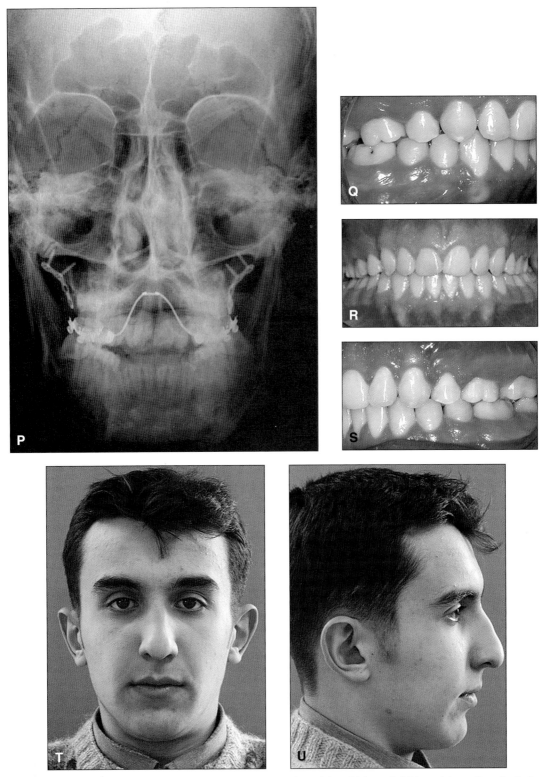

Fig. 14-14 *cont'd.* **P** Posteroanterior radiograph showing the locations of the miniplates. **Q-S** Intraoral views after orthodontic treatment is completed. **T** and **U** Extraoral views of the patient after treatment.   *Continued*

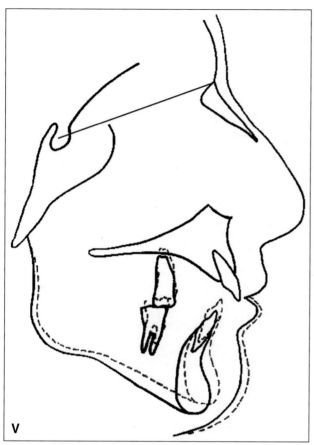

Fig. 14-14 *cont'd.* **V** Schematic illustration of the dental and skeletal changes related to treatment. Note the counterclockwise rotation of the mandible.

Evaluation of the Treatment Modality

This treatment method was found to be effective but some problems arose during the procedure:

- Surgical miniplates were bulky and created some hygiene problems and discomfort.
- Occlusal interferences prevented anterior rotation of the mandible.
- The transpalatal arch was not enough to prevent buccal tipping of the molars during intrusion.

Use of Multipurpose Implant in Open Bite Treatment

During the treatment of open bite, the MPI can be used as a stationary anchorage unit. The round bar is bent distally to form a hook at a level as high as possible after leaving the soft tissue. A 0.7 mm thick round bar is suitable as a stationary anchorage unit (Fig. 14-15A and B). The reduction in bar thickness will have a positive effect on the healing of the mucosa and patient comfort. To prevent buccal tipping of the molars during intrusion, MPIs are used in conjunction with an acrylic cap splint appliance with an open Hyrax screw (Fig. 14-15C). Nickel–titanium closed coil-springs are applied between the MPI and a hook embedded in the acrylic cap splint at the first molar region (Fig. 14-15D and E). The Hyrax screw is gradually closed to counteract the buccal tipping effect of the coil-springs.

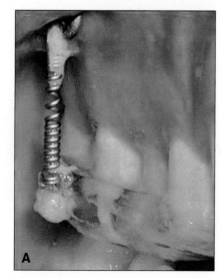
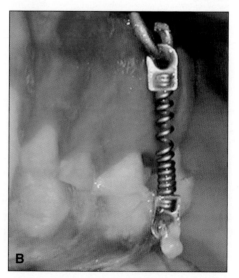

Fig. 14-15 **A** and **B** On both sides, 0.7 mm thick extension wire is bent distally to form a hook to which a nickel–titanium closed coil-spring can be attached.

Continued

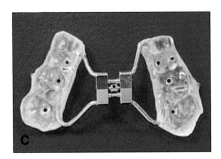
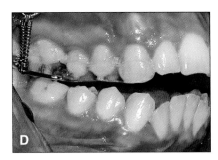
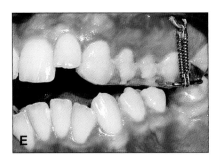

Fig. 14-15 *cont'd.* **C** An open Hyrax screw is incorporated in the cap splint to counteract the buccal tipping of the molars. **D** Right and **E** left side views of the intrusion appliance.

REFERENCES

1. Egolf RJ, Begole EA, Upshaw HS. Factors associated with orthodontic patient compliance with intraoral elastic and headgear wear. Am J Orthod 1990;97:336–348.
2. American Association of Orthodontists. Special bulletin on extra-oral appliance care. Am J Orthod 1975;75:457.
3. American Association of Orthodontists. Preliminary results of head gear survey. Bulletin 1982;1:2.
4. Bondemark L, Kurol J. Distalization of first and second molars simultaneously with repelling magnets. Eur J Orthod 1992;14:264–272.
5. Erverdi N, Koyuturk Ö, Kucukkeles N. Nickel–titanium coil springs and repelling magnets: a comparison of two different intra-oral molar distalization techniques. Br J Orthod 1997;24:47–53.
6. Fuhrmann R, Wehrbein H, Diedrich P. Anteriore Verankerungsqualitat der odifizierten Nance Apparatur bei der Molarendistalisierung, Fortschr Kieferorthop 1994;8:45–52.
7. Keles A, Sayinsu K. A new approach in maxillary molar distalization: Intraoral bodily molar distalizer. Am J Orthod Dentofacial Orthop 2000;117:39–48.
8. Ödman J, Lekholm U, Jemt T, Branemark P-I, Thilander B. Osseointegrated titanium implants–a new approach in orthodontic treatment. Eur J Orthod 1988;10:98–105.
9. Roberts WE, Smith R, Zilberman Y, Mozsary PG, Smith RS. Osseous adaptation to continous loading of rigid endosseous implants. Am J Orthod 1984;86:95–111.
10. Roberts WE, Helm FR, Marshall KJ, Gonglof RK. Rigid endosseous implants for orthodontic and orthopedic anchorage. Angle Orthod 1989;59:247–256.
11. Roberts WE, Marshall KJ, Mozsary PG. Rigid endosseous implant utilized as anchorage to protract molars and close an atrophic extraction site. Angle Orthod 1990;60:135–152.
12. Turley PK, Kean C, Sehur J, et al. Orthodontic force application to titanium endosseous implants. Angle Orthod 1988;58:151–162.
13. Van Roekel NB. The use of Branemark system implants for orthodontic anchorage: Report of a case. Int J Oral Maxillofac Implants 1989;4:341–344.
14. Chen J, Chen K, Garetto LP, Roberts WE. Mechanical response to functional and therapeutic loading of a retromolar endosseous implant used for orthodontic anchorage to mesially translate mandibular molars. Implant Dent 1995;4:246–258.
15. Melsen B, Lang NP. Biological reactions of alveolar bone to orthodontic loading of oral implants. Clin Oral Implant Res 2001;12:144–152.
16. Linder-Aronson S, Nordenram A, Anneroth G. Titanium implant anchorage in orthodontic treatment: an experimental investigation in monkeys. Eur J Orthod 1990;12:414–419.
17. Ödman, J, Grondahl K, Lekholm U, Thilander B. The effect of osseointegrated implants on the dento-alveolar development. A clinical and radiographic study in growing pigs. Eur J Orthod 1991;13:279–286.
18. Sennerby L, Ödman J, Lekholm U, Thilander B. Tissue reactions towards titanium implants inserted in growing jaws. A histological study in the pig. Clin Oral Implant Res 1993;4:65–75.
19. Smalley WM, Shapiro PA, Hohl TH, Kokich VG, Branemark P-I. Osseointegrated titanium implants for maxillofacial protraction in monkeys. Am J Orthod Dentofac Orthop 1998;94:285–295.
20. Thilander B, Ödman J, Grondahl K, Lekholm U. Aspects on osseointegrated implants inserted in growing jaws. A biometric and radiographic study in the young pig. Eur J Orthod 1992;14:99–109.
21. Haanaes HR, Stenvik A, Beyer Olsen ES, Tryti T, Faehn O. The efficacy of two-stage titanium implants as orthodontic anchorage in the preprosthodontic correction of third molars in adults: a report of three cases. Eur J Orthod 1991;13:287–292.
22. Ödman J, Lekholm U, Jemt T, Thilander B. Osseointegrated implants as orthodontic anchorage in the treatment of partially edentulous adult patients. Eur J Orthod 1994;16:187–201.
23. Thilander B, Ödman J, Grondahl K, Friberg B. Osseointegrated implants in adolescents. An alternative in replacing missing teeth? Eur J Orthod 1994;16:84–95.
24. Higuchi KW, Slack JM. The use of titanium fixtures for intraoral anchorage to facilitate orthodontic tooth movement. Int J Oral Maxillofac Implants 1991;6:338–344.
25. Abels N, Schiel HJ, Hery-Langer G, Neugebauer J, Engel M. Bone condensing in the placement of endosteal palatal implants: A case report. Int J Oral Maxillofac Implants 1999;14:849–852.
26. Glatzmaier J, Wehrbein H, Diedrich P. Die Entwicklung eines resorbierbaren Implantatsystems zur orthodontischen Verankerung, Fortschr Kieferorthop 1995;6:175–181.

27. Triaca A, Antonini M, Wintermantel E. Ein neues Titan-Flachschraubenimplantat zur Verankerung am anterioren Gaumen. Inf Orthod Orthop 1992;24:251–257.

28. Turley PK, Shapiro PA, Moffett BC. The loading of bioglass-coated aluminum oxide implants to produce sutural expansion of the maxillary complex in the pigtail monkey (*Macaca nemestrina*). Arch Oral Biol 1980;25:459–469.

29. Wehrbein H. Enossale Titanimplantate als orthodontische Verankerungselemente. Experimentelle Untersuchungen und klinische Anwendung. Fortschr Kieferorhop 1994;55:236–250.

30. Wehrbein H, Glatzmaier J, Mundwiller U, Diedrich P. The orthosystem: a new implant system for orthodontic anchorage in the palate. J Orofac Orthop 1996;57:142–153.

31. Higuchi KW. Ortho-integration: The alliance between orthodontics and osseointegration. In: Higuchi KW, ed. Orthodontic implications of osseointegrated implants. Hong Kong, Quitessence, 2000.

32. Bernhart T, Vollgruber A, Gahleitner A, Dörtbudak O, Haas R. Alternative to median region of the palate for placement of an orthodontic implant. Clin Oral Implant Res 2000;11:595–601.

33. Melsen B. Palatal growth studied on human autopsy material. Am J Orthod 1975;68:42–54.

34. Schlegel KA, Kinner F, Schlegel KD. The anatomic basis for palatal implants in orthodontics. Int J Adult Orthod Orthognath Surg 2002;17:133–139.

35. Keles A. Maxillary unilateral molar distalization with sliding mechanics: a preliminary investigation. Eur J Orthod 2001;23:507–515.

36. Keles A, Pamukcu B, Tokmak EC. Bilateral molar distalization with sliding mechanics: Keles Slider. World J Orthod 2002;3:57–66.

37. Keles A. Unilateral distalization of a maxillary molar with sliding mechanics: a case report. J Orthod 2002;29:97–100.

38. Keles A, Erverdi N, Sezen S. Bodily molar distalization with absolute anchorage. Angle Orthod 2003;73:471–482.

39. Tosun T, Keles A, Erverdi N. Method for the placement of palatal implants. Int J Oral Maxillofac Implants 2002;17:95–100.

40. Lawry DM, Heggie AA, Crawford EC, Ruljancich MK. A review of the management of anterior open bite malocclusion. Aust Orthod J 1990;11:147–160.

41. Rinchuse DJ. Vertical elastics for correction of anterior openbite, J Clin Orthod 28:284, 1994.

42. Kim YH. Anterior openbite and its treatment with multiloop edgewise archwire. Angle Orthod 1997;57:171–178.

43. Küçükkeleş N, Acar A, Demirkaya A, Evrenol B, Enacar A. Cephalometric evaluation of openbite treatment with NiTi archwires and anterior elastics. Am J Orthod Dentofac Orthop 1999;116:555–562.

44. Dellinger EL. A clinical assessment of the active vertical corrector. A nonsurgical alternative for skeletal open bite treatment. Am J Orthod Dentofacial Orthop 1986;89:428–436.

45. Kaira V, Burstone CJ, Nanda R. Effects of a fixed magnetic appliance on the dentofacial complex. Am J Orthod Dentofacial Orthop 1989;95:467–478.

46. Kiliaridis S, Egermark B, Thilander B. Anterior openbite treatment with magnets. Eur J Orthod 1990;12: 447–457.

47. İşcan HN, Sarısoy L. Comparison of the effects of passive bite blocks with different construction bites on the craniofacial and dentoalveolar structures. Am J Orthod Dentofacial Orthop 1997;112:171–178.

48. Stellzig A, Steegmayer G, Basdra EK. Elastic activator for treatment of openbite. Br J Orthod 1999;26:89–92.

49. Ohmae M, Saito S, Morohashi T, et al. A clinical and histological evaluation of titanium mini-implants as anchors for orthodontic intrusion in the beagle dog. Am J Orthod Dentofacial Orthop 2001;119:489–497.

50. Umemori M, Sugawara J, Mitani H, Nagasaka H, Kawamura H. Skeletal anchorage system for openbite correction. Am J Orthod Dentofacial Orthop 1999;115:166–174.

51. Erverdi N, Tosun T, Keles A. A new anchorage site for the treatment of anterior openbite. Zygomatic anchorage case report. World J Orthod 2002;43:417–153.

52. Sherwood K, Burch J, Thompson W. Closing anterior open bites by intruding molars with titanium miniplate anchorage. Am J Orthod Dentofacial Orthop 2002;122:593–600.

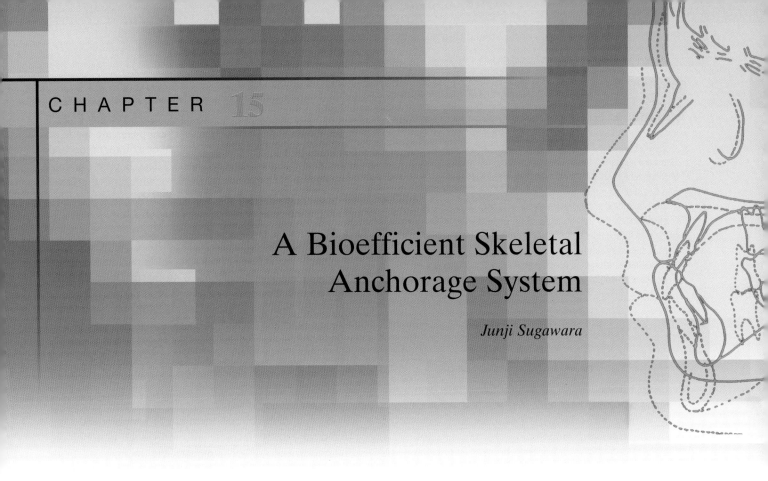

CHAPTER 15

A Bioefficient Skeletal Anchorage System

Junji Sugawara

Anchorage has long been one of the greatest problems in the field of orthodontics because teeth, even molars, move in response to orthodontic forces. Therefore, in maximal anchorage cases, patients have needed to wear headgear. Thus, reinforced anchorage with extraoral appliances has severe limitations because it requires excellent patient compliance.

In the intermaxillary fixation after jaw surgery, maxillofacial surgeons have also found that teeth do not make reliable anchor units. To solve this problem, surgeons proposed "skeletal anchorage" as an adjunct to tooth-borne anchorage. The maxillary teeth and bone were fixed with wires from the anterior nasal spine (ANS), infraorbital rim, or zygomatic arch. The mandibular teeth were anchored to the mandible with wires that circled the mandibular body in the anterior and posterior regions.

In 1983, Creekmore and Eklund[1] reported a severe deep bite case that was successfully treated with a surgical vitallium bone screw inserted just below the ANS to intrude the upper incisors. This was the first clinical report of "skeletal anchorage" for orthodontic tooth movement. A second case was reported by Jenner and Fitzpatrick[2] in 1985. They applied a large bone plate in the ramus to tip the mandibular molar distally with a leading wire and elastics.

Our research group noted that the osteosynthesis titanium miniplate had been thoroughly evaluated as an excellent biocompatible material in the field of maxillofacial surgery. In 1992, we first developed the skeletal anchorage system (SAS) utilizing titanium miniplates[3] and,

since then, SAS mechanics have been applied to various types of malocclusions in daily orthodontic practice.

The advantages and disadvantages of the SAS are listed in Boxes 15-1 and 15-2.

This chapter outlines the SAS and describes a typical case who was treated with the application of SAS.

Box 15-1	Advantages of skeletal anchorage system treatment

Anchor plates are made of pure titanium, making them very stable and safe

Anchor plates do not disturb any kind of tooth movement because they are placed outside the dentition. This is the most distinctive feature of SAS in comparison with the other implant systems currently being used in orthodontics

Molars can be moved easily as teeth in the anterior dentition can be moved. It is now possible to easily control the occlusal plane, and even the level of this plane

Patients are no longer required to wear uncomfortable extraoral appliances, i.e. the SAS can function like an invisible headgear.

Patient compliance is not necessary, except with regard to oral hygiene.

Orthodontic therapy based on treatment goals can go ahead with a very predictable outcome

The quality of orthodontic treatment is raised with SAS

The number of nonextraction cases can be significantly increased

The number of orthognathic surgery cases can be significantly decreased

Box 15-2	Problems with skeletal anchorage system treatment

Infection can be associated with anchor plate implantation. Better methods need to be established to prevent infection

There are limitations to the shapes and sizes of the anchor plates. Improvement in orthodontic anchor plate design is ongoing.

SAS treatment is a symptomatic, not a causative, treatment and, therefore, longterm evaluation is the only way to confirm its effectiveness

Guidelines for the differential diagnosis of the indications for SAS must be established

SAS mechanics has yet to become an established technique. The mechanics need to be continually refined and improved

New Orthodontic Anchor Plates

Because osteosynthesis titanium miniplates were not designed as orthodontic anchor plates and are not necessarily suitable for orthodontic treatment, they were noted to have the following shortcomings:

- The shape of the miniplate is not suitable for the application of orthodontic force.
- The surface of the arm portion which penetrates the mucoperiostium is roughly sandblasted and difficult to clean
- The size of the miniplate is relatively thick and large.

To solve those problems, our research group developed the new orthodontic anchor plates.[4]

Features

Figure 15-1 shows the newly developed anchor plates which are called SMAP (Super Mini Anchor Plate[R]; Dentsply-Sankin, Tokyo, Japan). These plates are made of pure titanium which is suitable for osseointegration and also tissue integration. In addition, Class II pure titanium is used, which is strong enough to withstand the usual orthodontic forces, and can also be bent with ease for fitting into the bone contour of the implantation site.

Figure 15-2 shows an example of the T-type anchor plate. The anchor plate consists of three portions: head, arm, and body. The head portion is intraorally exposed and positioned outside the dentition, so that it never disturbs any kind of tooth movement. Each head portion has three continuous hooks for easier application of orthodontic forces. As the need arises, it is possible to cut off the first and second hooks. There are two types of head portion which differ with regard to the direction of hooks, and which one is used depends on the manner of tooth movement.

The arm portion is transmucosal and has three graduated lengths—short (10.5 mm), medium (13.5 mm), and long (16.5 mm)—to compensate for individual morphologic differences and to accommodate the manner of tooth movement (Fig. 15-3).

The body portion is positioned subperiosteally. There are three basic types: T, Y, and I. The T-type plates are frequently used as L-type plates by cutting off one of the circles. The variations in shape mean that the surgeon can select the most appropriate anchor plate according to the bone contour of the implantation site.

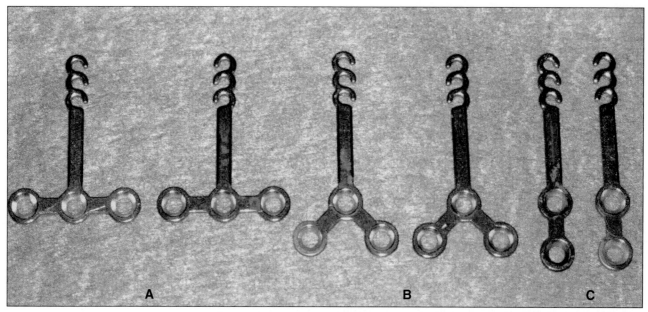

Fig. 15-1 Orthodontic anchor plates. **A** T-, **B** Y-, and **C** I-type.

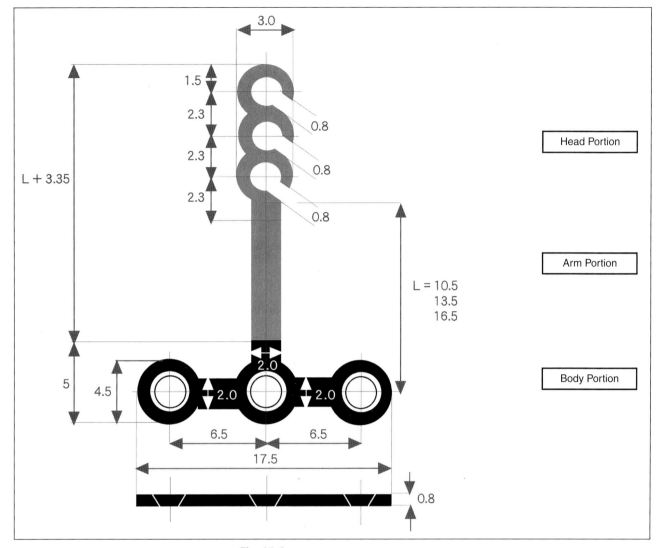

Fig. 15-2 Design of a T-type anchor plate.

In addition, the surface attached to the bone is sandblasted (Fig. 15-4) so that it is osseointegrated more readily. The other surfaces are polished with a mirror-like surface, so that they safely penetrate soft tissue and are effective in plaque control for preventing infection.

Positioning

The implantation site for the anchor plate must have sufficient depth of cortical bone (at least 2–3 mm) to allow it to be fixed with monocortical miniscrews. The screws are also made of pure titanium. Each screw has a head with a tapered inside square and self-tapping thread. The diameter of the screw is 2 mm, and the available lengths are 5 and 7 mm. If the screw becomes loose or bent, an emergency screw with a diameter of 2.2 mm is used.

Figure 15-5 shows the positioning of the orthodontic anchor plates. The Y-type plates are placed in the maxilla at the zygomatic buttress either to intrude or distalize the upper molars. Although the lateral wall of the maxilla is too thin to carry the screws for the anchor plates, the bone of the zygomatic buttress is thick enough. The I-type plates are mostly placed at the anterior ridge of the pyriform opening for intrusion of the upper anterior teeth and protraction of the upper molars. In fact, the areas where titanium screws can be implanted in the maxilla are limited to the zygomatic buttress and the pyriform rim.

The T- and L-type plates are usually placed with titanium miniscrews in the mandibular body to intrude, protract, and distalize the lower molars, or at the anterior border of the mandibular ramus to distalize the molars and tract the impacted second molars. The bone thickness of the lateral cortex in the mandible is sufficient to secure titanium screws at any points except around the foramen mentalis.

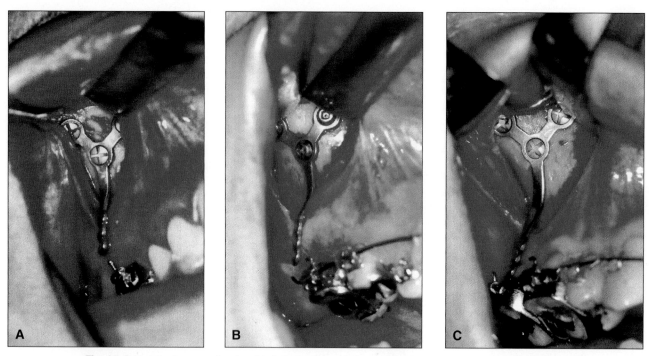

Fig. 15-3 Variation in arm portion (length). **A** Short (10.5 mm), **B** medium (13.5 mm), and **C** long type (16.5 mm).

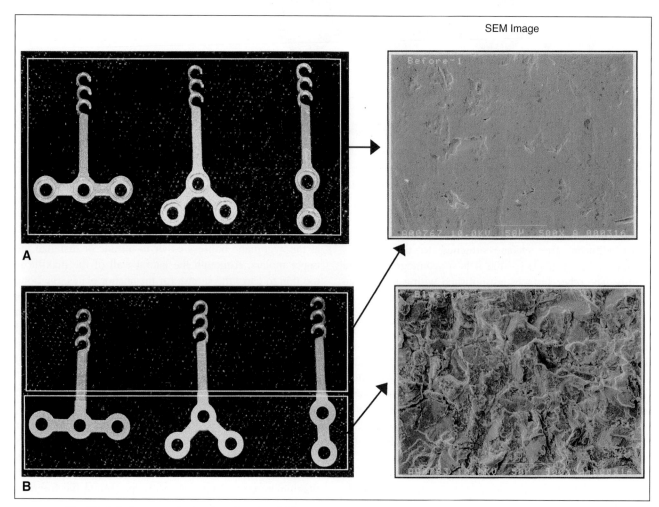

Fig. 15-4 Surface property of each anchor plate. **A** Mucous-attaching (mirror-like) and **B** bone-attaching surface (sandblasted).

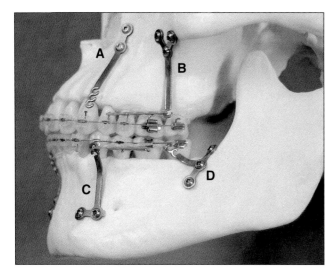

Fig. 15-5 Positioning of anchor plates. **A** I-, **B** Y-, **C** T-, and **D** L-type (modified T-type).

Surgical Procedures

The operation is carried out under local anesthesia administered with intravenous sedation. First, a mucoperiosteal incision is made at the buccal vestibular of the implantation site. A vertical incision is usually made in the maxilla, and a horizontal one in the mandible (Fig. 15-6A and B). The mucoperiosteal flap is elevated following the subperiosteal ablation and the surface of the cortical bone at the implantation site is exposed (Fig. 15-6C and D). Then, the appropriate type of anchor plate is selected according to the distance between the implantation site and the dentition. This should be quite clear from the panoramic X-ray film taken prior to surgery. The selected plate is contoured to fit the bone surface.

A pilot hole is drilled and one self-tapping and monocortical screw is inserted. With the insertion of the remaining screws, the anchor plate is firmly placed on the bone surface (Fig. 15-6E and F). At this moment it is important to make sure that the anchor plate does not disturb mandibular movement or adjacent soft tissues. The wound is finally closed and sutured with absorbable thread (Fig. 15-6G and H). The surgery takes about 10–15 min for each anchor plate.

Timing of Orthodontic Treatment

Most patients who undergo implantation surgery for SAS show mild-to-moderate facial swelling for a week after the operation. This is almost inevitable. In addition, infection occurs in about 10% of patients. Mild infections can be controlled with antiseptic mouth rinses and careful brushing. In more severe cases, antibiotics are needed. Practitioners must thoroughly instruct patients in home care, and professionally clean the plates every 3–4 weeks at routine appointments. This regimen has greatly reduced postsurgical infections.

Orthodontic force is usually applied about 3 weeks after implantation surgery, i.e. once postsurgical management is complete, but before the osseointegration of the titanium screws and plates. Figure 15-7 shows the osseointegration of titanium screws in SAS in an animal model.[5] As shown on the contact microradiograph (CMR) images, the thread of the bone screws is attached directly to the bone because of osseointegration. Loaded bone screws show a higher level of osseointegration than unloaded screws. The loaded bone screw is surrounded by smaller but much more numerous Harvasian system units, and the remodeling of this bone is more significant. This phenomenon suggests that orthodontic force application to the implants promotes higher levels of osseointegration.

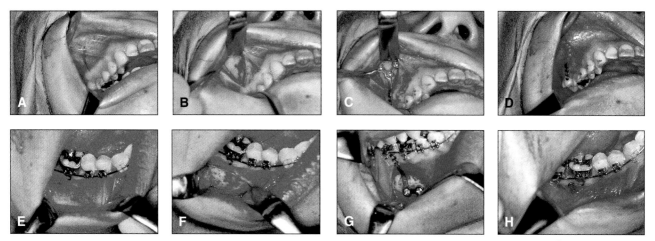

Fig. 15-6 Surgical procedures for implantation of anchor plates. **A-D** Maxilla: **A** incision line, **B** incision and exposure of the implantation site, **C** placement of anchor plates, and **D** suture. **E-H** Mandible: **E** incision line, **F** incision and exposure of the implantation site, **G** placement of anchor plates, and **H** suture.

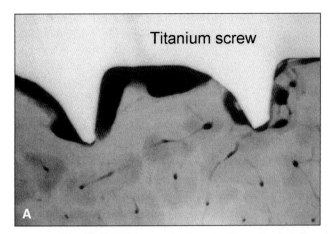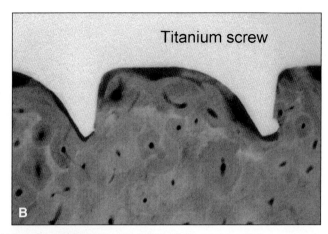

Fig. 15-7 CMR images showing osseointegration of titanium. **A** Unloaded and **B** loaded sample (orthodontic force was applied for 7 months). (Reproduced with permission from Daimaruya T, Nagasaka H, Umemori M, Sugawara J, Mitani H. The influences of molar intrusion on the inferior alveolar neurovascular bundle and root resorption by using anchorage system in dogs. Angle Orthod 2001;71:60–70.)

Removal

Immediately after orthodontic treatment, all anchor plates must be removed. First, a mucoperiosteal incision and subperiosteal ablation are performed at the implantation site (Fig. 15-8A). Then, the implanted anchor plate is exposed. The anchor plates are often observed to be covered with thin new bone (Fig. 15-8B). As shown in Figure 15-8C, even though the monocortical bone screws have been removed, the anchor plate is still firmly attached to the bone surface because of enhanced osseointegration.

After taking the anchor plate off, new bone formation can usually be observed surrounding the plate (Fig. 15-8D).

Skeletal Anchorage System Biomechancis for Molar Movement

Figure 15-9 shows the SAS mechanics for intrusion and distalization of the molars. The SAS has been applied to over 400 patients in our clinic, of whom about 85% needed one of these types of tooth movement.

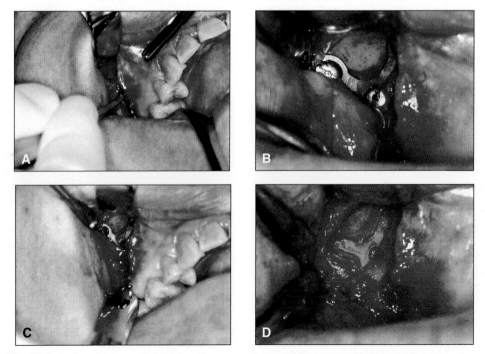

Fig. 15-8 Anchor plate removal. **A** Ablation, **B** exposure, **C** removal of screws, and **D** immediately before suture.

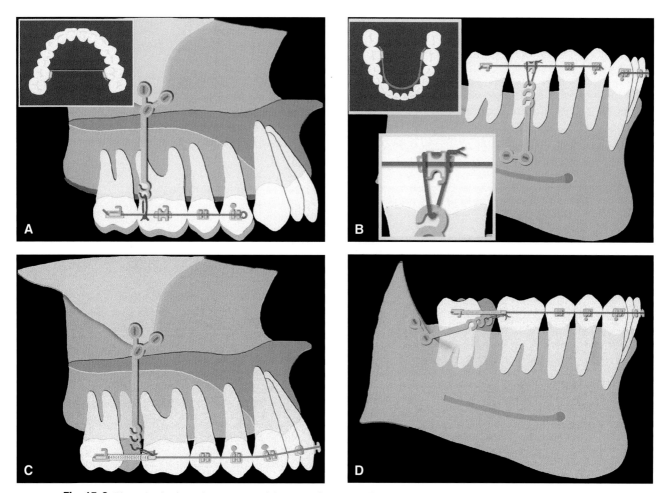

Fig. 15-9 Biomechanics for molar movement. **A** Intrusion of upper and **B** lower molars. **C** Distalization of upper and **D** lower molars.

It has been extremely difficult, if not impossible, to intrude the upper and lower molars with traditional orthodontic mechanotherapies. Impacting the lower molar region especially, even with orthognathic surgery, has posed real problems because of the risk of injuring the inferior alveolar nerve. SAS mechanics, however, can accomplish the intrusion of molars, making it possible to correct even severe open bite cases without orthognathic surgery and without iatrogenic side effects (Fig. 15-9A and B).[5–8]

Distalization of the upper or lower molars has long been considered a very difficult tooth movement even using headgear, and this is especially so in adult patients. However, using SAS mechanics to achieve distalization of the molars, it is now possible to correct even severe crowding, upper protrusion, anterior crossbite, and asymmetric dentition without premolar extraction and without the need for constant patient cooperation (Fig. 15-9C and D).[9,10]

CASE REPORT

Problem List

The patient was a 19-year-old Japanese girl who complained of anterior open bite, difficulty in incising, and temporomandibular joint disorders (TMD). She had mild facial asymmetry, a long face, and a large interlabial gap (Fig. 15-10). Intraorally, she showed severe anterior open bite, crowding of the upper and lower incisors, a narrow upper arch, and large overjet (Fig. 15-11). In addition, ankylosis was suspected in the lower left first molar

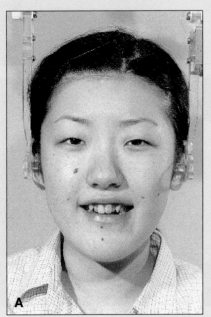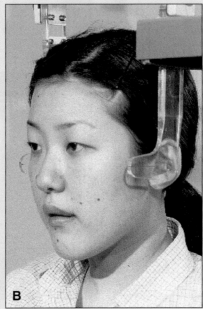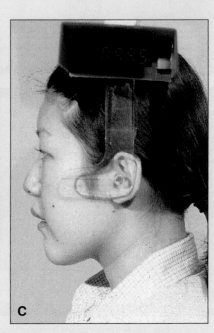

Fig. 15-10 Facial photographs at the initial examination. **A** Frontal, **B** 45°, and **C** side profile.

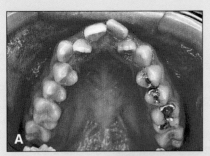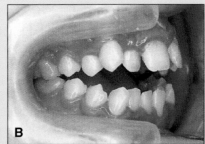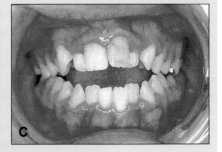

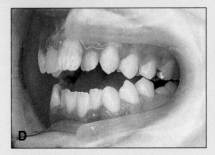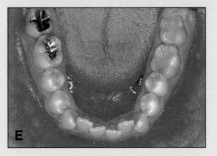

Fig. 15-11 A-E Intraoral photographs at the initial examination show a severe anterior open bite, crowding of the upper and lower incisors, a narrow upper arch, and a large overjet.

CASE REPORT

(Fig. 15-12). Figure 15-13 shows the results of her cephalometric template analysis, referred to as a craniofacial drawing standards (CDS) analysis,[11] compared to the Japanese norm. The major problems of her skeletal and soft tissue profiles were: (1) a large interlabial gap; (2) a short ramus; and (3) a vertical maxillary excess. It was obvious that these problems were closely associated with her excessive lower facial height. In addition to the orthodontic problems, she also exhibited TMD (pain and noise) and gingivitis in the lower incisors, and had a low lying tongue.

Treatment Options

Several treatment options are available to solve her orthodontic problems. The common, and perhaps most predictable response, would be to advise surgical orthodontics. Orthognathic surgery would be an excellent treatment option because it would be the most effective modality for the correction

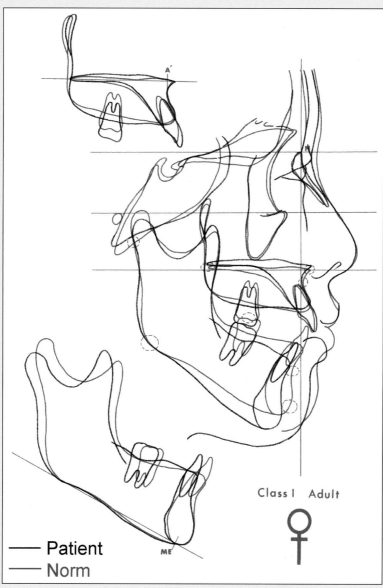

Fig. 15-12 CDS analysis. This case shows a long face, short ramus and vertical maxillary excess. (Reproduced with permission from Sugawara J, Soya T, Kawamura H, Kanamori Y. Analysis of craniofacial morphology using Craniofacial Drawing Standards (CDS): Application for orthognathic surgery. J Jpn Orthod Soc 1988; 47:394–408.)

CASE REPORT

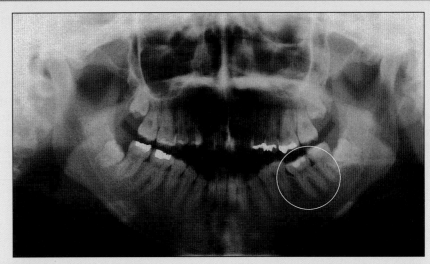

Fig. 15-13 Panoramic X-ray film at the initial examination. The lower left first molar (circled) was suspected of ankylosis.

of her vertical jaw disharmony. In fact, all her orthodontic problems could have been fixed with surgical orthodontics. It can be safely said that surgical orthodontic treatment would be the strategy most orthodontists would choose for this patient.[12]

What about other options? It may be possible to improve her anterior open bite, large overjet, and anterior crowding using a multibracket system, but clearly it would be very difficult to improve her skeletal profile using this approach. Therefore, the conventional multibracket system should probably be discarded as an option for this case.

Multiple loop edgewise archwire (MEAW) therapy[13] has been recognized as a viable modality for open bite correction. However, MEAW has almost no impact on jaw disharmony and the patient's severe vertical disharmony means that it is not the best option either.

SAS can solve most of this patient's orthodontic problems with the exception of her mild facial asymmetry. SAS makes it possible to voluntarily intrude the molars and significantly improve her vertical facial disproportion. In this case, SAS can address problems that are almost equivalent to those addressed by surgical orthodontic treatment. SAS was recommended to the patient as the first option based on a risk–benefit analysis.

Treatment Goal

The patient chose SAS treatment to intrude her upper and lower molars. Following intrusion of the molars, a counterclockwise rotation (autorotation) of

the mandible will occur automatically (Fig. 15-14A). Then, her excessive lower facial height and anterior open bite will simultaneously correct themselves. In addition, the upper and lower arches needed to be slightly expanded to coordinate her upper and lower dental arches. The intercuspation was checked with setup models made from the cephalometric and occlusogram predictions based on the treatment goals (Fig. 15-14B and C). The lower left first molar, which was suspected of ankylosis, was coincidently required neither to intrude nor distalize.

Implantation of Anchor Plates

To intrude the upper and lower molars, two orthodontic anchor plates were placed in the maxilla at the zygomatic buttress and another two plates were implanted in the mandible at the mandibular body (Fig. 15-15). After placing a rigid rectangular wire, elastic intrusive force was applied to the upper molars with Y-type anchor plates and the lower molars were tightly ligatured with L-type plates. The magnitude of the elastic intrusive force in the upper molars could be as high as 500 g on each side. A transpalatal arch was used in the upper molars (Fig. 15-15B and C) to prevent buccal flaring of the molars and to expand the upper arch with the distal rotation of the first molars.

Treatment Progress

Figure 15-16 shows the treatment progress of this patient. After completion of the expansion of the upper and lower arches, the brackets were bonded

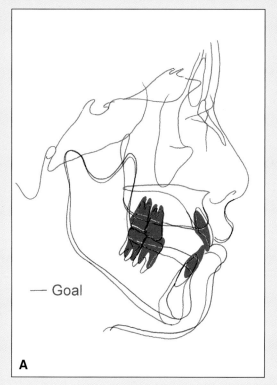
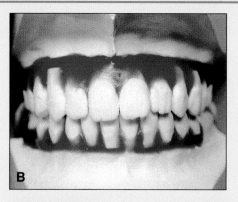
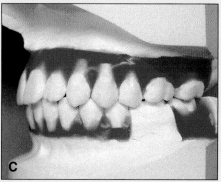

Fig. 15-14 Treatment goals. **A** Cephalometric prediction. **B** and **C** Setup model.

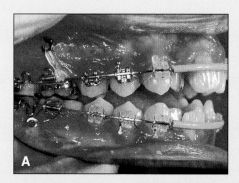
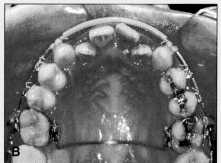
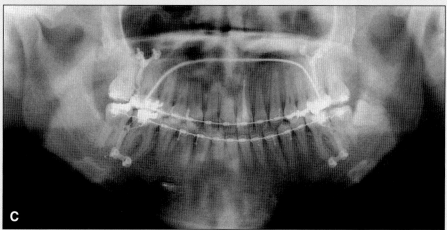

Fig. 15-15 Implantation of orthodontic anchor plates. **A** Intrusion of the upper and lower molars. **B** Transpalatal arch. **C** Y-type (zygomatic buttress) and L-type (mandibular body).

CASE REPORT

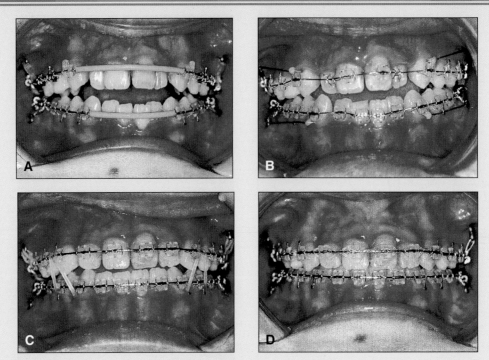

Fig. 15-16 Treatment progress. **A** Intrusion of the upper molars and expansion of the upper arch. **B** Leveling of the upper anteriors. **C** Intrusion of the upper molars. **D** Detailing and finishing.

at the incisors and leveling with continuous archwires was initiated (Fig. 15-16B). Leveling and aligning of the entire dentitions was completed but the intrusion of the upper molars was still in progress (Fig. 15-16C). Even at this early stage (7 months since SAS had been applied) the anterior open bite had significantly improved (Fig. 15-16D). At this detailing and finishing step, occlusal equilibrium was applied to stabilize the intercuspation.

Outcome

Figures 15-17 and 15-18 show the facial and oral photographs, respectively, taken at debonding after 11 months of treatment. She had a balanced profile and a functional occlusion. Her orthodontic problems at the initial diagnosis had been drastically corrected with the application of SAS treatment. After debonding, lingual bonded retainers from canine to canine were placed in the upper and lower dentitions.

Judging from the panoramic X-ray film which was taken immediately after debonding (Fig. 15-19), root parallelism was accomplished and no significant root resorption of the upper and lower molars

was observed following intrusion. In addition, no sinusitis was observed following significant intrusion of the upper molars. The orthodontic anchor plates were removed a month after debonding and the lower left third molar was extracted at the same time.

According to the pre- and post-treatment cephalometric superimposition, her anterior open bite was drastically corrected thanks to the radical intrusion of her upper and lower molars, and eventually her long face and large interlabial gap improved, because of the counterclockwise rotation of the mandible (Fig. 15-20). In fact, the amount of intrusion in the upper and lower second molars was 3.0 and 2.0 mm, respectively. Moreover, no significant change was observed in the clinical crown length. In other words, there was a significant decrease in the alveolar bone height, especially following intrusion of the upper molars. In addition, her large overjet was significantly improved following the distalization of the upper molars (4.0 mm) with the application of SAS. Figure 15-21 shows her oral photographs taken 1 year after debonding. She has maintained esthetic and functional occlusion.

CASE REPORT

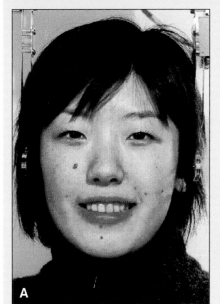
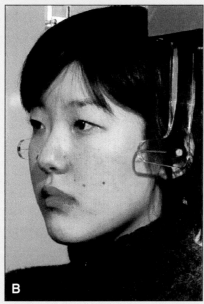
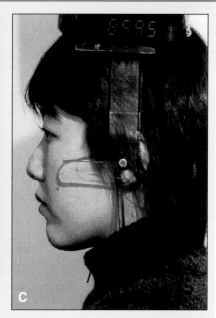

Fig. 15-17 Facial photographs immediately after debonding. **A** Frontal, **B** 45°, and **C** side profile.

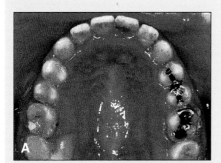
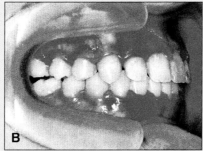
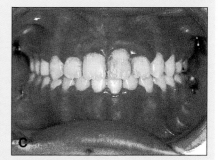

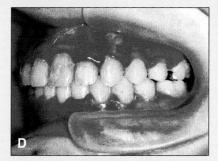
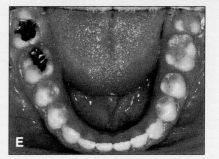

Fig. 15-18 **A-E** Intraoral photographs immediately after debonding show a balanced profile and a functional occlusion.

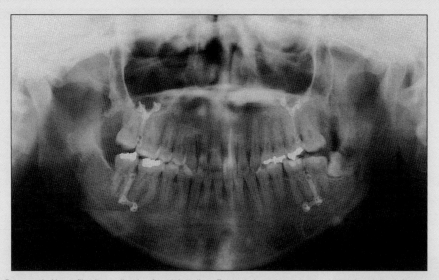

Fig. 15-19 Panoramic X-ray film immediately after debonding. Four anchor plates were removed and the left lower third molar was extracted after debonding.

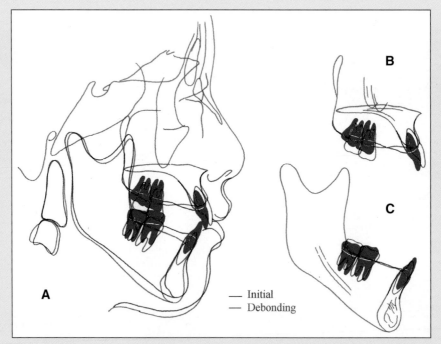

Fig. 15-20 Cephalometric superimposition. **A** Overall, **B** maxillary and **C** mandibular superimposition.

CASE REPORT

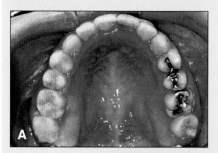
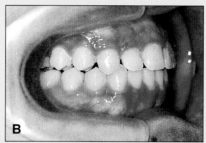
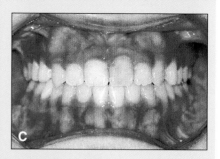
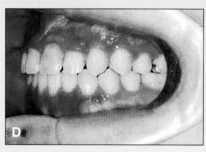
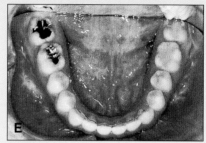

Fig. 15-21 A-E Intraoral photographs 1 year after debonding show that the patient is maintaining esthetic and functional occlusion.

Summary

Following the development of SAS, it has been possible to move the molars three-dimensionally. Therefore, the extent of camouflage treatment for the correction of crowding without premolar extraction, and skeletal malocclusions without orthognathic surgery, has drastically increased. Furthermore, SAS provides extremely effective biomechanics for second-phase treatment in developing patients, for patients with complex orthodontic problems, and for retreatment cases. SAS may extend the limits of orthodontic treatment.

REFERENCES

1. Creekmore TD, Eklund MK. The possibility of skeletal anchorage. J Clin Orthod 1983;17:226–269.
2. Jenner JD, Fitzpatrick BN. Skeletal anchorage utilizing bone plates. Aust Orthod J 1985;9:231–233.
3. Sugawara J. JCO interviews, Dr. Junji Sugawara on the skeletal anchorage system. J Clin Orthod 2000;33:689–696.
4. Sugawara J, Nagasaka H, Umemori M, et al. Skeletal Anchorage System (SAS). Dental Outlook 2002;99:397–406.
5. Daimaruya T, Nagasaka H, Umemori M, Sugawara J, Mitani H. The influences of molar intrusion on the inferior alveolar neurovascular bundle and root resorption by using anchorage system in dogs. Angle Orthod 2001;71:60–70.
6. Umemori M, Sugawara J, Mitani H, Nagasaka H, Kawamura H. Skeletal anchorage system for open-bite correction. Am J Orthod Dentofacial Orthop 1999;115:166–174.
7. Sugawara J, Baik UB, Umemori M, et al. Treatment and postreatment dentoalveolar changes following intrusion of mandibular molars with application of Skeletal Anchorage System (SAS) for open bite correction. Int J Adult Orthod Orthognath Surg 2002;17:243–253.
8. Daimaruya T, Takahashi I, Nagasaka H, Umemori M, Sugawara J, Mitani H. Effects of maxillary molar intrusion on the nasal floor and tooth root using skeletal anchorage system in dogs. Angle Orthod 2003;73:158–166.
9. Sugawara J, Umemori M, Mitani H, Nagasaka H, Kawamura H. Orthodontic treatment system for Class III malocclusion using a titanium miniplate as an anchorage. Orthod Waves 1998;57:25–35.
10. Sugawara J, Daimaruya T, Umemori M, et al. Distal movement of mandibular molars in adult patients with the skeletal anchorage system. Am J Orthod Dentofac Orthop 2004;125:130–138.
11. Sugawara J, Soya T, Kawamura H, Kanamori Y. Analysis of craniofacial morphology using Craniofacial Drawing Standards (CDS): Application for orthognathic surgery. J Jpn Orthod Soc 1988;47:394–408
12. Epker BN, Fish LC. Surgical–orthodontic correction of open bite deformity. Angle Orthod 1977;71:278–299.
13. Kim YH. Anterior openbite and its treatment with multiloop edgewise archwire. Angle Orthod 1987;57:290–321.

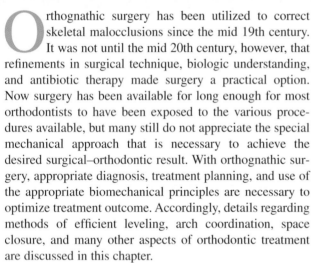

 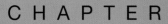
Biomechanical Factors in Surgical Orthodontics

Harry L Legan and R Scott Conley

Orthognathic surgery has been utilized to correct skeletal malocclusions since the mid 19th century. It was not until the mid 20th century, however, that refinements in surgical technique, biologic understanding, and antibiotic therapy made surgery a practical option. Now surgery has been available for long enough for most orthodontists to have been exposed to the various procedures available, but many still do not appreciate the special mechanical approach that is necessary to achieve the desired surgical–orthodontic result. With orthognathic surgery, appropriate diagnosis, treatment planning, and use of the appropriate biomechanical principles are necessary to optimize treatment outcome. Accordingly, details regarding methods of efficient leveling, arch coordination, space closure, and many other aspects of orthodontic treatment are discussed in this chapter.

Recent advances in orthopedic surgery are now being adapted to the craniofacial skeleton. Distraction osteogenesis, a biologic process designed to separate and manipulate two osteogenic fronts to extend or expand the jaws, is being applied to both the maxilla and mandible. While distraction is unlikely to replace traditional orthognathic surgery because, for example, it cannot be used in cases of excessive jaw growth, it offers a treatment alternative for correction of skeletal jaw deficiencies. Unfortunately, few papers describe the detailed biomechanical approach necessary to achieve the correct vectors and movements for optimal treatment results. Appliance placement, localizing the center of resistance of the osteotomized segments, and location of force application are vitally important to

minimize treatment complications and enhance treatment outcomes. The same efficient, effective, operator-determined biomechanical principles necessary to produce excellent orthodontic outcomes must be applied to distraction osteogenesis. The biomechanical principles are the same whether focusing on tooth-to-tooth movement or bony segment-to-bony segment movement, yet few recognize the merging of these disciplines. The mechanics of arch leveling, arch coordination, and space closure are extremely similar to those described for orthognathic surgery. Therefore, within the discussion below of distraction, emphasis will be given to vector selection for ideal dental and skeletal results.

Maxillary Orthognathic Surgery

Several reasons exist for surgical manipulation of the maxilla in all three planes of space. Surgical procedures include maxillary impaction, maxillary advancement, segmentalization of the maxilla, and more infrequently, maxillary inferior repositioning. In addition to the direction of movement, the level of the osteotomy must also be considered. The options range from LeFort I to LeFort III with several variations. With each type of surgical intervention, the pre- and post-surgical orthodontic mechanics must be appropriate for the type of surgery planned. Inappropriate mechanics can reduce the facial improvement and in some cases prevent the surgery from being able to be performed. Complete diagnostic records (lateral and posteroanterior cephalograph, models, photographs, hand–wrist X-ray, temporomandibular joint examination) must be obtained and examined in conjunction with a detailed clinical examination to accurately develop the surgical orthodontic database and determine the appropriate mechanics plan for each case. The orthodontic biomechanical considerations for several of the more common surgical procedures will be presented below.

Impaction

The most common indication for maxillary surgery is vertical maxillary excess. Some of the cephalometric indicators within the cephalometrics for orthognathic surgery (COGS) analysis,[1,2] include: an increased upper and lower facial height (N–ANS and ANS–Gn); increased mandibular plane angle (MP–HP); increased posterior facial height (N–PNS); increased gonial angle (Ar–Go–Gn); increased facial height ratio (N–ANS/ANS–Gn); and divergent occlusal planes. A typical clinical presentation includes an increased tooth-to-lip relation, increased gingival display, increased interlabial gap, and a relative mandibular deficiency. The patient will often have an anterior open bite, but this is not always present due to dentoalveolar compensations and hypereruption of the teeth.

Just as the surgical plan includes all three planes of space, the orthodontic biomechanics must also evaluate the patient's needs and plan the mode of correction in three dimensions. Of special consideration with vertical maxillary excess is minimizing the orthodontic extrusion that can occur quite rapidly with mechanics, such as the placement of low modulus continuous archwires. Segmented arch mechanics are an excellent way to predictably control the point of force application and magnitude of force applied, and to produce an operator-determined, not appliance-determined, force system. The segmented arch technique has the additional advantage of being able to level each arch without requiring additional arch length.[3]

When divergent occlusal planes exist, a treatment occlusal plane must be selected first and then the appropriate force system designed. Typically, a functional occlusal plane (perpendicular to the maxillary posterior teeth) is drawn. Once selected, the anterior teeth may be on, significantly above, or significantly below the treatment occlusal plane. Multiple options regarding arch leveling procedures exist. Should the arches be leveled before, during, or after surgery? Should the leveling be accomplished orthodontically, surgically, or using a combination of the two? The surgical approach to arch leveling will be discussed later in the section on maxillary arch segmentalization.

If the maxillary anterior teeth have erupted significantly beyond the treatment occlusal plane, an extremely efficient orthodontic mechanism for leveling the arch is the intrusive base arch. Two stainless steel posterior segments containing the second molar to the first premolar and an anterior stainless steel segment from the lateral incisor to the lateral incisor are fabricated. Either a 0.017 × 0.025 beta-titanium or a 0.017 × 0.025 stainless steel base arch with helices is activated to deliver approximately 20–25 g of intrusive force per maxillary incisor (Fig. 16-1). The extrusive forces in the posterior segment and the moment of the force created by the base arch are balanced by using a high-pull headgear oriented through a point above and in front of the center of resistance of the maxilla. Without the high-pull headgear setup to balance the adverse effects of the intrusive base arch, a significant steepening of the maxillary posterior occlusal plane can be observed, which can exacerbate the initial clinical presentation of a patient with vertical maxillary excess. In addition, no true anterior intrusion at the level of the center of resistance may occur. Once the anterior and posterior segments are oriented along the same plane (the treatment occlusal plane), a continuous archwire is placed to maintain the arch leveling.

In other vertical maxillary excess patients, the maxillary anterior segment may be more superiorly positioned than the posterior occlusal plane. In this situation the exact opposite orthodontic force system is designed. The segments of teeth are set up in the exact same orientation. The difference is that instead of an intrusive force being applied to the maxillary anterior teeth, an extrusive force of approximately 50 g per tooth is applied to extrude the anterior teeth to the level of the posterior occlusal plane. Once again, when all the teeth are oriented along the treatment occlusal plane, the extrusive base arch is removed, and a continuous stainless steel archwire is placed (Fig. 16-2).

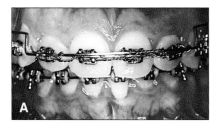 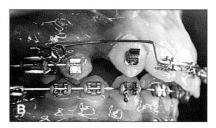 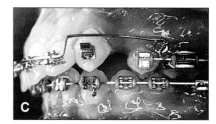

Fig. 16-1 0.017 × 0.025 stainless steel intrusive base arch (**A** frontal, and **B** and **C** lateral views) has two and a half helices immediately adjacent to the maxillary first molar. To minimize the side effect of incisal proclination resulting from the application of the intrusive force labial to the center of resistance of the tooth, the base arch is tied back with a stainless steel ligature to the molar band. A Dontrix gauge is used to accurately measure the force magnitude.

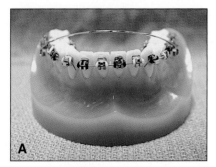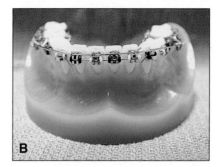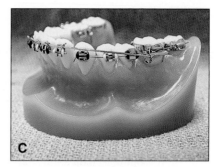

Fig. 16-2 Extrusive base arch is essentially the same as an intrusive base arch, merely turned upside-down. **A** Extrusive base arch activated, but not ligated to the anterior segment. **B** Ligated to the anterior segment. **C** Helices in a lateral view. The helix is made so that when the arch is activated, the loop is wound rather than unwound, which results in better load deflection and more constant force delivery.

Many surgeons will perform intermaxillary fixation, orienting the maxilla to the mandible and autorotating the entire maxillomandibular complex to the desired vertical position, and then use rigid fixation. This will typically cause a slight maxillary advancement in addition to the impaction. With vertical maxillary excess, the surgeon may or may not perform an osteotomy within the mandible, but attention must still be directed to the setup of the mandibular dental arch to assure appropriate arch co-ordination, arch form, and leveling. Within the mandible, attention is directed toward the depth of the curve of Spee, lower incisor–menton measurement, and the relative amount of prominence that is desired at both the soft and hard tissue pogonion. For specific information regarding leveling of the mandibular arch, see the section relating to mandibular surgery below.

Advancement

The main method of correction of any significant jaw deformity involved a mandibular osteotomy until the mid 1970s when Bell et al[4] performed a series of micro-angiographic studies. Those studies demonstrated the biologic basis for surgical manipulation of the maxilla. Since then, the maxilla has been diagnosed much more frequently than before as part of the etiology of Class III malocclusion. Some of the COGS analysis indicators of maxillary anteroposterior deficiency and normal mandibular position include glabella–subnasale (G–Sn), nasion–A point (N–A), nasion–B point (N–B), nasion–pogonion (N–Pg), and glabella–soft tissue pogonion (G–Pg'). Other clinical indications for performing a maxillary advance-ment rather than a mandibular setback include decreased pharyngeal airway, excessive submental adipose tissue, decreased malar convexity, and increased nasolabial grooves upon smiling. One way to clinically evaluate the patient involves using an object, such as a hand, fingers, or cardboard to "block out" the mid face and then examining the projection of the lower face relative to the clinically determined glabella vertical. If the chin position is

acceptable, it is most likely the patient has a maxillary anteroposterior deficiency.

Many patients with maxillary anteroposterior deficiency also exhibit varying degrees of transverse and vertical defi-ciency. Typically, a crossbite exists as part of the presenting Class III malocclusion. The crossbite should be evaluated critically to determine the magnitude and etiology. A posteroanterior cephalograph in addition to the clinical examination can assist in the diagnosis of transverse deficiency. In addition, the models should be evaluated not only in the position of the current malocclusion, but also the anticipated final occlusion. It is entirely possible that the crossbite may be a relative crossbite[5] and not need to be corrected once the maxilla is brought forward. If the patient exhibits an absolute crossbite,[5] or has a crossbite in both the presenting position as well as when placed in a Class I relationship, the magnitude and classification of transverse deficiency must be determined (skeletal versus dental). Skeletal crossbites are best corrected skeletally (rapid palatal expansion [RPE], transverse maxillary distraction osteogenesis, or segmented maxillary surgery), while dental crossbites may be corrected skeletally or den-tally (RPE, palatal arch, cross arch elastics, or expansion of the maxillary archwire).

Occlusogram analysis,[6,7] in addition to model analysis, can assist in the differential diagnosis of the transverse dimension. First, the occlusal aspect of the teeth is traced on a piece of acetate and articulated in the current anteroposterior occlusion. The maxillary member of the occlusogram is then brought forward the anticipated amount of the maxillary advancement surgery. Then, using the mandible as the template arch, the appropriate arch form, arch width, and arch length analysis is performed. The difference between the current and predicted arch width represents the required amount of maxillary expansion or mandibular constriction.

If the etiology of the crossbite is dental or small in magnitude, a transpalatal arch (TPA) provides an efficient method of dental arch expansion and does not require

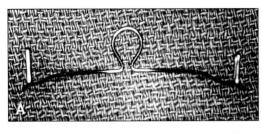

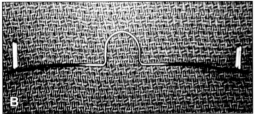

Fig. 16-3 A For expansion, a transpalatal arch (TPA) with an omega adjustment loop can be used. The loop introduces more flexibility to the TPA, but the advantage is that the wire can be maintained at the same depth within the palate after each activation. Without an adjustment loop, the TPA will be brought more occlusally after each activation and increase the potential for tongue irritation and alteration in speech. **B** Activated TPA.

patient compliance. The clinician needs to fabricate a 0.036" stainless steel heat-treated TPA (Fig. 16-3). The appliance should be first fitted passively to assure no unintended forces, moments, or vertical couples are present. To activate the TPA, the appliance should not only be expanded but also have buccal root torque placed. Because the expansive force is being applied occlusal to the center of resistance of the tooth, a significant buccal tip can be observed. To reduce the tipping tendency, buccal root torque is applied. It is essential to apply an equal amount of buccal root torque on the right and on the left or a significant vertical couple is produced. If left in place long enough, an iatrogenic occlusal plane cant can be created by extruding the side that has greater buccal root torque. Often the iatrogenic cant can only be resolved by differential vertical positioning of the maxilla as it is brought forward. Iatrogenic cant formation can make a straightforward maxillary advancement much more difficult for the surgeon and if undiagnosed can result in a post-treatment occlusal plane cant where the patient is unhappy with his/her appearance.

A similar TPA can be constructed for the patient with excess transverse dimension by placing a TPA with constriction. This is a much more efficient way of reducing arch width than using an archwire because the constricted archwire is much smaller in dimension and much of the constriction in the archwire is lost just in the act of inserting the wire into the buccal tubes. The TPA must be over-constricted as well, but the increased wire dimension as well as the heat treatment will prevent much of the activation from being lost upon insertion. In addition to the constriction, palatal root torque must be placed to

minimize tipping of the posterior teeth or posterior segments palatally.

Skeletal maxillary transverse deficiency is typically larger in magnitude and can be measured from the posteroanterior cephalograph by comparing the J point measurement to the midsagittal reference plane and the axial inclination of the posterior teeth. In a skeletally mature patient, the most stable method[8,9] of correction is maxillary transverse distraction osteogenesis (also referred to as surgically assisted RPE), or segmentalization of the maxilla (see below).

Some patients with maxillary anteroposterior hypoplasia will also have significant arch length deficiency. The above mentioned occlusogram analysis allows the clinician to accurately determine the amount of arch length deficiency and anchorage requirements. It is important to remember at this point that the occlusogram will provide different information regarding the anchorage requirements depending on where the upper member is placed. If the upper member is left in the pretreatment nonadvanced position, the anchorage requirements will often be exactly the opposite of what is required when the maxilla is advanced surgically. Extractions are performed in surgical orthodontic cases primarily for two reasons; to ideally position the teeth within the basal bone and to resolve significant arch length deficiency. The extraction mechanics typically should not be directed toward orthodontic correction of the molar classification or obtaining an ideal buccal segment relationship. Instead, the extractions should be directed toward making the occlusion reflect the magnitude of the skeletal discrepancy.

The type of extraction mechanics selected should be tailored to meet the specific needs of each case. Cases with significant maxillary anterior crowding where undesirable proclination of the anterior teeth will occur with placement of a continuous archwire are best managed by early extraction of the first bicuspids. The posterior segments are aligned and coordinated with the maxillary canines using a 0.017 × 0.025 stainless steel track. Once aligned, a segmental precalibrated 0.017 × 0.025 beta-titanium "A" anchorage "T" loop is placed from the first molar to the canine to perform initial canine retraction. "A" anchorage is achieved by placing four 30–40° moment activations in the posterior leg of the "T" loop and three moment activation bends in the anterior leg. The differential moments produce a moment/force ratio of 10:1 (translation) at the canine versus a moment/force ratio of 13:1 (root movement) at the posterior segment. In critical anchorage cases, a high-pull headgear and TPA will also be placed to assist in maintaining the position of the posterior teeth and to prevent anchorage loss. If all the extraction space is required for arch length resolution, the canine is brought back the entire distance and then the maxillary incisors are aligned. If the anchorage requirements are less stringent and some of the extraction space is intended to bring the maxillary posterior teeth forward, the canines are brought back

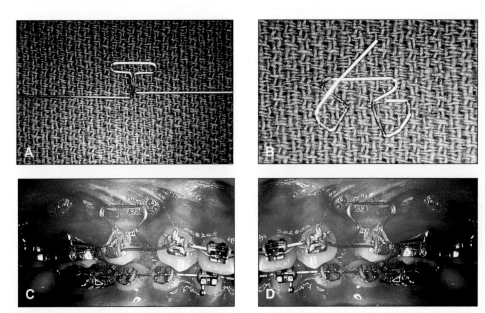

Fig. 16-4 **A** Preactivated 0.017 × 0.025 beta-titanium T loop. The anterior leg is more gingival due to the placement of a gingival horizontal tube on the canine. The loop is contoured to the arch and checked for passivity both anteriorly and posteriorly. **B** Then, depending on the anchorage requirements, the moments are placed within the anterior and posterior legs. **C** and **D** Clinical use of an active segmental T loop.

only enough to allow alignment of the maxillary anterior teeth. Once the anterior segment is aligned, the remaining spaces are closed with a new segmental "T" loop activated for "B" or "C" anchorage (Fig. 16-4).[10]

Inferior Repositioning (Down graft)

Vertical maxillary deficiency is much less common than its counterpart, vertical maxillary excess. Some of the cephalometric indicators within the COGS analysis include: decreased lower facial height (ANS–Gn); decreased mandibular plane angle (MP–HP); decreased gonial angle (Ar–Go–Gn); increased facial height ratio (N–ANS/ANS–Gn); and deep overbite. A typical clinical presentation includes a decreased tooth-to-lip relation, decreased gingival display, no interlabial gap, and a relative mandibular prognathism and/or prominent chin button.

Much like vertical maxillary excess, most attention is directed to the vertical relationship of the jaws. Instead of intruding maxillary and mandibular anterior teeth, posterior extrusion is the primary goal of the orthodontic biomechanics. Continuous low modulus archwires may be used to facilitate orthodontic eruption; however, in many of these short-face, low angle or convergent patients pre- or non-surgical orthodontic extrusion is extremely difficult to achieve. Extrusive force systems may be placed with continuous low modulus archwires, but often the heavy occlusal bite force of the patient will exceed the eruptive force delivered by the archwire. Two solutions are available. One method involves fabrication of extrusive base arches (see Fig. 16-2). These are designed to produce an extremely efficient eruptive force to the posterior maxillary

and/or posterior mandibular segments. The posterior extrusive base arch is fabricated in a similar manner to the intrusive base arch; the main difference is the level of activation. For intrusion, typically 15–25 g of force is used to intrude each anterior tooth. For extrusion of the posterior segments, a much higher force is applied, typically a minimum of 200 g. The force produces hyalinization of the anterior teeth, minimal to no anterior intrusion over the short term, and very efficient orthodontic eruption of the posterior segments.

With a Class III short-face malocclusion, the maxillary anterior teeth are often procumbent due to dentoalveolar compensations for the skeletal discrepancy. Additional benefits derived from the extrusive base arch force system include the possible arch length increase obtained as well as an uprighting force that can be applied to the maxillary anterior teeth. With an extrusive base arch, not only is a significant extrusive force present on the posterior segments, but also a crown distal or counterclockwise moment. If the arch is not tied back or is fabricated as a "split base arch", as the extrusion occurs, a space will develop between the segments (Fig. 16-5). Once leveling has occurred, this space can be used to retract the maxillary incisors using an "A" anchorage segmented arch "T" loop. The anterior crossbite will worsen presurgically, but the maxillary anterior teeth will be appropriately positioned and uprighted within the maxillary basal bone. The extrusive base arch can also be fabricated as a "split" base arch and the force can be applied behind the center of resistance of the maxillary anterior segment. This allows the maxillary incisors to be uprighted during the extrusion of the posterior

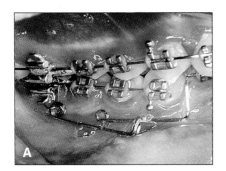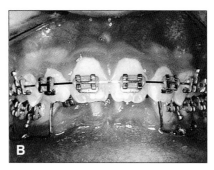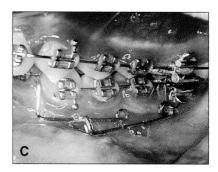

Fig. 16-5 A-C Split intrusive base arch allows for precise activation when intruding segments of teeth. The distal extension from the anterior segment allows the operator to place the intrusive force anterior to, at, or posterior to the center of resistance for the segment. This allows for simultaneous intrusion with proclination, intrusion with no axial change, or intrusion with simultaneous uprighting of the anterior segment for increased efficiency, respectively.

segments, even if the arch is tied back and spaces are not generated.

An alternative method that can be utilized involves performing the orthodontic leveling postsurgically. A significant mandibular curve of Spee is an excellent indication for postsurgical leveling. Postsurgically, the deepest part of the curve of Spee, the mid arch, is still present. Immediate postsurgical leveling is extremely effective because the teeth can be erupted into air rather than into heavy occlusal forces. Not only are the heavy occlusal forces absent because of the interocclusal space between the arches, but there is also decreased occlusion from the osteotomy itself. Postsurgically, due to a change in muscle fiber orientation, the mechanical advantage and thus the bite force may also decrease. In addition, due to the healing and increased vascularization, there is a regional accelerative phenomenon.[11] This combination of factors can cause extremely rapid and efficient orthodontic tooth movement. To assist eruption of the teeth, either a continuous light stainless steel archwire with vertical box elastics in the mid arch, segmented arch mechanics with an extrusive base arch, or an overlay extrusive base arch can be placed with a light continuous main archwire. Once complete arch leveling is obtained, a rigid continuous stainless steel archwire can be placed to maintain the arch leveling.

Segmentalization

Two main reasons exist for segmental maxillary osteotomies, one being multiple maxillary occlusal planes. The discrepant occlusal planes can be managed orthodontically or surgically, and the decision regarding which method is better is largely philosophical and based on the stability of the surgical intervention versus the stability of the vertical orthodontic movement.[12,13] When significantly different anterior and posterior occlusal planes are present, the treatment occlusal plane must be chosen prior to initiating surgical orthodontic treatment. Segmentalization allows for differing amounts of superior or inferior repositioning

of the segments surgically. When surgical closure of an anterior open bite is planned, orthodontic eruption of the maxillary anterior teeth is undesirable because this will build potential instability into the case and reduce the amount of vertical surgical repositioning. As a result, segmentalization of the maxilla for differing occlusal planes typically requires that segmental, not continuous, archwire mechanics be used. Placement of light continuous archwires will generally lead to unwanted extrusion of the maxillary anterior teeth, posterior teeth, or both. Instead, the teeth should be aligned in segments based on the location of the occlusal plane divergence. Typically, the maxillary arch is segmented either between the lateral incisor and the canine or between the canine and first premolar (Fig. 16-6). One advantage that a four-tooth incisor segment has over a six-tooth anterior segment is that the former can be set deeper surgically without the presence of the maxillary canine. Generally, there is also a natural root divergence between the maxillary canine and the lateral incisor. To augment the divergence, a segmental root spring can be placed from the molar to the canine to obtain the necessary root divergence for the osteotomy (Fig. 16-7). For segmental surgery, it is much less important to have space between the crowns than between the roots.[14]

One common mistake with continuous arch mechanotherapy is the placement of an open coil-spring to create an osteotomy space. The open coil-spring is effective in opening space at the level of the crown, but actually will bring the roots of the adjacent teeth into closer proximity and increase rather than decrease the risk of damage during the interdental osteotomy. Figure 16-8 clearly demonstrates that an open coil-spring places a separating force above the center of resistance of the two adjacent teeth. This results in a moment on both teeth which will act to converge, not diverge, the roots.

Another method for root divergence in the continuous arch method is to place a "V" bend with the apex of the "V" pointing apically instead of in the typical occlusal direction. If the "V" is centered between the teeth adjacent

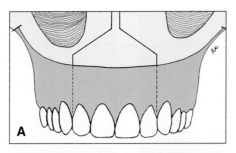 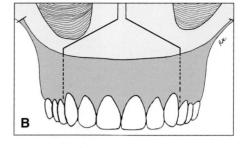

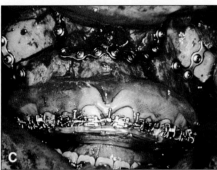

Fig. 16-6 Segmental maxillary procedures can be done in many ways and at many sites. The most common is the three-piece segmental LeFort I osteotomy either **A** between the lateral and canine, or **B** between the canine and first premolar. The figure demonstrates the approximate area of interdental osteotomy from the frontal view, looking from above the previously down fractured maxilla. It is important to note that the palatal mucosa must be carefully preserved to maintain adequate perfusion of the maxilla and dentition. **C** Clinical presentation after segmenting between the lateral incisors and canine and placing rigid internal fixation.

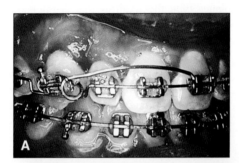 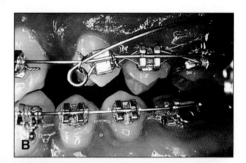

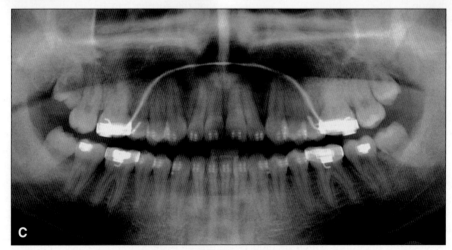

Fig. 16-7 Activated root spring is an efficient way to assist in developing an interdental osteotomy site. **A** Stainless steel main archwire can be stepped occlusally to minimize the extrusive effects of the spring, or **B** a light nickel–titanium archwire can be placed in the archwire slot. With the archwire in the slot, care must be taken to ensure that the archwire does not negate the effects of the root spring. **C** Panoramic radiograph must be viewed prior to performing the osteotomy to ensure that the clinical crown angulation is not demonstrating misleading root position. In this patient, the osteotomy was planned between the maxillary lateal and canine, and adequate divergence of the teeth was obtained. After surgery, the root position must be corrected to place the forces over the long axis of the teeth and to have parallel roots.

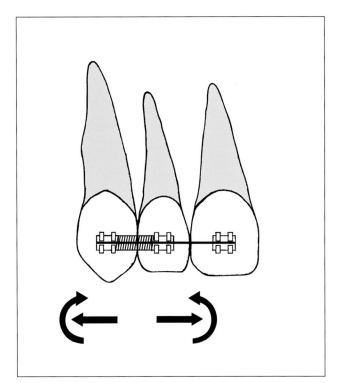

Fig. 16-8 Force system created by placing an open coil-spring between the crowns of the teeth is exactly the opposite of the desired force system. With an open coil-spring, the roots are brought closer together rather than further apart. An appropriate interdental osteotomy site may still be developed, but a greater than necessary amount of space may be created, causing inefficient postsurgical orthodontic finishing. The most important area in the interdental osteotomy is the divergence of the roots, not the crowns.

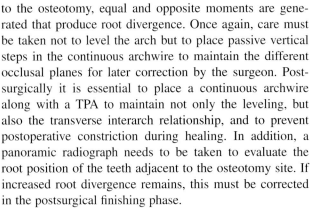

to the osteotomy, equal and opposite moments are generated that produce root divergence. Once again, care must be taken not to level the arch but to place passive vertical steps in the continuous archwire to maintain the different occlusal planes for later correction by the surgeon. Postsurgically it is essential to place a continuous archwire along with a TPA to maintain not only the leveling, but also the transverse interarch relationship, and to prevent postoperative constriction during healing. In addition, a panoramic radiograph needs to be taken to evaluate the root position of the teeth adjacent to the osteotomy site. If increased root divergence remains, this must be corrected in the postsurgical finishing phase.

The second reason for segmenting the maxilla relates to the maxillary transverse dimension. Skeletal crossbites that are more moderate in magnitude (no more than 5–7 mm) can be adequately addressed with segmental LeFort I osteotomy. The location of the segmental osteotomy depends on the location of the desired arch expansion (Fig. 16-9). If canine expansion is required when a three-piece maxillary osteotomy is planned, the canine must be in the posterior segment. If only molar and premolar expansion is desired,

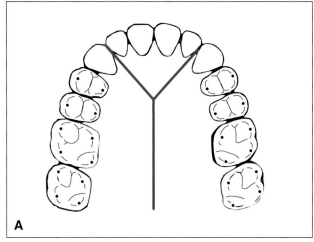

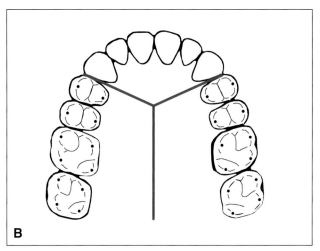

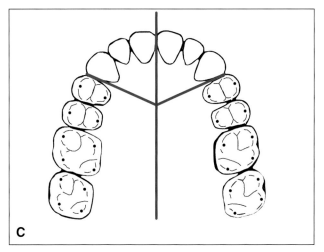

Fig. 16-9 Segmental maxillary procedures can be done in many ways and at many sites. The most common is the three-piece segmental LeFort I osteotomy either **A** between the lateral and canine or **B** between the canine and first premolar. **C** A less common option is the four-piece segmental LeFort I osteotomy, with segments in the midline and between the maxillary canine and first premolar. The segmentalization is shown here from the occlusal view to depict the ability to expand differentially within the arch.

the canine may be included in the anterior segment. When differing amounts of canine and molar expansion are treatment planned, a four-piece maxillary segmental osteotomy can be performed to increase not only the maxillary canine width, but also the maxillary molar width differentially. Here, the osteotomies are performed in the maxillary midline and between the maxillary canine and first premolar. Once again root divergence is essential to minimize the risk of damage to the teeth during the osteotomy. A two-piece maxillary osteotomy with a sagittal cut separating the maxilla into right and left segments may also be used when the cuspids as well as the buccal segments need to be expanded.

Presurgically, it is important not to make any attempts to increase the arch width with the TPA, archwires or cross arch elastics because this will introduce the possibility of orthodontic relapse into the surgical procedure, or the surgeon may underestimate the necessary amount of expansion. Intermaxillary fixation still takes 10–14 days, but postsurgically these patients are typically left in a "horseshoe" type splint with a palatal strut that is wired to the maxillary arch for approximately 6–8 weeks. As close to the day of splint removal as possible (and ideally the day the splint is removed), a continuous stainless steel maxillary archwire and either a TPA or labial overlay wire should be placed. The TPA or labial wire should be heat treated to prevent expansion from occurring over time from the memory of the wire. To maintain the labial overlay wire, a Coffin loop should be placed in the maxillary midline for ease of tying in place. Segmental expansion of the maxilla is among the less stable surgical moves and every effort orthodontically should be made to assist in maintaining the increased arch dimension throughout the remainder of treatment. In addition, these patients should be advised of the need for indefinite retention for best longterm results. Transverse discrepancies >6–7 mm in the skeletally mature patient are best managed with transverse maxillary distraction osteogenesis (see the section on distraction below).

Level of Osteotomy

The level of osteotomy is classified based on LeFort's trauma studies from the 19th century.[15]

1. LeFort I level osteotomies involve movement of only the dentoalveolar portion of the maxilla. Occasionally, patients will require anteroposterior augmentation of the malar area in addition to the maxilla. An intermediate surgical procedure is the "high" LeFort I osteotomy which goes slightly superior to the typical LeFort I and includes a portion of the zygomatic process of the maxilla and a small portion of the inferior aspect of the zygoma.
2. LeFort II osteotomies include the maxilla and nasal bones. One approach for the LeFort II level surgery is a subconjunctival approach. Another more extensive surgical approach involves use of a bicoronal flap.

3. LeFort III osteotomies include the maxilla, zygoma, and nasal bones, extending superiorly to the zygomaticofrontal suture as well as the frontomaxillary suture. The typical surgical approach for the LeFort III level surgery involves a bicoronal flap.

Most nonsyndromic patients requiring maxillary surgery typically have surgery that addresses the maxilla at a LeFort I or high LeFort I level when additional malar augmentation is desired. Many syndromic patients with Crouzon, Apert, Binders, Pfeiffer or other midfacial deficiencies will involve surgery at a LeFort II or III level. Others will even have frontal bone advancement (Monobloc procedure).

Maxillary Distraction Osteogenesis

Craniofacial distraction osteogenesis is still in its relative infancy when compared to orthognathic surgery. The first maxillary surgery was performed in the 1860s by Cheever to access a nasopharyngeal carcinoma.[16] The maxilla was down fractured, the carcinoma removed, and the maxilla replaced in its original position. Martin Wassmund[17] published one of the first examples of maxillary distraction osteogenesis. In the 1920s he reported on a total LeFort I osteotomy to which he later applied orthopedic traction in order to obtain the necessary movement. The most commonly cited person and "father of modern-day distraction osteogenesis" is Gavril Ilizarov, a Russian orthopedic surgeon who developed the contemporary distraction protocol.[18] His protocol, developed and refined in the 1950s and 1960s, requires a latency period of 1 week, with a specific rate (1 mm per day) and rhythm (0.25 mm four times per day). Ilizarov's main focus of attention was the long bones, particularly the femur, tibia, and fibula. Craniofacial distraction osteogenesis is much more recent, with McCarthy, Grayson, Chin, Molina, Guerrero[19–23] being among the major contributors throughout the 1990s. Maxillary and mandibular distraction have an advantage over orthognathic surgery in that not only is there a skeletal expansion, but potentially also a concomitant distraction histiogenesis that may produce an enhanced soft tissue response. A disadvantage of distraction osteogenesis is that it cannot be used to correct growth excesses, only deficiencies. Consequently, distraction osteogenesis is unlikely ever to completely replace orthognathic surgery as a means of correcting dentofacial deformities.

Maxillary Anterior Distraction

The orthodontic biomechanics for maxillary anteroposterior distraction osteogenesis are very similar to those already described for maxillary advancement surgery. The maxilla and mandible must be evaluated in all three planes of space to obtain the correct transverse, anteroposterior, and vertical relationship of the teeth to one another and with respect to the opposing arch. The first aspect that must be considered is the transverse relationship to assure that when the maxilla is distracted forward, it will be wide enough to accommodate the mandible. The second factor is the vertical relationship of the maxillary anterior and posterior teeth. It is difficult to fit the maxilla to the mandible until both arches are level. The same intrusive and extrusive mechanisms that are used in standard orthognathic surgery are applied to the distraction.

A major difference in distraction versus surgical advancement of the maxilla is vector control. Whereas in orthognathic surgery, the maxilla undergoes a single acute movement from its current to its final position all during one procedure, in distraction, the process is much more gradual. Precise and controlled movement of the maxilla is required to maximize occlusal contact and facial esthetics. To accomplish these precise movements, the location of the center of resistance of the maxilla is essential (Fig. 16-10).[24] Once the location is determined, the correct movement can then be planned using sound biomechanical diagnosis and treatment planning principles.

Maxillary distraction osteogenesis vector selection is very similar to procedures used for maxillary protraction headgear in growing patients. The primary difference is that the center of resistance in distraction will vary depending on the level of the osteotomy. The higher the osteotomy, the higher the center of resistance will be located. The result is that vector analysis will be unique for each patient. Previous research has localized the center of resistance of the maxilla in patients who have not had a surgical disjunction of the inferior portion of the maxilla from the cranium. Typically in the lateral cephalograph, the center of resistance is located halfway between the inferior aspect of the zygoma and the buccal cusp tip of the maxillary molar. In the posteroanterior cephalograph, the center of resistance is approximately 2 cm lateral to the malar base on the infraorbital portion of the zygoma.

After the center of resistance of the dentomaxillary portion of the mobilized maxilla is located, the direction of force application can be determined.[25] A patient with maxillary anteroposterior hypoplasia with an anterior open bite will be distracted using a vector through a point anterior to and above the center of resistance. This will produce both a protraction force as well as a clockwise moment that will act to bring the anterior maxilla downward and forward, increasing the amount of overbite and anteroposterior projection of the maxilla. A patient with maxillary anteroposterior deficiency but increased overbite will be distracted using a vector below the center of resistance of the maxilla to produce maxillary advancement, and posterior inferior positioning to decrease the amount of overbite. It is essential to closely monitor the distraction weekly as it is proceeding to assure that the desired vector of distraction is the actual vector of distraction that is obtained. Some patients will distort the distraction appliance and require modification of the original vector, or the center of resistance may be located slightly differently

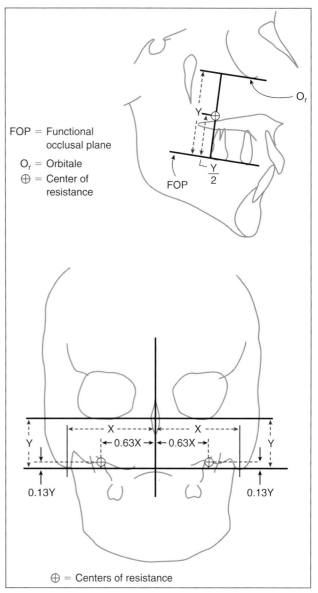

Fig. 16-10 Process for localizing the center of resistance of the maxilla. Remember, however, that the level of distraction will dictate the relative position of the center of resistance. The higher the level of osteotomy (high LeFort I, LeFort II, or LeFort III), the higher the center of resistance. The vector of distraction must be adjusted accordingly. (Reproduced with permission from Braun S, Bottrel JA, Lee KG, Lunazzi JJ, Logan HL. The biomechanics of rapid maxillary sutural expansion. Am J Orthod Dentofacial Orthop 2000;118:257–261.)

from originally calculated, due to factors such as soft tissue attachments and tonicity.

Multiple maxillary distraction appliances are currently available. The rigid external distractor (RED) appliance utilizes an orthopedic halo type of appliance that is anchored to the outer table of the cranium (Fig. 16-11). The halo serves multiple purposes. First, it is a fairly rigid anchorage device from which to advance the maxilla. Second, and of equal importance, is the fact that the halo serves as a

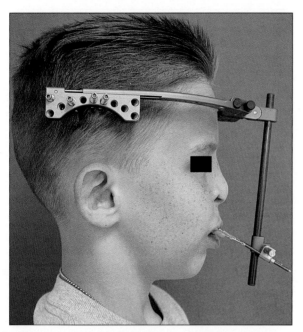

Fig. 16-11 Rigid external distractor (RED) appliance is extremely versatile. The halo is placed into the outer table of the cranium and serves as an extremely stable anchorage unit. The vertical pin allows for precise force vector application relative to the center of resistance of the mobilized maxilla.

constant reminder to the patient that the appliance must be worn to achieve the desired movement prior to consolidation of the osteotomy. Typically, a large labiolingual custom framework is fabricated and attached to the maxillary dentition. An extension is fabricated that is brought extraorally and superiorly to give the appropriate choice of vector. A connection from the extraoral wire to the vertical bar extending from the halo on the RED appliance is made with a stainless steel ligature wire. The vertical bar of the RED appliance can easily be moved superiorly, inferiorly, forward or backward during the distraction phase to alter the vector of distraction. Some surgeons have used a transcutaneous wire from the maxillary bone plates to the vertical rod in cases where the dentition is not a good option for a maxillary handle. A possible negative side effect of the transcutaneous approach is extraoral scarring.

Another appliance is the typical maxillary protraction face mask assembly (Fig. 16-12). Orthodontically, the face mask can be used with or without a facebow. Without a headgear bow, the direction of distraction is severely limited because the point of force application can only come from the level of the crowns of the teeth and pass through the commissure of the lips, which is often too low. With a headgear bow, the outer bow can be adjusted into countless different positions to produce the desired

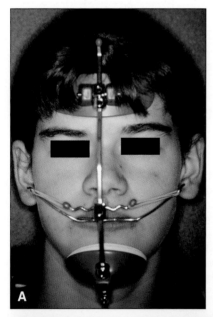

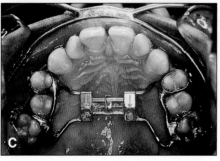

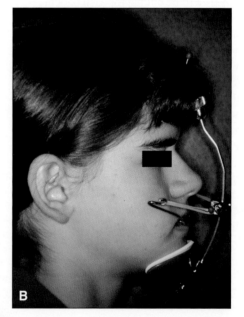

Fig. 16-12 Standard protraction headgear can be used when distracting the maxilla downward and forward. For best force application, a headgear bow is placed along the dentition, with the outer bow adjusted to deliver the intended vector of force. The force may be applied through the center of resistance to provide a pure translation of the maxilla. Alternatively, the outer bow may be adjusted above or below the center of resistance to provide either a clockwise or counterclockwise moment to assist in bite closing or opening.

direction of distraction. One disadvantage of the orthodontic face mask as a distractor is possible decreased patient compliance. Since the face mask is not fixated to the cranium, it may be removed, resulting in less use than a fixed appliance.

Maxillary Transverse Distraction Osteogenesis

In the mid 1970s, Bell[26] developed a technique for maxillary expansion of the skeletally mature patient. At the time, little was known about distraction osteogenesis, but the technique Bell utilized was very similar. At that time, a subtotal LeFort I osteotomy was performed. The same cuts were made as a standard LeFort I, including pterygoid plate disjunction; however, the inferior maxilla was not down fractured and separated from the superior aspect of the maxilla. In addition, a midsagittal cut was added to simulate the suture in a growing patient. Once the cuts were completed, the appliance was activated approximately 2 mm to ensure complete mobilization of the maxilla. Then, the patient was instructed to activate the appliance two turns in the morning and two turns in the evening until the desired expansion was achieved. This protocol is very similar to that of Ilizarov,[18] with one important distinction; there was no latency period. Because a soft callus was not allowed to form before activating the appliance, this protocol could not truly be called distraction osteogenesis.

The current protocol for maxillary transverse distraction osteogenesis utilizes a similar protocol as Bell's, but incorporates a latency period of approximately 1 week. In healthy, skeletally mature individuals, 1 week will allow for the formation of a fibrocartilaginous callus in the osteotomy sites. This callus can then be gradually separated, molded, and later stabilized to significantly augment the innate maxillary alveolus and basal bone (Fig. 16-13). Once the maxillary transverse distraction osteogenesis is completed, it is important to stabilize the teeth until there is radiographic evidence of bone formation. Premature movement of the teeth into the distraction gap can lead to a periodontal defect and possible loss of attachment. The teeth may be stabilized by stainless steel ligation, placement of a maxillary archwire with a passive open coil spring, or placement of two segments of wire. Once adequate consolidation has occurred, maxillary midline diastema closure can proceed along a stainless steel archwire track to minimize second-order tipping.

After anterior space closure, the mechanics required for the rest of the case can be initiated, such as intrusion/extrusion mechanics, space closure mechanics, and torquing arches. It is especially important to evaluate the torque of the maxillary anterior segment after significant transverse expansion. There is a tendency for the incisors to become much more upright which can cause difficulty in obtaining ideal overbite and overjet. If the maxillary incisors are too upright, they occupy a smaller arc and

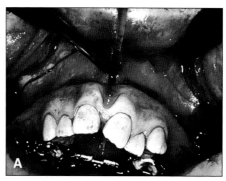
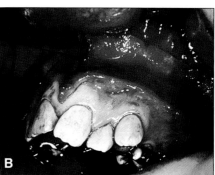
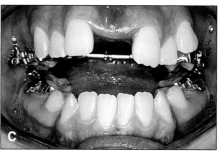

Fig. 16-13 Location of the osteotomy from the **A** frontal and **B** lateral view. The osteotomy is placed at the same time as the appliance is loaded to assist in propagating the midpalatal osteotomy. **C** Patient after completed maxillary transverse distraction osteogenesis. The total time since completion of the osteotomy is 3 weeks (1 week latency and 2 weeks of activation with two turns twice daily).

may not occlude correctly with the mandibular anterior segment. An efficient way to apply torque to the four incisors utilizes a high alpha torquing spring (Fig. 16-14). A full-dimension, rectangular stainless steel archwire is placed, filling the incisor bracket slots. The wire is then stepped gingivally and two helices are placed to deliver a crown labial/root palatal torque. The torquing spring must be tied back to prevent incisor proclination and ensure root movement. Care must be taken to minimize the force level to minimize the extrusive force anteriorly. If the spring extends posteriorly to approximately the first molar region and is brought up and hooked over the main archwire, a long moment arm is created, reducing the magnitude of the vertical forces. It is possible to obtain approximately a 2000–2500 g-mm moment with only 100 g of force. An incisal step is made in the main archwire distal to

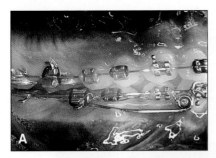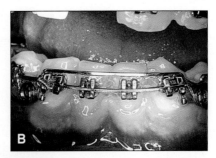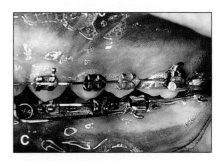

Fig. 16-14 A-C High alpha root spring utilizes a segmental approach to deliver a large moment without requiring a large vertical force. The root spring is placed into the slot of each of the anterior teeth, stepped gingivally, and then two and a half helices are wound with the extensions directed posteriorly and inferiorly. A hook is then fabricated so the spring can be placed over the main archwire in the posterior region. The longer the spring, the lower the force required, and the less chance that undesirable vertical forces will be produced.

the lateral incisors so that the wire can be placed on the underside of the incisal wings of the maxillary anterior brackets to further minimize the possible extrusive effect.

Maxillary transverse distraction osteogenesis can be performed as an isolated procedure, as a first surgical phase to obtain the necessary space for aligning the dentition and obtain adequate arch width prior to a second surgical phase to correct the anteroposterior jaw deformity, or in conjunction with mandibular symphyseal distraction osteogenesis.

Asymmetric Advancement/Inferior Distraction

Patients with both skeletal and soft tissue deficiencies (such as hemifacial microsomia) are ideal candidates for distraction osteogenesis. The results from distraction can in some cases reduce the need for additional esthetic surgery (e.g. buccal fat and alloplastic grafts) to address the associated soft tissue deficiencies. Diagnostically, the most important aspect is determining the amount of asymmetry from the clinical examination and standard orthodontic records. Particular attention should focus on the presence, location, and magnitude of any occlusal plane cant. The cant may be a frontal occlusal plane cant, posterior cant, or both. With only an isolated frontal occlusal plane cant, intrusive or extrusive base arches are excellent appliances to obtain the necessary correction. A rigid anterior segment can be placed, with the base arch tied only to the tooth or teeth that require intrusion. Once again, a high-pull headgear is placed with a short and elevated outer bow to prevent any posterior extrusion or posterior cant from developing. Once level, a continuous archwire can be placed to obtain coordinated maxillary and mandibular arches. Then, with level and coordinated arches, maxillary distraction can be initiated.

When the same amount of cant is present posteriorly and anteriorly, it is best addressed during the distraction phase. When distracting, extraoral appliances have a distinct advantage in that they are more easily activated, there is almost limitless choice of distraction vector, and space is plentiful. Unfortunately, patients are more self-conscious of an extraoral appliance, and the risk of significant extraoral scarring is much greater. The scars, if objectionable, can be revised by a plastic surgeon but this requires additional surgery. Intraoral appliances have the significant advantage of minimal risk of scarring; however, obtaining the correct vector of distraction is more difficult. Intraorally, there is limited space for appliance placement, fewer directional change options, and more difficult visualization. In addition, activation of the appliance is somewhat more complicated with only a finite number of adjustments that can be made. If the appliance is not placed along the correct line of action, very little substantive change can be made without performing surgery to change the orientation of the appliance. Interarch elastic traction[27] can be applied in a number of ways to assist in distraction vector refinement. Unfortunately, any time an elastic is placed on the teeth, dental rather than skeletal movement may be occurring. The end result may be a reasonable occlusion, but less correction of the skeletal asymmetry than anticipated or desired.

Mandibular Surgery

Mandibular Advancement

High Angle

When considering mandibular advancement, the clinician must determine if there is a true skeletal anteroposterior deficiency or if the deficiency is caused by a vertical maxillary excess and the mandible has rotated down and back. Some helpful cephalometric measurements to assist the diagnosis include: mandibular length (Go–Gn); facial height (N–ANS and ANS–Gn); gonial angle (Ar–Go–Gn); mandibular projection (N–B); chin projection (N–Pg); and angle of skeletal convexity (N–A–Pg). In the high-angle (steep mandibular plane, backward rotator, etc.) patient, often the effective chin projection is minimal and the mandibular incisors are extruded (lower incisor to mandibular plane distance measured perpendicular to the mandibular plane).

A true mandibular deficient patient with a normal face height but steep mandibular plane can often be treated with isolated mandibular surgery. On the other hand, the patient with increased facial height as well as a steep mandibular plane will often require two-jaw surgery with a maxillary impaction and mandibular advancement. Attempts at leveling the arch should be directed toward avoiding any additional backward rotation of the mandible caused by posterior extrusion, further reducing chin projection. If any mild extrusion is anticipated, it is important to do so prior to surgery. Any postsurgical extrusion would have the undesirable tendency to open the bite again. A better approach focuses on intrusion of the mandibular anterior teeth. In addition, leveling with a continuous archwire tends to produce incisor proclination. If the proclination is significant, the mandible may not be able to be advanced into a Class I relationship because the incisors take up a greater arc than they should.

True intrusion of the anterior teeth will require segmentalization of the mandibular arch and use of an intrusive base arch. If the arch length deficiency is minimal and the position of the mandibular incisors is reasonable (lower incisor to mandibular plane angle) then a rigid anterior segment and two rigid posterior segments are fabricated. A 0.017×0.025 stainless steel intrusive base arch is inserted into the auxiliary tube of the molar and tied either gingival to or just labial to the mandibular incisor brackets. It is important not to insert the wire directly into the incisor brackets as torque might be present which would produce an indeterminate force system. The torque could be additive, creating a larger intrusive effect, or negative, producing a smaller and clinically ineffective intrusive effect. Once the arch is level, a rigid stainless steel continuous archwire should be placed to maintain the overbite correction.

If the arch length deficiency is more significant or the lower incisors are proclined, a split intrusive base can be fabricated (see Fig. 16-5). The same posterior segments are used, but this time the anterior segment is stepped approximately 5 mm gingivally as the wire exits the mandibular lateral incisor. The wire is then contoured to the arch and extended distally with a stop at the distal extent of the segment. Then, a cantilever spring can be made (one on each side to deliver approximately 15 g of force per tooth to be intruded) and placed behind the center of resistance of the anterior segment of teeth. The applied force system produces simultaneous intrusion and uprighting of the anterior teeth.

By intruding the anterior teeth, not only can the mandible be advanced, but also rotated counterclockwise to increase the chin projection. In borderline genioplasty patients, the rotation at the time of surgery can negate the need for advancement genioplasty.

Low Angle

The low-angle (low mandibular plane, forward rotator, etc.) patient typically possesses a deep curve of Spee and decreased facial height. With short-face patients, the facial musculature (masseter, lateral, and medial pterygoids) is typically stronger, and posterior dental extrusion can be difficult to achieve and maintain due to high posterior bite force.[28] While the mandible may be deficient, the chin projection may be quite acceptable due to a large chin button. Class II, Division 2 patients often display these characteristics. One goal of treatment focuses upon increasing the facial height. One of the simplest approaches to lengthening the facial height is extrusion of the teeth and advancing the mandible "downhill" along the occlusal plane. This can be extremely easy with a steep maxillary occlusal plane, as the occlusal plane will dictate the relative amount of vertical and horizontal mandibular change in isolated mandibular advancement surgery. Unfortunately, many low-angle patients have a normal-to-flat occlusal plane, so additional techniques must be employed.

Timing of the leveling can dramatically increase the orthodontic efficiency. An extremely efficient way to obtain leveling is to perform the mandibular advancement surgery early in treatment prior to leveling the curve of Spee. Historically, prior to rigid fixation, the mandible was advanced to an edge-to-edge incisor relationship and occlusion on the second molars. The patient was fixated with an anterior and/or superior border wire and an interocclusal splint. After adequate healing time, the splint was removed and intermaxillary elastics in the mid arch were used. The maxilla would have a rigid archwire, with a relatively nonrigid mandibular wire, such as a 0.018 stainless steel wire. Once the elastics had leveled the mandibular arch, a more rigid mandibular wire was placed. Two processes may be occurring simultaneously to account for the efficiency in leveling. First, it is certainly easier to erupt teeth into air than into heavy bite forces and second, a regional accelerative phenomenon takes place in the time period shortly after surgery. It is speculated that this is due to the increased vascularization that occurs as part of normal wound healing.[12] Now, with rigid fixation, less immediate postsurgical relapse occurs, and the mandible does not need to be placed in an edge-to-edge "tripod" occlusion, but merely into Class I with a mid arch open bite. The fixation allows for elastic use almost immediately postsurgically, unlike with wire fixation. If heavy elastic traction is applied too quickly to the mid arch with wire fixation, "bending" of the bone can occur producing an inferior border notch. If the patient has too much chin projection and some facial lengthening is still desired, a vertical lengthening genioplasty with minimal advancement can be performed.

Mandibular Setback

Isolated mandibular setback procedures are less common today than in the past. More frequently, maxillary advancement with or without mandibular setback is employed. In addition, some advocate that there are few indications for mandibular setback due to a fear that it will cause obstructive sleep apnea. Cephalometric measurements that will assist in the diagnosis of mandibular hyperplasia include increased mandibular projection (N–B); chin projection (N–Pg), and a normal maxillary projection (N–A, and G'–Sn). Care must be directed in the diagnosis to evaluating the soft tissue drape of the lower face and neck, especially the lower face throat angle and lower face throat height/depth ratio. Both measurements can prevent inappropriate setback of the mandibular arch and avoid creating potential airway problems.

One of the most common findings with mandibular hyperplastic patients includes the dentally compensated, retroclined mandibular incisors. The lower incisor to mandibular plane angle can often be in the mid 70° range. In addition, the labial mucosa is often thin. Adequate decompensation of the lower incisors can be quite challenging. An efficient mechanism for lower incisor torque correction is the high alpha root spring (see Fig. 16-14). The root spring is an auxiliary full size archwire that is placed directly into the lower incisor brackets. The wire exits the brackets, is stepped gingivally, helices are placed bilaterally, and the activated distal archwire extension is then clipped over the main archwire as far posteriorly as possible. The longer the wire, the greater the moment generated, and the more efficient the root spring will be. With shorter root springs, significantly higher forces are required to generate the same moment, which has the tendency to cause unwanted mandibular incisor extrusion. To minimize the extrusive component, the main archwire is placed in the posterior brackets and then stepped incisally to rest on top of the tie wings of the mandibular incisor brackets. The extrusive force that is generated by the root spring will erupt the anterior teeth until the main archwire is contacted. Then the extrusion will cease. If labial crown torque of the incisors is desired, the high alpha root spring must be tied back to prevent the crowns of the lower anterior teeth from coming forward. If incisor proclination is desired, the root spring does not need to be tied back as tightly, but the force level should be reduced to prevent over proclination of the incisors.

Many Class III mandibular hyperplastic patients will present with minimal mandibular arch length deficiency and minimal curve of Spee. A crossbite may exist as well, but often the crossbite is relatively minor when the patient is placed in a Class I molar and canine position. Refer to the section regarding maxillary advancement for a further discussion regarding the transverse dimension.

The orthodontic treatment to remove the dental compensations should be the same whether a bilateral sagittal split ramus osteotomy (BSSRO) or an intraoral vertical ramus osteotomy (IVRO) is performed. Technically, the IVRO is a much simpler, faster, and less morbid procedure as compared to the BSSRO. When performing the setback, care must be directed toward proximal segment positioning. A critical error that occasionally occurs involves improper positioning of the condyle in the fossa and rigidly fixating the proximal and distal segment together. If the proximal segment has been surgically displaced posteriorly, when the patient is released from intermaxillary fixation, the mandible will rotate forward producing a more Class III relationship. If the proximal segment was not fully seated with the condyle in the fossa, but the condyle was distracted anteriorly, the patient will exhibit a Class II open bite malocclusion upon release from the intermaxillary fixation. Many surgeons prefer to perform the IVRO procedure with mandibular setback, involving longer intermaxillary fixation but without proximal and distal segment fixation. The result is that the proximal segment is allowed to assume a "physiologic" position that is determined by the musculature and not the surgeon.

Mandibular Distraction Osteogenesis

Mandibular Symphyseal Widening

Prior to distraction osteogenesis, attempts have been made to widen the mandibular arch by other means.[30,31] Most clinical research has suggested that nonsurgical attempts to widen the mandibular arch will not be successful long term.[32] Distraction offers new possibilities for expansion. Unfortunately, one recent paper describes incomplete resolution of the arch length by symphyseal distraction.[33] As a result, critics have suggested that distraction in the symphysis to widen the mandible and resolve arch length deficiencies has unnecessarily proclined the mandibular incisors. Others have suggested that extraction therapy is a more suitable treatment. Conceptually, distraction is the only mandibular expansion alternative that increases the mandibular basal and alveolar bone. The increase in bone can provide a suitable base for the dentition.

Many articles have described the diagnostic and treatment planning criteria regarding mandibular symphyseal distraction osteogenesis.[34,35] To summarize, the classic patient requiring mandibular widening presents with a buccal crossbite that completely encompasses a narrow mandible. Other individuals who would benefit from expansion include those with both a narrow maxilla and mandible. Expansion in the maxilla was previously limited by the mandibular arch width; now, both the maxilla and mandible can be widened simultaneously, producing additional basal and alveolar bone allowing for true skeletal bimaxillary expansion.

Presurgically, root divergence of the mandibular anterior teeth is required. Much like the interdental osteotomy in the maxilla, the midsagittal mandibular osteotomy requires adequate interradicular space.[36] A compressed open coil-spring will produce crown divergence, but can actually produce root convergence since the moment/force ratio is sufficient only to produce simple tipping with the center of rotation between the center of resistance and the root apex. One way to obtain the necessary root divergence preoperatively is by exaggerating the second-order bracket position. If this is done for all the mandibular incisors, care must be taken to avoid extrusion of the mandibular central incisors due to the excessive tip placed in the lateral brackets. In addition, a superelastic wire should not be used, because it cannot be stepped to minimize the incisor extrusion. Confirmation of the root divergence should be done with posteroanterior cephalometric, periapical, or panoramic radiographs. A second way to obtain the root divergence requires a vertical tube/slot in the incisor brackets and fabricating a modified root spring (see Fig. 16-7). The spring should exit the vertical slot, have a helix, and then extend posteriorly and clip over the archwire. This root spring will produce extrusion but also lateral root movement of the incisors. The force should be kept as low as possible to minimize the extrusive effects. Due to the long moment arm, the root spring will still be extremely efficient. Either way, once agreement between the surgeon and the orthodontist is reached, the osteotomy can be performed.

Postsurgically, a short (approximately 1 week) latency period is observed to allow for soft callus formation. Then the appliance is activated no more than 1 mm each day until the desired expansion has been obtained. The teeth are prevented from drifting toward the midline for approximately 30–60 days. After approximately 3 months or until radiographic evidence of new symphyseal bone is observed, the appliance can be removed and a passive 0.036" stainless steel lower lingual arch placed to maintain the expansion. At this point continuous stainless steel wires should be used as well. After appliance removal, the space is closed as it would be in any other arch length redundancy case.

An important consideration during distraction relates to the magnitude and direction of movement that occurs at the mandibular condyle.[37] A recent clinical study has shown that there appears to be translation at the condyle with no clinically significant effects or development of any joint symptoms.[38] As the procedure is performed more frequently, larger study groups will provide further information.

Mandibular Advancement

Some patients who have historically been treated with BSSRO advancements are now being treated utilizing distraction osteogenesis. While distraction itself is not new, adapting it to the craniofacial skeleton is a more recent application of the procedure. Codivilla first used distraction in 1924, but the process did not become popular until the early 1990s. Grayson and McCormick, Molina, and others have described distraction as an excellent mechanism for craniofacial anomalies such as hemifacial microsomia, Goldenhar syndrome, and Pierre–Robin sequence.[19–22]

When considering distraction, the principles of preparing the dentition are the same as those for standard orthognathic surgery. The main difference is that the mandibular skeletal change will be accomplished over a longer period of time using small incremental movements as opposed to an acute positional change in orthognathic surgery. The precise planning of the distraction vector presurgically is critical to obtain and control the correct shape and form of distraction callus.

Prior to orthognathic surgery, model surgery is performed, a custom splint is fabricated, and the amount and direction of the acute movement are determined. The interocclusal splint is then used intraoperatively to determine the final position of the mandible. With distraction, the direction of movement to obtain the desired occlusion is extremely important. Models should be taken to ensure that when the final distraction position is obtained the occlusion will be acceptable. Once the dental arches are coordinated, leveled, and fit is possible, the vector of distraction needs to be determined. Just as the amount and direction of force, and the location of force application are important in all orthodontic mechanics, these same principles apply to the process of distraction. Ideally, localization of the center of resistance of the distal and proximal segments should be performed. The center of resistance will depend on the age of the patient, geometry of the osteotomy, size and shape of the distal and proximal segments, bone density, and muscle strength and pull, among many other factors. It is likely impossible to describe one center of resistance for the mandibles of all distraction patients.

The correct appliance to deliver the appropriate vertical as well as horizontal distraction must be selected. The simplest distraction procedure is the uniplaner mandibular distraction where only anteroposterior distraction is needed. The appliance should most often be oriented to distract the proximal and distal segments parallel to the occlusal plane. Any distraction force applied in a direction other than parallel to the occlusal plane will produce rotation of the distal segment. The rotation could be counterclockwise or clockwise, either of which must be managed to avoid creating an iatrogenic malocclusion. Occasionally, the regenerate must be "molded" with extra- or intra-oral forces[27] to obtain the desired result due to anatomic restrictions limiting appliance placement. With a deep bite patient, it may be possible to orient the distractor above the level of the center of resistance in the distal segment. A moment will be generated that should produce a clockwise or bite-opening rotation. Too steep an angulation, however, could result in creating an open bite. Open bite patients may be able to have the same distractor placed, but below the level of the center of resistance of the distal segment. That way, a counterclockwise or bite closing rotation can be created. Any time the distractor is placed to produce rotation in addition to anteroposterior displacement, greater care and observation should be performed. An inadequately supervised distraction can quickly progress in an unanticipated direction with the rotation produced creating a need for mid-distraction correction.

Biplanar distraction is much more difficult to assess and obtain (Fig. 16-15). Fabrication of a plastic skull constructed from a three-dimensional CT can be a useful aid

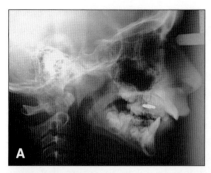
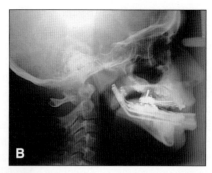
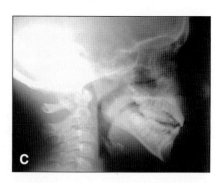

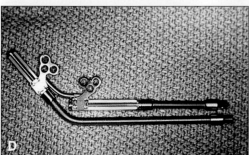

Fig. 16-15 Accurate and precise biplanar mandibular distraction is difficult to achieve due to the limitations of the intraoral appliances as well as the anatomic space limitations. The vector of distraction is just as important here as with maxillary distraction to achieve the optimal result. Here, the appliance is located to attempt to distract the mandible forward with a slight counterclockwise rotation to simultaneously correct the mandibular deficiency as well as reduce the open bite. No studies are available to determine the center of resistance of the proximal and distal segment so clinical judgment, relative size of the segments, and anatomic variation need to be considered to estimate the proper appliance placement. **A** Pretreatment, **B** immediately after appliance placement, and **C** post-treatment cephalographs. **D** Appliance used.

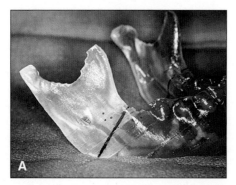
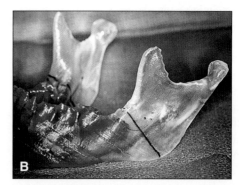

Fig. 16-16 To assist in localizing the center of resistance of the proximal and distal segments, a plastic reconstruction of the patient can be fabricated. The patient is sent for a three-dimensional CT, and the model precisely milled (**A** and **B**). The planned appliance placement can be attempted on the model for feasibility before proceeding to the operating room.

prior to surgery to determine the location of the appliance (Fig. 16-16). Then, the relative amount of vertical and horizontal distraction can be calculated with a predetermined activation schedule and sequence. Most importantly, the patient must be observed frequently to evaluate the distraction process to ensure that the protocol is delivering the desired result.

Just as a protraction headgear utilizing a headgear bow can deliver forces in many different directions relative to the center of resistance, the force from a transcutaneous distraction appliance can deliver similar adjustability. The mechanical advantage of the transmucosal appliances comes at a cost, namely the possibility of scar track formation. The scar tracks, if created, can be revised with plastic surgery procedures, but most patients elect to receive the less invasive, less morbid, intraoral appliances.

Occlusal Plane Change

Limited changes in the cant of the treatment occlusal plane can be performed with isolated maxillary or isolated mandibular surgery. Of course, the occlusal plane alteration is limited by the jaw which is not being surgically manipulated. To obtain an occlusal plane change with isolated mandibular or maxillary surgery, attention is directed to the position of the teeth in each arch relative to the current occlusal plane. High mandibular plane angle patients benefit facially from flattening of the occlusal plane. To accomplish this change, the mandible needs to be leveled with anterior intrusion rather than extrusion of the posterior teeth. The mandible can then be rotated counterclockwise, closing the gonial angle and flattening the mandibular occlusal plane. With maxillary advancement patients, the occlusal plane can be flattened or steepened, but extreme caution should be exercised with how the occlusal plane flattening occurs, due to stability concerns. The maxillary occlusal plane may be flattened if the anterior aspect of the maxilla is elevated, but it is unwise to inferiorly position the posterior maxilla. Such lengthening produces pterygomasseteric muscle stretch which is inherently unstable. The maxillary occlusal plane change is limited because it must still articulate with the unchanged mandible. Typically, when the maxillary occlusal plane is changed and no mandibular surgery is performed, a complete LeFort I (with or without segmentalization) is performed, the maxilla is placed in intermaxillary fixation and the entire complex is rotated to the desired position. In a Class I vertical maxillary excess patient, this requires a slight maxillary advancement along with the occlusal plane change.

For maximal occlusal plane change, two-jaw surgery is required. Then, the maxilla, mandible, and occlusal plane can be moved in all three planes of space, depending on the diagnostic and treatment planning goals for ideal stability, function, and esthetics.[14] As a general geometric rule, steepening the occlusal plane will take a patient who is dentally Class II and make him/her more Class I (Fig. 16-17). This is not unlike using a cervical headgear, Class II elastics, or some other type of functional appliance in the growing patient. However, steepening the occlusal plane will tend to make the facial profile more convex (i.e. more Class II).

Flattening the cant of the occlusal plane will have a tendency to take a Class III malocclusion and make the apical base discrepancy more Class I. However, flattening the occlusal plane with two-jaw surgery will make the facial profile less convex (i.e. flatter and more Class III). A common example of manipulating the cant of the occlusal plane to the patient's benefit is in the patient with a very convex profile, yet displaying a Class I malocclusion. Since the Class I bite limits the possible advancement of the mandible relative to the maxilla, a desirable change in the profile can be achieved by flattening the occlusal plane. In nongrowing individuals, changing the occlusal plane nonsurgically is usually unstable and will tend to revert to the original position. On the other hand, surgery, particularly to steepen the occlusal plane, can allow for significant occlusal plane changes that can be quite stable.

The most common two-jaw surgical patient displays vertical maxillary excess (Fig. 16-18). The goal of treatment typically focuses on steepening the occlusal plane by impacting the maxilla (usually more posteriorly than anteriorly as in an open bite patient) and allowing the mandible to autorotate. Then, either a mandibular advancement or setback is performed based on the occlusal result after maxillary impaction. Several practitioners have focused on flattening the occlusal plane in the same type of patient to produce greater gonial angle definition and chin augmentation. While the facial results appear excellent, the counterclockwise rotation of the dentomaxillary complex is inherently unstable and few, if any, practitioners routinely perform this type of osteotomy.

Other patients that benefit from occlusal plane changes include some of the Class III maxillary hypoplastic syndromic patients. Typical patients present with Apert or Crouzon syndrome, achondroplasia, or cleft lip and palate. All these patients to some degree would benefit from a clockwise rotation of the maxilla and mandible, and in some cases the frontal bone. The occlusion may be near Class I dentally, but skeletally presents as Class III. By rotating the entire complex clockwise, the relative mandibular projection is minimized, allowing greater projection of the frontal bone and maxilla. The initial dental malocclusion can be corrected orthodontically, and the occlusal change then maintained throughout.

Summary

Appropriate orthodontic biomechanics can be the difference between simply treating a patient and treating a patient successfully. When jaw surgery is combined with orthodontic tooth movement, greater care must be taken with the diagnosis and treatment plan as well as the treatment mechanics. Proper mechanics contribute efficiency, stability, enhanced esthetics, and better function to the surgical-orthodontic patient's result. The approach to orthodontic mechanics presented here is an attempt to provide an accurate, precise, planned and predictable operator-determined force system. In this manner, harmony among the dental, skeletal and soft tissue components may be achieved in all three planes of space.

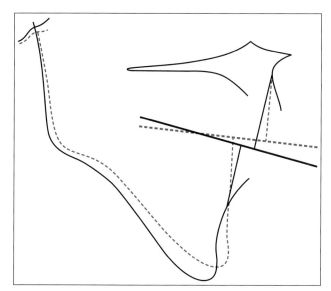

Fig. 16-17 Steepening the occlusal plane can assist in improving the apical base relationship, allowing the Class II dental relationship to be corrected. The clockwise mandibular rotation results in a more convex profile that can negatively impact facial esthetics.

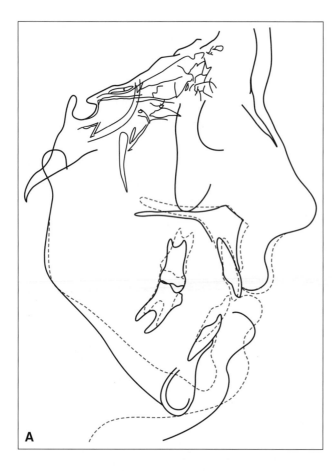

A

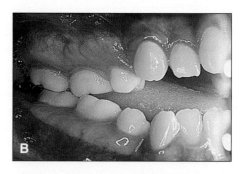

B

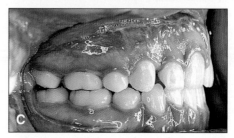

C

Fig. 16-18 A Superimposition depicts the entire surgical manipulation resulting from steepening the occlusal plane in an anterior open bite patient. **B** Pretreatment, a 9 mm anterior open bite was observed. The entire maxilla was impacted, with more impaction posteriorly than anteriorly. **C** Significant mandibular counterclockwise rotation was observed which assisted in closing the open bite.

REFERENCES

1. Burstone CJ, James RB, Legan HL, Murphy GA, Norton LA. Cephalometrics for orthognathic surgery. J Oral Maxillofac Surg 1978;36:269–277.
2. Legan HL, Burstone CJ. Soft tissue cephalometric analysis for orthognathic surgery. J Oral Surg 1980;38:744.
3. Braun S, Hnat WP, Johnson BE. The curve of Spee revisited. Am J Orthod Dentofacial Orthop 1996;110:206–210.
4. Bell WH, Fonseca RJ, Kenneky JW, Levy BM. Bone healing and revascularization after total maxillary osteotomy. J Oral Surg 1975:33:253–260.
5. Jacobs JD, Bell WH, Williams CE, Kennedy JW. Control of the transverse dimension with surgery and orthodontics. Am J Orthod 1980;77:284–306.
6. Marcotte WR. The use of the occlusogram in planning orthodontic treatment. Am J Orthod 1976:60:65–76.
7. Faber RD. Occlusograms in orthodontic treatment planning. J Clin Orthod 1992;26:389–401.
8. Bays RA, Greco JM. Surgically assisted rapid palatal expansion: an outpatient technique with long-term stability. J Oral Maxillofacial Surg 1992;50:110–113.
9. Phillips C, Medland WH, Fields HW Jr, Proffit WR, White RP Jr. Stability of surgical maxillary expansion. Int J Adult Orthod Orthognath Surg 1992;7:139–146.
10. Nanda R, Kuhlberg A. Biomechanical basis of extraction space closure. In: Nanda R, ed. Biomechanics in clinical orthodontics. Philadephia: WB Saunders, 1996.
11. Frost HM. Regional acceleratory phenomenon: a review. Henry Ford Hosp Med J 1983; 31:3–9.
12. Nemeth RB, Isaacson RJ. Vertical anterior relapse. Am J Orthod 1974:65:565–585.
13. Proffit WR, Turvey TA, Phillips C. Orthognathic surgery: a hierarchy of stability. Int J Adult Orthod Orthognath Surg 1996;11:191–204.
14. Legan HL. Orthodontic considerations. In: Peterson LJ, ed. Principles of orthognathic surgery. Philadelphia: JB Lippincott, 1992:1237–1278.
15. Gerlock AJ Jr, Sinn DP, McBride KL. Clinical and radiographic interpretation of facial fractures. Boston, Little, Brown and Company, 1981:99.
16. Moloney F, Worthington P. The origin of the LeFort I maxillary osteotomy. Cheever's operation. J Oral Surg 1981;39:731–734.
17. Wassmund, M. Lehrbuch der praktischen Chirurgie des Mundes und der Kiefer, vol 1. Leipzig, Meuser, 1935.
18. Ilizarov GA. Clinical application of the tension-stress effect for limb lengthening. Clin Orthop Rel Res 1990;250:8–26.
19. McCarthy JG, Stelnicki EJ, Mehrara BJ, Longaker MT. Distraction osteogenesis of the craniofacial skeleton. Plast Reconstr Surg 2001;107:1812–1827.
20. McCarthy JG, Stelnicki EJ, Grayson BH. Distraction osteogenesis of the mandible: a ten-year experience. Semin Orthod 1999;5:3–8.
21. Toth BA, Kim JW, Chin M, Cedars M. Distraction osteogenesis and its application to the midface and bony orbit in craniosynostosis syndromes. J Craniofac Surg 1998;9:100–113.

22. Molina F, Ortiz Monasterio F. Mandibular elongation and remodeling by distraction: a farewell to major osteotomies. Plast Reconstr Surg 1995;96:825–842.

23. Guerrero CA, Bell WH, Meza LS. Intraoral distraction osteogenesis: maxillar and mandibular lengthening. Atlas Oral Maxillofac Surg Clin North Am 1999;7:111–151.

24. Lee KG, Ryu YK, Park YC, Rudolph DJ. A study of holographic interferometry on the initial reaction of maxillofacial complex during protraction. Am J Orthod Dentofacial Orthop 1997;111:623–632.

25. Ahn JG, Figueroa AA, Braun S, Polley JW. Biomechanical considerations in distraction of the osteotomized dentomaxillary complex. Am J Orthod Dentofacial Orthop 1999;116:264–270.

26. Kennedy JW 3rd, Bell WH, Kimbrough OL, James WB. Osteotomy as an adjunct to rapid maxillary expansion. Am J Orthod 1976;70:123–137.

27. Hanson PR, Melugin MB. Orthodontic management of the patient undergoing mandibular distraction osteogenesis. Semin Orthod 1999;5:25–34.

28. Braun S, Bantleon HP, Hnat WP, Freudenthaler JW, Marcotte MR, Johnson BE. A study of bite force: Part II. Relationship to various cephalometric measurements. Angle Orthod 1995;65:373–377.

29. Bailey LJ, Proffit WR, White RP. Trends in surgical Class III treatment. Int J Adult Orthod Orthogn Surg 1995;10:108–118.

30. McDougall PD, McNamara JA Jr, Dierkes JM. Arch development in Class II patients treated with the Frankel appliance. Am J Orthod Dentofac Orthoped 1982;82:10–22.

31. Weinberg M, Sadowsky C. Resolution of mandibular arch crowding in growing patients with Class I malocclusion treated non-extraction. Am J Orthod Dentofac Orthoped 1996;110:359–364.

32. Little RM, Riedel RA, Stein A. Mandibular arch increase during the mixed dentition: Post retention evaluation of stability and relapse. Am J Orthod 1990;97:393–404.

33. Del Santo M, Guerrero CA, Buschang PA, English JD, Samchukov S, Bell WH. Midsymphyseal distraction osteogenesis for correcting transverse mandibular discrepancies. Am J Orthod Dentofacial Orthop 2002;121:629–638.

34. Conley RS, Legan HL. Mandibular symphyseal distraction osteogenesis: Diagnosis and treatment planning considerations. Angle Orthod 2003;73:3–11.

35. Contasti G, Guerrero C, Rodriguez AM, Legan HL. Mandibular widening by distraction osteogenesis. J Clin Orthod 2001;35:165–173.

36. Legan HL. Orthodontic planning and biomechanics for transverse distraction osteogenesis. Semin Orthod 2001;7:160–168.

37. Samchukov ML, Cope JB, Harper RP, Ross JD. Biomechanical considerations of mandibular lengthening and widening by gradual distraction using a computer model. J Oral Maxillofac Surg 1998;56:51–59.

38. Braun S, Bottrel JA, Legan HL. Condylar displacement related to mandibular symphyseal distraction. Am J Orthod Dentofacial Orthop 2002;121:162–165.

CHAPTER 17

Biomechanic Strategies for Optimal Finishing

Flavio Uribe and Ravindra Nanda

Orthodontic finishing is described as an "art" comprised of individual perceptions and small detailing. Its primary goals are to achieve excellent occlusion, proper alignment, and an esthetic smile.

Finishing is perhaps one of the most deceiving and difficult phases of orthodontic treatment. This is most likely due to:

1. The patient generally does not appreciate the clinical progress during this phase. The major orthodontic changes have already occurred during initial alignment and space closure and small tooth movements or root corrections are not easily observed or appreciated by the average patient.
2. When trying to achieve small corrections, adverse side effects may occur in segments of the dental arch that are already in an ideal position.
3. Occasionally, the treatment time of this stage exceeds that of the previous stages, especially when a substantial amount of root correction is required.
4. The majority of patients are eager to finish their treatment after alignment is obtained and space closure is completed.

Finishing is the last phase of "active" treatment and thus is heavily dependent upon the previous stages of treatment. It is extremely difficult, if not impossible, to achieve an acceptable end result when the treatment objectives have not been met and the mechanics have not been delivered properly. Major tooth movement, or macromechanics, should have been executed properly, so the minute tooth movements, or micromechanics (AJ Kuhlberg, personal communication), can be achieved with precision in the final finishing phase of treatment. When the treatment mechanics are less than optimal, the finishing stages often include indiscriminate use of intermaxillary elastics and quick-fix therapies like interproximal reduction. Although there are definite indications for these procedures, they should not be used routinely to compensate for deficiencies in treatment planning and/or application of mechanics.

Finishing distinguishes the true master of the profession from the average orthodontist (Fig. 17-1). It is the small details that make the difference and these details are the essence of finishing. Overall, the final stage of treatment is evaluated according to four major categories: intraoral, extraoral, radiographic, and functional objectives. Each category has specific objectives that must be met to obtain a desirable finish.

Intraoral Objectives

This category is arguably the most important of the four.[1] The intraoral objectives are classified into two subcategories: intra- and inter-arch objectives. The primary objective in both is to achieve ideal occlusion with well aligned arches. Most of these intraoral objectives are described in the American Board of Orthodontics (ABO) grading criteria.[3]

Intra-Arch Analysis

To understand the type of micromovements required in the arch during the finishing stage, each tooth must be

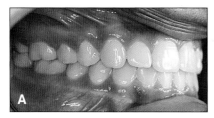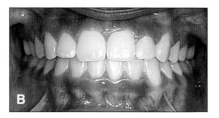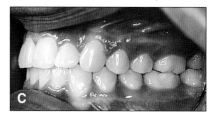

Fig. 17-1 A-C Frontal and lateral views of a finished patient with a good occlusal result.

evaluated with reference to its first-, second-, and third-order position. When evaluating the first order, teeth should have tight interproximal contacts and no rotations.[2] In addition, tooth morphology must be taken into consideration, and the cusp tips and fossae should follow the perfect arch form. An occlusal mirror is used to identify minor rotations and buccolingual displacement of teeth outside of the perfect arch form (Fig. 17-2). The upper first molar has special considerations regarding its first-order position. A mesial out rotation of the mesiobuccal cusp[3] is considered to be ideal. It has also been advocated that the buccal surface of the upper first molar should be parallel to the palatal suture (Fig. 17-3).[4]

In the second order, the root parallelism and marginal ridges are evaluated. The marginal ridges should be at the same level, particularly in the buccal segments. Often when marginal ridges between adjacent teeth coincide, root parallelism also will. Root correction of teeth in order to achieve root parallelism is important in longterm retention and stability. A panoramic X-ray is an adjunct to evaluate second-order discrepancies. Small adjustments in the second-order angulation of the anterior teeth (i.e. accentuating the distal tip) can help decrease any excess space in the anterior region (Fig. 17-4).[2]

The third order is most relevant to the interarch objectives (i.e. the occlusal relationship) and to the esthetics of the smile (an extraoral category which is discussed later). With regard to the intraoral objectives, a small curve of Monson between the buccal segments allows for proper occlusal function (i.e. adequate intercuspation without balancing interferences). An accentuated curve of Monson usually results in balancing interferences, especially in the second molar area.[5] This clinical situation is commonly encountered in adults after the dental correction of buccal crossbites without expansion of the basal bone/palatal suture (Fig. 17-5). Proper third-order angulation of anterior teeth is also important for good occlusion (Fig. 17-6). Furthermore, regarding the extraoral category, third-order angulation is important for good esthetics of the smile (Fig. 17-7).[2] Moreover, significant emphasis on the upper canine and first premolar third-order inclination has been

Fig. 17-2 Occlusal mirror as an aid to evaluating intra-arch discrepancies during finishing. This view is used to identify first-order rotations, spacing, and any arch form problems.

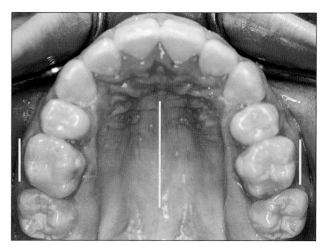

Fig. 17-3 Occlusal view of a finished case where the buccal surface of the upper first molar is parallel to the mid palatal raphe.

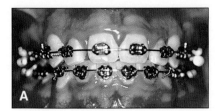
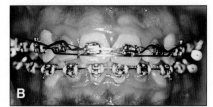
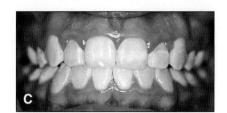

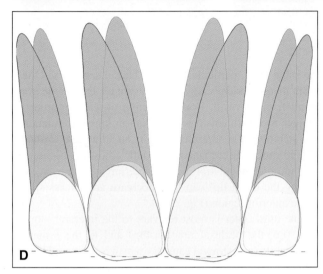

Fig. 17-4 A-C Patient shows no overjet but excess space between the incisors due to a Bolton discrepancy. These spaces can be closed or reduced by accentuating the distal root tip of the incisors, thereby increasing the interproximal contact distance. Incisal adjustments (enamoplasty) were done at the appliance removal visit. **D** Diagram showing the distal tip and enamoplasty required.

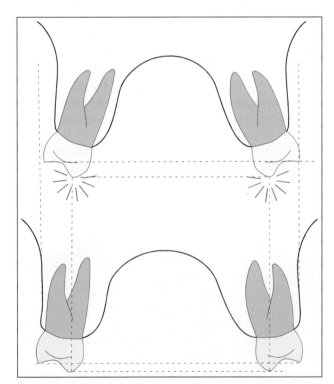

Fig. 17-5 Proper third-order angulation needed in the posterior buccal segments may not be achieved in adults after arch width expansion without surgery. Occlusal balancing contacts may result from the dental third-order compensation. The lower diagram shows the difference in skeletal width and vertical cusp position achievable with skeletal expansion.

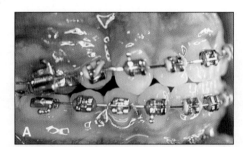
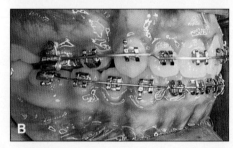

Fig. 17-6 A and **B** Patient shows an improvement in the occlusion after proper third-order angulation of the anterior teeth is obtained.

proposed by some clinicians.[6] In general, the buccal surfaces of these teeth should be close to parallel to the mid sagittal facial line in an ideal smile.

The final intra-arch objective is to achieve a gentle curve of Spee from the anterior teeth to the posterior buccal segments.[2] The magnitude of this curve will vary depending

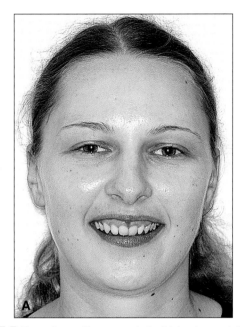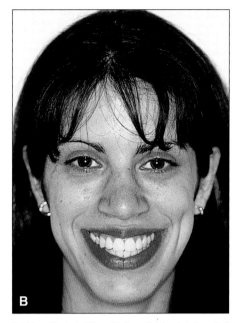

Fig. 17-7 Depending on the upper anterior third-order angulation, light is reflected differently from the frontal view. **A** Patient with retroclined incisors. Note the light reflected in the periodontal tissues. **B** Patient with proper incisor inclination. Note the light reflected in the middle third of the incisors. (Reproduced courtesy of Dr AJ Kuhlberg).

on the overbite (interarch relation) and incisor display (an extraoral finishing objective) which will be discussed later.

Inter-Arch Analysis

The first molars and canines are the most important teeth to evaluate regarding the interocclusal relationship. Traditionally, orthodontists have classified malocclusion in the anteroposterior dimension and thus the static analysis of the occlusion has primarily been based on the first molar relationship. Additionally, the canine is of prime importance if canine-guided functional occlusion is to be achieved. The main objective is to "seat" the canines into a Class I relationship and obtain good coupling with the antagonistic canines. This ideal interocclusal relationship is difficult to achieve when a significant tooth size discrepancy exists between the dental arches (i.e. a Bolton discrepancy).[7] The upper lateral incisors and lower second premolars are usually responsible for this interarch tooth size discrepancy,[8] as abnormal tooth morphology is more common in these teeth. This results in less than ideal occlusion that becomes apparent at the end of treatment (Fig. 17-8).

Two types of occlusion have been considered ideal: cusp-to-fossa relationship and cusp-to-interproximal space. In the natural dentition, a cusp-to-interproximal space is most characteristic.[3] The lingual cusps in the upper arch and the buccal cusps in the lower arch are primarily responsible for function. The buccal cusps of the upper premolars and the lingual cusps of the lower premolars should occlude in the interproximal space. In Class II patients, some of the anteroposterior correction can be achieved by over

rotation of the buccal cusps of the upper premolars distally to coincide with the lower interproximal spaces.[9,10] In the anterior segment, overbite and overjet are the most critical factors in achieving a proper interocclusal relationship. These two occlusal traits determine the disclusion of the posterior teeth during protrusive movements. More than 50% overbite may be excessive, as the contact of the lower incisors on the lingual surface of the upper incisors in these patients would not be on the cingulum (the most suitable portion to receive occlusal forces). Finally, it is important that the lingual surface of the upper incisors be properly inclined to allow the lower incisors to slide anteriorly in an angle that is in synchrony with the articular eminence.[11]

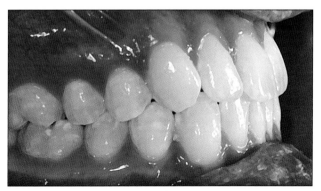

Fig. 17-8 Bolton discrepancy reflected in the occlusion in the finishing stage. There is a tendency to a Class II canine relationship due to the small upper laterals.

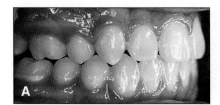 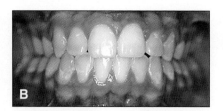 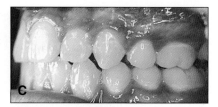

Fig. 17-9 A-C Midline discrepancy of approximately 2 mm to the right. A tendency towards a Class III canine occlusion is seen on the left side.

Arch coordination is also evaluated from the frontal view. This allows proper cusp seating to be visualized. The intercanine and intermolar widths should be coordinated to prevent excessive buccal overjet or a buccal crossbite tendency. The premolar area is also inspected transversely for proper coordination between the upper and lower arches.

Midlines are also used to evaluate interocclusal relationships. In the finishing phase of treatment, midlines should be coincident. Any discrepancy >2 mm should have been addressed in the macrodontic phases of treatment. Moreover, any discrepancy of 1–2 mm or more between the midlines will probably result in an inadequate occlusal relationship, at least in one of the buccal segments (Fig. 17-9). The midline objectives in the finishing stage are evaluated in the extraoral finishing category as well, particularly in the upper arch.

Extraoral Objectives

The extraoral objectives are based on esthetic concepts, with the majority of these concerning the smile. The key factors within the smile that need to be addressed are: smile arc, incisor display, gingival display, buccal corridors, incisal plane, midlines, upper incisor third-order angulations, and tooth morphology in the esthetic zone.

Smile Arc

The ideal smile arc is discussed in Chapter 3. In the finishing stage, little can be done to significantly affect the smile arc. Some small finishing bends can differentially extrude or intrude the anterior teeth, but that is about all that can be accomplished. The dilemma concerning these wire bends is the potential for antagonistic effects on the interocclusal finishing objectives. An example of this is seen when the overbite is perfect and the teeth need to be extruded to achieve an ideal smile arc. A choice between achieving an esthetic objective (ideal smile arc) and an occlusal objective (ideal overbite) is needed. A compromise might be the best decision. More importantly, a limit to the amount of compromise for each characteristic should be set (i.e. avoiding finishing with >50% overbite and a flat or reverse smile arc).

Incisor Display

On average, females show 2–3 mm of incisor at rest and 1 mm of gingiva when smiling.[12] Males show approximately 1 mm less of incisor for each of these lip relations. During the diagnosis and treatment planning phases, an appropriate plan for correction of any deviation is made. By the finishing phase of treatment, the vertical incisor objectives should have already been accomplished. Detailing in this area should be limited to proper alignment and leveling of the incisal edges (providing no restorations are needed). Attempting to significantly intrude or extrude the incisors may complicate and prolong treatment.

Open bite malocclusions with moderate-to-excessive incisor display present a challenge as they are difficult to correct. It is not unusual to find an open bite tendency still present by the finishing phase in this type of malocclusion. If no additional upper incisor display is desired, the overbite correction should be done by extruding the lower anterior teeth. This can be accomplished by accentuating the lower curve of Spee.

Gingival Display

The amount and characteristics of the gingival display (symmetry and height relationships of adjacent teeth) are important aspects to consider in a smile. Generally, males do not show any marginal gingiva when smiling and therefore the gingival height relationship of adjacent teeth is not as important. Females, on the other hand, display approximately 1 mm of gingiva upon smiling.[13] Thus, symmetry in the gingiva and proper gingival height relationships in the upper arch are important (Fig. 17-10).

During finishing, gingival display and symmetry can be altered within a narrow range of approximately 1 mm by selective intrusion or extrusion of any of the anterior teeth. Most frequently, the incisal edges will reflect gingival height asymmetries providing incisal wear is not present (Fig. 17-11). The overbite will be the limiting factor of the magnitude of the finishing bends. However, if wear is present, the gingival height relationship will determine the finishing movements of the anterior teeth in the vertical dimension, instead of being determined by the level of the incisal edges (Fig. 17-12).[14] The final incisal edge position, if there is significant incisal wear, is determined

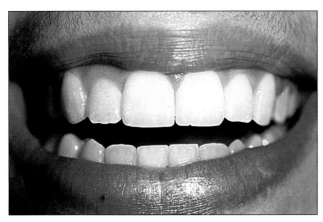

Fig. 17-10 Finished treatment in a young female patient who displays the upper gingiva on smiling. An asymmetry in the gingival heights of the lateral incisors is evident.

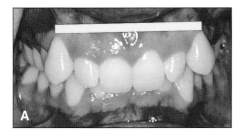

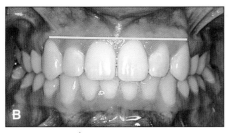

Fig. 17-11 A Incisal edges reflect the discrepancies in the gingival heights provided no incisal wear is present. **B** Correction of the incisal edges generally results in adequate gingival heights.

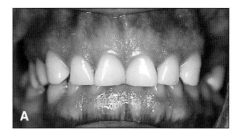

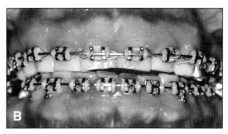

Fig. 17-12 A Inadequate gingival height in the upper anterior region with excessive overbite and worn incisors. **B** Intrusion mechanics of the four upper anterior teeth to obtain proper gingival heights. Restoration of the incisors is needed to achieve adequate proportions and overbite.

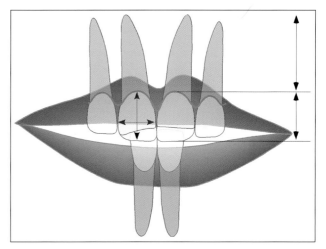

Fig. 17-13 Factors involved in the final incisal edge position. The interrelationship of gingival height, tooth proportions, lip to tooth relationship, crown/root ratio, and overbite determines the position of the upper incisor in space.

by proper tooth proportions, gingival heights, relationship to the upper lip, crown/root ratio, and overbite (Fig. 17-13).

Periodontal procedures should be considered as an adjunct to the esthetic objectives after finishing in patients with an excessive gingival display or asymmetric gingival heights. The periodontal procedures that can be considered are gingivectomy or crown lengthening (depending on the alveolar bone level) (Fig. 17-14). These procedures may also be combined with prosthetic alternatives in patients with worn incisal edges, or abnormally shaped incisors (i.e. peg laterals).

A common unesthetic result after gingivectomies or crown lengthening (performed exclusively in the anterior segment) is seen in the transition area from the canine to the premolars. Ideally, there should be a 1 mm step down in

gingival height between these teeth. When gingivectomies are not carried to the premolars, excess gingiva remains more pronounced in the corners of the smile (Fig. 17-15).[15]

In the literature little attention has been given to the gingival heights of the lower teeth. Symmetry and gingival height of the lower incisors in relation to the canines are important factors, especially in individuals over 30 years of age, as the lower gingival margin is more visible.[13] It is not uncommon to find a discrepancy in gingival heights between the lower incisors and the canines, particularly in deep bite patients (Fig. 17-16). In young patients, the gingival margin usually follows the incisal edges of the

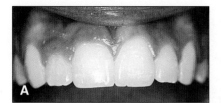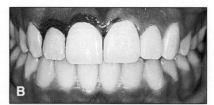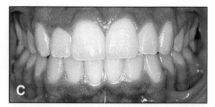

Fig. 17-14 Asymmetric gingival heights. **A** Upper right lateral incisor has a more coronal gingival height. The upper right central incisor also has a slight coronal relationship to the gingival margin compared with its contralateral tooth. **B** Gingivectomy performed on the upper right central and lateral incisors. **C** Post surgery.

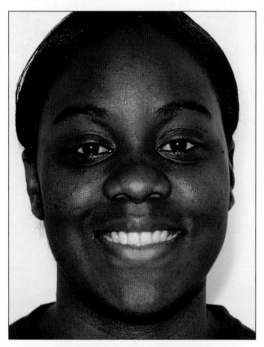

Fig. 17-15 Excess gingival show on the upper buccal segments. Gingival heights are adequate from canine to canine. A smoother transition from the canine to the first premolar can be obtained by periodontal surgical procedures.

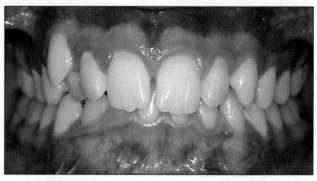

Fig. 17-16 Discrepancy between the gingival heights of the lower incisors and the canines. Supraeruption of the lower incisors is evident at the incisal edges and is reflected on the overbite.

lower anterior teeth. This problem is corrected as the canines and central incisors are leveled during the initial phases of orthodontic treatment. In the adult, wear facets can complicate the determination of where proper gingival heights should be located. As the incisors supra-erupt, a good incisal edge relationship with the canines will exist, but a significant discrepancy in the gingival height will develop. To correct this discrepancy, a decision must be made from the following choices: gingivectomy/crown lengthening to match gingival heights with no restorations; gingivectomy/crown lengthening and restorations (composites or veneers or crowns); intrusion of the four anterior teeth to level the gingival heights (no surgery) and restorations (composites or veneers or crowns). A very important additional factor in deciding between these alternatives is the crown/root ratio. Any osseous resective periodontal procedure (crown lengthening) increases this ratio; there-

fore, a good assessment of the eventual remaining root structure is required (Fig. 17-17).

Buccal Corridors

The esthetic objective of widening the narrow buccal corridors, if indicated (see Ch. 3), should have been achieved long before the finishing stage. Any type of arch expansion during the finishing stages is difficult to achieve and unstable in the long term.

Incisal Cant

From the frontal view, a cant in the upper incisor segment is sometimes found during finishing procedures. This cant may be limited to the incisor segment or involve the entire maxillary arch. The incisal cant can be the result of improper bonding techniques (i.e. incorrect bracket positioning), asymmetric mechanics, or a true maxillary skeletal cant which was undetected during diagnosis due to dental compensations. Therefore, a differential diagnosis between a dental or a skeletal incisal cant is important.

Patients who have an incisal cant due to a skeletally canted maxilla generally present with uneven heights between the labial commissure and the occlusal surfaces of the premolars (Fig. 17-18). This can also be identified by an uneven gingival display between the left and right sides when smiling. Care must be taken when developing a differential diagnosis between a true maxillary cant (skeletal etiology) and an asymmetric smile (soft tissue

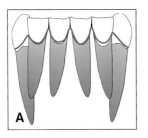
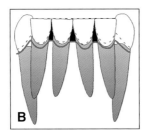
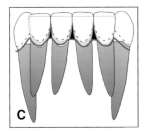
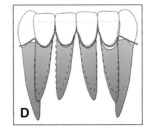

Fig. 17-17 **A** Significant attrition with supraeruption of the lower incisors. Different treatment modalities include: **B** Gingivectomy/crown lengthening to match the gingival heights. As the gingival margin is brought down a more tapered crown morphology is observed. Black triangles may result with this alternative; **C** gingivectomy/crown lengthening with additional restorations (crowns or veneers). The crown morphology is restored to normal tooth proportions and the crown/root ratio is increased; and **D** orthodontic intrusion plus restorative procedures. The crown/root ratio is more favorable.

etiology). A true maxillary cant is difficult to correct, and when the discrepancy is excessive, a maxillary LeFort osteotomy may be the best treatment. Other alternatives may involve periodontic and prosthodontic options to camouflage the cant (Fig. 17-18B).

In patients where the cant only involves the anterior teeth, corrections in the finishing stages are difficult but possible. An option is to place an intrusive force on the area that needs to be intruded (Fig. 17-19).[17] If the rotation of the anterior segment needs to be around the center of resistance, two cantilevers (with equal and opposite forces that produce a couple) may be placed to achieve intrusion of one side and extrusion of the opposite side (Fig. 17-20A). A second method to achieve rotation around the center of resistance is to place a cantilever in an auxiliary tube of the anterior segment (Fig. 17-20B).

Midlines

A discrepancy between the upper and lower dental midlines is generally most noticeable at the end of treatment. Coincidentally, it is also at this time that this problem is most difficult to correct. To achieve coincident midlines during finishing, the range of correction for each arch is approximately 1 mm to each side. Tipping is the major type of tooth movement that can be used to correct midlines at the finishing stage. It is important to stress that a slight discrepancy between the upper midline is esthetically acceptable[18-20] and generally does not have any occlusal implications.

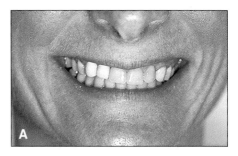
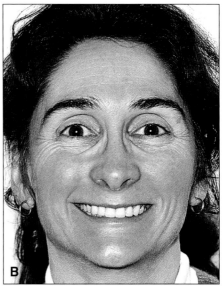

Fig. 17-18 Occlusal cant of the maxilla evidenced on the left side. Gingiva is only displayed on the left side in relation to the labial commissure. **B** Cant was camouflaged by prosthodontic work. Crowns were elongated on the right side and shortened on the left. Interproximal contacts were made more parallel to the facial midline.

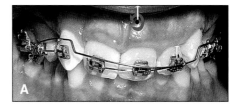
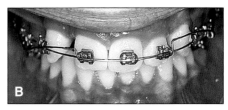

Fig. 17-19 Asymmetric intrusion arch placed to correct the incisal cant. **A** 0.017 × 0.025 nickel–titanium intrusion arch is tied to the distal of the upper left lateral incisor. A continuous 0.017 × 0.025 stainless steel segment from the upper right central incisor to upper left lateral incisor is tied into the brackets of these teeth. The force system produces an intrusive force and a moment at the center of resistance of the anterior segment. **B** Correction seen 1 month later. The cant was corrected and the midline discrepancy had improved.

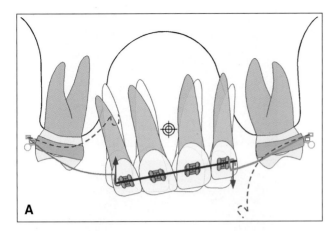

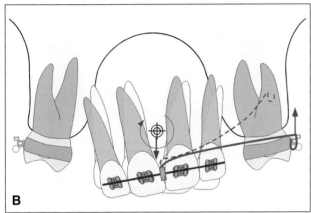

Fig. 17-20 A Moment produced by two cantilevers with the same amount of force in opposite directions. **B** Moment produced by a cantilever with the single couple tied to an auxiliary tube in the anterior segment. A transpalatal arch is used in both situations for a solid anchor unit to minimize the side effects.

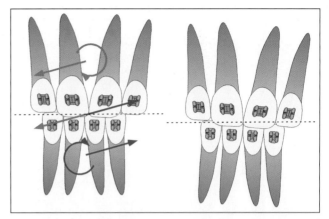

Fig. 17-21 Vertical effects produced by an anterior cross elastic. The vertical component of the elastic force to correct midline discrepancy may produce canting of the incisal plane.

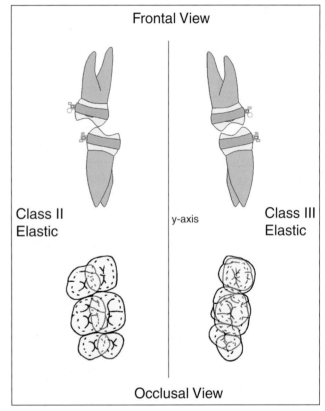

Fig. 17-22 Class II and Class III elastics produce rotation around the y axis. Brodie bite tendency is seen on the Class III elastic side and a cross bite tendency on the Class II elastic side.

On occasion there is a relationship between an incisal cant and a midline discrepancy. By correcting the incisal cant, the midline problem may be improved (see Fig. 17-19), although in some instances the midline discrepancy might be accentuated. It is important to consider all the smile characteristics together; correction of one characteristic should maintain, if not improve, the other.

The techniques used to correct midline problems during the finishing phase mainly rely on the use of anterior cross elastics. In some instances a combination of Class II elastics on one side and Class III on the other can be used. This method seems easy, but can result in serious problems if used indiscriminately. The orthodontist must watch for the side effects that may occur in the vertical and transverse planes with this manner of longterm elastic use. In the vertical direction, canting of the occlusal planes as a result of the vertical component of the anterior cross elastic force may occur (Fig. 17-21). In the transverse plane, rotation of the dental arches around the y axis with the use of Class II/Class III elastics may result in a crossbite tendency on one buccal segment and a Brodie bite tendency on the other (Fig. 17-22).[21]

A final method to correct the dental midline in the finishing stages is the use of a cantilever with the active force along the x axis. The upper anteriors are treated as a segment and a force is applied at the bracket level of this segment. The anchor unit (posterior segment) is made up of the molars and premolars. A palatal arch is used to prevent the rotational moment and lingual force on the

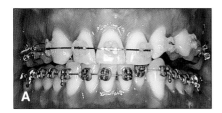
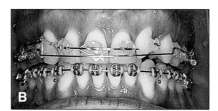
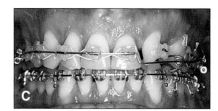

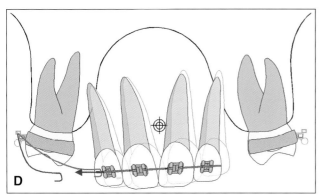

Fig. 17-23 Method for correction of small midline deviations. **A** Upper incisors tipped to the left with a midline deviation of approximately 2 mm. **B** Force system in place (see **D** for explanation). A transpalatal arch offsets the moment on the posterior segment (mesial in). A continuous base arch bypassing the incisors aids in preventing their extrusion as they tip. The cantilever can be tied directly to the anterior segment. An elastic was placed for patient comfort. **C** Force from the cantilever tips the teeth in the direction of the midline correction. **D** Force system.

anchor unit where the cantilever (couple side) is inserted (Fig. 17-23.).

Upper Incisor Third-Order Inclination

Esthetic considerations of the upper incisal inclination are not only important from the profile view, but also from the frontal view. A common occurrence in the final stages of treatment, particularly in extraction cases, is excessive lingual crown torque. Although this is easily visualized from a lateral view, it can also be appreciated from the frontal view.[22] Third-order tooth corrections are difficult and time consuming movements. Extensive bone remodeling needs to occur as root correction is pursued and side effects such as upper molar mesial migration become common. Perhaps the best way to approach this objective is by maintaining a proper moment/force ratio during the retraction phase in extraction cases.[23] Some of the alternative mechanics in the finishing phase include auxiliary torquing springs (Fig. 17-24). Care must be taken to prevent the incisors from flaring if only root correction is needed. This can be achieved by cinching the archwires

or lacing together the entire arch. The clinician must also be aware of the rowboat effect that is generated with root correction (Fig. 17-25).[24] Simultaneous use of Class II elastics is recommended to prevent this effect. Additionally, a mild bowing of the anterior segment with the torquing spring is expected due to the intrusive lateral forces on the posterior segment.

Tooth Morphology

Tooth morphology in the anterior or esthetic zone is of prime importance. The upper lateral incisors most often exhibit abnormal morphology in this zone. It is less common to find abnormally shaped central incisors. Preliminary planning regarding the space distribution for restoring teeth with abnormal morphology should be accomplished during the diagnosis and treatment planning phase. Involving a restorative dentist and a periodontist during the treatment planning phase is good practice. In the finishing phase, communication within the team is crucial and will help determine any precise finishing orthodontic tooth movements needed. Many of the

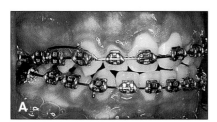
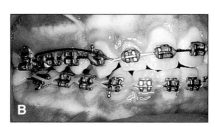
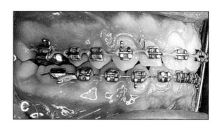

Fig. 17-24 A Upright upper incisors with anterior crossbite tendency. The torquing spring produces an anterior moment and an extrusive force needed in the anterior segment. The upper arch is laced together in order to prevent anterior spacing. **B** Correction seen after 1 month. **C** Final correction achieved in approximately 3 months.

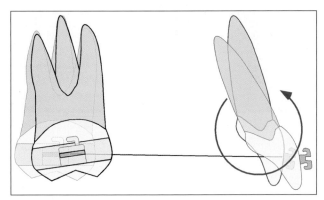

Fig. 17-25 Rowboat effect produced by the lingual root correction moment (facial crown movement).

restorative procedures should be done in conjunction with periodontal procedures to achieve the best tooth proportions.

Tooth proportions are influenced by the position of the gingival margin, as well as the width and height of the tooth. These factors can be affected by the restorative dentist in conjunction with the periodontist. The shape of the incisor and the restorative option (composite buildup, veneers or crowns) will determine the position of the abnormally shaped lateral incisor within the dental arch.[15] It is of primary importance in achieving excellent esthetic results that good communication is maintained with the restorative dentist.

Slight contouring of the incisal edges of the upper anterior teeth, especially the canines, has been recommended at the end of treatment for most patients.[25] The incisal edges of the anterior teeth with a small incisal edge fracture can also be contoured after previous extrusion. The gingival height relation to the adjacent tooth may be altered with the extrusion of the incisor; thus, an additional gingivectomy or crown lengthening procedure may be indicated if the patient displays gingiva upon smiling.

In patients congenitally missing lateral incisors treated by canine substitution, the alteration of canine morphology to mimic a lateral incisor is usually done in the early stages of treatment, with small detailing left for the finishing stages (Fig. 17-26). The premolars that substitute for

canines also need to be contoured on the lingual cusps to avoid balancing interferences.

The final situation in which abnormalities in tooth morphology are considered during finishing is the pronounced lingual fossae of the upper incisors. This abnormal crown morphology is found most frequently in Asian and African populations.[26] In these patients the mesial and distal ridges adjacent to the fossa are pronounced and prevent a good intercuspation in the buccal segments. It is recommended that the height of these ridges should be reduced to achieve better posterior occlusion.

Radiographic Objectives

Just before starting the finishing stage of treatment, it is always recommended that a panoramic radiograph be taken to evaluate root angulation and root parallelism. Problems in second-order angulation of the upper lateral incisors, lower premolars, and teeth adjacent to the extraction sites are commonly found (Fig. 17-27). Clinically, marginal ridge discrepancies are also a good method to detect possible root angulation discrepancies. However, the panoramic radiograph provides better evidence of root position, angulation, and parallelism.

Root angulation problems observed in the finishing panoramic radiograph might be also related to abnormal tooth morphology and/or bracketing errors. This is especially evident in the buccal segments where it is difficult to gain access for bracket placement and premolars with abnormal crown morphology are common.

Root parallelism is important for three reasons. First, the occlusal load of the forces will be transmitted properly across the longitudinal axis of the tooth. Second, in patients where only the crown has been tipped and the root is not in its proper position, there is a greater potential for relapse.[27] Finally, there is a potential for periodontal problems due to root proximity. However, the rationale for this last statement is not well supported by the literature; no deleterious effects on the periodontium have been found in finished orthodontic cases with root proximity.[28]

The finishing panoramic radiograph is also helpful in evaluating root resorption. If external apical root resorption is observed, the orthodontist may want to decrease the length of time spent on the finishing stage. Although

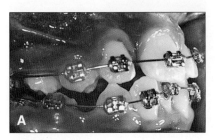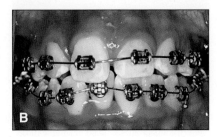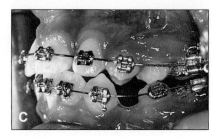

Fig. 17-26 A-C Early contouring of the canines to resemble lateral incisor morphology.

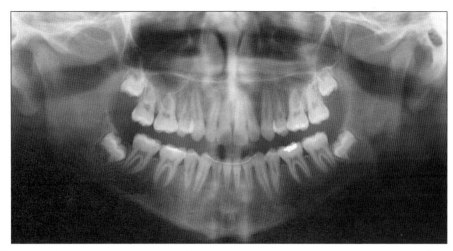

Fig. 17-27 Finished four premolar extraction (upper first and lower seconds) patient with poor root alignment of the lower first premolars and upper laterals.

monitoring for root resorption has been recommended during the first 6 months of treatment,[29,30] usually it is noticed on the finishing panoramic radiograph.

Finally, two other important pieces of information can be obtained from a panoramic radiograph: evidence of any deterioration in periodontal health, and the eruption angle of the third molars. If the eruption of the second molars is delayed, or the orthodontic treatment is being finished before complete eruption of the second molars, it is important to evaluate their position and the eruption pattern (Fig. 17-28).

Periapical radiographs are usually only indicated in the finishing stages to obtain a more detailed view of any significant findings observed in the panoramic radiograph such as: extensive root resorption, root parallelism between adjacent teeth to an implant site, or evidence of periodontal bone loss.

Functional Considerations

A proper functional occlusion is the goal in every orthodontic treatment. However, as mentioned in Chapter 3, the definition of an ideal functional occlusion is not completely clear. In general, a mutually protected occlusion is considered to be the ideal goal.

To achieve this ideal occlusion during the finishing stages, it is important to have the maximum amount of normal occlusal contacts during maximum intercuspation. Although a coinciding centric relation with centric occlusion is the goal proposed by some clinicians, a small

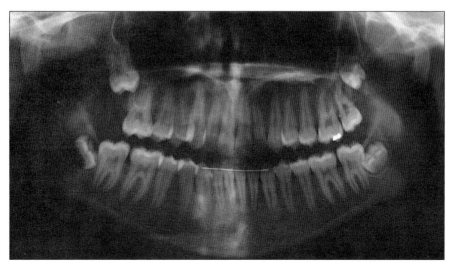

Fig. 17-28 Panoramic X-ray should be taken before appliance removal to evaluate root apices, root parallelism, and status of unerupted teeth. This panoramic X-ray reveals an abnormally erupting second molar, noticed only after appliance removal.

discrepancy between these two occlusal relationships is acceptable (long centric).[12]

With lateral movements of the jaw, a canine disclusion is the standard, although group function is acceptable. More importantly, no balancing contacts should be present. Canine disclusion is also a major protective factor in patients who receive any type of anterior esthetic restorations (veneers, composites, porcelain crowns). Finally, the anterior teeth should disclude the posterior teeth during protrusive movements. All these movements should be evaluated during the finishing stage and proper adjustments in crown angulations (relative to tip and torque) should be achieved. Small adjustments can be made after appliance removal, e.g. occlusal adjustments with rotary instruments; however, these should be minimal as there is a limit to the amount of tooth structure that can be removed.

Overcorrection

During finishing, the concept of overcorrection can be applied to the alignment (first order corrections) and to certain malocclusions.[11,31–33] It is believed by some that overcorrection of rotated teeth, especially in the antero-inferior segment of teeth, may be necessary for stability. Since the amount of, and to a certain extent the direction of, rotational relapse is unpredictable,[34] this practice may not be indicated. However, overcorrection in some malocclusions may be more applicable, e.g. problems in the vertical dimension, especially open bites, may have better longterm stability if overcorrected.

Unusual Finishing Situations

Lower Incisor Extraction
Finishing in patients treated with a lower incisor extraction is challenging. If no tooth size discrepancies are present (i.e. excessive tooth mass in the lower arch), the patient will generally finish with either a Class I canine relationship with excessive overjet, or with ideal overjet and a Class III canine tendency relationship (Fig. 17-29). Generally, when an excessive tooth mass exists in the lower arch compared to the upper arch, a good occlusal intercuspation with ideal overjet is seen at the end of treatment.

Another problem frequently observed with incisor extractions is that the patient ends up with black interproximal triangles in the lower incisor segment (Fig. 17-30). To solve this problem, slight interproximal enamel reduction and root reproximation on the lower teeth is done to move the contact more gingivally and to decrease the size of these black triangles. To some degree this procedure will accentuate the overjet because more tooth structure is removed from the lower anterior incisors, thus increasing the interarch tooth size discrepancy. Finally, major efforts should be made to coordinate the arches as the lower incisor extraction space is closed. Lower incisor extraction also results in a decrease in the intercanine distance,[35] and thereby an excessive canine overjet results (see Figs 17-29B and 17-30).

Finishing with Primary Teeth
Finishing is also challenging when the succedaneous permanent tooth is congenitally missing from the primary teeth, and particularly when the primary tooth without a successor is the first or second molar. Some advocate extraction of the primary molar and closure of the space, while others believe the primary molar should be kept for as long as possible and be restored with an implant or bridge on its eventual loss.[36]

Bypassing Debilitated Teeth During Finishing
In certain clinical situations, after taking a finishing panoramic radiograph, there may be evidence of localized root resorption. Two options are available: minimize the time spent on the finishing stage, or bypass the affected tooth in order to avoid any force that will perpetuate the root resorption. Figure 17-31 illustrates the latter option during finishing. Sound biomechanic principles should be used to achieve the desired tooth movement with the minimum of side effects (the ideal objective during finishing).

Substitution of Missing Lateral Incisors
When canines replace lateral incisors, it is difficult to adjust their morphology to resemble that of lateral incisors. Ideally, the majority of the canine contouring should have been accomplished in the early phases of treatment. During

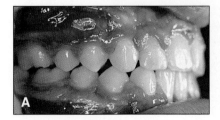
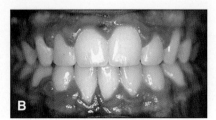
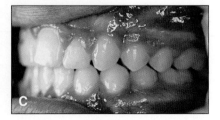

Fig. 17-29 A-C Patient with a lower incisor extraction finished with an ideal overjet but with a Class III tendency on the right side and poor interdigitation. Gingival contours are not ideal, especially in the area of incisor extraction.

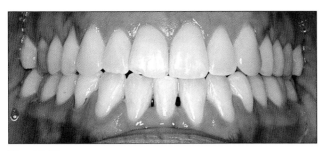

Fig. 17-30 Black triangles are often seen in adult patients having lower incisor extraction. The canine overjet is excessive.

finishing, only minor contouring should be done in consultation with the restorative dentist.

One of the most challenging esthetic concerns for the restorative dentist in these situations is the gingival heights. In ideal esthetic situations, the premolar that is replacing the canine will have a 1–1.5 mm greater incisal gingival height than the canine, and the canine's gingival height is usually at the same level as that of the central incisor. To achieve proper gingival heights, the canine substituting the lateral incisor morphology should be extruded slightly (approximately 0.5–1.0 mm), and for the premolar replacing the canine, the only option is a periodontal resective procedure. However, this periodontal procedure needs to be done with caution as the anatomic crown height of the premolar is much smaller than that of the canine and such procedure may end up exposing the cementum on the facial aspect of the premolar.

Another challenge with canine substitution concerns lingual cusp contouring of the upper first premolar. This cusp should be reduced mainly for functional reasons to avoid balancing interferences during disclusion. Care should be taken not to remove excessive amounts of tooth structure in order to avoid postoperative sensitivity.

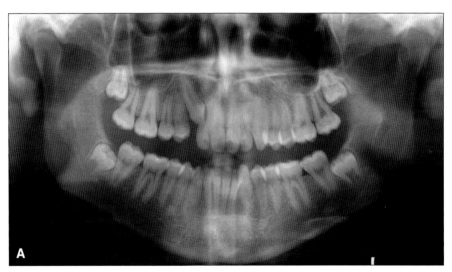

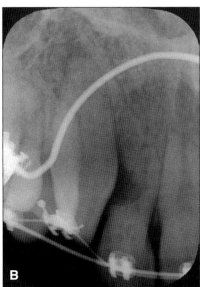

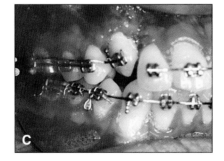

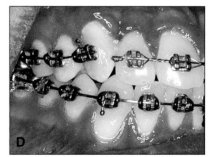

Fig. 17-31 **A** and **B** Patient with extensive root resorption on the upper right lateral tooth. **C** This tooth was bypassed using segmental mechanics to position the canine in the arch. A 0.017 × 0.025 stainless steel segment was placed from the upper right first molar to the first premolar. A transpalatal arch (not seen) connected this segment to the other side of the arch. A 0.017 × 0.025 CNA beta-titanium segment was tied from the molar to the canine. The resultant geometry of the two couple system produced a distal crown tip and intrusive force on the canine in the second order. The intrusive force was counteracted by a vertical elastic. **D** Canine correction in 4 weeks. Finishing detailing for the canine was done by sectioning the wire without engaging the upper right lateral.

Edentulous Site for an Implant

One of the most common mistakes when an edentulous space is prepared to receive an implant is to leave inadequate space. The minimum space that should be opened for an implant is approximately 6 mm. This measurement derives from 3.5 mm of mesiodistal width of the fixture and 1 mm mesial and distal space to the fixture for a papilla in the interproximal space.[37]

It is not only a space problem at the coronal level that is encountered by the restorative dentist, but also a root angulation problem of the adjacent teeth to the implant site at the apical level. Since the space is usually achieved by a push coil mechanism at the coronal level, the roots of the teeth tip into the implant space (Fig. 17-32). During finishing, adequate moments for root correction should be placed in these adjacent teeth to achieve the minimum 6 mm distance throughout the entire implant site. It is important to note that new developments in implant fixture shape (anatomically shaped implants), allow more leeway in this respect (Fig. 17-33).

Stripping During Finishing

Interproximal tooth reduction generally has been advocated where tooth size discrepancies exist and in some instances it has been recommended during finishing. This procedure is used to achieve a better occlusal relationship in the finishing stages.[25] Since the amount of interproximal enamel reduction is limited, it should be noted that tooth size discrepancies should be evaluated during the diagnosis phase so as to avoid last minute quick-fix solutions in the finishing stages. Thus a slight interproximal reduction of certain teeth with abnormal morphology contributing to

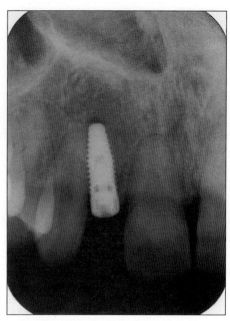

Fig. 17-33 Anatomically shaped implants may allow fixture placement in sites where adjacent roots converge.

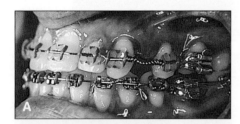
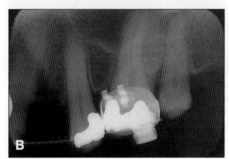

Fig. 17-32 A Push coil mechanism pushes the crown apart and the roots together. **B** X-ray depicts the root convergence with no space in the apical portion to place an implant.

the discrepancy, usually between the upper lateral incisors and the lower second premolars,[9] can be selectively done, instead of reducing teeth indiscriminately as a result of inappropriate diagnosis and treatment planning.

Finishing with Class II Mechanics

Usually, in Class II mechanics using elastics or interarch Class II appliances, correction of the malocclusion is achieved by rotating the occlusal plane in a clockwise direction. As a result, the maxillary incisors finish with a retroclined angulation (Fig. 17-34). To address this problem, torque needs to be applied to the anterior teeth. This can be accomplished using a bracket prescription with an excessive amount of torque for the anteriors (i.e. 16° or more), or by applying buccal crown torque to the archwire (via individual bends or adding a gentle curve of Spee). Another method involves using a torquing spring that adds a moment to the teeth that will correct the root angulation (see Fig. 17-24).

Finishing Sequence

Third-order objectives during finishing should be addressed first since these usually take the most time to correct. The buccolingual inclination of the upper anterior segment is important in the finishing stage for two reasons: occlusal and esthetic. Proper incisor inclination is a key factor in achieving good buccal occlusion and an esthetic smile.

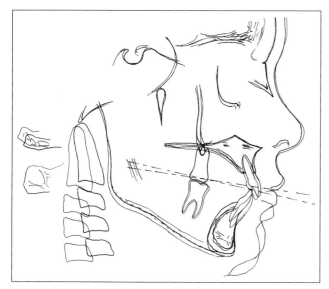

Fig. 17-34 Treatment changes with Class II mechanics. Occlusal plane changes and retroclined and extruded upper incisors (treatment changes in blue) are seen.

with a medium-to-low load deflection rate (such as a 0.017 × 0.025 beta-titanium CNA)* can be selected. For example, if a patient has a lingual inclination of the crowns of the upper incisors, a counterclockwise moment given by the coupling between the wire and the bracket is needed to achieve a proper buccolingual inclination. If there is slop between the two (Table 17-1), the option is to increase the dimension of the rectangular wire, while trying to maintain a medium load deflection (achieving the desired moment), or adding bends to the existing archwire to create the couple. Other options include selecting the proper prescription for patients in whom loss of third-order control in the incisors is anticipated, or to change from a 0.22 slot to a 0.018 slot in the anterior segment.

In the straight wire appliance, proper third-order angulation can be achieved through rectangular archwires engaged into prescription brackets that can then express the torque of the appliance. For additional third-order correction on specific teeth, a 0.016 × 0.022 beta-titanium CNA* is recommended. Third-order bends are placed in this archwire which provides an adequate load–deflection rate[38] to achieve proper buccolingual inclination.

After the third-order objectives are met, second-order movements are addressed. Adjustments in this plane also take a significant amount of time because they also involve root correction. To achieve second-order objectives, either the same 0.016 × 0.022 beta-titanium CNA* or a 0.016 steel round archwire can be used, providing all the third-order objectives have been met. This allows for marginal

The major factors involved in achieving this proper anterosuperior incisor inclination are the bracket and wire coupling. Therefore, depending on the existing buccolingual inclination of the tooth and the relation of the bracket to the occlusal plane, a specific archwire

| Table 17-1 | Relationship between slot and wire dimensions in third order (Personal communication Dr AJ Kuhlberg.) |

Slot size 0.022 in

Wire height (in)	Wire depth (in)	Max. wire dimension (in)	Angle wire/bracket (degrees)	Angle (degrees)	Slop (degrees)
0.016	0.022	0.0272	36.03	53.97	17.95
0.017	0.025	0.0302	34.22	46.69	12.48
0.018	0.025	0.0308	35.75	45.57	9.82
0.019	0.025	0.0314	37.23	44.48	7.24
0.021	0.025	0.0326	40.03	42.36	2.33
0.022	0.025	0.0333	41.35	41.35	0.00

Slot size 0.018 in

Wire height (in)	Wire depth (in)	Max. wire dimension (in)	Angle wire/bracket (degrees)	Angle (degrees)	Slop (degrees)
0.016	0.016	0.0226	45.00	52.70	7.70
0.016	0.022	0.0272	36.03	41.43	5.40
0.017	0.025	0.0302	34.22	36.54	2.32
0.018	0.025	0.0308	35.75	35.75	0.00

*Ortho Organizers Inc, San Marcos, CA

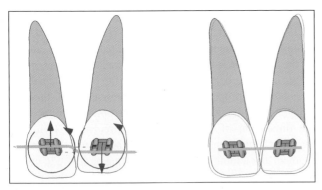

Fig. 17-35 Step bends on the finishing wires can produce undesirable side effects.

ridge discrepancies and root parallelism problems to be corrected.

The final step in finishing is the correction of first-order problems. Usually these problems are obvious clinically and can be corrected quickly. In many instances, only small correction bends in the archwire are needed. Correction can also be achieved with auxiliary plastic rotation wedges on the brackets, or by making small bends in either the 0.016 × 0.022 beta-titanium CNA* or 0.016 steel archwire.

All the finishing bends placed in an archwire will result in either a V or step bend.[39] Care must be taken as all these bends will have vertical side effects and rotational tendencies on the adjacent teeth (Fig. 17-35).

Interarch objectives are the last to be addressed in the finishing stage. In many instances, the intra-arch adjustments mentioned above will result in a good occlusion. To achieve good final intercuspation of the buccal segments, vertical elastics may be worn for a short period of time, usually 2–3 weeks.

It is important to note that although some orthodontists expect a settling of the occlusion to occur during retention, the amount of settling is unpredictable,[40] and in some patients does not occur. Care must also be taken with the elastics in the finishing stages. Prolonged wear of vertical elastics with light or no archwires may result in deformation of the arch form and/or lingual inclination of the teeth (Fig. 17-36) as a result of the elastic force applied buccally to the center of resistance (Fig. 17-36C).

Summary

The literature addressing the topic of orthodontic finishing is scarce. Most of the studies and theories on finishing are anecdotal and subjective in nature. This supports the idea that orthodontic finishing is predominantly an art, rather than a science. The common consensus on guidelines to evaluate finishing are described by the ABO standards. The evaluation is based on intraoral criteria and does not incorporate esthetic or functional objectives. This chapter provides a general overview of the most important aspects of finishing using solid biomechanic principles. The goals for each of the four categories (intraoral objectives, extraoral objectives, radiographic objectives, and functional objectives) have been described. The key to good orthodontics relies heavily on the diagnosis, treatment planning, and application of good mechanics. The key to excellence in orthodontics lies in the ability to identify and correct the small details needed for a perfect smile with an ideal occlusion.

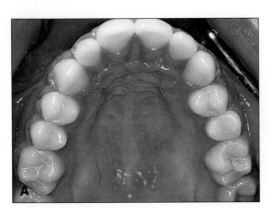
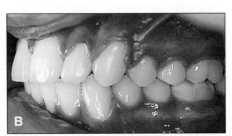
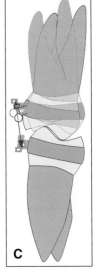

Fig. 17-36 A Longterm (6 weeks or more) vertical elastics with no or very light wires used to seat the occlusion may affect the upper arch form. **B** Good buccal occlusion obtained at the expense of the arch form and the third order of the upper left first premolar (**C**).

*Ortho Organizers Inc, San Marcos, CA

REFERENCES

1. Casko JS, Vaden JL, Kokich VG et al. Objective grading system for dental casts and panoramic radiographs. American Board of Orthodontics. Am J Orthod Dentofacial Orthop 1998;114:589–599.
2. Andrews LF. The six keys to normal occlusion. Am J Orthod 1972;62:296–309.
3. Bennett JC, McLaughlin RP. First molars. In: Bennett JC, McLaughlin RP, eds. Orthodontic management of the dentition with preadjusted appliance. London: Mosby, 2001:281-310.
4. McNamara JA. Transpalatal arches. In: McNamara JA, Brudon WL, eds. Orthodontics and dentofacial orthopedics. Ann Arbor: Needham Press, 2001:199–209.
5. McNamara JA. The transverse dimension. In: McNamara JA, Brudon WL, eds. Orthodontics and dentofacial orthopedics. Ann Arbor: Needham Press, 2001:97–110.
6. Zachrisson BU. Making the premolar extraction smile full and radiant. World J Orthod 2002;3:260–265.
7. Bolton W. The clinical application of a toothsize analysis. Am J Orthod 1962;48:504–529.
8. Smith SS, Buschang PH, Watanabe E. Interarch tooth size relationships of 3 populations: "does Bolton's analysis apply?" Am J Orthod Dentofacial Orthop 2000;117:169–714.
9. Swartz M. Comprehensive fixed appliance therapy. In: McNamara JA, Brudon WL, eds. Orthodontics and dentofacial orthopedics. Ann Arbor: Needham Press, 2001:149–168.
10. Zachrisson BU. JCO/interviews Dr. Bjorn U. Zachrisson on excellence in finishing. Part 1. J Clin Orthod 1986:20(7):460–482.
11. Ramfjord A. Occlusion, 4th edn. Philadelphia: WB Saunders, 1995.
12. Vig RG, Brundo GC. The kinetics of anterior tooth display. J Prosthet Dent 1978;39:502–504.
13. Tjan AH, Miller GD, The JG. Some esthetic factors in a smile. J Prosthet Dent 1984;51:24–28.
14. Kokich VG, Spear FM. Guidelines for managing the orthodontic–restorative patient. Semin Orthod 1997;3:3–20.
15. Poling R. A method of finishing the occlusion. Am J Orthod Dentofacial Orthop 1999;115:476–487.
16. van Steenbergen E, Nanda R. Biomechanics of orthodontic correction of dental asymmetries. Am J Orthod Dentofacial Orthop 1995;107:618–624.
17. Johnston CD, Burden DJ, Stevenson MR. The influence of dental to facial midline discrepancies on dental attractiveness ratings. Eur J Orthod 1999;21:517–522.
18. Kokich VO, Kiyak HA, Shapiro PA. Comparing the perception of dentists and lay people to altered dental esthetics. J Esthet Dent 1999;11:311–324.
19. Beyer JW, Lindauer SJ. Evaluation of dental midline position. Semin Orthod 1998;4:146–152.
20. Burstone CJ. Diagnosis and treatment planning of patients with asymmetries. Semin Orthod 1998;4:153–164.
21. Peluso C, Kuhlberg A. The axial inclination of central incisors and its effects on the perception of the facial profile. Annual American Dental Association Meeting, Scientific Program, Memphis, 2002.
22. Uribe F, Nanda R. Treatment of class II, division 2 malocclusion in adults: biomechanic considerations. J Clin Orthod 2003;37:599–606.
23. Shroff B. Root correction during orthodontic therapy. Semin Orthod 2001;7:50–58.
24. McNamara JA, Nolan PJ, West KS. Finishing and retention. In: McNamara JA, Brudon WL, eds. Orthodontics and dentofacial orthopedics. Ann Arbor: Needham Press, 2001:453–474.
25. Kharat DU, Saini TS, Mokeem S. Shovel-shaped incisors and associated invagination in some Asian and African populations. J Dent 1990;18:216–220.
26. Hatasaka HH. A radiographic study of roots in extraction sites. Angle Orthod 1976;46:64–68.
27. Artun J, Kokich VG, Osterberg SK. Long-term effect of root proximity on periodontal health after orthodontic treatment. Am J Orthod Dentofacial Orthop 1987;91:125–130.
28. Levander E, Bajka R, Malmgren O. Early radiographic diagnosis of apical root resorption during orthodontic treatment: a study of maxillary incisors. Eur J Orthod 1998;20:57–63.
29. O'Hea CM. A prospective investigation of maxillary central incisor root resorption incident to orthodontic therapy. Thesis. Department of Orthodontics, University of Connecticut, Farmington, 1999:151.
30. Joondeph D. Retention and relapse. In: Graber TM, Vanarsdall RL, eds. Orthodontics: current principles and techniques. Mosby: St Louis, 2000:985–1012.
31. Proffit WR. The third stage of comprehensive treatment: Finishing. In: Proffit WR, ed. Contemporary orthodontics. St Louis: Mosby, 2000.
32. McLaughlin R, Bennett J. Finishing with the preadjusted orthodontic appliance. Semin Orthod 2003;9:165–183.
33. Little RM, Riedel RA, Artun J. An evaluation of changes in mandibular anterior alignment from 10 to 20 years postretention. Am J Orthod Dentofacial Orthop 1988;93:423–428.
34. Faerovig E, Zachrisson BU. Effects of mandibular incisor extraction on anterior occlusion in adults with Class III malocclusion and reduced overbite. Am J Orthod Dentofacial Orthop 1999;115:113–124.
35. Kokich VO Jr. Congenitally missing teeth: orthodontic management in the adolescent patient. Am J Orthod Dentofacial Orthop 2002;121:594–595.
36. Spear FM, Mathews DM, Kokich VG. Interdisciplinary management of single-tooth implants. Semin Orthod 1997;3:45–72.
37. Johnson E. Relative stiffness of beta titanium archwires. Angle Orthod 2003;73:259–269.
38. Burstone CJ, Koenig HA. Creative wire bending—the force system from step and V bends. Am J Orthod Dentofacial Orthop 1988;93:59–67.
39. Parkinson CE, Buschang PH, Behrents RG, Throckmorton GS, English JD. A new method of evaluating posterior occlusion and its relation to posttreatment occlusal changes. Am J Orthod Dentofacial Orthop 2001;120:503–512.

Interrelationship of Orthodontics with Periodontics and Restorative Dentistry

Vincent G Kokich and Vincent O Kokich

Today, orthodontics is not just for children and adolescents. For the past two decades, increasing numbers of adults have been referred to orthodontists to correct their malocclusions. Adults are usually wonderful patients, because they are cooperative, clean their teeth, show up for appointments, and are appreciative of the clinician's efforts. However, adults may have problems other than malposed teeth and jaws that make their orthodontic treatment more challenging. Whereas children and adolescents have intact dentitions with few restorations and a healthy periodontium, adults may have old failing restorations, edentulous spaces, abraded teeth, periodontal bone defects, gingival level discrepancies, hopeless teeth, and a variety of other restorative and periodontal problems that could compromise the orthodontic result. In the past, orthodontists made all the decisions about the treatment plan for a child or adolescent. However, in the compromised adult malocclusion, a team of orthodontist, oral and maxillofacial surgeon, periodontist, endodontist, and restorative dentist must interact to make prudent treatment decisions for the patient.

This chapter will elucidate the dilemmas encountered in the orthodontic patient with multidisciplinary problems, and describe a series of 10 guidelines to help manage the interrelationship of orthodontics with periodontics and restorative dentistry.

Generate Realistic Treatment Objectives

The first step in any type of dental therapy is to establish the treatment objectives. It is impossible to achieve the correct end result if the appropriate goals or objectives have not been identified before treatment. In nonrestored, adolescent patients with complete dentitions, orthodontic treatment objectives tend to be idealistic. After all, if patients have intact dentitions without restorations, it is appropriate to expect that ideal esthetic and occlusal treatment should be attainable, if the patient cooperates. Because of this tendency, most orthodontists are trapped into applying these same idealistic treatment objectives to adult patients with missing teeth, abraded teeth, old restorations, or other restorative and periodontal complications. Idealistic treatment objectives may not be appropriate for the ortho-perio-restorative patient. For these patients, it is important to establish realistic, not idealistic, treatment objectives. Realistic treatment objectives generally should be economically realistic, occlusally realistic, periodontally realistic, and restoratively realistic.[1]

If an adult orthodontic patient is missing several teeth, the edentulous spaces created during orthodontic treatment will require restoration after the removal of the orthodontic appliances. Several restorative alternatives may exist for replacing the missing teeth. The cost of these restorative treatment plans may differ widely. Furthermore, each type of restoration may require slightly different tooth positioning. Therefore, it is mandatory for the team to establish a treatment plan that is economically realistic for each patient. If the team fails to establish economically realistic objectives, the patient might not complete the restorative treatment following orthodontic therapy.

In young patients it is important to establish ideal occlusal objectives, such as an Angle Class I canine relationship with normal overbite and overjet relationships. When planning occlusal treatment for young patients, the orthodontist is missing two critically important pieces of information: (1) because of their young age, there is no occlusal history; and (2) the orthodontist unfortunately cannot predict the future habits or problems that a young patient will encounter during his/her lifetime. Therefore, in these situations it is appropriate for the orthodontist to create an ideal occlusion. However, in the adult patient, orthodontists often overlook the most valuable piece of information, i.e. the patient's dental history. Has the

adult patient demonstrated parafunctional occlusal habits, evidence of temporomandibular disorders, cracked teeth or restorations, wear facets, abraded incisors, or other signs and symptoms that would suggest that the treatment plan should alter the existing occlusion? Not all existing occlusions in adult patients need to be corrected to an adolescent ideal (Fig. 18-1). In all adult patients, the dental history, as well as the future restorative requirements, play a greater role in determining the final occlusion (Fig. 18-2). For example, it may not be necessary to correct posterior crossbites in adults who have no occlusal interferences and no shift of the mandible, and who can be restored adequately in a posterior crossbite relationship (Fig. 18-3).

If patients are missing many teeth, it may not be prudent to establish idealistic occlusal objectives. An ideal Angle Class I posterior occlusion is achievable in a patient with a complete nonrestored, nonabraded dentition. However, if the patient is missing several teeth and will require extensive restorative treatment after orthodontics, it may be more prudent to establish treatment objectives that are occlusally realistic for the specific patient. For example, if the patient

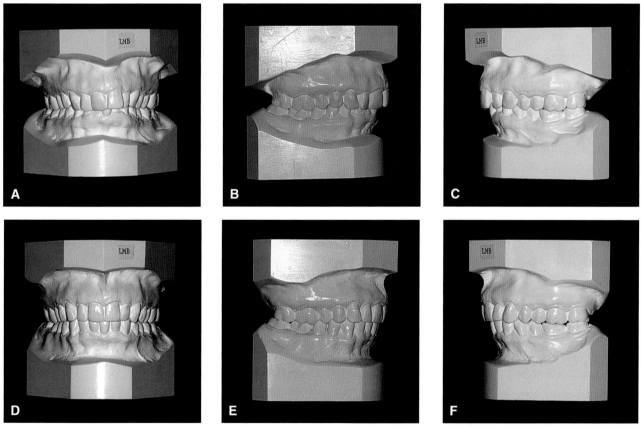

Fig. 18-1 This 68-year-old female had a deep anterior overbite (**A**) with Class I molar and canine relationships on the right (**B**) and Class II molar and canine relationships on the left (**C**). She had no temporomandibular joint symptoms and a healthy periodontium. **D** Treatment objectives included alignment of teeth in both arches and reduction of the deep overbite. Because of an anterior tooth-size discrepancy, proclined mandibular incisors, and upright maxillary incisors, her treatment objectives did not include correction of the Class II molar and canine relationships on the left. **E** and **F** At the end of treatment all treatment objectives were achieved, including maintaining the original posterior occlusal relationships.

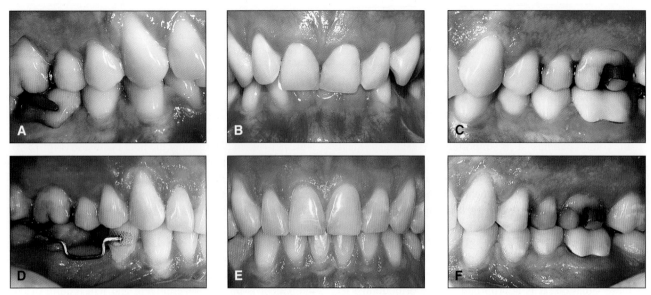

Fig. 18-2 This 52-year-old male had a bilateral Class II, Division 2 malocclusion with a deep anterior overbite (**A**), retroclined maxillary incisors (**B** and **C**), a missing mandibular second premolar, and a mandibular dental midline that deviated to the right. The patient had no temporomandibular joint symptoms, and the periodontium was healthy. Treatment objectives included reduction of the deep overbite (**D**), opening space for the missing premolar, correction of the dental midline, and establishing normal overjet. Because of the inclination of the anterior teeth and the anterior tooth-size relationships, a Class I canine relationship was established on the right (**E**), and a Class II relationship was maintained on the left (**F**). The objectives were achieved without correcting the Class II canine relationship on the right side.

will require extensive restorations after orthodontic treatment, the restorative dentist may suggest altering an Angle Class I occlusion to facilitate restoration of the teeth (Fig. 18-4). It is critical for the orthodontist to be aware of these alterations before bracket placement to achieve an occlusally realistic relationship for the restorative patient.[1]

A common occlusal treatment objective in children is to align the marginal ridges of the posterior teeth in order to produce a uniform vertical relationship between the maxillary and mandibular posterior teeth.[2] In a nonabraded, periodontally healthy adolescent dentition, aligning the marginal ridges helps to establish even contact of the posterior teeth, when they are brought into occlusion. However, in the adult patient with interproximal bone loss and uneven wear of the posterior teeth, the marginal ridges are poor guides for positioning the posterior teeth.[3] In these patients, the periodontal objectives outweigh the occlusal objectives. The role of the orthodontist in the periodontal patient is to level the bone during orthodontic treatment. This could require equilibration and reshaping of the posterior teeth in order to maximize the occlusal contacts. In most of these situations, the teeth that have been equilibrated will require restoration anyway after orthodontic treatment.

Certain types of restorations require specific positioning of adjacent or opposing teeth. As a result, orthodontists must not establish idealistic treatment objectives for patients who will require extensive restoration. If teeth are worn or abraded, it may be more important to position the teeth in a restoratively realistic location to facilitate the appropriate restoration.

Create the Vision

After an orthodontist has treated several hundred adolescent patients with complete dentitions, it is easy for him/her to visualize or foresee the final orthodontic result before beginning treatment. However, some adult orthodontic patients may be missing several permanent teeth. If teeth have been absent for several years, the remaining teeth may have drifted. In other situations it may be necessary to position teeth in unusual situations. These patients may require a combination of orthodontics and restorative dentistry to rehabilitate their occlusion. In these patients it may be difficult for the orthodontist to visualize or foresee the final result as he/she may not be aware of the restorative requirements or the eventual restorative treatment plan. Similarly, it may be difficult for the restorative dentist to visualize the final result as he/she may be unaware of the orthodontic possibilities.

However, it is possible to predetermine the final occlusal and restorative outcome by completing a diagnostic wax setup for these types of patients. A diagnostic setup is mandatory for any patient who is missing multiple permanent teeth[4] and will require a combination of orthodontics and restorative dentistry (see Fig. 18-4). In addition,

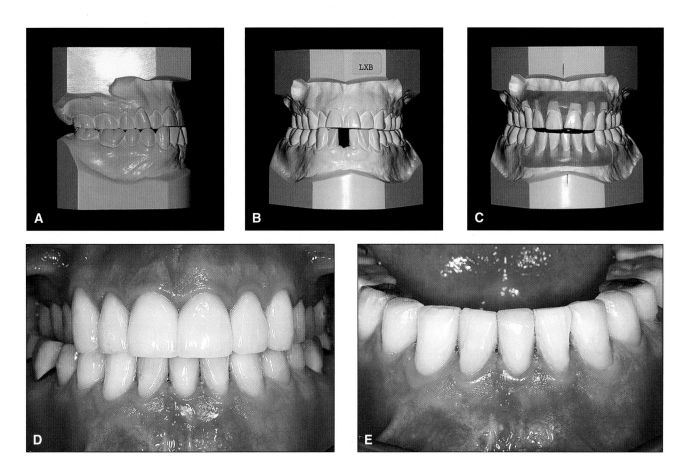

Fig. 18-3 This 57-year-old male had a Class III end-to-end posterior occlusion with an anterior dental crossbite (**A**), a missing mandibular incisor (failed endodontic therapy), severe wear of the maxillary incisors, and bilateral posterior dental crossbites with no lateral shift of the mandible (**B**). He had no temporomandibular joint symptoms, and the periodontium was healthy. Treatment objectives included correction of the anterior crossbite to create an overjet to restore the abraded maxillary incisors. Correction of the bilateral dental crossbites was not a treatment objective. **C** A diagnostic setup showed that the mandibular space could be closed to create restorative space. The final photographs of the **D** restored maxillary and **E** mandibular incisors show that correction of the posterior crossbites was not necessary to achieve the restorative objectives.

patients who will have implants used first for orthodontic anchorage and later for restorative abutments will require a diagnostic setup[5] to position the implants properly prior to the beginning of orthodontics (Fig. 18-5). The orthodontist should never make the restorative decisions, but should consult with the restorative dentist when planning treatment for these types of patients. In that way, the orthodontist may reposition the teeth to simulate realistic orthodontic objectives that will be in harmony with the patient's restorative requirements. Both practitioner and patient can visualize the result. The diagnostic wax setup is the blueprint for treatment in these types of patients.

A diagnostic wax setup is also necessary for patients who have unusual combinations of missing teeth, and in whom the orthodontist is planning to substitute one tooth for another. For example, if a patient were missing maxillary lateral incisors, and the orthodontist were planning canine substitution, a diagnostic wax setup would be mandatory to determine if the occlusion will fit properly

and if the teeth can be shaped accordingly. Occasionally, a patient is missing a central incisor,[6] and a treatment option could be to restore the opposite lateral incisor as a central incisor in order to avoid an implant or fixed bridge (Fig. 18-6). A diagnostic wax setup would be necessary to determine if the tooth arrangement will be both esthetic and functional.

Finally, adult malocclusions with significant mandibular incisor crowding occasionally are treated with extraction of a single mandibular incisor.[7] This type of extraction improves longterm stability, easily eliminates the crowding, simplifies the mechanics, preserves facial esthetics, and improves periodontal health in certain adults. However, before extracting the incisor, the orthodontist must know if the occlusion will fit properly, especially in the canine and incisor region (Fig. 18-7). A diagnostic wax setup will give the clinician the appropriate information to make the correct decision when planning incisor extraction in crowded adult malocclusions.

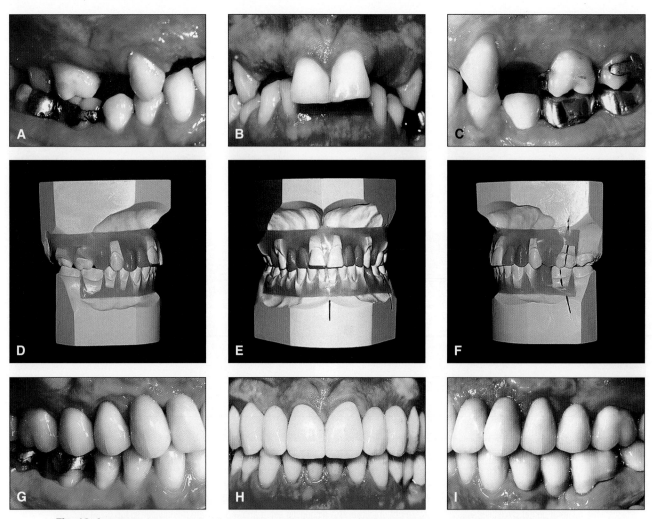

Fig. 18-4 A-C This 32-year-old female had a Class II, Division 1 malocclusion with a deep anterior overbite. She was congenitally missing both maxillary lateral incisors and all four maxillary premolars. The restorative dentist wanted the maxillary canines positioned in the first premolar positions in order to restore the maxillary arch with three segments of fixed restorations connected at the canines with a semirigid connector. **D-F** A diagnostic wax setup provided the guide for the orthodontist to position the canines in their appropriate position. **G-I** After the final restorations were placed, the widths of the pontics and abutments in the maxillary arch were functionally and esthetically correct, because the vision was created with the diagnostic setup.

Establish the Sequence of Treatment

Many orthodontic–restorative patients also require adjunctive periodontal therapy and orthognathic surgery. As the number of dentists involved in a patient's treatment increases, the complexity of the treatment also increases. In many of these situations, different specialists must interact at varying intervals during the patient's overall treatment. Therefore, the team of specialists must not only establish a realistic plan of treatment, but should also determine the sequence of interaction between the different specialists (Fig. 18-8).

This critical step is often overlooked. It requires that the team members meet to discuss the patient's treatment before the initiation of therapy. After the sequence of intervention has been determined, it should be recorded by one of the clinicians.[1] A copy of the treatment sequence should be given to each of the participating dentists and to the patient. Then, at any time during treatment, any of the team members can review the sequence, determine his/her point of interaction, and feel secure that the plan is proceeding properly. In addition, the patient is aware of the pathway toward completing treatment. The importance of this step in interdisciplinary treatment cannot be overemphasized. The success in treating a patient with complex restorative, periodontal, orthognathic, and orthodontic problems is dependent on not only the correct plan of treatment, but also the correct sequence of interaction among different practitioners during the course of treatment.

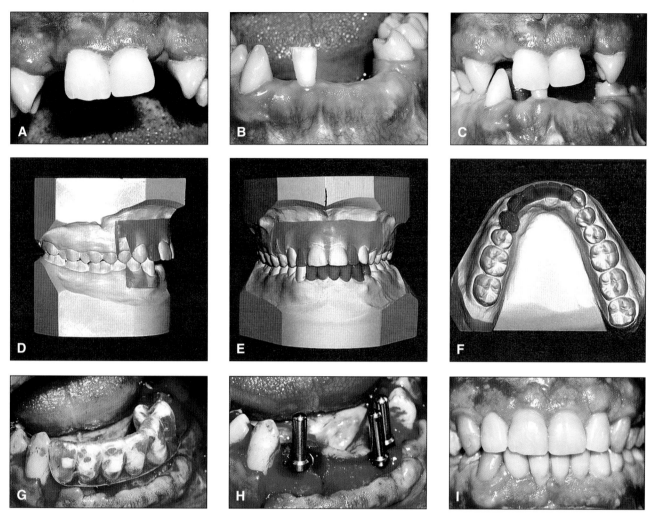

Fig. 18-5 This 24-year-old male was the victim of a robbery during which he was shot in the face and lost **A** his maxillary lateral incisors and **B** most of his mandibular anterior teeth. The restorative plan involved single-tooth implants in the maxilla and an implant-supported bridge in the mandible to replace the missing teeth. The implants were also to be used as anchors to intrude the mandibular right canine and first premolar. **D-F** A diagnostic setup was constructed to determine the appropriate implant position prior to orthodontics. A placement guide (**G**) was constructed from the setup so the surgeon could guide the placement of the implants (**H**). **I** After orthodontics, the same implants that were used as orthodontic anchors were used to restore the missing teeth.

Identify Who Will Correct the Periodontal Defects

Many adult orthodontic patients have underlying periodontal defects that will need to be resolved before, during, or after the orthodontic therapy. It is mandatory that the orthodontist and periodontist discuss the management of these patients to determine who will be responsible for correcting the periodontal problems.[8] These problems are generally divided into two categories: soft tissue or gingival discrepancies; and hard tissue or bony defects. Gingival discrepancies include recession, lack of attached gingiva, and open gingival embrasures. Bony alveolar defects include interproximal craters, one-, two-, and three-wall

defects, furcation defects, and generalized or localized horizontal bone loss secondary to periodontal disease. Each of these defects must be discussed prior to the initiation of orthodontic bracketing to determine who will be responsible for correcting them.

Gingival recession and inadequate attached gingiva often will require the placement of a connective tissue graft. In some cases it is best to perform the grafting prior to orthodontic treatment. This is especially important when the adult patient has pre-existing recession and dental crowding, and will be treated without the extraction of teeth.[3] If there is a dehiscence labial to the tooth, and recession has already occurred, it could get worse during orthodontic treatment. Therefore, the periodontist will

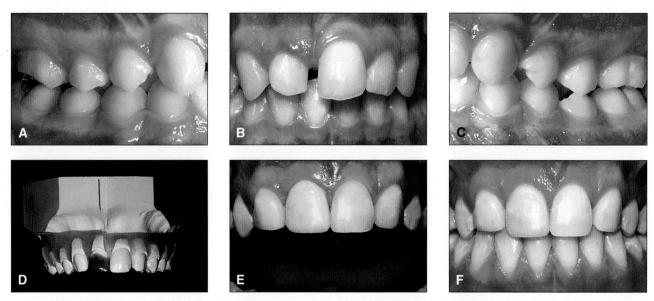

Fig. 18-6 A-C This 14-year-old female lost her maxillary right central incisor in a horse-back riding accident as a child. No treatment was done at the time, and the edentulous space had closed partially. She had a bilateral Class II malocclusion, no crowding in either dental arch, and a good facial profile. Although various treatment options were considered initially, the final plan involved extraction of the left lateral incisor, restoration of the right lateral as a central incisor, and bilateral canine substitution. **D** A diagnostic wax setup was necessary to confirm that this plan would satisfy the objectives. The setup helped the orthodontist to achieve an excellent **E** esthetic and **F** occlusal result.

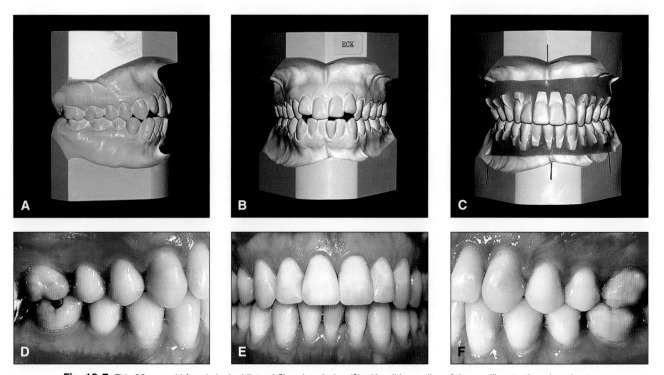

Fig. 18-7 This 32-year-old female had a bilateral Class I occlusion (**A**) with mild crowding of the maxillary teeth and moderate crowding of the mandibular incisors (**B**). **C** A diagnostic setup was constructed to determine if extraction of a mandibular incisor would eliminate the crowding and permit satisfactory overbite and overjet. **D-F** The setup was invaluable in creating the vision and allowing the orthodontist to achieve a well-interdigitated occlusal result.

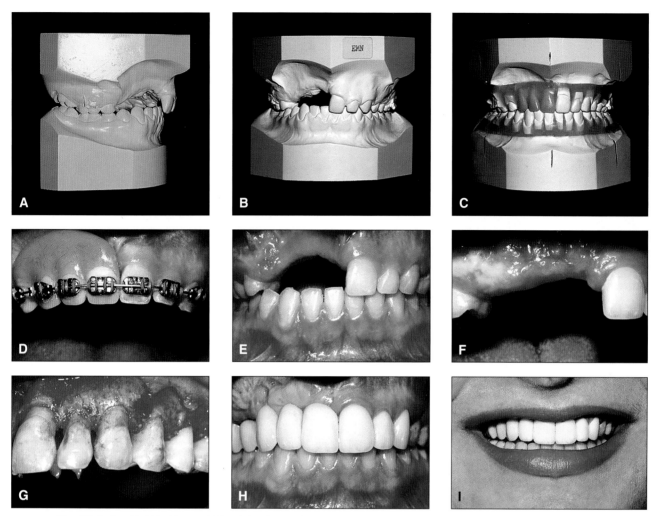

Fig. 18-8 A and **B** This 14-year-old female lost her maxillary anterior teeth in a water skiing accident, which left a huge void in the maxillary alveolus. **C** A diagnostic setup was constructed to create the vision for the practitioners and patient. Several treatment options were discussed, but the final plan involved orthodontics (**D** and **E**), segmental maxillary jaw surgery, sagittal split ramus osteotomy, autogenous soft tissue ridge grafting (**F**), crown lengthening (**G**), provisionalization, and final restoration (**H** and **I**). Because of the complexity of the treatment plan, the four practitioners on her team established the sequence of treatment before beginning therapy. Having the flow chart or treatment sequence facilitated the smooth treatment of this complicated case by keeping all practitioners aware of the timing of each of the steps along the way.

probably place a connective tissue graft prior to the orthodontic therapy to insure that the recession will not progress, and to cover the exposed root with gingiva.

Open gingival embrasures often occur during orthodontic therapy. If not corrected, these dark spaces between the teeth create an esthetic compromise after orthodontic therapy. The presence of a space above the central incisor interproximal contact may be caused by one of three factors.[9] The first possible cause is diverging roots of the maxillary central incisors. This is usually the result of improper bracket placement (Fig. 18-9). In patients with overlapping and abraded maxillary central incisors, brackets may be placed inadvertently at an angle that is not perpendicular to the long axis of the central incisor. As the teeth are aligned, the roots may diverge distally.

To identify this cause, the clinician should evaluate a periapical radiograph. If the roots diverge, the brackets should be removed and repositioned with the bracket slots perpendicular to the long axes of the roots. As the roots align, the interproximal contact lengthens and moves apically toward the papilla. Usually, the distal–incisal corners of the centrals also move apically. This reflects the amount of incisal wear that may have occurred before orthodontic treatment. These teeth usually require an incisal restoration to restore proper incisal contour.

A second possible cause of space above the interproximal contact of the central incisors is abnormal tooth shape.[9] In some patients, the crowns of the centrals are much wider at the incisal edges than at the cervical region (Fig. 18-10). In these situations the contact between the incisors is

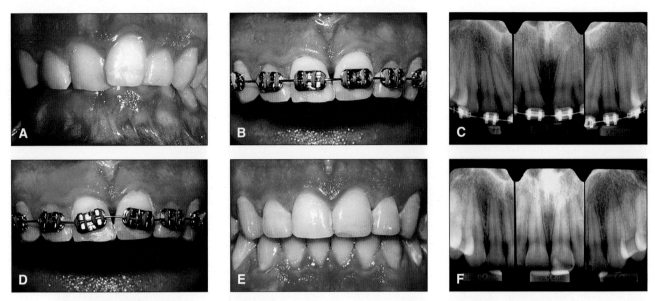

Fig. 18-9 A This young adult male had a Class II deep overbite malocclusion with mild crowding in both arches. **B** During alignment of his overlapped maxillary incisors, an open embrasure developed between the maxillary central incisors. **C** Progress periapical radiographs showed that the central incisor roots were diverted distally, causing the open embrasure. **D** Therefore, the teeth were rebracketed with the bracket slot perpendicular to the long axis of the roots. **E** and **F** This permitted uprighting of the central incisor roots, which moved the contact gingivally and the papilla incisally to close the open embrasure.

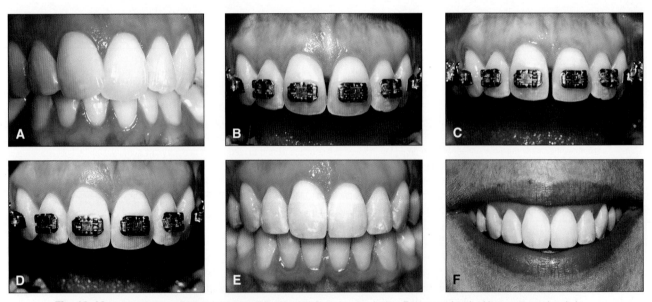

Fig. 18-10 A This 28-year-old female had a mildly crowded Class I malocclusion. Four premolars had been extracted early in her life, but no orthodontic treatment had been performed. The objectives were to align the teeth and reduce the overbite. **B** During alignment an open embrasure developed between the central incisors. The papilla height was normal, but the contact between the centrals was too low, due to the triangular shape of the maxillary central incisors. The mesial surfaces of both centrals were reshaped with a diamond disc (**C**), and the space was closed (**D**), moving the contact gingivally toward the normal papilla. **E** and **F** After orthodontics the open embrasure had been eliminated, and the occlusion and esthetics were satisfactory.

located in the incisal 1 mm between the two centrals. This is an unusual contact relationship as the contact should occupy about half the distance between the gingival margin and the incisal edge. One method of correcting this problem is to recontour the mesial surfaces of the central incisors

and close the space (Fig. 18-10). The other method is to restore the contact with either a composite or porcelain laminate restoration. If recontouring of the tooth will make it too narrow, then restoration is appropriate. In all other cases, recontouring of the teeth and space closure is the easiest way to correct the open embrasure. The amount of enamel that must be removed from each tooth is equal to half the distance between the mesial surfaces of the incisors at the level of the tip of the papilla. Usually this will be about 0.5–0.75 mm and does not penetrate into the dentin. After this diastema has been created, the space between the teeth is consolidated. As this occurs, the contact lengthens and moves toward the papilla.

In patients with advanced generalized or localized periodontal disease and destruction of the crestal bone between anterior teeth, the papilla may be absent. This produces an unesthetic large gap after orthodontics. Several methods may be needed to resolve this problem (Fig. 18.11). In some cases, reshaping the adjacent teeth, altering the root angulation, eruption of the adjacent teeth, and restoration will be necessary to move the bone coronally and to squeeze the gingival tissue between the adjacent crowns to establish a papilla between adjacent teeth after orthodontic therapy.

Adult orthodontic patients may also have osseous defects that could compromise the patient's ability to clean his/her teeth adequately and that require correction prior to or during orthodontic therapy.[8] These osseous defects

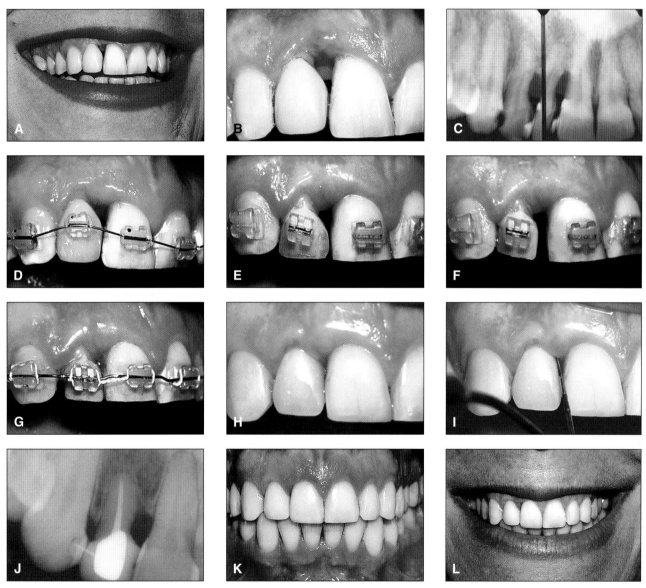

Fig. 18-11 This adult female had a significant open embrasure between the maxillary right central and lateral incisors (**A** and **B**), caused by a periodontal abscess with resultant interproximal bone loss (**C**). The correction required moving the papilla coronally by **D** placing brackets nearer the gingival margins of the incisors and **E** erupting the two teeth. Then, in order to correct the contact problem, the bracket was repositioned (**F**), the mesial of the lateral was reshaped, and the space was closed (**G**). A provisional crown was placed after orthodontics (**H**), and the sulcular depth was reduced significantly (**I**). **J** The post-treatment radiograph shows the amount of bone that was created by erupting the tooth incisally. **K** and **L** The final restoration looked much more esthetic after the open embrasure had been closed by orthodontics, periodontics, endodontics, and restorative dentistry.

include interproximal craters, one-, two-, and three-wall defects, furcation defects, and horizontal defects. Interproximal craters can be the most volatile intrabony defects in the orthodontic patient. These are two-wall defects, where the remaining walls are the buccal and lingual walls. Attachment loss occurs on the mesial and distal surfaces of the adjacent roots. Orthodontic movement cannot improve interproximal craters.[8] If the crater is mild to moderate, but the patient cannot maintain the area adequately, it may require resective bone removal and recontouring prior to orthodontic bracketing.

One-wall defects are treated most efficiently by the orthodontist.[10] In these situations, periodontal pathogenic bacteria have destroyed the attachment on three of the four interproximal walls, leaving one wall remaining. These defects are difficult for a periodontist to manage, because resective surgery could be too destructive, and regenerative therapy is inappropriate. However, orthodontic eruption of the tooth will eliminate the defect (Fig. 18-12). In these situations, the orthodontist must place the bracket more apically on the facial surface of the crown and perpendicular to the long axis of the root of the tooth. As the tooth erupts, the orthodontist must equilibrate the crown to avoid premature contact with teeth in the opposing arch, and increased mobility of the erupting tooth. The orthodontist should evaluate a progress periapical radiograph to determine when the tooth has erupted sufficiently. When the interproximal bone is flat between adjacent teeth, and the one-wall defect has been eliminated, then the extrusion of the tooth is complete. Most of these erupted and equilibrated teeth will require a crown to cover the dentin that may have been exposed during the eruption process.

Two-wall defects are best treated with orthodontics and periodontal surgery.[8] When two walls remain in an interproximal region, and the patient cannot maintain the area, it is difficult for a periodontist to completely resolve the defect with resective or regenerative treatment. These defects often require orthodontic eruption of the affected tooth, followed by crown lengthening to improve the

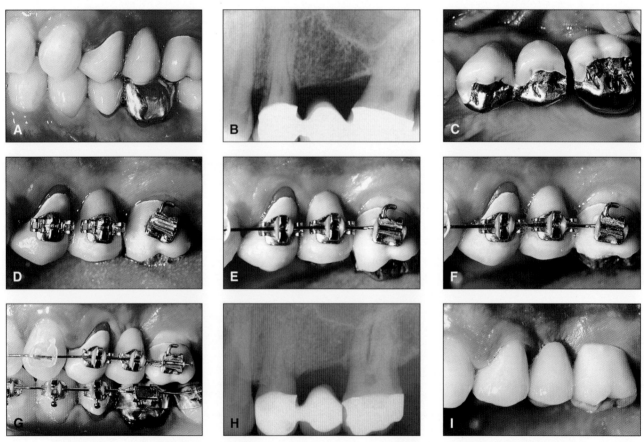

Fig. 18-12 A This 43-year-old veterinarian had a 6 mm bleeding pocket on the mesial surface of the maxillary left first molar. This tooth was an abutment for an existing three-unit bridge. **B** The periapical radiograph shows the one-wall defect that was present mesial to the tipped first molar. The treatment plan involved sectioning of the bridge (**C**), placing the molar bracket perpendicular to the long axis of the root (**D**), and inserting an archwire to upright and erupt the tooth (**E**). Because the crown had been overcontoured, the occlusal surface was equilibrated (**F**) to establish satisfactory occlusal contact (**G**). The post-treatment radiograph shows the amount of molar extrusion that was accomplished in order to eliminate the one-wall defect (**H**), so the final bridge could be placed on a periodontally healthy tooth (**I**).

restorability of the tooth. *Three-wall defects* are not resolvable with orthodontics. If the patient cannot maintain a three-wall defect during orthodontic therapy, it must be resolved prior to bracket placement. These defects are generally treated with regenerative therapy, using either autogenous or alloplastic bone grafts in the affected area.[8] Generally, orthodontic tooth movement can begin a short time after placement of the bone graft in order to enhance the fibroblastic and osteoblastic turnover that is necessary to heal the defect and move the adjacent teeth.

Furcation defects are typically divided into three classifications: class 1, 2 and 3. Class 1 furcation defects are typically very shallow and do not enter the molar furcation deeply, and usually are observed or monitored during orthodontic therapy. Class 2 furcation defects extend into the furcation but do not communicate with the opposite side or interproximal region of the tooth. If the patient cannot maintain a class 2 furcation defect, and the tooth is necessary for the occlusal and restorative treatment plan, then the periodontist must treat the furcation prior to orthodontics. Treatment most likely will involve a regenerative approach[8] using membranes to isolate the defect in order to promote regeneration of the periodontal membrane, while the membrane blocks the ingrowth of the epithelium which would recreate the furcation defect. Class 3 furcation defects are typically not maintainable by patients during orthodontic therapy and decisions about their outcome must be made during the treatment planning process before beginning orthodontics. In the past, hemisection, root amputation, and root separation using orthodontics have been attempted.[3] In some cases these techniques worked nicely. However, today clinicians are more interested in the longterm outcome of treatment and, therefore, most significant class 3 furcations are treated with extraction of the affected tooth and replacement with an implant.[8]

A common periodontal problem among adult orthodontic patients is generalized horizontal bone loss in the anterior region of the mouth. In these situations, if significant bone loss has occurred on all anterior teeth, then often the teeth have disproportionate crown/root ratios. The orthodontist must recognize this problem prior to bracket placement (Fig. 18-13). It may be appropriate in these situations to reduce the clinical crown lengths of these teeth to achieve

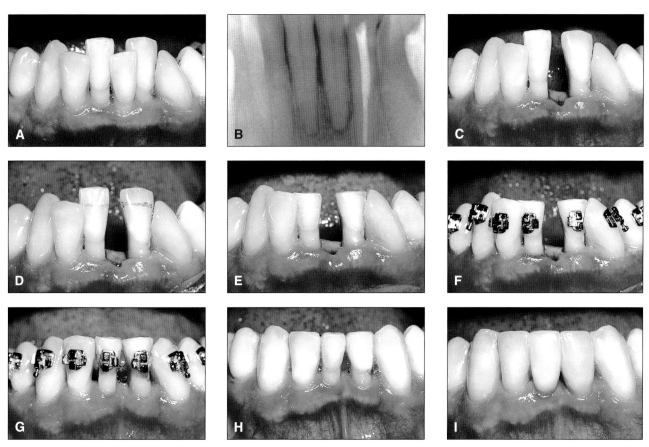

Fig. 18-13 This 61-year-old female had **A** severe crowding of her mandibular incisors and **B** significant horizontal bone loss around her mandibular incisors. **C** A diagnostic wax setup showed that the mandibular left lateral incisor could be extracted to eliminate the crowding. Since the bone levels were flat, the incisal edges were equilibrated prior to bracket placement (**D** and **E**), in order to maintain a flat bony architecture during orthodontics (**F-H**). **J** After bracket removal, the restorative dentist placed porcelain veneers on the teeth to close the open embrasures.

two objectives.[3,8] First, if the crown length is reduced, then the crown/root ratio will improve, and the mobility of the tooth after orthodontic therapy will be reduced. Second, if horizontal bone loss has occurred in only one area, then reduction of crown length will avoid the creation of bony defects between adjacent teeth as the teeth are aligned. The orthodontist should draw on the tooth with a pencil or pen to identify how much crown length must be removed (Fig. 18-13). Then tooth removal should be accomplished slowly with water spray to avoid damaging the pulp of the tooth.[11] Once the new incisal edge has been established, then the orthodontist can use this surface of the tooth as a reference for bracket placement. At the end of treatment, the mobility of the teeth will be improved, and the periodontal defect will be eliminated.

Negotiate the Extraction of Hopeless Teeth

Occasionally, adults present for orthodontic treatment with teeth that are either periodontally or restoratively hopeless and which require extraction at some point during interdisciplinary treatment (Fig. 18-14). In these situations it is important for all members of the team (restorative dentist, periodontist, orthodontist, and oral and maxillofacial surgeon) to participate in the decision regarding timing of the extraction.[1] If the tooth has a periodontal or pulpal infection that cannot be maintained by the patient, dentist or periodontist during treatment, then the tooth may require extraction before orthodontic bracketing. However, orthodontic treatment becomes more complicated with each edentulous space that is created prior to orthodontics, especially if that space must be maintained during and after orthodontic therapy. In addition, the mechanics could be more complicated if several teeth must be removed prior to orthodontic treatment. The fewer teeth the patient has, the more difficult it is to anchor the remaining tooth movement. If possible, it is advantageous for the orthodontist to maintain hopeless teeth in the dental arch during orthodontic treatment (Fig. 18-14). They provide anchorage and space maintenance for the orthodontist, and occlusal function and intraoral comfort for the patient. Therefore, it is desirable to extract hopeless teeth after orthodontic treatment as long as the periodontal health of adjacent teeth can be maintained.

Reshape/Rebuild Teeth with Unusual Crown Form

Some orthodontic–restorative patients have small, malformed teeth that will require restoration after the completion of orthodontic treatment. In some of these situations, the orthodontist must create additional space to restore these teeth. In other situations, the malformed teeth are too large, and must be reduced in width. Ideally, restoration of these small or malformed teeth should be performed before the initiation of orthodontic therapy. However, often there is not enough space to restore the tooth before bracket

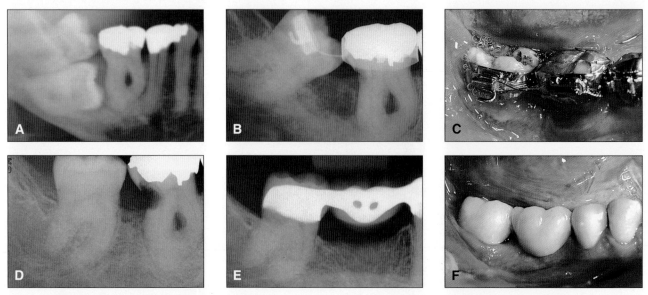

Fig. 18-14 This 55-year-old female had an impacted mandibular right second molar (**A**), and the third molar had erupted over the occlusal surface. The first molar had severe bone loss on the distal root, a Class 3 furcation defect, and was considered hopeless. The second molar was extracted (**B**), and the first molar was used as an anchor to upright the third molar (**C** and **D**). Although the first molar would eventually be extracted, the timing of the extraction was delayed until after the orthodontics, and a bridge was chosen to restore the edentulous space (**E** and **F**). Timing the extraction of hopeless teeth until after orthodontics can help to facilitate difficult tooth movement.

placement. The team must decide how much space to create for these restorations and the timing of restoring these small or malformed teeth. Two situations are common: retained primary teeth and peg-shaped lateral incisors.

When patients are congenitally missing their mandibular second premolars, the primary second molar may be unrestored, caries free, not submerged, and not ankylosed. If the patient will not have an implant placed for several years after orthodontics because of the potential for further jaw growth, then it may be advantageous to reduce and retain the primary molar during orthodontics.[12] After all it will maintain the width of the alveolar bone, prevent supereruption of opposing teeth, and help to maintain mesiodistal width after orthodontics. However, these teeth are too wide and must be reduced to the size of a premolar (Fig. 18-15). After reduction, these teeth have exposed cementum on the mesial and distal surfaces, so it is often advantageous to build-up these teeth with composite. These temporary, inexpensive restorations will help to prevent interproximal caries and provide a better-shaped buccal

surface for bonding of an orthodontic bracket.[12] If the primary molar roots do not resorb excessively during orthodontics, these primary teeth may remain for several years until the patient is old enough to have an implant placed.

Another common orthodontic–restorative problem is peg-shaped or malformed maxillary lateral incisors. In some patients, the best choice for treating a peg-shaped lateral incisor is to restore the malformed tooth to its correct dimension. If sufficient space exists, a composite restoration may be placed before orthodontic treatment (Fig. 18-16). However, in most situations, there is insufficient space to restore the malformed lateral incisors. Therefore, orthodontics is often necessary to create space to build-up peg-shaped lateral incisors. The space is usually acquired by placing open coil-springs on either side of the tooth.[1] This will create space on the mesial and distal surfaces for future restoration. It is generally advantageous to position the tooth closer to the central incisor than the canine, so the emergence profile of the restoration on the mesial surface is rather flat and matches the adjacent

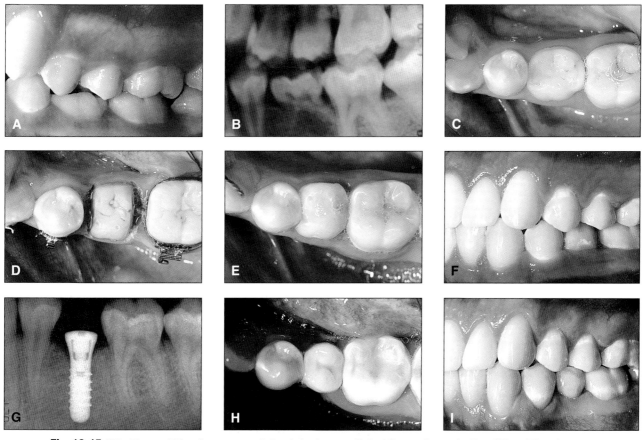

Fig. 18-15 This 15-year-old female was congenitally missing her mandibular left second premolar (**A** and **B**), and the primary second molar was retained (**C**). The restorative plan was to replace the missing tooth with an implant. To maintain the alveolar ridge width for the implant, but to create the appropriate space for the implant crown, the width of the primary tooth was reduced significantly (**D**), and the exposed dentin was restored with composite. Two years later, at the end of orthodontics, the primary molar was still present and helped to maintain the intra-arch space (**E**) and provide an occlusal stop for the opposing premolar (**F**). One year later, the primary molar was extracted, an implant was placed (**G**), and 6 months later it was restored with a porcelain crown (**H** and **I**).

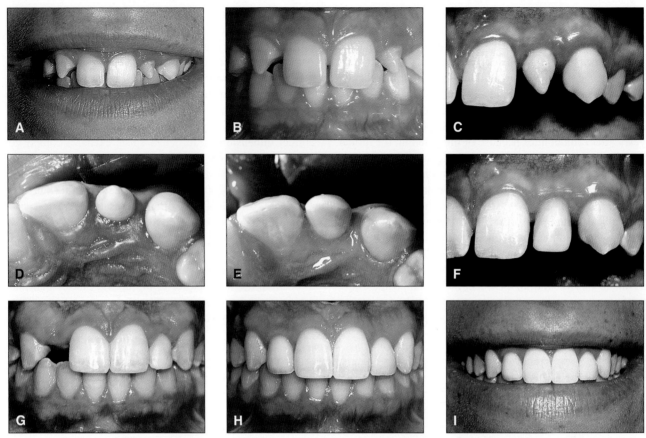

Fig. 18-16 This 12-year-old female was congenitally missing her maxillary right lateral incisor (**A** and **B**), and the left lateral was cone shaped (**C** and **D**). The restorative plan involved replacing the missing tooth with an implant and restoring the malformed lateral incisor with a porcelain crown. A diagnostic wax setup was constructed to determine the appropriate size of the temporary restoration of the malformed lateral incisor (**E** and **F**) and facilitated the orthodontic correction of the malocclusion (**G**). When the patient completed facial growth 3 years later, an implant was placed, and porcelain crowns were placed on the implant and malformed lateral incisors (**H** and **I**).

incisors. In this way, most of the overcontouring is on the distal surface, which is less obvious esthetically. In addition, the gingival margin of the peg-shaped tooth should be aligned with the contralateral lateral incisor in order to create symmetric gingival levels and crown lengths after restoration. If these principles are followed, the restored peg-shaped lateral incisor will match the contralateral lateral incisor in size and shape.

Position Teeth to Facilitate Restorative Dentistry

In the nonrestored adolescent patient, orthodontic positioning of teeth is determined by the size and shape of the teeth. Ideally, if the sizes of all teeth are compatible, then a Class I occlusion with complete interdigitation is possible. However, in the orthodontic–restorative patient, it may not be prudent to position teeth ideally. If restorations are planned for the patient, it may be advantageous to position

teeth to facilitate this restorative treatment. Specific restorations require different types of tooth positioning.

A common orthodontic–restorative situation involves the patient who is congenitally missing one or two maxillary lateral incisors and will have implants to replace the missing tooth or teeth after orthodontic therapy. If the patient were missing one maxillary lateral incisor, the contralateral lateral incisor would determine the amount of space for the implant and crown. However, in some patients the existing lateral incisor may be peg shaped (see Fig. 18-16). In other situations, both lateral incisors are congenitally absent (Fig. 18-17), and the amount of space is determined by two factors[12]: esthetics and occlusion (Fig. 18-17). An esthetic relationship exists between the size of the maxillary central and lateral incisors. The size relationship has been called the "golden proportion".[13] Ideally, the maxillary lateral incisor should be about two-thirds the width of the central incisor.[14] Since most central incisors are about 9 mm wide, the width of the lateral incisor space should be no less than 6 mm. Today the narrowest implants

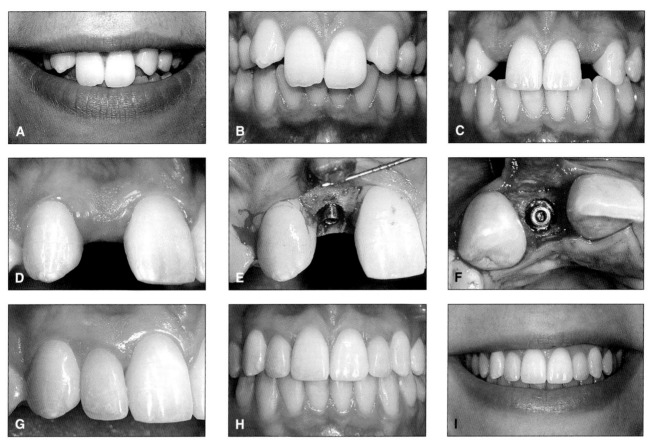

Fig. 18-17 **A** and **B** This 14-year-old female was congenitally missing both maxillary lateral incisors. **C** The treatment plan involved opening space for two implants and two crowns. **D** The labial sulcus depths of the central incisor and canine were 1 mm, there was no incisal wear of either tooth, and the width-to-length proportions of these teeth were normal. **E** and **F** Therefore, the position of the head of the implant was determined by the future gingival margin of the lateral incisor implant crown. When the implant crown was placed (**G**), the gingival margin level was positioned correctly relative to the adjacent teeth as well as the contralateral incisor (**H** and **I**).

are about 3.2 mm in diameter. If the edentulous space were 6 mm wide, then about 1.4 mm would exist between the implant and the adjacent roots (Fig. 18-17). Previous studies have documented that narrower distances between the implant and adjacent root are more likely to show a reduction in bone height over time.[15,16] So at least 1 mm between implant and adjacent root is desirable.

However, in some situations, the orthodontist may create less than the ideal width for a lateral incisor implant and crown because of the patient's occlusal relationships. The orthodontist should assess the posterior intercuspation as well as the appropriate amount of overbite and overjet. If the correct occlusion has been achieved, and the space for the implant crown is too narrow, the orthodontist should remove interproximal enamel from the central incisors and canines to provide additional width for the lateral incisor implant. In some cases, if the interproximal surfaces of the canines and central incisors are already flat, then the orthodontist must remove enamel interproximally from the premolars.[17] The maxillary premolars generally have

tapered crowns with sufficient thickness of enamel, so they can be reduced without penetrating the dentin interproximally. By reducing the widths of adjacent anterior or posterior teeth, the orthodontist can create sufficient space for lateral incisor implants.

Another method for temporarily replacing congenitally missing maxillary lateral incisors is a resin-bonded bridge. Although this type of restoration has a high incidence of failure caused by debonding, it is a conservative means of replacing a missing maxillary lateral incisor, until an implant can be placed at a later time. If the teeth are in the proper position, the life of a resin-bonded bridge can be increased, and the tendency for debonding may be decreased. Since a resin-bonded bridge depends on surface coverage for retention,[18,19] the greater the area of coverage on the lingual of the teeth, the greater the retention (Fig. 18-18). It is therefore important to position anterior teeth with appropriate overjet and overbite relationships. The anterior overbite should not be excessive, but enough to provide disocclusion of the posterior teeth,

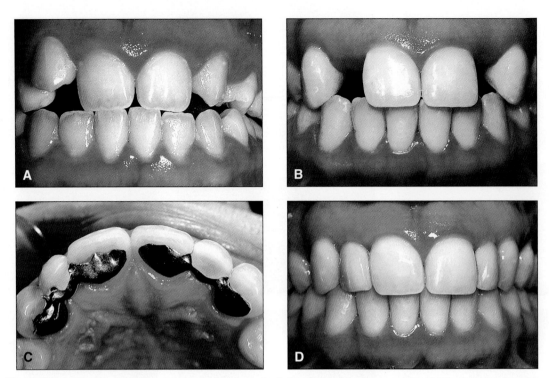

Fig. 18-18 A This 22-year-old female was congenitally missing both maxillary lateral incisors. The orthodontic–restorative plan involved opening space (**B**) for bilateral resin-bonded bridges (**C**). To enhance retention and provide sufficient space for bonding of the metal connectors, the overbite should be minimal (**B**), and only sufficient to permit posterior disocclusion in protrusive function. Seven years later (**D**), the original bridge was still in place, and the esthetic appearance was satisfactory.

when the mandible is protruded forward. The anterior overjet should produce contact of the maxillary and mandibular incisors in centric occlusion. The angulation of the maxillary anterior teeth should be upright and oriented more vertically after orthodontic treatment. This will produce a shear force on the major connector of the resin-bonded bridge, which will enhance retention and stability of the bridge.[20] If incisors are proclined, the force on the bonded metal connector will be a tensile force, which could cause debonding of the bridge.

Another common problem in the adult orthodontic patient is wear or abrasion of the maxillary incisors causing uneven gingival levels and unequal crown length of adjacent central incisors (Fig. 18-19). Treatment for this problem could consist of periodontal crown lengthening to level the gingival margins, orthodontic extrusion of the longer central incisor, or intrusion and restoration of the short tooth or teeth. To diagnose this problem adequately, the clinician must first evaluate the labial sulcular depth of the maxillary incisors.[21] If the sulcular depths are uniformly 1 mm, then the discrepancy in gingival margins may be due to uneven wear or trauma of the incisal edges of the anterior teeth. In these situations, the clinician must decide if the amount of gingival discrepancy will be noticeable (Fig. 18-19). If so, bracketing and alignment of these teeth must be accomplished in a way that improves the esthetics and restorability of the abraded teeth. In these

situations, the gingival margins are used as a guide in tooth positioning, not the incisal edges.[22] As the gingival margins are aligned, the discrepancy in the incisal edges becomes more apparent (Fig. 18-19). These incisal discrepancies are restored temporarily with composite restorations, and then restored permanently with porcelain veneer restorations after the teeth have stabilized. If the gingival margin discrepancies are corrected by leveling the gingival margins orthodontically, these tooth positions should be maintained for at least 6 months to avoid relapse. As teeth are intruded, the orientation of the periodontal fibers changes and becomes more oblique.[23] It typically takes at least 6 months for these fibers to reorient themselves in the horizontal position and to stabilize the tooth position.

Mandibular incisal edge abrasion is also a common problem in the adult orthodontic–restorative patient (Fig. 18-20). When this occurs, the mandibular incisors typically erupt in order to maintain contact. This presents a restorative dilemma for the general dentist, because it leaves no space to place the incisal restoration. Without orthodontics to intrude the lower incisors and create restorative space, the patient would require periodontal crown lengthening with bone removal and apical positioning of the gingival margin. If severe wear has occurred, this could also require root canal therapy and a post and coping on the short and abraded mandibular incisors. However, orthodontics is of tremendous benefit for restorative

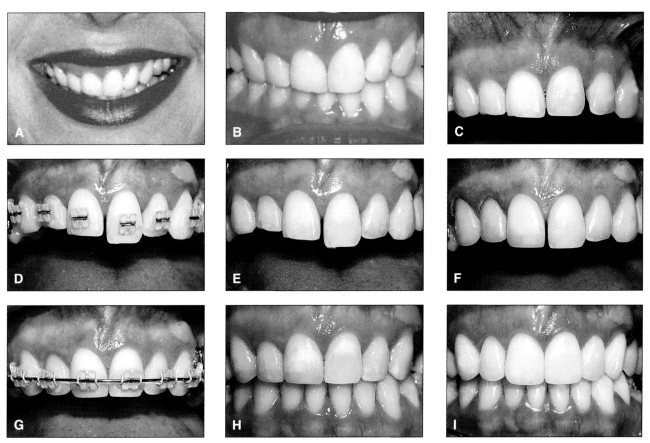

Fig. 18-19 A-C This 29-year-old female had crown length discrepancies between the maxillary right and left central and lateral incisors and canines. The labial sulcular depths of all anterior teeth were 1 mm, and the cementoenamel junctions were at the bottom of the sulcus. The anterior teeth on the right had been abraded, and the teeth had continued to erupt. Therefore, the correct treatment plan involved intrusion of the right central and lateral incisors and canine (**D**), temporary restoration of these teeth with composite (**E** and **F**), and replacement of the orthodontic brackets (**G**) for 6 months to stabilize the intruded teeth. **H** At the end of orthodontics the lengths of the right and left anterior teeth were equivalent. **I** Two years later, after final restoration with porcelain veneers, the intruded position of the anterior teeth was stable.

patients with significant wear of their mandibular incisors. By intruding the lower incisors (Fig. 18-20), the orthodontist can create space for the restoration, avoid gingival surgery, eliminate the need for endodontic treatment, and thereby simplify the restoration of the abraded teeth.

When patients are congenitally missing their mandibular permanent second premolars, the clinician must monitor the vertical position of the primary second molar. Occasionally, the mandibular primary second molar will become ankylosed and fused to the alveolus (Fig. 18-21). In these situations, leaving the primary molar may result in a significant vertical bone defect in the edentulous ridge. If an implant is planned in the edentulous site, the vertical defect may be difficult to implant. If an ankylosed primary molar is not extracted early enough, and a vertical ridge defect is produced, one option is to place a bone graft in the area either at the same time or prior to implant placement. Another option is to move the mandibular first premolar into the second premolar position[20] and to place the implant

in the first premolar position (Fig. 18-21). Previous studies have shown that it is possible, within limits, to move a tooth into a narrower edentulous ridge[24,25] in order to create an implant site. The bone that is created behind the moving tooth typically will be as wide as the root of the tooth that was moved. This type of orthodontic movement (called orthodontic implant site development) may eliminate the need for a bone graft in the edentulous site.

Consider Implants to Facilitate Difficult Tooth Movement

In recent years, dental implants have become an accepted method of replacing missing teeth.[26] Today millions of implants are placed annually to rehabilitate and re-establish patients' occlusions. In many of these individuals, the teeth may be in a less than ideal position to accept the integration of a single implant or groups of implants with

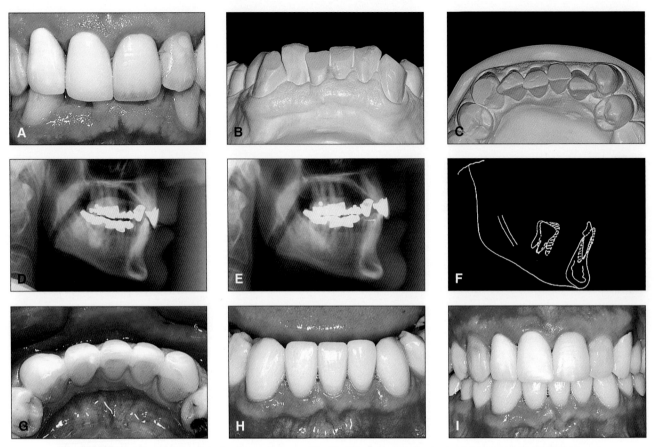

Fig. 18-20 This 52-year-old male had a deep anterior overbite (**A**) and a protrusive bruxing habit that produced significant wear of the mandibular incisors (**B** and **C**). **D** There was no space for the restorative dentist to restore these teeth. Orthodontic treatment was initiated to intrude the mandibular incisors (**E** and **F**), so they could be restored with porcelain veneers (**G** and **H**). **I** Not only was the deep overbite corrected, but also the orthodontic intrusion had permitted the restoration of esthetics and function to this debilitated dentition.

the remaining teeth. These patients could benefit from orthodontics to reposition malposed teeth and enhance the overall occlusal scheme.[27] However, if significant numbers of teeth are missing, the orthodontist is at a disadvantage, because of the lack of anchorage to effect the desired tooth movement.

Several types of implant systems are available to provide anchors for tooth movement. These include subperiosteal implants,[28–30] interproximal transitional implants,[31] palatal implants,[32–34] mini-implants,[35–37] and titanium plates.[38–40] These auxiliaries are typically placed between the roots of teeth, apical to the roots of teeth, or in the retromolar regions of the maxilla and mandible. Although they are efficient anchors for tooth movement and are very versatile, they are also expendable. Usually they are removed after orthodontic treatment and discarded. Although this may be an extra expense for the patient, in a completely dentulous patient, this technology may be appropriate. However, in a partially edentulous patient, where implants will be used as anchors to restore the occlusion, these restorative implants could be used initially for orthodontic anchorage,

and later as restorative abutments after orthodontics has been completed.[27]

The indications[27] for using a restorative implant as an orthodontic anchor include: intra-arch intrusion of teeth that have overerupted; intra-arch retraction of teeth that are proclined; and intra-arch protraction of teeth that are positioned distally (Fig. 18-22). In each of these situations, the implant must be placed prior to orthodontic bracketing. However, the implant must be positioned appropriately, so it will not only satisfy the orthodontic requirements, but also be in a suitable position for the final restoration. The orthodontist must construct a diagnostic wax setup, after consultation with the restorative dentist and surgeon. The diagnostic wax setup must be constructed in a series of specific steps to ensure accuracy. These steps have been documented elsewhere.[27,41,42] The diagnostic wax setup permits construction of a placement guide for the surgeon to provide accurate positioning of implants.

After placement the implants must integrate with the bone prior to orthodontic loading. The timing of implant loading for single implants is determined by the amount

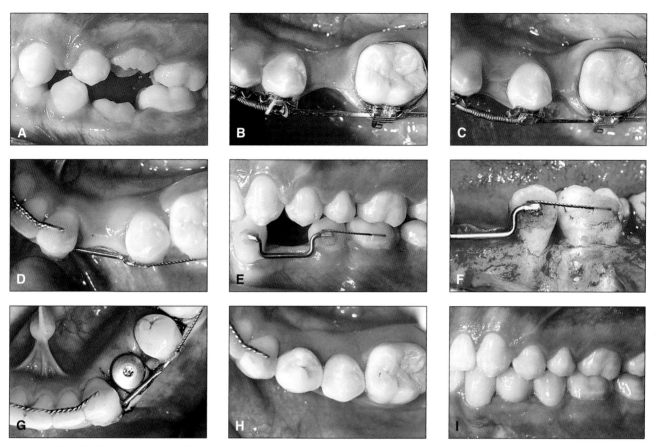

Fig. 18-21 **A** This 16-year-old female was congenitally missing the mandibular left second premolar, and the primary molar had ankylosed and was submerged. **B** After extraction of the primary molar, the alveolar ridge width decreased significantly. To create adequate ridge width for placement of an implant, the first premolar was moved distally into the second premolar position (**C-E**), and the implant was placed in the first premolar position (**F** and **G**). **H** and **I** The process of "orthodontic implant site development" is an excellent method to facilitate implant placement in sites with deficient bone.

of time required by the bone adjacent to the implant to undergo secondary osteon (remodeling) formation around the implant.[43] If multiple implants are placed at the same time, they are often loaded immediately after placement, using a provisional prosthesis. Even though the bone around the implant has not completely remodeled, the rigidity supplied by cross-arch splinting allows for integration to occur around the functioning implants.[44] Recent research has shown that when implants are loaded with static or continuous load in the same direction, the bone on the implant surface develops more rapidly.[45,46] However, when a dynamic load is applied to the implant (not continuous and in different directions), much less bone develops on the implant surface.[46] When the implant is loaded continuously, the same biomechanic message is delivered to the bony surface, which is to stimulate bone formation on the compressed surface, in order to form more supporting bone. When the force on the implant is dynamic or intermittent, the biomechanic message is not clear, and less bone is formed. Therefore, if implants are to be used for orthodontic anchorage, they could be loaded

immediately, since an orthodontic load is continuous and in the same direction.

Animal studies have shown that when implants are loaded, more bone develops on the pressure or compressive side of the implant.[47] This is the opposite of what happens around teeth. When the periodontal ligament of a tooth is loaded with a compressive force, bone resorbs on the pressure side and deposits on the tension side. However, implants do not have a periodontal ligament, and therefore the bone that forms on the pressure side of the implant is referred to as *buttressing bone*, which develops in response to implant loading.

After the implant has been uncovered, a provisional restoration must be placed so that the orthodontic force can be attached to the implant. The type of provisional restoration varies, depending on the type of orthodontic mechanics.[27] In some situations, a tooth-shaped plastic restoration is required. However, in other situations, a metal abutment is sufficient to provide the anchorage. In general, if orthodontic brackets are not to be used, a simple metal cap can be placed on top of the implant. In most situations,

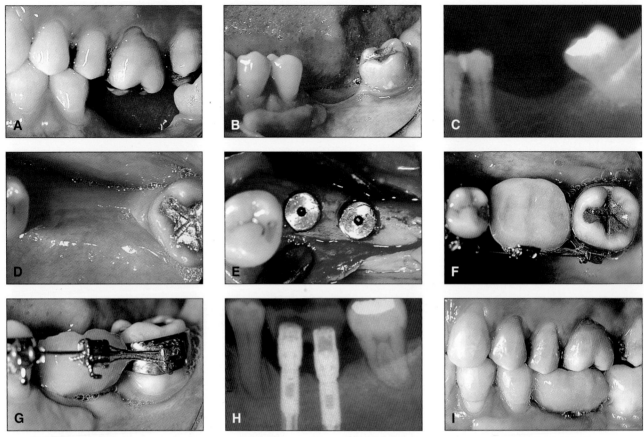

Fig. 18-22 A This adult female had lost her mandibular left first and second molars due to dental caries, and the maxillary first molar had supererupted. **B-D** In addition, the mandibular third molar had tipped mesially. **E** The restorative plan was to place two premolar implants to replace the missing teeth. The implants would be used as anchorage to upright the third molar and move the tooth (**F** and **G**) and roots (**H**) mesially. **I** By using the implants as anchorage, the posterior occlusion was maintained, and the implants were restored to provide occlusion for the maxillary left first molar.

if the teeth adjacent to the implant are to be moved toward the implant, a provisional plastic restoration is necessary to permit accurate positioning of these teeth during the orthodontic process. In these situations, the size of the provisional crown can be ascertained from the diagnostic wax setup used to create the placement guide.

Evaluate Tooth Position Prior to Bracket Removal

If an orthodontic patient will not require restorations, it is appropriate that the orthodontist makes the final decisions regarding tooth position and appliance removal. However, if the patient will require restorations after orthodontics, the restorative dentist should play a part in the finishing process. It is advantageous to request input from the restorative dentist during final tooth positioning, and the patient should be referred back to the restorative dentist during the final 6 months of treatment. A note or letter should be sent asking for input from the restorative dentist

or periodontist about final tooth positioning, especially in areas where restorations are planned. Not only does the patient benefit from having several individuals evaluate the final result, but also the orthodontist will learn from this interaction about the individual requirements of certain types of restorative patients.

In most orthodontic patients, aligning the crowns of the teeth will produce proper root angulation. Ideally, the roots of the teeth should not be in close interproximal contact. In that way, sufficient bone will be present between the roots of each of the teeth. Proper root angulation may be even more important for the orthodontic–restorative patient. When implants are planned for missing maxillary lateral incisors, it is important to create adequate space for the implant between adjacent roots.[12] As the central incisor and canine are pushed apart, the apices of the roots move toward one another (Fig. 18-23). During orthodontic finishing, radiographs must be taken to assess whether or not proper root angulation has been achieved. If not, the archwire must be removed, and the teeth should either be rebracketed or bends placed in the archwire to achieve

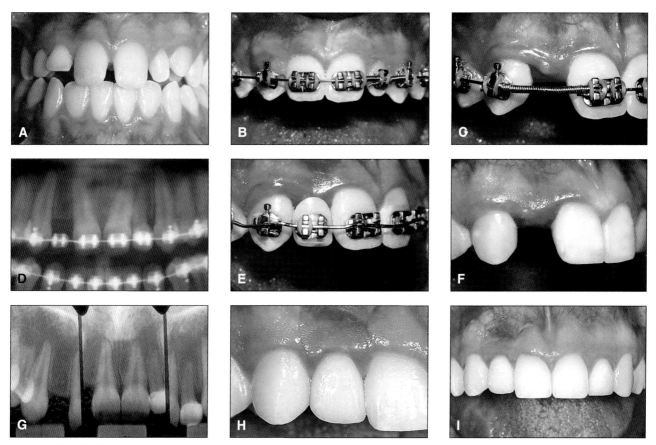

Fig. 18-23 **A** This 16-year-old female was congenitally missing her maxillary right lateral incisor, and the left lateral incisor was malformed. The restorative plan involved restoration of the malformed left lateral incisor and placement of an implant and crown to replace the missing right lateral incisor. After aligning the teeth (**B**) and opening space (**C**) for the implant, a progress radiograph (**D**) was indispensable in determining the appropriate tooth and root movement (**E**) necessary to create the correct final crown (**F**) and root (**G**) position prior to implant placement and restoration (**H** and **I**).

proper root angulation. If the roots are too close together, an implant cannot be placed.

Determine the Appropriate Type of Retention

Fixed and/or removable retainers are used routinely to maintain tooth position immediately after removal of orthodontic appliances. In most orthodontic patients, removable retainers include either maxillary and mandibular Hawley appliances or custom-fit Essix retainers. Fixed retainers typically consist of braided or solid stainless steel or gold wires that are bonded to the lingual surfaces of the maxillary or mandibular anterior teeth. In some patients it is beneficial to place combinations of fixed and removable retainer types. If patients wear their retainers for a sufficient time, the teeth will stabilize. However, the adult orthodontic patient may be missing one or more teeth. In addition, an adult restorative patient may have had prior bone loss, and the periodontally involved teeth could be significantly mobile. If so, the purpose of retention is not only to stabilize the teeth and reduce mobility, but also to maintain posterior and anterior edentulous spaces, until they are restored with either bridges or implants.

If a patient is missing three or more adjacent anterior or posterior teeth after orthodontic treatment, fixed retention is probably unlikely. Therefore, a removable retainer with prosthetic teeth will be necessary to help stabilize the remaining teeth in that arch, as well as to provide an occlusal stop for teeth in the opposing arch (Fig. 18-24). However, when constructing the removable retainer, occlusal stops are necessary, in order to prevent occlusal loads from damaging the edentulous ridge. These stops are constructed from wire and/or acrylic and can cover the cingula of the anterior teeth or insert onto the occlusal surfaces of posterior teeth.

If one tooth is missing, and an implant or bridge is planned to restore the edentulous space, a fixed bonded wire is more desirable for several reasons (Fig. 18-24). First, the fixed retainer does not require patient compliance. Second, it can stop the opposing occlusion from overerupting.

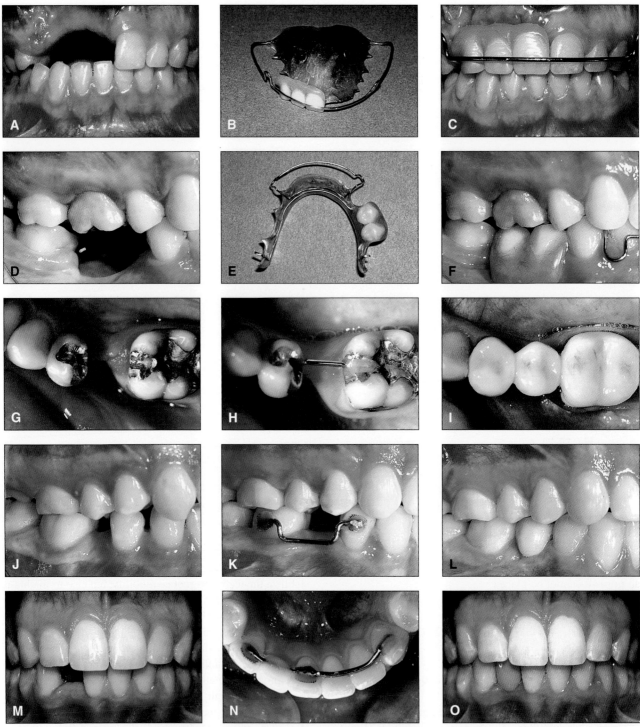

Fig. 18-24 An important step in any interdisciplinary treatment plan is to select the appropriate method of retaining the orthodontic tooth movement prior to restoration. In patients who are missing several maxillary (**A-C**) or mandibular (**D-F**) teeth after orthodontic treatment, it may be prudent to maintain tooth position with a removable retainer with prosthetic teeth to establish satisfactory esthetics and function. If the patient is to have a posterior fixed bridge placed after orthodontic treatment, an intracoronal wire and acrylic splint (**G-I**) is an excellent method to prevent supereruption of teeth in the opposing arch, and to rigidly maintain tooth position prior to bridge construction. If an implant is to be used to replace a missing mandibular second premolar after orthodontic treatment, it is advantageous to place an extracoronal wire and acrylic splint (**J-L**) to maintain the space rigidly during implant placement, osseointegration, and final restoration. If a mandibular incisor is missing, and the space is to be maintained after orthodontics (**M-O**) a fixed mandibular lingual retainer with an attached tooth is a convenient method of retaining the space until the bridge or implant is placed.

Third, teeth can be attached to the bonded wire in order to provide an esthetic temporary replacement for the patient. Whatever the choice of retainer, the important step is to make a decision about the responsibility for retention in perio-restorative patients prior to orthodontic treatment. It is much easier to coordinate the appointments and appliances if the team members make the decisions collectively, so the patient will be provided with the optimum method of retention for his/her specific ortho-perio-restorative situation after appliance removal.

Summary

This chapter has discussed and illustrated a series of 10 guidelines for managing the orthodontic patient with periodontal or restorative complications. One of the most important steps is to generate realistic treatment objectives that will fit the patient's needs, desires, and financial capabilities, and the goals of the team members. Then, a visual representation of the final result must be created in the form of a diagnostic wax setup. This provides the blueprint or endpoint of treatment for the entire team. Next, the sequence of treatment must be established for patients who will require several steps performed by multiple team members at varying points during their treatment. This structured list of steps and responsibilities becomes the roadmap for treating the patient. Then, the periodontal problems must be identified, and the person responsible for the treatment of these soft tissue or osseous defects must be determined. If certain teeth are hopeless, the timing of extraction must be sequenced to facilitate the needs of all practitioners on the team. Prior to appliance placement, any malformed, abraded, or broken-down teeth should be built up to facilitate bracketing. The future position of teeth should be determined by the specific restorative or periodontal needs of the patient. If insufficient anchorage exists for tooth movement, implants could be considered for orthodontic as well as restorative anchorage during and after tooth movement. Prior to appliance removal, the orthodontist should ask the restorative dentist and/or periodontist to evaluate the patient's tooth position in order to achieve appropriate crown and root position for restorative treatment, and to determine the type of retention necessary, especially for missing teeth prior to appliance removal. If the team of periodontist, surgeon, orthodontist, and restorative dentist follows these 10 guidelines, the management of ortho-perio-restorative patients will be simplified, predictable, and pleasurable.

REFERENCES

1. Kokich V, Spear F. Guidelines for managing the orthodontic–restorative patient. Semin Orthod 1997;3:3–20.
2. Casko J, Vaden J, Kokich V, et al. American Board of Orthodontics grading system for dental casts and panoramic radiographs. Am J Orthod Dentofac Orthop 1999;114:18–23.
3. Mathews D, Kokich V. Managing treatment for the orthodontic patient with periodontal problems. Semin Orthod 1997;3:21–38.
4. Kokich V. Anterior dental esthetics: An orthodontic perspective. III. Mediolateral relationships. J Esthet Dent 1993;5:18–22.
5. Kokich V. Managing complex orthodontic problems: The use of implants for anchorage. Semin Orthod 1996;2:153–160.
6. Kokich V, Nappen D, Shapiro P. Gingival contour and clinical crown length: Their effects on the esthetic appearance of maxillary anterior teeth. Am J Orthod 1984;86:89–94.
7. Kokich VG, Shapiro PA. Extraction of a mandibular incisor to facilitate orthodontic treatment. Angle Orthod 1984;54:139–153.
8. Kokich V. The role of orthodontics as an adjunct to periodontal therapy. In: Newman MG, Takei HH, Carranza FA, eds. Clinical periodontology, 9th edn. Philadelphia: WB Saunders, 2002:704–718.
9. Kokich V. Esthetics: the orthodontic–periodontic–restorative connection. Semin Orthod 1996;2:21–30.
10. Ingber J. Forced eruption: Part I. A method of treating isolated one and two wall infrabony osseous defects—rationale and case report. J Periodontol 1974;45:199–206.
11. Zachrisson B, Mjor I. Remodeling of teeth by grinding. Am J Orthod 1975;68:543–553.
12. Spear F, Mathews D, Kokich V. Interdisciplinary management of single-tooth implants. Semin Orthod 1997;3:35–74.
13. Lombardi R. The principles of visual perception and their application to dental esthetics. J Prosthet Dent 1973;29:359–382.
14. Rufenacht C. Structural esthetic rules. In: Rufenacht C, ed. Fundamentals of esthetics. Chicago: Quintessence Publishing, 1992:67–134.
15. Esposito M, Ekkestube A, Grondahl K. Radiological evaluation of marginal bone loss at tooth surfaces facing single-tooth implants. Clin Oral Implant Res 1993;4:151–157.
16. Thilander B, Odman J, Grondahl K, Friberg B. Osseointegrated implants in adolescents. An alternative in replacing missing teeth? Europ J Orthod 1994;16:84–95.
17. Kokich V. Single-tooth implants: Planning with the aid of orthodontics. J Oral Maxillofac Surg 2004;62:48–56.
18. Creugers N, Kayser A, Van't Hof M. A seven-and-a-half year survival study of resin-bonded bridges. J Dent Res 1992;71:1822–1825.
19. Boyer D, Williams V, Thayer K, Dennehy G. Analysis of debond rates of resin-bonded bridges. J Dent Res 1993;72:1244–1248.
20. Kokich V. Orthodontic–restorative management of the adolescent patient. In: McNamara JA Jr, ed. Orthodontics and dentofacial orthopedics. Ann Arbor: Needham Press, 2001:425–452.

21. Kokich V. Anterior dental esthetics: An orthodontic perspective. I. Crown length. J Esthet Dent 1993;5:19–23.

22. Kokich VG, Kokich VO, Spear F. Maximizing anterior esthetics: An interdisciplinary approach. In: McNamara JA Jr, Kelly K Jr, eds. Frontiers in dental and facial esthetics. Ann Arbor, Needham Press, 2001:1–18.

23. Reitan K. Clinical and histologic observations of tooth movement during and after orthodontic treatment. Am J Orthod 1967;53:721–745.

24. Stepovich M. A clinical study of edentulous closing spaces in the mandible. Angle Orthod 1979;49:277–283.

25. Hom B, Turley P. The effects of space closure on the mandibular first molar area in adults. Am J Orthod 1984;85:475–489.

26. ADA Council on Scientific Affairs. Dental endosseous implants: An update. J Am Dent Assoc 2004;135:92–97.

27. Kokich V. Comprehensive management of implant anchorage in the multidisciplinary patient. In: Hiiguchi K, ed. Orthodontic application of osseointegrated implants. Chicago: Quintessence, 2000:21–32.

28. Block M, Hoffman D. A new device for absolute anchorage for orthodontics. Am J Orthod Dentofac Orthop 1995;107:251–258.

29. Kluemper GT, Spalding PM. Realities of craniofacial growth modification. Atlas Oral Maxillofac Surg Clin North Am 2001;9:23–51.

30. Armbruster PC, Block MS. Onplant–supported orthodontic anchorage. Atlas Oral Maxillofac Surg Clin North Am 2001;9:53–74.

31. Gray JB, Smith R. Transitional implants for orthodontic anchorage. J Clin Orthod 2000;34:659–666.

32. Keles A, Erverdi N, Sezen S. Bodily distalization of molars with absolute anchorage. Angle Orthod 2003;73:471–482.

33. Giancotti A, Greco M, Docimo R, Arcuri C. Extraction treatment using a palatal implant for anchorage. Aust Orthod J 2003;19:87–90.

34. Celenza F. Implant-enhanced tooth movement: Indirect absolute anchorage. Int J Periodontics Restor Dent 2003;23:533–541.

35. Ohmae M, Saito S, Morohashi T, et al. A clinical and histological evaluation of titanium mini-implants as anchors for orthodontic intrusion in the beagle dog. Am J Orthod Dentofac Orthop 2001;119:489–497.

36. Kyung SH, Choi JH, Park YC. Mini-screw anchorage used to protract lower second molars into first molar extraction sites. J Clin Orthod 2003;37:575–579.

37. Cheng SJ, Tseng IY, Lee JJ, Kok SH. A prospective study of the risk factors associated with failure of mini-implants used for orthodontic anchorage. Int J Oral Maxillofac Implants 2004;19:100–106.

38. Chung KR, Kim YS, Linton JL, Lee YJ. The miniplate with tube for skeletal anchorage. J Clin Orthod 2002;36:407–412.

39. Sherwood KH, Burch J, Thompson W. Intrusion of supererupted molars with titanium miniplate anchorage. Angle Orthod 2003;73:597–601.

40. Sugawara J, Daimaruya T, Umemori M, et al. Distal movement of mandibular molars in adult patients with the skeletal anchorage system. Am J Orthod Dentofac Orthop 2004;125:130–138.

41. Smalley W. Implants for orthodontic tooth movement: Determining implant location and orientation. J Esthet Dent 1995;7:62–72.

42. Smalley WM, Blanco A. Implants for tooth movement: A fabrication and placement technique for provisional restorations. J Esthet Dent 1995;7:150–154.

43. Roberts WE, Smith R, Zilberman Y, et al. Osseous adaptation to continuous loading of rigid endosseous implants. Am J Orthod 1984;86:95–111.

44. Tarnow DP, Emtiaz S, Classi A. Immediate loading of threaded implants at stage 1 surgery in edentulous arches: Ten consecutive case reports with 1 to 5-year data. Int J Oral Maxillofac Implants 1997;12:319–324.

45. Piatelli A, Corigliano M, Scarano A, Costigliola G, Paolantonio M. Immediate loading of titanium plasma-sprayed implants: An histologic analysis in monkeys. J Periodontol 1998;69:321–327.

46. Duyck J, Ronold HJ, Van Oosterwyck H, Naert I, Vander Sloten J, Ellingsen JE. The influence of static and dynamic loading on marginal bone reactions around osseointegrated implants: An animal experimental study. Clin Oral Implants Res 2001;12:207–218.

47. Turley P, Shapiro P, Moffett B. The loading of bioglass coated aluminum oxide implants to produce sutural expansion of the maxillary complex in the pigtail monkey. Arch Oral Biol 1980;25:459–464.

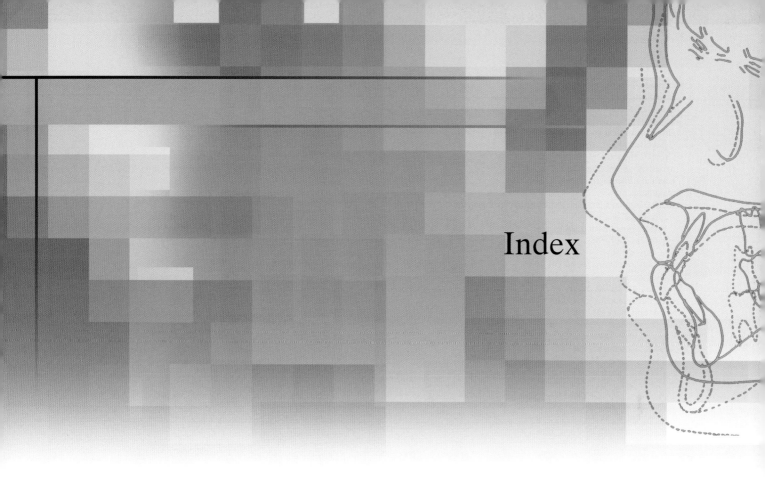

Index

QM Medical Libraries

24 1018414 7

Barts and The London
Queen Mary's School of Medicine and Dentistry

WHITECHAPEL LIBRARY, TURNER STREET, LONDON E1 2AD
020 7882 7110

4 WEEK LOAN

Books are to be returned on or before the last date below,
otherwise fines may be charged.

- 8 JAN 2007		
1 6 APR 2007		
1 3 AUG 2008		
30/11/08		
1 4 JUL 2009		

WITHDRAWN
FROM STOCK
QMUL LIBRARY